NOVEL APPROACHES AND STRATEGIES FOR BIOLOGICS, VACCINES AND CANCER THERAPIES

NOVEL APPROACHES AND STRATEGIES FOR BIOLOGICS, VACCINES AND CANCER THERAPIES

Edited by

MANMOHAN SINGH, MAYA SALNIKOVA

Novartis Vaccines, Holly Springs, NC, USA

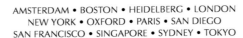
AMSTERDAM • BOSTON • HEIDELBERG • LONDON
NEW YORK • OXFORD • PARIS • SAN DIEGO
SAN FRANCISCO • SINGAPORE • SYDNEY • TOKYO
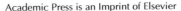
Academic Press is an Imprint of Elsevier

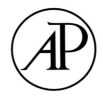

Academic Press is an imprint of Elsevier
32 Jamestown Road, London NW1 7BY, UK
225 Wyman Street, Waltham, MA 02451, USA
525 B Street, Suite 1800, San Diego, CA 92101-4495, USA

British Library Cataloguing-in-Publication Data
A catalogue record for this book is available from the British Library

Library of Congress Cataloging-in-Publication Data
A catalog record for this book is available from the Library of Congress

ISBN : 978-0-12-416603-5

For information on all Academic Press publications
visit our website at http://store.elsevier.com/

Typeset by Thomson

Printed and bound in United States of America

13 14 15 16 17   10 9 8 7 6 5 4 3 2 1

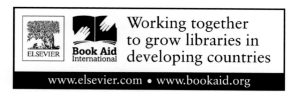

**Working together
to grow libraries in
developing countries**

www.elsevier.com • www.bookaid.org

Contents

List of Contributors

Reinaldo Acevedo Research and Development vice-presidency of Finlay Institute, Havana, Cuba

Juan C. Almagro CTI-Boston, Pfizer, Inc., Boston, MA, USA

Manal Alsaadi University of Tripoli, Faculty of Pharmacy, Tripoli, Libya

Chantal C.M. Appeldoorn to-BBB Technologies B.V., Leiden, The Netherlands

Alexandra Beumer Sassi Biopharm R&D, GlaxoSmithKline, King of Prussia, PA, USA

Akhilesh Bhambhani Merck Research Laboratories, Bioprocess R&D, Formulation Development, West Point, PA, USA

Catherine M. Bollard Children's National Health System, Washington DC, USA

Kim Braz-Gomes Mercer University, College of Pharmacy, Vaccine Nanotechnology Laboratory, Atlanta, GA, USA

Randall J. Brezski Principal Scientist, Biologics Research, Janssen R&D, LLC, USA

Andrew Buchanan Antibody Discovery and Protein Engineering, MedImmune, Cambridge, UK

Danilo Casimiro Merck Research Laboratories, Vaccine Research, West Point, PA, USA

Divya Chandra Howard P. Isermann Department of Chemical and Biological Engineering, Rensselaer Polytechnic Institute, Troy, New York, USA

Maurizio Chiriva-Internati Texas Tech University, Health Science Center, Lubbock, TX, USA

Beth-Ann Coller Merck Research Laboratories, Vaccine Research, Global Clinical Development, North Wales, PA, USA

Conrad Russell Y. Cruz Children's National Health System, Washington DC, USA

Marco de Boer to-BBB Technologies B.V., Leiden, The Netherlands

Robert De Rose Department of Microbiology and Immunology, The University of Melbourne, at the Peter Doherty Institute for Infection and Immunity, University of Melbourne, Melbourne, Australia

Sucheta D'Sa Mercer University, College of Pharmacy, Vaccine Nanotechnology Laboratory, Atlanta, GA, USA

Bernadette D'Souza Department of Pharmaceutical Sciences, McWhorter School of Pharmacy, Social and Administrative Sciences, Samford University, Birmingham, AL, USA

Marissa D'Souza Mercer University, College of Pharmacy, Vaccine Nanotechnology Laboratory, Atlanta, GA, USA; Georgia Institute of Technology, Biomedical Engineering Program, Atlanta, GA, USA

Martin J. D'Souza Mercer University, College of Pharmacy, Vaccine Nanotechnology Laboratory, Atlanta, GA, USA

Nigel D'Souza Mercer University, College of Pharmacy, Vaccine Nanotechnology Laboratory, Atlanta, GA, USA

Mauro Ferrari Houston Methodist Research Institute, Houston, TX, USA; Weill Cornell Medical College, New York, NY, USA

Valerie A. Ferro University of Strathclyde, Strathclyde Institute of Pharmacy and Biomedical Science, Glasgow, UK

Pieter J. Gaillard to-BBB Technologies B.V., Leiden, The Netherlands

Rikhav P. Gala Mercer University, College of Pharmacy, Vaccine Nanotechnology Laboratory, Atlanta, GA, USA

Deborah A. Garside Imperial College London, Faculty of Medicine, London, UK

Ayman Gebril University of Strathclyde, Strathclyde Institute of Pharmacy and Biomedical Science, Glasgow, UK

Werner Gladdines to-BBB Technologies B.V., Leiden, The Netherlands

Ana Maria Gonzalez-Angulo Department of Breast Medical Oncology, Department of Systems Biology, The University of Texas M.D. Anderson Cancer Center, Houston, TX, USA

Paul Hamblin Biopharm R&D, GlaxoSmithKline, King of Prussia, PA, USA

Qing-Yu He   Key Laboratory of Functional Protein Research of Guangdong Higher Education Institutes, Institute of Life and Health Engineering, College of Life Science and Technology, Jinan University, Guangzhou, China

Jon Heinrichs   Merck Research Laboratories, Vaccine Research, West Point, PA, USA

Erica Jackson   College of Medicine, University of South Florida, Tampa, FL, USA

Pankaj Karande   Howard P. Isermann Department of Chemical and Biological Engineering, Rensselaer Polytechnic Institute, Troy, New York, USA

Stephen J. Kent   Department of Microbiology and Immunology, The University of Melbourne, at the Peter Doherty Institute for Infection and Immunity, University of Melbourne, Melbourne, Australia

Sreekumar Kodangattil   CTI-Boston, Pfizer, Inc., Boston, MA, USA

Dimitrios Lamprou   University of Strathclyde, Strathclyde Institute of Pharmacy and Biomedical Science, Glasgow, UK

Kenneth Lundstrom   Pan Therapeutics, Lutry, Switzerland

Sara Movassaghian   Center for Pharmaceutical Biotechnology and Nanomedicine, Northeastern University, Boston, MA, USA

Nihal S. Mulla   Mercer University, College of Pharmacy, Vaccine Nanotechnology Laboratory, Atlanta, GA, USA

Alexander B. Mullen   University of Strathclyde, Strathclyde Institute of Pharmacy and Biomedical Science, Glasgow, UK

Radhika Nagarkar   Biopharmaceutical Development, KBI Biopharma, Inc., Durham, NC, USA

Lakshmy Nair   Department of Breast Medical Oncology, Department of Systems Biology, The University of Texas M.D. Anderson Cancer Center, Houston, TX, USA

Natalie Nimmo   University of Strathclyde, Strathclyde Institute of Pharmacy and Biomedical Science, Glasgow, UK

Ashwin C. Parenky   Mercer University, College of Pharmacy, Vaccine Nanotechnology Laboratory, Atlanta, GA, USA

Brianna Oliver   College of Medicine, University of South Florida, Tampa, FL, USA

Ernesto Oviedo-Orta   Novartis Vaccines and Diagnostics, Vaccines Research, Siena, Italy

Teresa Ramirez-Montagut   Genomics Institute of the Novartis Research Foundation, San Diego, CA, USA

Charani Ranasinghe   John Curtin School of Medical Research, Australian National University, Canberra, Australia

Arie Reijerkerk   to-BBB Technologies B.V., Leiden, The Netherlands

Jefferson D. Revell   Antibody Discovery and Protein Engineering, MedImmune, Cambridge, UK

Jaap Rip   to-BBB Technologies B.V., Leiden, The Netherlands

Haifa Shen   Department of Nanomedicine, Houston Methodist Research Institute, Houston, TX, USA; Weill Cornell Medical College, New York, NY, USA

Hatem Soliman   Moffitt Cancer Center and Research Institute, Women's Oncology and Experimental Therapeutics, Tampa, FL, USA

Bin Sun   Southern Medical University; Key Laboratory of Functional Protein Research of Guangdong Higher Education Institutes, Institute of Life and Health Engineering, College of Life Science and Technology, Jinan University, Guangzhou, China

Krishna Suri   Houston Methodist Research Institute, Houston, TX, USA

Jan ter Meulen   Immune Design, Seattle, WA, USA

Vladimir P. Torchilin   Center for Pharmaceutical Biotechnology and Nanomedicine, Northeastern University, Boston, MA, USA

John Philip Trasatti   Chemistry and Chemical Biology, Rensselaer Polytechnic Institute, Troy, NY, USA

Ruhi V. Ubale   Mercer University, College of Pharmacy, Vaccine Nanotechnology Laboratory, Atlanta, GA, USA

Corine C. Visser   to-BBB Technologies B.V., Leiden, The Netherlands

Trinh Phuong Vo   Mercer University, College of Pharmacy, Vaccine Nanotechnology Laboratory, Atlanta, GA, USA

Joy Wolfram   Houston Methodist Research Institute, Houston, TX, USA; National Center for Nanoscience and Technology of China, Beijing, China

Preface

Recent advances in human gene profiling have led to improved understanding of disease mechanisms and the discovery of new molecular targets. Specific disease targets, such as for cancer, are now being treated by novel modalities of biologics and immunotherapies. Currently, exciting new approaches and therapies have evolved from academia and industry, where new ideas have been evaluated and tested over years of persistent research and development. Some of these novel therapies have now moved into clinical evaluation to establish safety, proof of concept, and therapeutic effectiveness. Upon rigorous clinical testing, only a few therapies have found success and have been adapted for treatment of patients. In spite of these developmental challenges, there is a growing number of novel therapies that now cure serious diseases, reduce pain, and improve the quality of life.

In this book, we present an overview of these emerging trends in such novel approaches as gene therapy, nanotechnology, non-parenteral delivery of biologics, and delivery to the central nervous system. These novel strategies are being explored for biologics (newer and diverse antibodies), therapeutic proteins, and biobetters. The book also covers topics on new vaccines against novel targets and evolving pathogens and discusses novel cancer therapies such as personalized therapy, immunotherapy, and advanced approaches for small molecules.

Among novel therapies, gene therapy represents a novel approach that is being fueled by advanced understanding of genomics, epigenomics, and innovative research on various fronts of vector development and discovery of new therapeutic agents. Recently, the delivery of new therapeutic agents through physiological barriers has been enabled by nanotechnology, where multifunctional delivery vehicles are being designed for biophysical and molecular targeting. Additionally, unique challenges are overcome when delivering biologics to the central nervous system by utilizing natural transport pathways, vector-mediated delivery systems, stem cells, and nanomaterials. Moreover, the delivery of the novel biotherapeutic agents has been showing promise in enhancing effectiveness and reducing side-effects when administered *via* non-parenteral routes such as oral, transdermal, and pulmonary.

Due to the complexity of some of the novel targets for treating diseases, the majority of novel therapies are now based on biological agents such as monoclonal antibodies and therapeutic proteins. The design of these unique antibodies is often based on next-generation sequencing. Remarkably, the new generation of antibodies includes molecular modalities beyond natural antibodies with bi- and multispecific functions. Furthermore, novel therapeutic proteins include Kunitz-type domains, ankyrin repeat proteins, fibronectin scaffolds, lipocalins, and avimers; novel peptides include constrained, hydrocarbon-stapled, and lactamized peptides. A new trend of improving the performance of marketed biologics has been demonstrated by *biobetters*, a new class of biosimilar pharmaceutical molecules developed by formulation modifications and changes in the molecular profile through chemical, structural, or functional optimization.

Novel vaccines have the potential to significantly improve prevention of non-infectious diseases by encompassing novel targets such as allergen, addiction, and fertility regulating proteins in order to control conception and hormone-induced conditions. New vaccines include targets in neurodegenerative diseases such as Alzheimer's and Parkinson's diseases, stress, and depression. Meanwhile, evolving infectious pathogens such as influenza, dengue, HIV, and pneumococcal diseases are being targeted with novel platforms and universal vaccines. Prominently, HIV vaccines are being developed by utilizing vaccination strategies of priming with viral vectors or DNA and boosting with antigens in order to elicit HIV-specific T- and B-cell avidity.

A special consideration has been given in this book to advances in novel therapies for cancer. Cancer, being one of the prevalent diseases, is now been treated by a creative approach of personalized therapy, where each patient has custom-tailored treatment based on that person's unique clinical, genetic, genomic, and environmental information. Additionally, molecular cancer targets are now being identified based on proteomics tools, where the mechanisms of action for anticancer agents and novel targets are being elucidated via chemical proteomics.

New immunotherapies have been inspired based on the ability of a patient's immune system to recognize and reject cancerous tissue. Therapeutic cancer vaccines are developed in order to activate immune-cells to recognize and kill malignant cells. Recently, immune cell-based therapies have been developed by utilizing T-cells and their ability to direct cytotoxicity (cell death) toward their targets as well as their ability to orchestrate immune responses via cytokine secretion. Many immunostimulators and immunomodulators activate an effective anti-tumor response or reverse tumor-mediated immunosuppression through manipulation of key regulatory pathways. Additionally, significant advances have been made in improving the performance of small-molecule-based cancer therapies by enabling long circulation and delivery through the blood–brain barrier.

Overall, this book highlights the most recent and up-to-date advances in the field of biologics, vaccines, and cancer therapies. This book will greatly help researchers and students to enhance their understanding of these novel trends and approaches.

NOVEL THERAPEUTIC APPROACHES

Clinical Considerations in the Design, Evaluation, and Development of Novel Therapies

Ernesto Oviedo-Orta

Novartis Vaccines and Diagnostics, Vaccines Research, Siena, Italy

INTRODUCTION

Today's healthcare landscape turns around not only on diseases and medical needs that continue to be unmet but also on a political and public perception background totally different than what was encountered 20 years ago. The new challenges in drug development are therefore focused on parallel routes that are very closely scrutinized: (1) the production of new and more effective and safer drugs, and (2) the tightened regulatory environment driven by public and political influences. Regulatory bodies, especially in the United States but also in Europe, are dictating the pace at which medicines are being trialed and approved beyond their borders, and we can say now that a pathway toward global harmonization may no longer be a dream but an achievable and not so distant goal. Technically speaking, the

Novel Approaches and Strategies for Biologics, Vaccines and Cancer Therapies. DOI: 10.1016/B978-0-12-416603-5.00001-8

development and testing of pharmaceutical compounds today represent a dynamic and self-improving environment that has achieved a level of globalization and sophistication that makes licensed products almost flawless. However, to attain such a level of sophistication clinical researchers have had to develop, and are continuing to develop, innovative and in many cases riskier strategies to make sure that during the process of assessment the data derived clearly answer the most critical questions related to safety, tolerability, and efficacy for each compound. Nevertheless, in certain diseases we have come to the realization that a personalized approach may be more effective despite the costs and the time and effort associated with the chosen therapeutic strategy.

This chapter provides a general and critical overview of the current process for the design, evaluation, and testing of pharmaceutical compounds destined to treat or prevent diseases in humans. First, we will look at how new scientific discoveries are shaping the discovery and speed of development of pharmaceutical compounds before moving on to describe how the clinical evaluation pathway has been adapted to address more refined scientific questions and to meet stringent regulatory and financial constraints. The chapter concludes with questions and challenges that must be addressed.

SCIENTIFIC CHALLENGES IN THE DESIGN OF EFFECTIVE PHARMACOLOGICAL AND BIOLOGICAL COMPOUNDS

In the quest to identify and license a pharmaceutical product most of us will agree that science most follow medicine. Although this axiom has traditionally been the norm it is being applied less frequently today. Compounds are generally developed for specific, targeted diseases or disorders; however, there are many examples of cross-disease usage of drugs. In light of recent developments, especially in bioinformatics and computational biology, new approaches to drug discovery are being implemented. The identification of common pathways and processes for the synthesis, metabolism, and degradation of certain natural or synthetic compounds has aided scientists in the discovery, design, and modification of drugs targeting various diseases. Also, biological or clinical observations during experimental or medical usage of drugs have proven useful. Such observations, supported by an extensive body of research discoveries, are helping to solve the dilemma of an increasingly narrowing product pipeline within the pharmaceutical industry. Novel scientific breakthroughs are becoming more difficult to achieve, even in the early stages of clinical development, in part because of cross-over, paradoxically, to common physiological and metabolic pathways that their specificity targets.

Indisputably, the pharmaceutical industry has come to the realization that their relationship with academia is evolving into a long-awaited marriage. As we look deeper into the causes of diseases, we have come to realize that, even though the industry has developed the infrastructure and practical and financial foundations required to allow the development and licensing of new drugs, it will still come up short in the race toward discovery when academia can provide quicker and more affordable answers. Partnerships between industry and academia today are fundamental to breaking the discovery bottlenecks that are limiting the pipeline and providing a business model opportunity to support and sustain basic research.

From the clinical perspective, addressing as early as possible the predictability of side and adverse effects is one of the greatest challenges for scientists. In many cases, the scientific evidence accumulated today provides us with sufficient information to make qualified predictions; however, as our scientific methods develop further and disease targets are refined, new challenges will inevitably emerge. Animal models have served as a platform for obtaining safety evidence for drug usage, but intrinsic biological differences between humans and some of the animal species used as models (e.g., mouse, rabbit) raise questions about the reliability of results obtained. History has demonstrated that we cannot continue to rely on this classical approach. The sad reality is that there are currently no prediction tools or technologies available to provide us with reliable information at a molecular level with regard to the safety of a compound before it is tested in humans. It is hoped that eventually humanized animal models and *ex vivo* human tissue systems, together with advanced systems biology applications, can be utilized but such information is still limited and unreliable. Moreover, genetic diversity will continue to be the main hurdle for many disease targets in terms of response and drug metabolism further adding to the uncertainty.

Scientific challenges derive from specific elements of experimental analysis; for example, it has been postulated that methods for measuring the free energy of binding small molecules to random molecules, including nucleic acids and proteins, are still inaccurate. Such a lack of knowledge substantially hinders the design and validation of prediction algorithms that can model specific responses and shed light on the behavioral characteristics of these molecules in different artificial and biological environments. Protein–ligand interactions are at the core of the mechanisms of action of many drugs, and these interactions are important to the tissue distribution, metabolism, and excretion of drugs. From very early in the process of discovery great attention is given to the product formulation and the behavior of the discovered new molecules in different solvents that can be used as vehicles for administration. It seems that we are still a long way from finding the platforms necessary to understand and subsequently optimize these interactions, especially for complex mixtures in which the only available solution is to maintain the compounds separately until the moment of administration. Such considerations have important clinical relevance to assessing not only the safety but also the efficacy of a drug.

On the other hand, we have gained extraordinary knowledge regarding the modification and engineering of biological compounds in order to make them more suitable for use, such as eliminating bioactive deleterious fragments, using molecular fusion to enhance the biological effect, and targeting mutations to increase or decrease degradation. Still, biologicals continue to present new challenges associated with their size, molecular interactions *in vivo*, and, most importantly, their recognition by the immune system, which can potentially trigger a myriad of proinflammatory or suppressor reactions. Biologicals such as monoclonal antibodies and vaccines represent a significant number of all therapeutics used today and are among the most promising to consider for further development. Their use spans inflammatory chronic diseases, cancer, autoimmunity, infectious diseases, and allergies.

The use of biomarkers that provide data on the effect of these interventions is as important as the compound that is being evaluated. No clinical study using small bioactive molecules or biologicals is conducted without the use of an accompanying set of biomarkers that monitors either the safety or the efficacy of the intervention. This is a field that has received enormous investment and has taken center stage in the relationship between academia and the industry.

The use of biomarkers spans the entire process of drug discovery and clinical evaluation. During early clinical phases of evaluation, biomarkers are critical tools to assess functional responses, safety and toxicity data used to support go/no-go decisions, and eventually dose selection. As such, their application changes in later phases of drug development, where they are mostly used to provide data on specific disease-related parameters and pharmacokinetics and to understand inter-patient variability. Such information is critical to enhancing the strength of a regulatory dossier submission. Fundamental characteristics of biomarkers used in clinical research are that they must be reliable and accurate for the purpose of aiding decision making. These biomarkers should comply with analytical validation requirements specific for the stage of drug development process being assessed and, after implementation, they must be subjected to revalidation to guarantee their quality and performance.

CHANGES IN THE CURRENT LANDSCAPE OF CLINICAL DEVELOPMENT EVALUATION FOR NOVEL THERAPIES

In 2012, a new program was announced by the U.S. Food and Drug Administration (USFDA) aiming to strengthen global regulatory capacity by working with the World Health Organization (WHO) to support new, innovative approaches to clinical trial designs for vaccine products and post-marketing pharmacovigilance. The program states that, "Adequate regulatory oversight throughout the vaccine development life cycle is essential in assuring the safety, purity, and potency of vaccines and other biological. ... With the globalization of markets, the volume of vaccines and biological medicinal products crossing national borders continues to rise, making it even more critical that regulatory knowledge and experience be shared as appropriate to do so, and that global monitoring to ensure product safety be harmonized to the greatest extent possible." Both the USFDA and WHO are proposing entering into an agreement to investigate new approaches to designing clinical trials for vaccines. "In the case of early phase clinical trials, new approaches can more rapidly determine whether novel vaccine candidates are likely to be safe and efficacious, and better approaches to optimizing allocation of study participants between late phase clinical trials and post-marketing safety studies could lead to more rapid access to lifesaving vaccines, while still obtaining the data necessary to ensure vaccine safety." The main goals of the project are to minimize the number of ineffective candidate vaccines entering into Phase IIb and Phase III clinical trials, to identify promising vaccines candidates early on in the development cycle for accelerated testing, to establish "correlates of protection" more quickly, and to promote the efficient use of clinical trial resources. It is also recognized that special attention should be paid to pharmacovigilance, particularly for "rare adverse events" that are not being caught during clinical trials and that it is "essential to continue monitoring of vaccine safety throughout the product life cycle and to obtain and analyze any additional safety information in 'real time.' The project targets the improvement of adverse event data reporting and evaluation and the interoperability of global pharmacovigilance systems approaches to clinical trials in low- and middle-income countries and how social media and mobile communication devices can be used to promote vaccine safety. The project would also seek to develop a mathematical simulation of a vaccine's development life cycle to better anticipate what constitutes "acceptable vaccine risk."

In recent years, many changes have been made to the regulatory aspects of clinical trials. Most changes derive from the introduction of good clinical practices (GCPs), good manufacturing practices (GMPs), and the Clinical Trials Directive, which is based on GCPs and GMPs. The main documents include the following:

- International Conference on Harmonisation (ICH) Directive 75/318/EEC on GCPs[1]
- European Union (EU) Directive 2001/20/EC on clinical trials[2]
- *EudraLex—The Rules Governing Medicinal Products in the European Union*, Volume 4[3,4] and Annexes, especially Annexes 1,[5] 13,[6] and 16[7]
- European Commission Directive 2003/94/EC on GMPs for medicinal products and ideal medical practices (IMPs)[8]
- European Commission Directive 2005/28/EC on GCPs[9]
- European Medicines Agency's *Guideline on Strategies to Identify and Mitigate Risks for First-in-Human Trials with Investigational Medicinal Products* (EMEA/CHMP/SWP/28367/07).[10]

The Statutory Instrument (SI) 2004/1031 has since been amended on an annual basis. Its aims are

- To simplify and harmonise clinical trials across Europe
- To give better protection to subjects who take part in clinical trials
- To enforce by law the principles of GCPs and GMPs.

The European Commission has published a set of guidelines covering a range of clinical trial aspects (*EudraLex*, Volume 10).[3] The *EudraLex* is a 10-volume set of regulations and guidelines governing medicinal products in the European Union.

The scope of the Clinical Trials Directive is wide; it covers all commercial and academic clinical trials of IMPs and marketed medicines, apart from trials of marketed medicines prescribed in the usual way. The types of IMPs are as follows:[11]

- Chemical entities
- Biotechnology products
- Cell therapy products
- Gene therapy products
- Plasma-derived products
- Other extractive products
- Immunological products, such as vaccines, allergens, and immune sera
- Herbal products
- Homeopathic products
- Radiopharmaceutical products.

Exploratory clinical studies are those intended to be conducted early in Phase I and that involve limited human exposure, have no therapeutic or diagnostic intent, and are not intended to examine maximum tolerated dose. First-time-in-man (FTIM) studies have been pursued more and more due to the common inability to predict the safety and pharmacological behavior of new medicines by animal models. Although the assumption of prediction of nontoxic effects and molecular behavior should always be supported by assessment in preclinical animal models as required by the regulatory authorities, these are not an absolute guarantee due to species differences and diverse genetic makeups, among other reasons. The Committee for Medical Products for Human Use (CMPHU) set up the ICH M3 in order to harmonize the general requirements for nonclinical support for human clinical trials in the European Union. These guidelines apply to all new chemical and biological investigational medicinal products except gene and cell therapy medicinal products and cover nonclinical issues for consideration prior to the first administration in humans and the design and conduct of such trials. Most recently, these guidelines have been revised and are required to be applied to all FTIM studies and not just to those compounds classified as "higher risk."

Current development of novel pharmaceutical products requires not only innovative testing but also lower costs and less time to distinguish earlier in the drug development process those candidates that hold promise from those that do not. A new section added to the revised M3, referred to as "Exploratory Clinical Studies," recognizes that in some cases human physiology/pharmacology insights may be necessary to expand knowledge of a drug candidate's characteristics and therapeutic target relevance to disease. Such knowledge will benefit greatly from access to earlier human data and exploratory approaches.

The ICH M3[12] states five clinical approaches that can be supported by more limited nonclinical testing programs. The approaches imply a more thorough characterization of the pharmacology using *in vivo* and/or *in vitro* disease models in support of human dose selection.

Microdose Studies

The first approach would involve a total dose of not more than 100 μg that can be divided among up to five doses in any subject. These uses could be supported by an extended single-dose toxicity study in one species, usually rodent, by the clinical route of administration, together with appropriate characterization of pharmacology. The second microdose approach is one that involves fewer than five administrations with a maximum of 100 μg per administration (a total of 500 μg per subject). This approach could be supported by a 7-day toxicity study in one species, usually rodent, by the clinical route of administration, together with further pharmacological characterization. The guideline also suggests the use of clinical microdose studies using the intravenous (i.v.) route on a product intended for oral administration and for which an oral nonclinical toxicology package already exists. But, it only recommends that approach for investigations of i.v. local tolerance if the dose is above 100 μg.

Single-Dose Studies up to Subtherapeutic or Intended Therapeutic Range

The third approach involves a single dose within the subtherapeutic (pharmacological) or therapeutic range in subjects. The maximum allowable dose should be derived from the nonclinical data. It can be further limited based on clinical information obtained during a single-dose study in humans. This approach could be supported by extended single-dose toxicity studies in both rodent and non-rodent species, an assessment of genotoxic potential (Ames test), appropriate characterization of pharmacology, and a core battery of safety pharmacology studies.

Multiple-Dose Studies

The fourth and fifth approaches involve up to 14 days of dosing for determination of pharmacokinetics and pharmacodynamics in humans and are not intended to support the determination of maximum tolerated clinical dose. These involve 2-week repeated-dose toxicity studies in rodents and non-rodents where dose selection is based on exposure multiples of anticipated area under the curve (AUC) at the maximum clinical dose. In the absence of toxicity in both species, clinical dosing up to 1/10th the lower exposure in either species at the highest dose tested in the animal studies would be considered appropriate. The fifth approach involves a 2-week toxicity study in a rodent species up to a maximum tolerated dose and a confirmatory non-rodent study that seeks to demonstrate that the no observed adverse effect level (NOAEL) in the rodent is also not a toxic dose in the non-rodent. The duration of the non-rodent study should be a minimum of 3 days and at least equivalent to the number of intended administrations in the clinical trial.

It is important to point out that other approaches not described in the ICH M3 guidance may be acceptable and should be discussed with the appropriate regulatory authorities. The amount of nonclinical supporting data appropriate in these situations will be dependent on the extent of proposed human exposure, with respect to both the maximum clinical dose used and the duration of dosing. These studies contribute to making better informed decisions as to whether or not to progress with a compound but cannot be taken as confirmatory evidence.

The USFDA published a guidance entitled *Guidance for Industry. Oversight of Clinical Investigations —A Risk-Based Approach to Monitoring*,[13] which is intended to support the process of clinical monitoring during clinical trials. In addition to being a sponsor's responsibility, the effective monitoring of clinical investigations is critical to the protection of human subjects and the conduct of high-quality studies. The USFDA believes that sponsors of clinical investigations involving human drugs, biological products, medical devices, and combinations thereof are required to provide oversight to ensure adequate protection of the rights, welfare, and safety of human subjects and the quality of the clinical trial data submitted to the USFDA. The USFDA's regulations require sponsors to monitor the conduct and progress of their clinical investigations.[14] The USFDA regulations are not specific about how sponsors are to conduct such monitoring and are therefore compatible with a range of approaches to monitoring that will vary depending on multiple factors.

The USFDA guidelines state that the dramatic growth in the complexity of clinical trials has created novel challenges to clinical trial oversight, particularly increased variability in clinical investigator experience, site infrastructure, treatment choices, and standards of health care,[15] as well as challenges related to geographic dispersion. In parallel, the use of electronic systems and records and improvements in statistical assessments has created opportunities for alternative monitoring approaches (e.g., centralized monitoring) that can improve the quality and efficiency of sponsor oversight of clinical investigations. The USFDA encourages sponsors to develop monitoring plans that manage important risks to human subjects and data quality and that address the challenges of oversight in part by taking advantage of the innovations in modern clinical trials.

The USFDA document clearly states that a risk-based approach to monitoring does not suggest any less vigilance in the oversight of clinical investigations. Rather, it focuses sponsor oversight activities on preventing or mitigating important and likely risks to data quality and to processes critical to human subject protection and trial integrity. Moreover, the USFDA affirms that a risk-based approach is dynamic, more readily facilitating continual improvement in trial conduct and oversight.

This USFDA guidance assists sponsors of clinical investigations in developing risk-based monitoring strategies and plans for investigational studies of medical products, including human drug and biological products, medical devices, and combinations thereof. The objective of the guidance is to enhance human subject protection and the quality of clinical trial data by focusing sponsor oversight on the most important aspects of study conduct and reporting. The guidance makes clear that sponsors can use a variety of approaches to fulfill their responsibilities for monitoring clinical investigator (CI) conduct and performance in investigational new drug (IND) studies conducted under 21 CFR 312 or investigational device exemption (IDE) studies conducted under 21 CFR 812. The guidance describes strategies for monitoring activities that reflect a modern, risk-based approach that focuses on critical study parameters and relies on a combination of monitoring activities to oversee a study effectively. The guidelines describe the FDA current thinking on a topic and shouldn't be viewed only as recommendations, unless specific regulatory or statutory requirements are cited. The use of the word "guidance" means that something is suggested or recommended but not required.

Finally, another area of human experimentation that is closely monitored not just by regulatory authorities but also, and most importantly, by ethics considerations is the case of human challenge studies. Human challenge studies are not new; however, their use becomes more and more relevant in today's clinical research in order to obtain refined scientific answers to questions that cannot be addressed in animal models. One of the first recorded use of a "human challenge" was carried out by Edward Jenner when he used the pus from cowpox sores to infect a healthy boy, James Phipps. History says that 6 weeks later Jenner inoculated Phipps with the pus from smallpox sore and Phipps did not develop smallpox, thus giving birth to what is now considered vaccination. Other examples exist, such as the work of Walter Reed and the Yellow Fever Commission, which investigated the theory that mosquitoes were responsible for the spread of yellow fever. The volunteers were warned of the possibility of death from yellow fever and were each paid a $100 gold piece for their participation in the study.[16] It has been known for many years that the U.K. Medical Research Council's Common Cold Unit challenged healthy volunteers with common cold viruses (rhinovirus) in order to study both the natural history of the disease and the effectiveness of potential treatments, such as antiviral agents.[17-20] Another example has been the use of human challenge in the development of malarial vaccines where the detailed study of both the clinical and immune responses of healthy volunteers to inoculation with candidate vaccines, followed by challenge with the infective organism, is a critical step toward assessing the efficacy of the test vaccine.[21-24]

Other recent examples include challenge with cholera bacilli to evaluate novel vaccines[25-27] and challenge studies with pneumococcus to assess correlates of protection against nasopharyngeal colonization.[28] Human challenge studies are used to study the pathogenesis, transmission, and disease course of a particular infectious agent and to test the efficacy of candidate prophylactic or therapeutic agents. It is argued that incomplete reporting of the methodology of studies involving human challenge experiments may prevent other researchers from repeating those studies and learning how to improve the challenge study methodology over time. It is mandatory that any literature reporting challenge clinical trials with human volunteers must provide readers with enough detail so they can judge the reliability and validity of the study's findings or extract data for systematic reviews. Most importantly, as with all animal and human experimentation, the smart design and execution of each study are essential to conducting ethical research in this field. In 2005, the Academy of Medical Sciences (AMS) published guidelines for conducting microbial challenge studies on human volunteers.[29] These guidelines cover safety and ethical considerations, transparency, and accountability; recruitment of volunteers; consent and confidentiality; and legal issues. The AMS also recommends the formation of a National Expert Advisory Committee and enhanced institutional safety monitoring to ensure the safety and welfare of human subjects participating in human challenge studies.

INFLUENCING AND CHANGING THE *STATUS QUO*: CONSIDERATIONS IN THE CLINICAL DEVELOPMENT OF FUTURE THERAPIES

Many efforts have been made over the last decade toward developing a harmonization process for the regulation and design of clinical trials, including those made by the USFDA and the European Medicines Agency. The influence of the regulatory bodies created by these two major institutions is growing, as other large bodies such as the State Food and Drug Administration (SFDA) in China are following a similar trend. Although they provide a statutory framework, such guidelines should not be seen as a rigid mandates. Scientists know that the process of scientific discovery, the technological advances that accompany it, and their influence on ethics consideration surrounding such investigations continue to evolve. Moreover, it is now accepted that the assessment of clinical effects on human volunteers may require additional scientific and technological support to minimize risk while at the same time speeding up the process of drug assessment and registration.

One important element that clinical scientists have today at their disposal is the availability of large databases that can be interrogated extensively and can provide us with novel or confirmatory information with high predictable value. To accomplish this, current bioinformatics tools require similar harmonization processes that may only be achievable within the academic sector with financial support from governments and global nonprofit organizations that can guarantee their impartiality and accessibility to the scientific and medical communities.

Technological developments can also alleviate the burden of expenses linked to data acquisition from patients in controlled studies. It can also positively affect the expansion of data acquisition to geographically remote areas, where it has not been possible to conduct complex trials, through the use of telemetric technologies for data collection and transmission, thus further reducing the cost of the trials.

Most important, though, is the transparency of clinical trials. Competition is intense, and the rush to be first to market is hindered by the daunting process of target drug discovery. New business models are needed to attract more academic partnerships to improve this process, and perhaps a reassessment of what "discovery" means may be necessary. Sustaining the process of finding new and better drugs to fight diseases is imperative. Despite the setbacks we all are used to, we realize that failure to continue will seriously hinder our quality of life.

Finally, genetic differences may be winning the battle, and the concept of personalized medicine should perhaps be better pondered. Also, the influence of patients and how they influence the process of development should be considered. There are encouraging signs for public registries of drugs, as well as proposals for trial feed-forward mechanisms,[30] in which patients will be allowed to choose between various medicines whose efficacies have been determined in different ways. It has also been speculated that the use of pricing controls may encourage drug developers to move forward toward more progressive trial designs.[31]

The scenario is complex and the pathway forward will require more intelligence than numbers. Only through the realization of the changes that we are experiencing will we be able to propose effective strategies of growth.

References

1. International Conference on Harmonisation (ICH). *Good Clinical Practice*, Directive 75/318/EEC, 1990, http://ec.europa.eu/health/files/eudralex/vol-10/3cc1aen_en.pdf.
2. European Parliament and Council of the European Union. *Directive 2001/20/EC of the European Parliament and of the Council of 4 April 2001*, 2001, http://eur-lex.europa.eu/LexUriServ/LexUriServ.do?uri=OJ:L:2001:121:0034:0044:en:PDF.
3. European Commission. *EudraLex—The Rules Governing Medicinal Products in the European Union*, 2nd ed. Vol. 10. *Clinical Trial Guidelines*, 1992, http://ec.europa.eu/health/documents/eudralex/vol-10/index_en.htm.
4. European Commission. *EudraLex—The Rules Governing Medicinal Products in the European Union*, 2nd ed. Vol. 4. *Good Manufacturing Practice (GMP) Guidelines*, 1992, http://ec.europa.eu/health/documents/eudralex/vol-4/index_en.htm.
5. European Commission. *EudraLex—The Rules Governing Medicinal Products in the European Union*, 2nd ed. Vol. 4. *Good Manufacturing Practice (GMP) Guidelines*. Annex 1: *Manufacture of Sterile Medicinal Products*, 2008, http://ec.europa.eu/health/documents/eudralex/vol-4/index_en.htm.
6. European Commission. *EudraLex—The Rules Governing Medicinal Products in the European Union*, 2nd ed. Vol. 4. *Good Manufacturing Practice (GMP) Guidelines*. Annex 13 *Investigative Medical Products*, 2008, http://ec.europa.eu/health/files/eudralex/vol-4/2009_06_annex13.pdf.
7. European Commission. *EudraLex—The Rules Governing Medicinal Products in the European Union*. Vol. 4. *Good Manufacturing Practice (GMP) Guidelines*. Annex 16: *Certification by a Qualified Person and Batch Release*, 2001, http://ec.europa.eu/health/files/eudralex/vol-4/pdfs-m/v4_an16_200408_en.pdf.
8. European Commission. *Commission Directive 2003/94/EC of the European Parliament and of the Council of 8 October 2003*, 2003, http://ec.europa.eu/health/files/eudralex/vol-1/dir_2003_94/dir_2003_94_en.pdf.
9. European Commission. *Commission Directive 2005/28/EC of the European Parliament and of the Council of 8 April 2005*, 2005, http://eur-lex.europa.eu/LexUriServ/LexUriServ.do?uri=OJ:L:2005:091:0013:0019:en:PDF.
10. European Medicines Agency. *Guidelines on Strategies to Identify and Mitigate Risks for First-in-Human Clinical Trials with Investigational Medicinal Products*. London: Committee for Medicinal Products for Human Use, European Medicines Agency, 2007, http://www.ema.europa.eu/docs/en_GB/document_library/Scientific_guideline/2009/09/WC500002988.pdf.
11. European Medicines Agency. *Non-Clinical Safety Studies for the Conduct of Human Clinical Trials and Marketing Authorization for Pharmaceuticals*. Step 4. *Note for Guidance on Non-Clinical Safety Studies for the Conduct of Human Clinical Trials and Marketing Authorization for Pharmaceuticals*, CPMP/ICH/286/95. London: Committee for Medicinal Products for Human Use, European Medicines Agency, 2009, http://www.tga.gov.au/pdf/euguide/ich028695enfinal.pdf.
12. European Medicines Agency. *Non-Clinical Safety Studies for the Conduct of Human Clinical Trials and Marketing Authorization for Pharmaceuticals*. Step 3. *Note for Guidance on Non-Clinical Safety Studies for the Conduct of Human Clinical Trials and Marketing Authorization for Pharmaceuticals*, CPMP/ICH/286/95. London: Committee for Medicinal Products for Human Use, European Medicines Agency, 2008, http://www.ema.europa.eu/docs/en_GB/document_library/Scientific_guideline/2009/09/WC500002941.pdf.

13. USFDA. Guidance for Industry: Oversight of Clinical Investigations—A Risk-Based Approach to Monitoring. Silver Spring, MD: U.S. Food and Drug Administration; 2013, http://www.fda.gov/downloads/Guidances/UCM269919.pdf.

14. USFDA. *Code of Federal Regulations Title 21: Food and Drugs.* Chapter 1: Food and Drug Administration Department of Health and Human Services. Subpart D: Responsibilities of Sponsors and Investigators. Washington, DC: Food and Drug Administration; 2013, http://www.gpo.gov/fdsys/pkg/CFR-2011-title21-vol5/pdf/CFR-2011-title21-vol5-sec312-50.pdf.

15. Glickman SW, McHutchison JG, Peterson ED, Cairns CB, Harrington RA, Califf RM, et al. Ethical and scientific implications of the globalization of clinical research. New Engl. J. Med. 2009;360(8):816–23.

16. Hope T, McMillan J. Challenge studies of human volunteers: ethical issues. J. Med. Ethics. 2004;30(1):110–6.

17. Callow KA, Parry HF, Sergeant M, Tyrrell DA. The time course of the immune response to experimental coronavirus infection of man. Epidemiol. Infect. 1990;105(2):435–46.

18. Higgins PG, Barrow GI, Tyrrell DA, Isaacs D, Gauci CL. The efficacy of intranasal interferon alpha-2a in respiratory syncytial virus infection in volunteers. Antiviral Res. 1990;14(1):3–10.

19. Al-Nakib W, Higgins PG, Barrow I, Tyrrell DA, Lenox-Smith I, Ishitsuka H. Intranasal chalcone, Ro 09-0410, as prophylaxis against rhinovirus infection in human volunteers. J. Antimicrob. Chemother. 1987;20(6):887–92.

20. Smith AP, Tyrrell DA, Al-Nakib W, Coyle KB, Donovan CB, Higgins PG, et al. Effects of experimentally induced respiratory virus infections and illness on psychomotor performance. Neuropsychobiology 1987;18(3):144–8.

21. Crompton PD, Moebius J, Portugal S, Waisberg M, Hart G, Garver LS, et al. Malaria immunity in man and mosquito: insights into unsolved mysteries of a deadly infectious disease. Annu. Rev. Immunol. 2014;32:157–87.

22. White MT, Bejon P, Olotu A, Griffin JT, Riley EM, Kester KE, et al. The relationship between RTS,S vaccine-induced antibodies, CD4(+) T cell responses and protection against *Plasmodium falciparum* infection. PloS ONE 2013;8(4):e61395.

23. Richie TL, Charoenvit Y, Wang R, Epstein JE, Hedstrom RC, Kumar S, et al. Clinical trial in healthy malaria-naive adults to evaluate the safety, tolerability, immunogenicity and efficacy of MuStDO5, a five-gene, sporozoite/hepatic stage *Plasmodium falciparum* DNA vaccine combined with escalating dose human GM-CSF DNA. Hum. Vaccin. Immunother. 2012;8(11):1564–84.

24. Sheehy SH, Duncan CJ, Elias SC, Choudhary P, Biswas S, Halstead FD, et al. ChAd63-MVA-vectored blood-stage malaria vaccines targeting MSP1 and AMA1: assessment of efficacy against mosquito bite challenge in humans. Mol. Ther. 2012;20(12):2355–68.

25. Shirley DA, McArthur MA. The utility of human challenge studies in vaccine development: lessons learned from cholera. Vaccine (Auckl) 2011;2011(1):3–13.

26. Garcia L, Jidy MD, Garcia H, Rodriguez BL, Fernandez R, Ano G, et al. The vaccine candidate *Vibrio cholerae* 638 is protective against cholera in healthy volunteers. Infect. Immun. 2005;73(5):3018–24.

27. Pitisuttithum P, Migasena S, Suntharasamai P, Supanaranond W, Desakorn V, Prayurahong B. Immune responses following killed whole vibrio-B subunit oral cholera vaccine in human volunteers. Southeast Asian J. Trop. Med. Public Health 1989;20(2):201–5.

28. Gritzfeld JF, Wright AD, Collins AM, Pennington SH, Wright AK, Kadioglu A, et al. Experimental human pneumococcal carriage. J. Vis. Exp. 2013;72.

29. AMS. Medical Challenge Studies of Human Volunteers. London: Academy of Medical Sciences; 2005. www.acmedsci.ac.uk/download.php?i=13495&f=file.

30. Hvitfeldt H, Carli C, Nelson EC, Mortenson DM, Ruppert BA, Lindblad S. Feed forward systems for patient participation and provider support: adoption results from the original US context to Sweden and beyond. Qual. Manag. Health Care 2009;18(4):247–56.

31. Madden BJ. Free to Choose Medicine. Chicago, IL: Heartland Institute; 2010.

I. NOVEL THERAPEUTIC APPROACHES

New Era in Gene Therapy

Kenneth Lundstrom

Pan Therapeutics, Lutry, Switzerland

INTRODUCTION

Gene therapy, defined as genetic modifications and gene delivery in medical interventions, has seen a wide variety of applications during the last 20 years. Typically, both non-viral and viral delivery systems have been used, from basic research to clinical trials. The key issues to address have been the lack of efficiency of gene delivery, inefficient targeting of action tissue, intermittent duration of therapeutic effect, and obviously unknown long-term safety of the whole procedure. Although *in vitro* models and preclinical studies in rodent models demonstrated high therapeutic efficacy, disappointing results have been obtained in primates and particularly in patients in clinical trials. However, intensive vector development and formulation activities such as application of different vectors and strategies have presented real improvement and have brought breakthroughs to gene therapy of various diseases. Recently, targeted deliveries of therapeutic genes and

Novel Approaches and Strategies for Biologics, Vaccines and Cancer Therapies. DOI: 10.1016/B978-0-12-416603-5.00002-X gene silencing molecules have begun to demonstrate therapeutic effects in both animal models and human patients.

Since the late 1990s, gene therapy has gone from being considered the "medicine of the future" to the "failure in drug discovery." Early development of gene therapy combined with the knowledge obtained from sequencing the complete human genome were perhaps naively thought to bring a revolution to modern medicine. However, as was to be discovered the hard way, major obstacles mostly related to delivery, efficacy, and safety had to be overcome. In hindsight, it was therefore not a surprise that at the height of the hype mistakes were made. Typically, researchers with little experience in clinical trials set off to test their favorite vectors in patients. Most tragically, the application of an adenovirus vector to treat a non-life-threatening disease, ornithine transcarbamylase deficiency, resulted in the death of an 18-year-old male.[1] Although definitely seen as a success, the treatment of children with severe combined immunodeficiency (SCID) resulted in leukemia due to retrovirus integration into the LMO2 protooncogene region.[2,3] This clearly demonstrated the necessity of more basic research and vector development to provide efficient and safe therapeutic intervention.

Gene therapy can be defined as the application of heterologous genetic material or replacement of malfunctioning genetic information with functional counterparts to obtain a therapeutic effect in animal models and human individuals. Generally, non-viral and viral vectors have been employed for the delivery of genetic material; however, gene therapy applications must be further expanded to the use of oligonucleotides and RNAi sequences.[4] Due to the broad range of potential applications, various vectors have been evaluated for a large spectrum of indications, including different types of cancer, hemophilia, muscular dystrophy, ophthalmological diseases, and immunodeficiency as summarized in Table 2.1. The aim of this chapter is to give an overview of current development in gene therapy with an emphasis on cancer therapy.

NON-VIRAL VECTORS

Gene delivery based on non-viral vectors has attracted much attention due to their universal application range and high safety level of delivery.[5] A number of nanoparticle delivery systems based on polymers and liposomes have been developed. Furthermore, physical approaches including, for example, electroporation and gene gun have provided the means for plasmid DNA and other forms of nucleic acid delivery.

Polymers and Dendrimers

Microsphere polymer formulations have been engineered to generate micro- and nanoparticle systems for subcutaneous and intramuscular injections. In this context, poly(lactic acid) (PLA) and poly(lactic-co-glycolic acid) (PLGA) have provided enhanced and slow release of drugs.[6,7] Furthermore, biodegradable semicrystalline poly-ε-caprolactone (PLC) polyesters have demonstrated slow degradation and sustained drug release.[8] Additionally, polyphosphoesters, polyanhydrides, and polyorthoesters have frequently been used for drug delivery.[5] Particularly block co-polymers have been used for extended release of interleukin-2 (IL-2) in renal carcinoma patients.[9] Moreover, several cationic polymers such as polyethylenimine

TABLE 2.1　Gene and Drug Delivery Methods

Delivery	Cargo	Indication	Observation	Refs.
POLYMERS				
PLA	Paclitaxel, 5-FU	Cancer	High encapsulation efficiency	Gupte and Ciftci[6]
Block copolymer	IL-2	Renal cancer	Sustained release	Chan et al.[9]
Poly(β-amino ester)	Minicircle DNA	*In vitro* delivery	Improved gene delivery	Keeney et al.[11]
Bioreducible polymer	Plasmid DNA	Liver cancer	Hepatoma cell specific expression	Kim et al.[12]
DENDRIMERS				
Bioreducible polymer	Plasmid DNA	Gene delivery carrier	Enhanced cellular uptake	Nam et al.[14]
PAMAM-EGF	Plasmid DNA	Cancer	Tumor targeting	Yin et al.[15]
Triazine dendrimers	DNA, RNA, drugs	Gene delivery carrier	Promising *in vivo* activity	Lim and Simanek[16]
LIPOSOMES				
Stealth liposomes	Doxorubicin	Cancer	Enhanced delivery	Cattel et al.[23]
Cationic liposomes	Cisplatin	Cancer	Reduced cytotoxicity	Stathopoulos and Boulikas[24]
Cationic/anionic liposomes	Plasmid DNA	Tumors	Tumor accumulation	Chen et al.[25]
Liposomes + folate receptor	Gene delivery	Ovarian cancer	Targeted delivery	He et al.[26]
Liposomes + PSA/PSMA	siRNA	Prostate cancer	Targeted delivery	Xiang et al.[27]
Dendrosomes	Plasmid DNA	HeLa cells	Delivery	Movassaghian et al.[28]
Lipid–polymer hybrids	Plasmid DNA, drugs	Cancer cells	Improved delivery	Hadinoto et al.[29]
ELECTROPORATION				
Subcutaneous	Plasmid DNA	Cancer, neuro	Immunotherapy	Fioretti et al.[31]
Intradermal	Plasmid DNA	Cancer	Tumor protective antigen	Ligtenberg et al.[32]
Intratumoral	DNA (IL12)/cisplatin	Melanoma	B16 tumor regression	Kim and Sin[33]
Retinal	Plasmid DNA/rAAV	Eye diseases	Retinal delivery	Venkatesh et al.[34]
Electroporation	Plasmid DNA	Cell delivery	Restricted transport to nuclei	Dean[35]
Electroporation	Plasmid DNA	Alzheimer	DNA vaccine	Aravindaram and Yang[38]

(Continued)

I. NOVEL THERAPEUTIC APPROACHES

TABLE 2.1   Gene and Drug Delivery Methods *(cont.)*

Delivery	Cargo	Indication	Observation	Refs.
GENE GUN				
Gene gun	DNA/gold particles	Schistosomiasis	DNA vaccine	Cao et al.[37]
Gene gun	Plasmid DNA	Alzheimer	DNA vaccine	Daytyan et al.[38]
Subcutaneous	Plasmid DNA	Sarcoma	Fibrosarcoma suppression	Abe et al.[39]
Gene gun	HPV E7, 6, 5 DNA	Cancer	Enhanced antitumor effect	Smahel et al.[40]
ADENOVIRUS				
Ad5	Therapeutic genes	Various cancers	Tumor regression *in vitro/in vivo*	Matthews et al.,[46] Ekblad and Halden,[47] Fu et al.[48]
Ad5T*F35++	TIMP-3	Vascular cells	Targeted delivery	White et al.[49]
Man-Ad5-PTEN	β-Galactosidase	Cancer	Tumor-specific cell killing	Liu et al.[50]
Ad RPL23/p53	RPL23-p53	Gastric cancer	Tumor suppression	Zhang et al.[51]
Oncolytic adenovirus	shRNA	Cancer	Increased tumor regression	Choi et al.[53]
Oncolytic adenovirus VRX-007	Luciferase	Cancer	Reduced tumor growth	Young et al.[54]
Oncolytic Ad5	hTERT	GI cancer	Improved delivery	Fujiwara[55]
Oncolytic adenovirus	Combined radiotherapy	Cancer	Improved tumor growth inhibition	Young et al.[56]
Oncolytic adenovirus	E1A	Cancer	Tumor-specific replication	Wang et al.[44]
ADENO-ASSOCIATED VIRUS (AAV)				
AAV	Factor IX	Hemophilia	Long-term therapeutic FIX expression	Chuah et al.[64]
AAV9	Sulfamidase	MPS IIIA CNS	Treatment of MPS IIIA in mice	Haurigot et al.[65]
AAV	IFN-γ	Retinoblastoma	Antitumor effect	Shih et al.[60]
AAV2	VEGF	Pulmonary cancer	Prevention of 4T1 metastases	Lu et al.[61]
AAV1/2	EGFP	Lung cancer cells	High transduction efficiency	Chen et al.[62]

TABLE 2.1   Gene and Drug Delivery Methods *(cont.)*

Delivery	Cargo	Indication	Observation	Refs.
AAV3-HGFR	Reporter gene	Hepatoblastoma	Improved transduction	Ling et al.[66]
AAV	Apoptin-IL-24	Liver cancer	Apoptosis, tumor regression	Yuan et al.[67]
AAV5/6	neu	Breast cancer	Oral delivery, better survival	Steele et al.[68]
HERPES SIMPLEX VIRUS				
HSV-1	Various genes	CNS targets	Parkinson's, Alzheimer's	Jerusalinsky et al.[70]
HSV-1 RH2	Lytic virus	Human SCC	Tumor suppression	Meshii et al.[71]
HSV-1	miRNA-145	NSCLC	Reduced cell proliferation	Li et al.[72]
HSV	hNIS	Prostate cancer	Tumor eradication	Li et al.[73]
RETROVIRUS				
MLV	γ-Chain	SCID-X1	Successful treatment	Cavazzano-Calvo et al.[74]
Retrovirus	iNOS	Cancer	Tumor growth inhibition	Khare et al.[76]
Retrovirus	TRAIL	Ovarian cancer	Tumor activity	Li et al.[77]
HERV	HERV-K Env Abs	Melanoma	Tumor growth inhibition	Cecolon et al.[78]
LENTIVIRUS				
HIV-1	INS-FUR	Hepatocytes	Normoglycemia in mice	Ren et al.[81]
HIV-1	shRNA, siRNA	AIDS, HIV	Cell-based therapy	Liu et al.,[86] DiGiusto et al.[87]
HIV-1	GDNF	Parkinson's	Primate model	Kordower et al.[88]
HIV-1	CNTF	Huntington's	Quinolinic acid rat model	de Almeida et al.[90]
HIV-1	PSCA	Prostate cancer	Vaccine	Xiao et al.[91]
HIV-1	IFN-γ	Pancreatic cancer	Prevention of cancer progression	Ravet et al.[85]
HIV-1	shRNA	Liver cancer	Inhibition of proliferation	Zhang et al.[92]
HIV-1	Livin	Lung cancer	Reduced tumor proliferation	Chen et al.[93]

(Continued)

I. NOVEL THERAPEUTIC APPROACHES

TABLE 2.1   Gene and Drug Delivery Methods *(cont.)*

Delivery	Cargo	Indication	Observation	Refs.
HIV-1	Livin	Lung cancer	Oral delivery	Minai-Tehrani et al.[94]
HIV-hydrogels	Reporter genes	Cell lines	Improved delivery	Seidlits et al.[95]
HIV-nanofibrils	Reporter genes	Cell lines	Enhance gene transfer	Yolamanova et al.[96]
ALPHAVIRUS				
SFV RNA	β-gal RNA	Cancer	Tumor regression, prevention	Ying et al.[101]
SIN DNA	TRP-1 DNA	Melanoma	Tumor protection	Leitner et al.[102]
SFV	IL-12 p40/p35	Melanoma	Tumor regression	Asselin-Paturel et al.[104]
Oncolytic SFV	EGFP	Melanoma	Tumor regression	Vähä-Koskela et al.[105]
Oncolytic SFV	EGFP	Osteosarcoma	Improved survival	Ketola et al.[106]
Oncolytic SFV	EGFP	Lung cancer	Improved survival	Määttä et al.[107]
SFV DNA	ePNP	Cancer	Oral delivery, tumor regression	Chen et al.[108]
SIN	Luciferase, IL-12	Cancer	Natural tumor targeting	Tseng et al.[110]
SFV-liposomes	β-gal, IL-12	Cancer	Target delivery	Lundstrom and Boulikas[111]
POXVIRUS				
Vaccinia	Mutant TK–VGF	Cancer	Tumor-specific replication	Zeh and Bartlett[113]
Vaccinia	IL-2/IL-12	C6 glioma	Antitumor activity	Chen et al.[115]
Oncolytic vaccinia	GLV-1h68	Colorectal cancer	Tumor growth inhibition	Ehrig et al.[116]
Oncolytic vaccinia	GLV-1h68	Salivary gland	Tumor regression	Chernichenko et al.[117]
Oncolytic vaccinia	Anti-VEGF scAb	Canine cancer	Tumor growth inhibition	Patil et al.[118]
Oncolytic vaccinia	GLV	XP-cancer	Long-term tumor resolution	Brun et al.[119]
Oncolytic vaccinia	GLV-1h68	Sarcomas	Complete tumor regression	He et al.[120]

TABLE 2.1   Gene and Drug Delivery Methods *(cont.)*

Delivery	Cargo	Indication	Observation	Refs.
BACULOVIRUS				
Baculovirus	Reporter gene	Colorectal cancer	Tumor delivery	Paul et al.[125]
Baculovirus	hEA	Prostate cancer	Anti-angiogenic activity	Luo et al.[126]
Baculovirus	Nitroreductase	Glioma	Tumor growth inhibition	Zhao et al.[128]

Abbreviations: 5-FU = 5 fluorouracil; anti-VEGF scAb = anti-vascular epidermal growth factor single-chain antibody; CNTF = ciliary neurotrophic factor; EGFP = enhanced green fluorescent protein; ePNP = *E. coli* purine nucleoside phosphorylase 2; GDNF = glial cell line-derived factor; hEA = human endostatin–angiostatin fusion; HERV = human endogenous retrovirus; HPV = human papilloma virus; hNIS = human sodium iodide symporter; hTERT = human telomerase reverse transcriptase; IFN-γ = interferon-γ; IL-2 = interleukin-2; IL-12 = interleukin-12; IL-24 = interleukin-24; iNOS = inducible nitric oxide synthase; INS-FUR = furin-cleavable insulin; PSCA = prostate stem cell antigen; RPL23-p53 = ribosomal protein 23-p53; SFV = Semliki Forest virus; SIN = Sindbis virus; TIMP-3 = tissue inhibitor of matrix metalloproteinase 3; TK–VGF = thymidine kinase–Vaccinia growth factor; TRAIL = TNF-related apoptosis-inducing ligand; TRP-1 = TYR-related protein 1; XP = xeroderma pigmentosum.

(PEI), poly-L-lysine (PLL), chitosan, and poly(amidoamine) (PAMAM) have been used for gene delivery.[10] In general, the delivery efficacy is lower than that obtained for viral vectors, although some improvements have been achieved through PEGylation and combination and multifunctional modifications of cationic polymeric vectors.

Recently, biodegradable nanoparticles based on poly(β-amino ester) (PBAE) were generated for efficient delivery of minicircle DNA.[11] The PBAE-based delivery was more efficient than Lipofectamine® 2000 in HEK293 cells and mouse embryonic fibroblasts. Additionally, high transgene expression was observed after intraperitoneal injections *in vivo*. In another study, a novel hypoxia and hepatoma dual-specific gene expression system was engineered.[12] The bioreducible PAM-ABP polymer was employed for the delivery of plasmid DNA hosting an alphafectoprotein (AFP) promoter and enhancer for hepatoma tissue for luciferase reporter gene expression. Furthermore, the erythropoietin (Epo) enhancer was introduced for hypoxic cancer-specific gene expression, which resulted in increased reporter gene expression in transfected hepatoma cells under hypoxic conditions. Moreover, introduction of herpes simplex virus thymidine kinase (HSV-TK) enhanced cancer cell death in the presence of ganciclovir.

Dendrimers have been developed as complex nanocarriers for a number of biomedical applications.[13] For example, arginine-grafted bioreducible poly(disulfide amine) (ABP) incorporated into the PAMAM dendrimer showed efficient packaging of plasmid DNA.[14] The cellular uptake of these compact polyplexes was superior to ABP alone and may provide a promising gene delivery system. In another study, epidermal growth factor (EGF)-conjugated PAMAM dendrimers exhibited enhanced transfection of EGFR-positive cells, decreased cytotoxicity, and EGFR-positive tumor targeting *in vivo*.[15] Furthermore, triazine dendrimers have been applied for drug delivery with an emphasis on DNA and RNA delivery but also drugs such as paclitaxel, camptothecin, brefeldin A (BFA), and desferrioxamine (DFO).[16]

Formulation of polypseudorotaxane (PPRX)-grafted α-cyclodextrin/polyamido amine dendrimer provided sustained release of plasmid DNA.[17] The release occurred for at least 72 hours *in vivo* but retarded when the volume of dissolution medium decreased. Sustained transfection efficiency lasted for at least 14 days after intramuscular injection. PAMAM dendrimers have also found applications. Furthermore, lactosylated dendrimer (G3)/α-cyclodextrin conjugates (Lac-α-CDE(G$_3$)) have been developed as carriers for siRNA molecules for targeting familial amyloidotic polyneuropathy (FAP) caused by the deposition of variant transthyretin (TTR).[18] Hepatocyte-selective siRNA has been evaluated both *in vitro* and *in vivo*. Another approach involved structurally flexible fifth-generation triethanolamine (TEA)-core PAMAM dendrimers (G$_5$) for delivery of sticky siRNA with long complementary sequence overhangs.[19] It was demonstrated that the gene silencing efficacy of siRNA molecules depended on the length, nature, and flexibility of overhangs. Moreover, siRNA interaction with the dendrimer vectors presented an impact on delivery efficacy and thereby gene silencing. Cross-linked neutral PAMAM dendrimers with hydrazide groups and *N*-acetylgalactosamine (GalNAc) ligands were applied for siRNA delivery.[20] Uptake and gene silencing experiments demonstrated efficient interaction with HepG2 cells and significantly decreased luciferase reporter gene expression. Dendrimer-based delivery of short hairpin RNA (shRNA) targeting human telomerase reverse transcriptase (hTERT) for oral cancer was evaluated *in vitro* demonstrating hTERT silencing, growth inhibition, and apoptosis.[21] Moreover, administration of shRNA dendriplex *in vivo* resulted in attenuated tumor growth in a murine xenograft model.

Liposomes

Liposomes have frequently been used for the delivery of drugs and nucleic acids.[22] For example, doxorubicin formulated in stealth liposomes provided a more efficient drug delivery in cancer patients.[23] Moreover, improved tumor targeting and prolonged presence in circulation was obtained for cisplatin encapsulated in liposomes.[24] Recently, complexes containing 3β-[N-(N′,N′-dimethylaminoethane) carbamoyl] cholesterol (DC-Chol) and dioleoylphosphatidyl ethanolamine (DOPE) liposomes and pH-sensitive liposomes composed of cholesteryl hemisuccinate (CHEMS) and DOPE were prepared.[25] These formulations provided high plasmid DNA transfection efficiency and tumor accumulation *in vivo*. In another study, the overexpression of folate receptors on ovarian cancer cells was explored for targeted delivery by engineering folate-modified cationic liposomes (F-PEG-CLPs).[26] Liposome/plasmid DNA complexes (F-targeted lipoplexes) showed protection against DNase degradation and transfected human ovarian carcinoma SKOV-3 cells. Complete inhibition was observed by addition of free folic acid. Furthermore, human oral carcinoma KB cells and human liver carcinoma HepG2 cells were susceptible to F-targeted lipoplexes. Also, a dual-modified liposome with prostate-specific antigen (PSA) and prostate-specific membrane antigen (PSMA) elements provided enhanced tumor targeting and improved delivery of siRNA.[27] This approach elevated cellular uptake and enhanced apoptosis in prostate tumor cells. Moreover, the dual-modified liposomes showed improved accumulation, retention, and knockdown of PLK-1 tumor cells, as well as strong inhibition of tumor growth *in vivo*.

An interesting approach has been to formulate dendromers, which are lipid vesicles containing entrapped PAMAM dendrimer–DNA complexes.[28] Generated dendrosomes were evaluated for transfection efficiency and toxicity in HeLa cells, which suggested that this could provide an alternative gene delivery approach *in vivo*. In another approach, lipid–polymer hybrid nanoparticles, comprised of polymer cores encapsulated by lipid–PEG shells, showed superior *in vivo* cellular delivery efficacy in comparison to polymeric nanoparticles and liposomes.[29] This approach has allowed delivery of not only single drugs for anticancer therapy but also combinatorial and targeted drugs, genetic materials, vaccines, and diagnostic imaging agents.

Electroporation and Gene Gun

Electroporation has provided the means for less invasive drug delivery.[30] It has become a common procedure for DNA delivery in treatment of cancer and neurodegenerative diseases.[31] No adverse effects have been associated with electroporation, and the method has been approved for various clinical applications. Electroporation has been applied for DNA vaccinations with plasmids encoding tyrosine-related protein 2 (TRP2) and ovalbumin (OVA) of mice lacking different signaling components.[32] Antigen-specific CTL responses were obtained in vaccinated animals, and suppression of lung metastasis was observed. Furthermore, intratumoral electroporation of cisplatin in combination with intramuscular electroporation of interleukin-12 (IL-12) cDNA has been evaluated in tumor-bearing mice.[33] Both electroporated cisplatin and IL-12 cDNA resulted in tumor growth inhibition, and combination therapy demonstrated a synergic effect. In another study, electroporation was applied for retinal plasmid DNA delivery.[34] In attempts to provide cell-specific targeting of electroporation-mediated gene delivery, selective plasmid nuclear import has been applied in living animals.[35]

The gene gun technology has been frequently used for DNA delivery for cancer vaccines.[36] In this context, a broad range of somatic cells including established cell lines and primary cultures has been successfully subjected to gene gun-based DNA delivery. For example, BALB/c mice were immunized with a DNA vaccine based on thioredoxin glutathione reductase of *Schistosoma japonicum* (SjTGR) by applying gene gun delivery.[37] All animals vaccinated developed significant specific anti-SjTGR antibodies and splenocyte proliferative responses in the form of increased interferon-γ (IFN-γ) and IL-4 levels. Moreover, protective efficacy against the parasite was obtained. Similarly, the gene gun approach was used for intradermal delivery of an Alzheimer's disease DNA vaccine, which resulted in strong anti-amyloid-β (Aβ) antibody and T-cell responses.[38] Furthermore, the anti-Aβ antibodies demonstrated binding to amyloid plaques in brain tissue and to toxic forms of the Aβ42 peptide.

The gene gun technology has proven successful for skin vaccination against melanoma using human tumor-associated antigen (TAA) gp100.[36] Furthermore, Flt3 ligand DNA-coated gold particles were delivered to C57BL/6J mice previously intradermally injected with MCA205 tumor cells, which resulted in a significant inhibition of tumor growth due to enhanced dendritic cell mobilization and induction of suppressive immunity.[39] In another study, the immune response of gene gun-based DNA vaccines was evaluated by systemic co-administration of two conventional adjuvants (synthetic oligodeoxynucleotide carrying CpG motifs and levamisole).[40] DNA immunizations directed against E7 oncoprotein of human papillomavirus (HPV) type 16 or the BCR-ABL1 oncoprotein reduced activation of mouse splenic CD8+ T-lymphocytes, but the overall antitumor effect was superior. Another DNA vaccine based on HPV type 16 E7, E6, and E5 proteins fused to herpes simplex virus glycoprotein D was administered intradermally using the gene gun approach.[41] A single dose induced strong activation of IFN-γ-producing CD8⁺ T cells and provided full prophylactic antitumor protection in vaccinated mice. Furthermore, tumor growth was inhibited in 70% of mice with established tumors.

VIRAL VECTORS

In addition to non-viral gene delivery, viral vectors have been commonly subjected to both preclinical and clinical gene therapy applications.[42] Generally, viral vectors possess a naturally high susceptibility for a broad range of host cells and capacity to provide high levels of transgene expression. However, different viruses show variations in foreign gene packaging potential, tropism, and gene expression profiles. For this reason, different types of viral vectors can be applied for specific indications. Naturally, the drawback of using viral vectors has been the potential safety risks, but during the last few years much attention has been paid to addressing this issue.

Adenoviruses

One of the most commonly used viral vector types is based on adenoviruses,[43] which have been subjected to numerous preclinical and clinical studies. Obviously, the setback due to the unfortunate fatality in the treatment of a patient suffering from ornithine transcarbamylase deficiency caused serious concern and rethinking of the application of adenovirus vectors for gene therapy. Recent development has included novel adenovirus vectors with improved biosafety profiles.[44]

Adenoviruses have been applied in numerous gene therapy applications to treat cancer.[45] A common approach has been to utilize specific therapeutic genes that cause death of cancer cells. Employment of cancer and tissue specific promoters has further aimed at improving the efficacy.[45] In this context, adenovirus vectors have been subjected to treatment of ovarian[46] and prostate[47] cancer as well as brain tumors.[48] Much attention has also been paid to targeting of adenoviruses. For example, the vascular transduction capacity was improved by modification of the adenovirus capsid structure.[49] The modified vector Ad5T*F35++ expressing tissue inhibitor of matrix metalloproteinase-3 (TIMP-3) as the therapeutic gene showed improved binding and transduction of human vascular cells resulting in reduced smooth muscle cell metabolic activity and migration *in vivo*. Furthermore, preexisting neutralizing antibodies were less prevalent to Ad5T*F35++ than to Ad5 in human serum. In another study, the polysaccharide mannan (polymannose) was conjugated to the adenovirus surface, and the generated Man–Ad5–PTEN was assessed *in vitro* for β-galactosidase reporter gene expression in hepatocellular carcinoma cell lines.[50] Furthermore, the antitumor effect was evaluated after intraperitoneal injection of H22 tumor-bearing mice. No cell growth suspension was observed in normal hepatocyte cells, whereas tumor-selective killing was discovered in tumors.

In another approach, a bicistronic adenovirus was engineered to express the ribosomal protein L23 (RPL23) and p53 to treat gastric cancer.[51] Because induction of murine double minute 2 (MDM2) expression generates resistance to p53 gene therapy and RPL23 can inhibit MDM2, co-expression of RPL23 should enhance p53-based therapy. The tumor-suppressor activity in human gastric cancer was significantly higher after treatment with Ad–RPL23/p53 than with Ad–p53 alone. Moreover, antitumor responses were observed for MKN45 cells initially resistant to p53 gene transfer. Additionally, survival benefit was obtained in an orthotopic nude mouse model for human gastric cancer.

One issue in gene therapy approaches has been cancer cell heterogeneity, which has hampered the efficacy of treatment and resulted in drug resistance. To address this problem, adenovirus vectors have been modified to replicate in a cancer-specific manner and the regulation of gene expression has been targeted to tumor heterogeneity.[52] Approaches have included a combination of prodrug-activation gene therapy in combination with novel conditionally replicating and tumor targeting oncolytic vectors. Especially employment of oncolytic adenoviruses has become an attractive approach in cancer therapy due to the selective infection and replication in tumor cells.[53] However, in most cases the adenovirus-based oncolytic antitumor activity is insufficient, but a number of vector improvements have been introduced such as incorporation of shRNAs, cytokines, and matrix-modulating proteins. Furthermore, the adenovirus surface has been modified with polymers, liposomes, and nanoparticles to extend circulation time and reduce immunogenicity, resulting in increased antitumor potency and reduced liver accumulation and toxicity.[53] In a recent study, oncolytic adenovirus expressing luciferase (VRX-007-Luc) was verified for tumor growth inhibition in Syrian hamsters after intratumoral injections.[54] Tumor growth inhibition was similar when cyclophosphamide (CP), an immunosuppressive and chemotherapeutic agent, was administered before or after VRX-007-Luc injections, suggesting independent antitumor activity for the two therapies. As human telomerase is highly active in more than 85% of primary cancers, an attenuated Ad5 vector with the human telomerase reverse transcriptase (hTERT) promoter element was engineered.[55] Intratumoral administration in an orthotopic human esophageal tumor model showed effective *in vivo* purging of metastatic tumor cells. Moreover, regional irradiation induces a strong antitumor effect due to tumor-cell-specific radiosensitization. In another study, tumor-specific irradiation of subcutaneous tumors was combined with treatment with oncolytic adenovirus (VRX-007) and cyclophosphamide in a Syrian hamster tumor model.[56] The combination treatment enhanced tumor growth inhibition, although no increase of viral replication occurred in tumors. Furthermore, similar results were obtained for irradiation one week before or after virus administration, suggesting independent antitumor effect from radiation and adenovirus therapy. Oncolytic adenovirus vectors have been engineered for induced expression of the E1A from the bladder-tissue-specific uroplakin II (UPII) promoter.[44] Intratumoral injections into subcutaneous xenografts in nude mice revealed virus replication only in tumor cells and therefore demonstrated high biosafety of the oncolytic adenovirus approach.

Adeno-Associated Viruses

Adeno-associated virus (AAV) vectors have been frequently used for gene therapy applications due to the lack of pathogenicity and toxicity, ability to infect both dividing and non-dividing cells, and long-term transgene expression profiles.[57] Furthermore, the safety profile in various clinical trials has been good. One shortcoming with using AAV has been the immune response against the vector observed after readministration.[58] However, this issue has been addressed by applying different AAV serotypes for repeated injections. Another detail is the relatively limited packaging capacity of foreign genes in AAV vectors.[59] AAV vectors have been subjected to gene therapy applications for cystic fibrosis and Parkinson's disease,[57] Gaucher disease, hemochromatosis, porphyria,[58] and a number of cancers.[57,60–62] Furthermore, AAV vectors expressing mitochondria-targeted catalase have been evaluated for life extension and prevention of aging-related pathology in mice.[63] One of the most promising applications for AAV has been the treatment of hemophilia, described in more detail below.[64] In another approach, AAV serotype 9 vectors expressing sulfamidase were shown to correct both CNS and somatic pathology in mucopolysaccharidosis type IIIA (MPS IIIA) mice.[65] The treatment increased enzymatic activity throughout the brain and serum, which resulted in whole-body correction of glucosaminoglycan (GAG) accumulation and lysosomal pathology.

In the context of cancer therapy, AAV vectors were employed for interferon-γ (IFN-γ) treatment of retinoblastoma.[60] Intravitreal administration led to efficient delivery and sustained production of IFN-γ in the eye with a potent antitumor effect. In another study, AAV serotype 2 was applied for expression of vascular endothelial growth factor (VEGF), a signaling protein and mediator in tumor growth and metastasis.[61] In this case, AAV2 with the high-affinity soluble decoy receptor (VEGF-Trap) was administered intravenously in a mouse model, which resulted in sustained expression and prevention of pulmonary metastases of 4T1 tumors. Furthermore, five AAV serotypes were evaluated for transduction efficiency in a number of lung cancer cell lines by reporter gene expression as a potential approach for lung cancer therapy.[62] AAV2/1 showed the best transduction efficacy (30 to 50% at multiplicity of infection [MOI] 100).

It was recently discovered that the AAV serotype 3 efficiently transduced hepatoblastoma (HB) and hepatocellular carcinoma (HCC) cell lines due to the utilization of a human hepatocyte growth factor receptor as a co-receptor for binding and cell entry.[66] Reporter gene expression demonstrated efficient delivery to human liver cancer cells. Furthermore, to target hepatocellular carcinoma, AAV vectors were used for combination therapy with the p53-independent Bcl-3-insensitive apoptotic protein apoptin and the immunostimulatory cytokine IL-24.[67] AAV-based therapy resulted in induction of apoptosis and suppression of cell growth in HepG2 cells. Similarly, in xenograft nude mice, apoptosis was observed in tumor cells and tumor growth was significantly reduced. AAV vectors have also been applied for oral and intramuscular vaccination.[68] For example, AAV serotypes 5 and 6 expressing a truncated form of the neu oncogene were evaluated in a neu-positive murine TUBO breast cancer model. A single oral administration significantly improved survival and was more efficient than applying the intramuscular route. Moreover, AAV6–neu vaccinations showed longer survival in comparison to AAV5–neu. Long-lasting tumor protection was obtained, with 80% of mice orally treated with AAV6–neu surviving rechallenges with TUBO cells at 120 and 320 days post-vaccination.

Herpes Simplex Viruses

Due to its long-term interaction with infected host cells characterized by lytic and latent infections herpes simplex virus type 1 (HSV-1) has become an attractive gene therapy vector.[69] Deletion of toxic HSV genes has provided a non-pathogenic vector with very high transgenic capacity of large pieces of foreign DNA, attenuated oncolytic activity, and establishment of life-long latent infection in neurons. In this context, three classes of vectors have been derived: replication-competent attenuated vectors, replication-deficient recombinant vectors, and defective helper-dependent amplicon vectors. HSV vectors have found a number of applications in neuroscience.[70] The wide tropism allows delivery to several cell types, including glial cells, and the absence of chromosomal integration means that no insertional mutagenesis is induced. Gene therapy applications have focused on inherited neuronal genetic diseases such as ataxias and neurodegenerative diseases including Parkinson's and Alzheimer's disease. Furthermore, complex neural functions such as neuroplasticity, anxiety, learning, and memory have been investigated.

Herpes simplex virus vectors have been applied for a number of applications in cancer therapy. For example, RH2 is an HSV-1 vector with a lytic ability in human squamous cell carcinoma (SCC) cells.[71] The effect of HSV-1 RH2 was examined in a syngenic C3H mouse model, where SCCVII cells first decreased but then recovered with time, indicating limited RH2 replication. Moreover, the growth of contralateral tumors of RH2-treated mice was significantly suppressed. In another study, oncolytic HSV-1 vectors were evaluated for selective killing of human non-small cell lung cancer (NSCLC) cells.[72] In this approach, four copies of microRNA-145 target sequences were incorporated into the 3'-end untranslated region of the HSV-1 essential viral gene ICP27. The HSV-1 amplicon vector carrying the miRNA-145 copies selectively reduced cell proliferation and prevented colony formation of NSCLC cells. Furthermore, combination with radiotherapy was significantly more potent in killing cancer cells than individual therapies alone. Oncolytic HSV has also been engineered to express human sodium iodide symporter (NIS) to increase its antitumor efficacy.[73] The HSV–NIS efficiently concentrated radioactive iodine in human prostate LNCap cells. Furthermore, LNCap xenografts in nude mice were efficiently eradicated after intratumoral administration of HSV-NIS. Likewise, systemic administration prolonged the survival of tumor-bearing mice, which was further enhanced by administration of the ^{131}I isotope.

Retroviruses and Lentiviruses

The application of retroviruses in gene therapy was significantly boosted by the preliminary success in treating children with severe combined immunodeficiency (SCID).[74] However, the random unfortunate integration of the therapeutic gene in the *LMO2* oncogene resulted in several cases of leukemia in retrovirus treated patients,[2,3] which emphasized the need for improved targeted integration events. This has indeed been reflected in development of safer retrovirus vectors and helper cells.[75] A recombinant bifunctional retrovirus vector displaying an scFV antibody to carcinoembryonic antigen (CEA) and expressing the iNOS gene has been subcutaneously injected into SCID mice with CEA-expressing MKN-45 cells.[76] The growth of MKN-45 tumors was significantly inhibited, demonstrating a 70% reduction in tumor size after 50 days. In another study, retrovirus vectors encoding the tumor necrosis factor (TNF)-related apoptosis-inducing ligand (TRAIL) gene were demonstrated to transduce drug-resistant A2780/DDP ovarian carcinoma cells *in vitro*.[77] Exposure of retrovirus transduced cells to cisplatin resulted in higher antitumor activity *in vitro* as well as in xenograft A2780/DDP tumors in nude mice. Interestingly, although human endogenous retroviruses (HERVs) express low levels of antigens by the host, HERV-K has been associated with different types of tumors.[78] Abnormal HERV-K expression can therefore contribute to morphological and functional cellular modifications implicated in melanoma maintenance and progression as well as other tumors such as sarcoma, lymphoma, bladder, and breast cancer. Furthermore, monoclonal and single-chain antibodies against the HERV-K Env protein have been shown to block the proliferation of human breast cancer cells *in vitro* and inhibit tumor growth in murine xenograft models.

Although classified as retroviruses, lentiviruses have received special attention as gene delivery vectors due to their minimal toxicity and capacity of transducing non-dividing cells.[79,80] Lentiviral vectors have been applied for different indications such as diabetes,[81] AIDS,[82] neurological disease,[83] and cancer.[84,85] For the treatment of diabetes, a lentivirus vector expressing furin-cleavable human insulin (INS-FUR) was delivered to mice liver.[81] Long-term transduction of hepatocytes restored normoglycemia for the entire time of monitoring (150 days) and re-established normal glucose tolerance. Liver function remained normal and no intrahepatic inflammation or autoimmune destruction of the liver tissue was observed. Obviously, natural targets for lentivirus-based therapy have been AIDS and HIV, which have prompted several approaches. For instance, lentiviral vectors with single or multiple RNAi-inducing cassettes have been designed.[86] Furthermore, lentiviruses expressing anti-HIV moieties (tat/rev short hairpin RNA, TAR decoy, and CCR5 ribozyme) were transduced into peripheral blood-derived CD34+ hematopoietic progenitor cells.[87] Persistent expression in multiple cell lineages was obtained for up to 24 months at low levels and therefore supports development of an RNA-based cell therapy platform for HIV.

Lentivirus vectors expressing glial cell line-derived neurotrophic factor (GDNF) was subjected to administration to the striatum and substantia nigra in nonhuman primate models of Parkinson's disease.[88] Extensive GNDF expression was detected in all injected animals, which provided augmented dopaminergic function. In monkeys treated with 1-methyl-4-phenyl-1,2,3,6-tetrahydropyridine (MPTP), lenti-GDNF reversed functional deficits and completely prevented nigrostriatal degeneration. Furthermore, overexpression of wild type rat parkin from lentivirus vectors demonstrated protection against the toxicity of mutated human A30P alpha-synuclein in a rat model for Parkinson's disease.[89] Also, lentivirus vectors expressing human ciliary neurotrophic factor (CNTF) were evaluated in a quinolinic acid rat model for Huntington's disease,[90] which revealed significantly diminished striatal damage.

In cancer therapy approaches lentivirus vectors encoding prostate stem cell antigen (PSCA) have been directed to dendritic cells as a novel tumor vaccine mouse model for prostate cancer.[91] It was shown that the lentivirus vector preferentially delivered the PSCA antigen to DC-SIGN-expressing 293T cells and bone marrow-derived dendritic cells. In an adenocarcinoma mouse prostate cell line (TRAMP-C1) synergetic tumor model, protection against lethal challenges was obtained in a prophylactic model, and tumor growth was significantly slower in animals with established tumors. Furthermore, tumor metastases were inhibited in the B16-F10 melanoma model. In another study, self-inactivated lentivirus vectors showed 90% transduction efficiency of pancreatic cancer-derived cell lines.[85] Furthermore expression of human interferon-β (hIFN-β) from lentivirus vectors inhibited cell proliferation and induced apoptosis. In mice, hIFN-β expression prevented pancreatic cancer progression for up to 15 days and induced tumor regression in 50% of treated animals. Lentivirus vectors have also been subjected to targeting of liver tumors. In this context, recombinant lentivirus vectors expressing the Wtp53-pPRIME-miR30-shRNA were delivered to AFP-positive liver cancer cells.[92] Both *in vitro* and *in vivo* studies demonstrated improved efficacy of inhibition of proliferation in Hep3B cells of these targeted lentivirus vectors.

In another approach, shRNA for Livin, an inhibitor of apoptosis protein, was delivered by lentivirus vectors into established xenograft tumors from the lung adenocarcinoma cell line SPC-A-1 in BALB/C nude mice.[93] Livin-shRNA downregulated Livin expression efficiently, induced apoptosis in tumor cells, and reduced tumor proliferation and growth dramatically. Furthermore, Livin gene silencing induced G_0/G_1-phase cell cycle arrest and cyclin D_1 downregulation. Lentivirus vectors have also been subjected to oral administration for treatment of lung cancer.[94] In this context, osteopontin (OPN), suggested for involvement in cancer development, was introduced into a lentivirus vector. Aerosols of lentivirus carrying a triple mutant of OPN were delivered to the lungs of K-ras (LA1) mice through a nose-only inhalation chamber three times a week for four weeks. The treatment resulted in inhibition of lung tumorigenesis and inhibition of the OPN-mediated Akt signaling pathway.

Further development of vector delivery has included the entrapment of lentivirus particles in hydrogels[95] to preserve lentivirus activity and shielding from host immune responses. Another approach has dealt with the application of artificial nanofibrils that self-assemble to enhance lentivirus gene transfer.[96] Furthermore, the nanofibrils facilitate concentration of lentiviruses by conventional low-speed centrifugation. Recently, a platform for insertional mutagenesis has been developed based on lentivirus vectors.[97] This approach allowed efficient induction of hepatocellular carcinoma in three different mouse models and further resulted in the identification of four previously unknown liver cancer-associated genes. Much effort dedicated to the production and purification of lentivirus has dealt with improved virus titers and limited degradation during the purification procedure.[98]

Alphaviruses

Single-stranded RNA alphaviruses have been commonly used for recombinant protein expression and in neuroscience but they have also found applications in gene therapy.[99] Typically, alphaviruses have been used for vaccine development to protect against challenges with lethal doses of viruses and tumor cells.[100] In this context, immunization of mice with Semliki Forest virus (SFV) RNA carrying the *lacZ* gene resulted in tumor regression and protection against tumor challenges.[101] Furthermore, antitumor activity and immune protection against melanomas were observed in mice vaccinated with Sindbis virus plasmid DNA expressing the tyr-related protein-1 gene.[102] Moreover, SFV vectors have been applied for intratumoral injections. For example, SFV–GFP vectors provided tumor regression in immunodeficient mice implanted with human lung carcinoma cells.[103] Likewise, SFV particles expressing the p40 and p35 subunits of interleukin-12 resulted in significant tumor regression and inhibition of tumor blood vessel formation in a B16 melanoma tumor model.[104]

Oncolytic replication-competent alphaviruses were recently engineered to improve *in vivo* distribution and prolong transgene expression. The avirulent SFV A7(74) strain provided efficient infection and lysis of cancer cell lines monitored by EGFP expression.[105] A single injection of SFV VA7–EGFP resulted in significant tumor regression in SCID mice grafted with human melanomas. Furthermore, the VA7–EGFP vector was evaluated in a nude mouse model with human osteosarcoma xenografts where SFV treatment extended survival despite the highly aggressive tumor growth.[106] In another study, the oncolytic VA7–EGFP vector increased survival rates significantly in an orthotypic lung cancer tumor model in nude mice.[107] Recently, a human telomerase reverse transcriptase promoter-driven SFV-based DNA vector (pShT–ePNP) providing high expression of the *Escherichia coli* purine nucleoside phosphorylase-2 showed significant inhibitory effect on tumor cells. Oral administration with the aid of live attenuated *Salmonella typhimurium* 7207 exerted powerful therapeutic efficacy, including reduced tumor growth and prolonged lifespan of tumor-bearing mice.[108]

The broad host range of alphaviruses has posed some concerns about targeting and safe delivery of vectors for gene therapy applications. Efforts have been made to target alphavirus particles to the cell or tissue of choice by engineering IgG binding domains of protein A in the E2 envelope structure.[109] However, Sindbis virus was discovered to possess natural targeting of tumors.[110] Intraperitoneal administration provided specific luciferase reporter gene expression in implanted tumors in mice. Additionally, the tumor load was reduced to 6.2% of control mice after daily subcutaneous injections of SIN–IL12. In contrast, no natural targeting has been described for SFV particles, which triggered the development of another targeting approach by encapsulation of virus particles in liposomes.[111] Encapsulated SFV–LacZ particles showed targeted β-galactosidase expression in tumors after systemic delivery in SCID mice.

Poxviruses

Poxviruses are large double-stranded DNA viruses that replicate in the cytoplasm and have been subjected to engineering of replication-deficient expression vectors.[112] Tumor-selective replication-competent poxvirus vectors have shown high efficiency of *in vivo* replication, and intradermal injection caused a dermal zone of necrosis in non-human primates that was directly related to cellular destruction by viral replication.[113] Introduction of a mutant virus with deletions in the thymidine kinase (TK) and vaccinia growth factor (VGF) genes caused no damage to normal cells, but allowed efficient replication in tumor cells. Furthermore, recombinant poxviruses providing expression of cytokines and other immunostimulatory antigens can enhance immune recognition of tumors.[114] In another study, attenuated vaccinia virus vectors carrying either the IL-2 or IL-12 gene were administered into a C6 glioma mouse model.[115] The observed antitumor activity correlated with the number of killer T cells in the spleen and local induction of IFN-γ and TNF-α. Furthermore, the oncolytic vaccinia virus GLV-1h68 was evaluated in both cell cultures and subcutaneous tumor models.[116] Cell lines such as Colo 205, HCT-15, HCT-116, HT-29, and SW-20, derived from all four stages of human colorectal cancer, showed efficient vaccinia replication and cell lysis. Moreover, a single intravenous injection of the GLV-1h68 vaccinia virus significantly inhibited tumor growth of two human colorectal tumor xenografts in athymic nude mice, leading to improved survival rates. The treatment was well tolerated and viral replication confined to tumor cells. The GLV-1h68 vaccinia virus was also assessed for human salivary gland carcinoma.[117] Among five tested human salivary gland carcinoma cell lines three showed exquisite sensitivity to GLV-1h68 infection. A single intratumoral injection induced significant tumor regression in flank and parotid tumor models. Moreover, the oncolytic vaccinia virus GLV-1h109 expressing the anti-VEGF single-chain antibody (scAb) GLAF-1 was evaluated for canine cancer therapy.[118] *In vitro* GLV-1h109 showed efficient infection, replication, and killing of canine cancer cell lines. Systemic administration to two different xenograft models resulted in significant tumor growth reduction and continued production of functional scab GLAF-1, which further inhibited angiogenesis. Vaccinia virus vectors have found another application in tumor-bearing xeroderma pigmentosum (XP) patients, who cannot be treated with conventional DNA damaging therapies.[119] It was demonstrated that vaccinia virus was 10- to 100-fold more cytotoxic to tumor-derived cells from XP patients than non-tumor control cells. *In vivo*, local or systemic delivery of vaccinia virus vectors provided long-term tumor resolution in xenograft and genetic models of XP. Oncolytic vaccinia virus GLV-1h68 has further been evaluated for selective targeting of human bone and soft-tissue sarcoma cell lines *in vitro* and *in vivo*.[120] Robust transgene expression was observed in fibrosarcoma HT-1080, osteosarcoma U-2OS, fibrohistiocytoma M-805, and rhabdomyosarcoma HTB-82 cell lines. Furthermore, intratumoral GLV-1h68 injection of mice with HT-1080 xenograft flank tumors resulted in localized intratumoral luciferase activity without spread to normal tissue and complete tumor regression within 28 days. The novel vaccinia virus vector GLV-1h151, which has genetic modifications enhancing cancer specificity, has been tested in several human cancer cell lines from breast, lung, pancreatic, and colorectal origin.[121] Efficient infection and replication occurred in several cancer cell types leading to high-level killing. Intravenous or intratumoral administration of GLV-1h151 confirmed replication in tumors and a good biosafety profile.

Baculoviruses

Although originally applied for recombinant protein expression in insect cells,[122] certain modifications has allowed additional targeting of mammalian cells.[123] These modified baculovirus vectors have demonstrated local delivery to rat brain with specific transduction of cuboid epithelium of the choroid plexus in ventricles with a higher efficacy than observed for adenoviruses.[124] These findings suggest that baculovirus vectors could be used for local intracerebral gene therapy.

Baculovirus vectors have been assessed for a number of cancer therapy applications. In this context, baculovirus vectors were tested for delivery to colorectal cancer cells. The results suggested that baculovirus-based delivery holds great promise for colorectal cancer therapy and also other major carcinomas such as breast, pancreas, and brain.[125] Furthermore, baculovirus vectors have been exploited for anti-angiogenesis-based cancer therapy.[126] Expression of the fusion protein of human endostatin and angiostatin (hEA) from a baculovirus vector containing AAV inverted terminal repeats (ITRs) demonstrated cell proliferation, migration, and tubule network formation. Intratumoral injection into a prostate cancer mouse model generated strong anti-angiogenic effects. Furthermore, a number of prostate cancer models were analyzed for the potential of baculovirus-based therapy.[127] It was demonstrated that baculovirus preferentially transduced invasive malignant prostate cancer cell lines. Furthermore, primary patient-derived prostate cancer cells were susceptible to baculovirus. In addition, baculovirus vectors were able to penetrate three-dimensional structures such as *in vitro* spheroids and *in vivo* orthotopic xenografts. When baculovirus vectors expressing a nitroreductase gene were combined with the prodrug CB1954, efficient tumor cell killing was observed. In another approach, baculovirus-mediated transgene expression of thymidine kinase in neural stem cells (NSCs) opposite the tumor site in the cerebral hemisphere provided growth inhibition of human glioma xenografts in the presence of ganciclovir.[128]

GENOMICS AND EPIGENOMICS IN DRUG DISCOVERY

In addition to direct effects on the contents of the genome, epigenomic modifications have more recently been demonstrated to have a major impact on therapeutic efficacy and therefore also on gene therapy approaches.[129] The most common epigenetic modifications are characterized by DNA methylations, histone modifications, and RNA interference.[130] Dysregulation of epigenetic function can cause upregulation and downregulation of enzymes as well as gene amplification, providing the conditions for cancer development.[131] In this context, mutations in regulatory regions such as miRNA and DNA methyltransferase coding regions or environmental factors such as smoking and famine could result in aberrations of epigenetic function. Recent discoveries point to a genome-scale epigenomic disruption, which involves DNA hypomethylation, mutations in epigenetic modifier genes and heterochromatin alterations in cancer, thus suggesting potential novel approaches for cancer diagnostics and therapy.[132] In this context, DNA methylation and histone acetylation have been targeted as therapeutic strategies in lung cancer.[133] Furthermore, epigenetic changes in non-small-cell lung cancer were evaluated by using inhibitors against DNA methyltransferases (DNMTs) and histone deacetylases (HDACs) to promote re-expression of silenced tumor suppressor genes.[134]

Recently, the epigenetic modifications associated with cancer have been demonstrated to be affected by the dietary composition as means of acting as cancer prevention agents.[135] In this context, sulforaphane and green tea polyphenols have been suggested to provide chemoprevention against modulation of DNA methylation and histone modification in skin cancer. The potential reversibility of epigenetic modifications triggered by nutrition and bioactive food components may further provide the link between susceptibility genes and environmental factors in the etiology of cancer.[136]

A common epigenetic abnormality in many cancers is the loss of imprinting (LOI) of the insulin-like growth factor 2 (IGF2) gene regulated by differentially methylated domains (DMDs) in the control region.[137] Adenoviral vectors driven by H19 enhancer–DMD-H19 promoter carrying EGFP and E1A genes were verified for tumor growth *in vitro* and *in vivo*. HRT-18 and HT-29 cancer cells with LOI showed high EGFP expression, whereas HCT-116, MCF-7, and GES-1 with maintenance of imprinting (MOI) provided only weak EGFP expression. Moreover, Ad-E1A decreased cell viability only in HRT-18 and HT-29 cells. Furthermore, HRT-18 and HT-29 xenografts in nude mice showed substantial tumor regression after Ad-E1A administration. In another study, CD34+ cells *ex vivo* transduced with lentivirus vectors induced genome-wide epigenetic modifications and may provide new biomarkers for the optimization of gene and cell therapy protocols.[138]

CLINICAL TRIALS

Despite the setbacks experienced in gene therapy in the first years of the century and the recent global economic struggles, the number of annual clinical trials has remained steady. According to one source,[139] more than 1800 gene therapy trials have been conducted or are currently in progress. Another source suggests that close to 2000 clinical trials have been completed or are ongoing.[140] Not surprisingly, the large majority of trials have taken place

TABLE 2.2   Clinical Trials Applying Gene Therapy

Country	No. of Trials	Indication	No. of Trials	Vector	No. of Trials	Gene Type	No. of Trials
United States	1235	Cancer	1264	Adenovirus	476	Antigen	417
United Kingdom	204	Monogenic	176	Retrovirus	388	Cytokine	349
Germany	82	Infectious	162	Plasmid DNA	359	Tumor suppressor	158
Switzerland	50	Cardiovascular	160	Vaccinia	159	Suicide	156
France	48	Neurological	37	Lipofection	112	Deficiency	156
China	34	Ocular	28	Adeno-associated virus	105	Receptor	149
Netherlands	33	Inflammatory	13	Poxvirus	97	Growth factor	143
Australia	30	Other	28	Lentivirus	67	Replication inhibitor	87
Canada	23	Gene marking	50	HSV	62	Marker	54
Belgium	22	Healthy volunteers	51	Other	137	Other	250
Other	131	×					
Multi-country	78	×					

in the United States, followed by United Kingdom and other highly developed countries such as Germany and Switzerland (Table 2.2). Moreover, logically cancer is clearly the most studied partly due to the straightforward, albeit difficult, task to kill tumor cells. Infectious diseases have also been high on the list. The importance of efficient treatment of neurological diseases is reflected by 37 clinical trials despite difficulties in delivery and the sustained therapeutic effect required. Interestingly, viral vectors seem to have gained in popularity at the cost of non-viral delivery methods. Adenovirus-based gene therapy tops the list with 476 trials. Lentivirus vectors have seen a rapid increase in number of trials ($n = 67$), particularly as the first trial was only initiated in 2005.[141] The selection of therapeutics naturally reflects the indications targeted but also the ease of expression and production. For this reason, antigens ($n = 417$) and cytokines ($n = 349$) are the most frequently employed, followed by tumor suppressors ($n = 156$) and suicide drugs/genes ($n = 156$). Obviously, Phase I ($n = 1171$) and Phase I/II ($n = 376$) represent the majority of clinical trials, but encouragingly 326 have reached Phase II, 20 Phase II/III, 72 Phase III, and 2 Phase IV.

CONCLUSION AND FUTURE PROSPECTS

Gene therapy has seen recent success on several fronts. This is due to better understanding of targeting and delivery of therapeutic agents as well as plenty of experience with a number of conducted clinical trials. The delivery vehicles vary from non-viral vectors based on polymers to liposomes with targeting peptides or other agents engrafted on the surface to provide cell/tissue specific delivery. A large number of different viral vectors have also been employed. These include retrovirus vectors for treatment of SCID with a strong emphasis on safe chromosomal integration to avoid unwanted oncogene activation. Adenoviruses have been applied for various indications, such as the approval of Gendicine® on the Chinese market for adenovirus-based p53 expression to treat cancer. Furthermore, AAV vectors have seen some remarkable development in the treatment of hemophilia, as well as other indications. Herpes simplex viruses are attractive delivery vectors due to their life-long expression capacity. Furthermore, more recent viruses such as lentivirus, alphavirus, and poxviruses have found applications in HIV, cancer, and other areas.

The therapeutic agents present as much variation as the delivery systems. Classic approaches in cancer therapy include overexpression of cytotoxic (suicide) genes, tumor suppression genes, and anti-angiogenesis genes. Furthermore, immunostimulatory genes including cytokines have been commonly used for cancer therapy to stimulate the tumor cell killing process. A number of antigens, including monoclonal and single-chain antibodies, have been employed as vaccines in attempts to provide protection against challenges with lethal doses of infectious agents or tumor cells. More recent approaches include gene silencing. Although antisense and ribozyme applications have been used for years, RNA interference and especially microRNA-based therapeutic applications have widened the opportunities for drug development. Recent developments in gene therapy bode well for their finally living up to the promise as medicines of the future.

References

1. Raper SE, Chirmule N, Lee FS, et al. Fatal systemic inflammatory response syndrome in a ornithine transcarbamylase deficient patient following adenoviral gene transfer. Mol Genet Metab. 2003;80:148–58.
2. McCormack MP, Rabbitts TH. Activation of the T-cell oncogene *LMO2* after gene therapy for X-linked severe combined immunodeficiency. New Engl. J. Med. 2004;350:913–22.
3. Hacein-Bey-Abina S, Garrigue A, Wang GP, et al. Insertional oncogenesis in 4 patients after retrovirus-mediated gene therapy of SCID-X1. J. Clin. Invest. 2008;118:3132–42.
4. Martinez T, Wright N, Lopez-Fraga M, et al. Silencing human genetic diseases with oligonucleotide-based therapies. Hum. Genet. 2013;132:481–93.
5. Lundstrom K. Delivery Technologies for Biopharmaceuticals: Peptides, Proteins, Nucleic Acids, Vaccines In: Jorgensen L, Moerck Nielsen H, editors. Nanocarriers for the delivery of peptides and proteins. London: John Wiley & Sons; 2009. p. 193–205.
6. Gupte A, Ciftci K. Formulation and characterization of paclitaxel, 5-FU and paclitaxel + 5-FU microspheres. Int. J. Pharm. 2004;276:93–106.
7. Cui F, Cun D, Tao A, et al. Preparation and characterization of melittin-loaded poly(D,L-lactic acid) or poly(D,L-lactic-co-glycolic acid) microspheres made by the double emulsion method. J. Control. Release 2005;107:310–9.
8. Sinha VR, Bansal K, Kaushik R, et al. Poly-epsilon-caprolactone microspheres and nanospheres: an overview. Int. J. Pharm. 2004;278:1–23.
9. Chan Y-P, Meyrueix R, Kravtzoff R, et al. Review on Medusa®: a polymer-based sustained release technology for protein and peptide drugs. Exp. Opin. Drug Deliv. 2007;4:441–51.
10. Sun X, Zhang N. Cationic polymer optimization for efficient gene delivery. Mini Rev. Med. Chem. 2010;10:108–25.
11. Keeney M, Ong SG, Padilla A, et al. Development of poly(β-amino ester)-based biodegradable nanoparticles for nonviral delivery of minicircle DNA. ACS Nano. 2013;7(8):7241–50.
12. Kim HA, Nam K, Lee M, et al. Hypoxia/hepatoma dual specific suicide gene expression plasmid delivery using bio-reducible polymer for hepatocellular carcinoma therapy. J. Control. Release 2013;171:1–10.

13. Gardikis K, Micha-Screttas M, Demetzos C, et al. Dendrimers and the development of new complex nanomaterials for biomedical applications. Curr. Med. Chem. 2012;19:4913–28.
14. Nam HY, Nam K, Lee M, et al. Dendrimer type bio-reducible polymer for efficient gene delivery. J. Control. Release 2012;160:592–600.
15. Yin Z, Liu N, Ma M, et al. A novel EGFR-targeted gene delivery system based on complexes self-assembled EGF, DNA, and activated PAMAM dendrimers. Int. J. Nanomedicine 2012;7:4625–35.
16. Lim J, Simanek EE. Triazine dendrimers as drug delivery systems: from synthesis to therapy. Adv. Drug Deliv. Rev. 2012;64:826–35.
17. Motoyama K, Hayashidi K, Higashi T, et al. Polypseudorotaxanes of pegylated α-cyclodxtrin/polyamidoamine dendrimer conjugate with cyclodextrins as a sustained release system for DNA. Bioorg. Med. Chem. 2012;20: 1425–33.
18. Hayashi Y, Mori Y, Higashi T, et al. Systemic delivery of transthyretin siRNA mediated by lactosylated dendrimer/α-cyclodextrin conjugates into hepatocyte for familial amyloidotic polyneuropathy therapy. Amyloid 2012;19(Suppl. 1):47–9.
19. Posocco P, Liu X, Laurini E, et al. Impact of siRNA overhangs for dendrimer-mediated siRNA delivery and gene silencing. Mol. Pharm. 2013;10:3262–73.
20. Liu J, Zhou J, Luo Y. SiRNA delivery system based on neutral cross-linking dendrimers. Bioconjug. Chem. 2012;23:174–83.
21. Liu X, Huang H, Wang J, et al. Dendrimers-delivered short hairpin RNA targeting hTERT inhibit oral cancer growth *in vitro* and *in vivo*. Biochem. Pharmacol. 2011;82:17–23.
22. Lundstrom K, Boulikas T. Viral and non-viral vectors in gene therapy: technology development and clinical trials. Technol. Cancer Res. Treatment 2003;2:471–85.
23. Cattel L, Ceruti M, Dosio F. From conventional to stealth liposomes: a new frontier in cancer chemotherapy. Tumori 2003;89:237–49.
24. Stathopoulos GP, Boulikas T. Lipoplatin formulation review article. J. Drug. Deliv. 2012;581363.
25. Chen Y, Sun J, Lu Y, et al. Complexes containing cationic and anionic pH-sensitive liposomes: comparative study of factors influencing plasmid DNA gene delivery to tumors. Int. J. Nanomedicine 2013;8:1573–93.
26. He Z, Yu Y, Zhang Y, et al. Gene delivery with active targeting to ovarian cancer cells mediated by folate receptor alpha. J. Biomed. Nanotechnol. 2013;9:833–44.
27. Xiang B, Dong DW, Shi NQ, et al. PSA-responsive and PSMA-mediated multifunctional liposomes for targeted therapy of prostate cancer. Biomaterials 2013;34:6976–91.
28. Movassaghian S, Moghimi HR, Shirazi FH. Dendrosome–dendriplex inside liposomes: as a gene delivery system. J. Drug Target 2011;19:925–32.
29. Hadinoto K, Sundaresan A, Cheow WS. Lipid–polymer nanoparticles as a new generation delivery platform: a review. Eur. J. Pharm. Biopharm. 2013;85(3 Pt. A):427–43.
30. Elsabahy M, Foldvari M. Needle-free gene delivery through the skin: an overview of recent strategies. Curr. Pharm. Des. 2013;19(41):7301–15.
31. Fioretti D, Iurescia S, Fazio VM, et al. *In vivo* DNA electrotransfer for immunotherapy of cancer and neurodegenerative diseases. Curr. Drug. Metab. 2013;14:279–90.
32. Ligtenberg MA, Rojas-Colonelli N, Kiessling R, et al. NF-κB activation during DNA vaccination is essential for eliciting tumor protective antigen-specific CTL responses after intradermal DNA electroporation. Hum. Vaccin. Immunother. 2013;9(10):2189–95.
33. Kim H, Sin JI. Electroporation driven delivery of an interleukin-12 expressing plasmid and cisplatin synergizes to inhibit B16 melanoma tumor growth through an NK cell mediated tumor killing mechanism. Hum. Vaccin. Immunother. 2012;8:1714–21.
34. Venkatesh A, Ma S, Langellotto F, et al. Retinal gene delivery by rAAV and plasmid DNA electroporation. Curr. Protocol. Microbiol. 2013. Chapter 14, Unit 14D.4.
35. Dean DA. Cell-specific targeting strategies for electroporation-mediated gene delivery in cells and animals. J. Membr. Biol. 2013;246(10):737–44.
36. Aravindaram K, Yang NS. Gene gun delivery systems for cancer vaccine approaches. Methods Mol. Biol. 2009;542:167–78.
37. Cao Y, Zao B, Han Y, et al. Gene gun bombardment with DNA-coated golden particles enhanced the protective effect of a DNA vaccine based on thioredoxin glutathione reductase Schistosoma japonicum. Biomed. Res. Int. 2013;2013:952416.

I. NOVEL THERAPEUTIC APPROACHES

38. Daytyan H, Ghochikyan A, Moysesyan N, et al. Delivery of a DNA vaccine for Alzheimer's disease by electropo-ration versus gene gun generates potent and similar immune responses. Neurodegener. Dis. 2012;10:261–4.

39. Abe A, Furumoto H, Yoshida K, et al. Gene gun-mediated skin transfection with FL gene suppressed the growth of murine fibrosarcoma. J. Med. Invest. 2011;58:39–45.

40. Smahel M, Polakova I, Sobotkova I, et al. Systemic administration of CpG oligodeoxynucleotide and levami-sole as adjuvants for gene gun-delivered antitumor DNA vaccines. Clin. Dev. Immunol. 2011;2011:176759.

41. Diniz MO, Ferreira LC. Enhanced antitumor effect of a gene gun-delivered DNA vaccine encoding the human papillomavirus type 16 oncoproteins genetically fused to the herpes simplex virus glycoprotein D. Braz. J. Med. Res. 2011;44:421–7.

42. Lundstrom K. Latest development in viral vectors for gene therapy. Trends Biotechnol. 2003;21:117–22.

43. Schiedner G, Morral N, Parks RS, et al. Genomic DNA transfer with a high-capacity adenovirus vector results in improved *in vivo* gene expression and decreased toxicity. Nat. Genet. 1998;18:180–3.

44. Wang F, Wang Z, Tian H, et al. Biodistribution and safety assessment of bladder cancer specific oncolytic adenovirus in subcutaneous xenografts tumor model in nude mice. Curr. Gene Ther. 2012;12:67–76.

45. Fukazawa T, Matsuoka J, Yamatsuji T, et al. Adenovirus-mediated cancer gene therapy and virotherapy (re-view). Int. J. Mol. Med. 2010;25:3–10.

46. Matthews KS, Alvarez RD, Curiel DT. Advancements in adenoviral-based virotherapy for ovarian cancer. Adv. Drug Deliv. Rev. 2009;61:836–41.

47. Ekblad M, Halden G. Adenovirus-based therapy for prostate cancer. Curr. Opin. Mol. Ther. 2009;12:421–31.

48. Fu YJ, Du J, Yang RJ, et al. Potential adenovirus-mediated gene therapy of glioma cancer. Biotechnol. Lett. 2010;32:11–8.

49. White KM, Alba R, Parker AL, et al. Assessment of a novel, capsid-modified adenovirus with an improved vascular gene transfer profile. J. Cardiothorac. Surg. 2013;8:183.

50. Liu Z, Ke F, Duan C, et al. Mannan-conjugated adenovirus enhanced gene therapy effects on murine hepatocellular carcinoma *in vitro* and *in vivo*. Bioconjug. Chem. 2013; 24(8):1387-97.

51. Zhang YF, Zhang BC, Zhang AR, et al. Co-transduction of ribosomal protein L23 enhances the therapeutic ef-ficacy of adenoviral-mediated p53 gene transfer in human gastric cancer. Oncol. Rep. 2013;30:1989–95.

52. Doloff JC, Waxman DJ. Adenoviral vectors for prodrug activation-based gene therapy for cancer. Anticancer Agents Med. Chem. 2013;14(1):115–26.

53. Choi JW, Lee JS, Kim SW. Evolution of oncolytic adenoviruses for cancer treatment. Adv. Drug Deliv. Rev. 2012;64:720–9.

54. Young BA, Spencer JF, Ying B, et al. The role of cyclophosphamide in enhancing antitumor efficacy of an adeno-virus oncolytic vector in subcutaneous Syrian hamster tumors. Cancer Gene Ther. 2013;20(9):521–30.

55. Fujiwara T. A novel molecular therapy using bioengineered adenovirus for human gastrointestinal cancer. Acta Med. Okoyama 2011;65:151–62.

56. Young BA, Spencer JF, Ying B, et al. The effects of radiation on antitumor efficacy of an oncolytic adenovirus vector in the Syrian hamster model. Cancer Gene Ther. 2013;20(9):531–7.

57. Park K, Kim WJ, Cho YH, et al. Cancer gene therapy using adeno-associated virus vectors. Front. Biosci. 2008;13:2653–9.

58. Mingozzi F, High KA. Immune responses to AAV vectors: overcoming barriers to successful gene therapy. Blood 2013;122:23–36.

59. Grieger JC, Samulski RJ. Packaging capacity of adeno-associated virus serotypes: impact of larger genomes on infectivity and postentry steps. J. Virol. 2005;79:9933–44.

60. Shih CS, Laurie N, Holzmacher J, et al. AAV-mediated local delivery of interferon-beta for the treatment of retinoblastoma in preclinical models. Neuromolecular Med. 2009;11:43–52.

61. Lu L, Luo ST, Shi HS, et al. AAV2-mediated gene transfer of VEGF-Trap with potent suppression of pri-mary breast tumor growth and spontaneous pulmonary metastases by long-term expression. Oncol. Rep. 2012;28:1332–8.

62. Chen C, Akerstrom V, Baus J, et al. Comparative analysis of the transduction efficiency of five adeno-associated virus serotypes and VSV-G pseudotyped lentiviral vector in lung cancer cells. Virol. J. 2013;10:86.

63. Li D, Duan D. Mitochondria-targeted anti-aging gene therapy with adeno-associated virus vectors. Methods Mol. Biol. 2013;1048:160–80.

64. Chuah MK, Evens H, Vandendriessche T. Gene therapy for hemophilia. J. Thromb. Haemost. 2013;11 (Suppl. 1):99–110.

65. Haurigot V, Marco S, Ribera A, et al. Whole body correction of mucopolysaccharidosis IIIA by intracerebrospinal fluid gene therapy. J. Clin. Invest. 2013. July 1 [Epub ahead of print].

66. Ling C, Lu Y, Cheng B, et al. High efficiency transduction of liver cancer cells by recombinant adeno-associated virus serotype 3 vectors. J. Vis. Exp. 2011;22:2538.

67. Yuan L, Zhao H, Zhang L, et al. The efficacy of combination therapy using adeno-associated virus co-expression of apoptin and interleukin-24 on hepatocellular carcinoma. Tumour Biol. 2013;34(5):3027–34.

68. Steele JC, Di Pasquale G, Ramlogan CA, et al. Oral vaccination with adeno-associated virus vectors expressing the Neu inhibits the growth of murine breast cancer. Mol. Ther. 2013;21:680–7.

69. Epstein AL, Marconi P, Argnani R, et al. HSV-1-derived recombinant and amplicon vectors for gene transfer and gene therapy. Curr. Gene Ther. 2005;5(5):445–58.

70. Jerusalinsky D, Baez MV, Epstein AL. Herpes simplex virus type 1-based amplicon vectors for fundamental research in neurosciences and gene therapy of neurological diseases. J. Physiol. Paris 2012;106:2–11.

71. Meshii N, Takahashi G, Okunaga S, et al. Enhancement of systemic tumor immunity for squamous cell carcinoma cells from oncolytic herpes simplex virus. Cancer Gene Ther. 2013;20(9):493–8.

72. Li JM, Kao KC, Li LF, et al. MicroRNA-145 regulates oncolytic herpes simplex virus-1 for selective killing of human non-small lung cancer cells. Virol. J. 2013;10:241.

73. Li H, Nakashima H, Decklever TD, et al. HSV-NIS, an oncolytic herpes simplex virus type 1 encoding the human sodium iodine symporter for preclinical prostate cancer radiovirotherapy. Cancer Gene Ther. 2013;20: 478–85.

74. Cavazzano-Calvo M, Hacein-Bey S, de Saint Basille G, et al. Gene therapy of human severe combined immunodeficiency (SCID)-X1 disease. Science 2000;288:669–72.

75. Hu WS, Pathak VK. Design of retroviral vectors and helper cells for gene therapy. Pharmacol. Rev. 2000;52: 493–511.

76. Khare PD, Liao S, Hirose Y, et al. Tumor growth suppression by a retroviral vector displaying scFv antibody to CEA and carrying the iNOS gene. Anticancer Res. 2002;22:2443–6.

77. Li F, Guo Y, Han L, et al. *In vitro* and *in vivo* growth inhibition of drug-resistant ovarian carcinoma cells using a combination of cisplatin and a TRAIL-encoding retrovirus. Oncol. Lett. 2012;4:1254–8.

78. Cecolon L, Salata C, Wiederpass E, et al. Human endogenous retroviruses and cancer prevention: evidence and prospects. BMC Cancer 2013;13:4.

79. Vigna E, Naldini L. Lentiviral vectors: excellent tools for experimental gene transfer and promising candidates for gene therapy. J. Gen. Med. 2000;2:308–16.

80. Kay MA, Glorioso JC, Naldini L. Viral vectors for gene therapy: the art of turning infectious agents into vehicles of therapeutics. Nat. Med 2001;7:33–40.

81. Ren B, O'Brien BA, Byrne MR, et al. Long-term reversal of diabetes in non-obese diabetic mice by liver-directed gene therapy. J. Gen. Med. 2013;15:28–41.

82. Chung J, Rossi JJ, Jung U. Current progress and challenges in HIV gene therapy. Future Virol. 2011;6:1319–28.

83. Deglon N, Aebischer P. Lentiviruses as vectors for CNS diseases. Curr. Top. Microbiol. Immunol. 2002;261: 191–209.

84. Guo SW, Che HM, Li WZ. Antitumor effect of lentivirus-mediated gene transfer of alphastatin on human glioma. Cancer Sci. 2011;102:1038–44.

85. Ravet L, Lulka H, Gross F, et al. Using lentiviral vectors for efficient pancreatic cancer gene therapy. Cancer Gene Ther. 2010;17:315–24.

86. Liu YP, Westerink JT, ter Brake O, et al. RNAi-inducing lentiviral vectors for anti-HIV-1 gene therapy. Methods Mol. Biol. 2011;721:293–311.

87. DiGiusto GL, Krishnan A, Li L, et al. RNA-based gene therapy for HIV lentiviral vector-modified CD34(+) cells in patients undergoing treatment for AIDS-related lymphoma. Sci. Transl. Med. 2010;2:36r43.

88. Kordower JH, Emborg ME, Bloch J, et al. Neurodegeneration prevented by lentiviral vector delivery of GDNF in primate models of Parkinson's disease. Science 2000;290:267–73.

89. Lo Bianco C, Schneider BL, Bauer M, et al. Lentiviral vector delivery of parkin prevents dopaminergic degeneration in an alpha-synuclein rat model of Parkinson's disease. Proc. Natl. Acad. Sci. USA 2004;101:17510–5.

90. de Almeida LP, Zala D, Aebischer P, et al. Neuroprotective effect of a CNTF–lentiviral vector in a quinolinic acid rat model of Huntington's disease. Neurobiol. Dis. 2001;8:433–46.

91. Xiao L, Joo KI, Lim M, et al. Dendritic cell-directed vaccination with a lentivector PSCA for prostate cancer in mice. PLoS ONE 2012;7:e48866.

I. NOVEL THERAPEUTIC APPROACHES

92. Zhang YW, Niu J, Lu X, et al. Multi-target lentivirus specific to hepatocellular carcinoma: *in vitro* and *in vivo* studies. J. Hepatol. 2013;58:502–8.

93. Chen YS, Li HR, Miao Y, et al. Local injection of lentivirus-delivered livinshRNA suppresses lung adenocarcinoma growth by inducing a G_0/G_1-phase cell cycle arrest. Int. J. Clin. Exp. Pathol. 2012;5:796–805.

94. Minai-Tehrani A, Chang SH, Kwon JT, et al. Aerosol delivery of lentivirus-mediated *O*-glycosylation mutant osteopontin suppresses lung tumorigenesis in K-ras (LA1) mice. Cell Oncol. (Dordr.) 2013;36:15–26.

95. Seidlits SK, Gower RM, Shepard JA, et al. Hydrogels for lentiviral gene delivery. Expert Opin. Drug Deliv. 2013;10:499–509.

96. Yolamanova M, Meier C, Shaytan AK, et al. Peptide nanofibrils boost retroviral gene transfer and provide a rapid means for concentrating viruses. Nat. Nanotechnol. 2013;8:130–6.

97. Ranzani M, Cesana D, Bartolomae CC, et al. Lentiviral vector-based insertional mutagenesis identifies genes associated with liver cancer. Nat. Methods 2013;10:155–61.

98. Segura MM, Mangion M, Gaillet B, et al. New developments in lentiviral vector design, production and purification. Expert Opin. Biol. Ther. 2013;13:978–1011.

99. Lundstrom K. Biology and application of alphaviruses in gene therapy. Gene Ther. 2005;12:S92–7.

100. Lundstrom K. Alphaviruses in gene therapy. Viruses 2009;1:13–25.

101. Ying H, Zaks TZ, Wang RF, et al. Cancer therapy using a self-replicating RNA vaccine. Nat. Med. 1999;5:823–7.

102. Leitner WW, Hwang LN, deVeer MJ, et al. Alphavirus-based DNA vaccine breaks immunological tolerance by activating innate antiviral pathways. Nat. Med. 2003;9:33–9.

103. Murphy AM, Morris-Downes MM, Sheahan BJ, et al. Inhibition of human lung carcinoma cell growth by apoptosis induction using Semliki Forest virus recombinant particles. Gene Ther. 2000;7:1477–82.

104. Asselin-Paturel C, Lassau N, Guinebretiere JM, et al. Transfer of the murine interleukin-12 *in vivo* by a Semliki Forest virus vector induces B16 tumor regression through inhibition of tumor blood vessel formation monitored by Doppler ultrasonography. Gene Ther. 1999;6:606–15.

105. Vähä-Koskela MJ, Kallio JP, Jansson LC, et al. Oncolytic capacity of attenuated replicative Semliki Forest virus in human melanoma xenografts in severe combined immunodeficient mice. Cancer Res. 2006;66:7185–94.

106. Ketola A, Hinkkanen A, Yongabi F, et al. Oncolytic Semliki Forest virus vector as a novel candidate against unresectabe osteosarcoma. Cancer Res. 2008;68:8342–50.

107. Määttä AM, Mäkinen K, Ketola A, et al. Replication competent Semliki Forest virus prolongs survival in experimental lung cancer. Int. J. Cancer 2008;123:1704–11.

108. Chen CH, Huang GL, Tu YQ, et al. Dual specific antitumor effects of Semliki Forest virus-based DNA vector carrying suicide *Escherichia coli* purine nucleoside phosphorylase gene via *Salmonella*. Int. J. Oncol. 2013;42:2009–18.

109. Ohno K, Sawai K, Iijima Y, et al. Cell-specific targeting of Sindbis virus vectors displaying IgG-binding domains of protein A. Nat. Biotechnol. 1997;15:763–7.

110. Tseng JC, Levin B, Hurtado A, et al. Systemic tumor targeting and killing by Sindbis viral vectors. Nat. Biotechnol. 2004;22:70–7.

111. Lundstrom K, Boulikas T. Breakthrough in cancer therapy: encapsulation of drugs and viruses. Curr. Drug Discov. 2002;11:19–23.

112. Kwak H, Honig H, Kaufmann HL. Poxviruses as vectors for cancer immunotherapy. Curr. Opin. Drug Discov. Devel. 2003;6:161–8.

113. Zeh HJ, Bartlett DL. Development of a replication-selective oncolytic proxvirus for the treatment of human cancers. Cancer Gene Ther. 2002;9:1001–12.

114. Mastrangelo MJ, Lattime EC. Virotherapy clinical trials for regional disease: *in situ* immune modulation using recombinant poxvirus vectors. Cancer Gene Ther. 2002;9:1013–21.

115. Chen B, Timiryasova TM, Haghighat P, et al. Low-dose vaccinia virus-mediated cytokine gene therapy of glioma. J. Immunother. 2001;24:46–57.

116. Ehrig K, Kilinc MO, Chen NG, et al. Growth inhibition of different human colorectal cancer xenografts after a single intravenous injection of oncolytic vaccinia virus GLV-1h68. J. Transl. Med. 2013;11:79.

117. Chernichenko N, Linkov G, Li P, et al. Oncolytic vaccinia virus therapy of salivary gland carcinoma. JAMA Otolaryngol. Head Neck Surg. 2013;139:173–82.

118. Patil SS, Gentschev I, Adelfinger M, et al. Virotherapy of canine tumors with oncolytic vaccinia virus GLV-h109 expressing an anti-VEGF single-chain antibody. PLoS ONE 2012;7:e47472.

119. Brun J, Mahoney DJ, Le Boeuf F, et al. Oncolytic Vaccinia virus safely and effectively treats skin tumors in mouse models of xeroderma pigmentosum. Int. J. Cancer 2013;132:726–31.

120. He S, Li P, Chen CH, et al. Effective oncolytic vaccinia therapy for human sarcomas. J. Surg. Res. 2012;175:e53–60.
121. Haddad D, Chen N, Zhang Q, et al. A novel genetically modified vaccinia virus in experimental models is effective against a wide range of human cancers. Ann. Surg. Oncol. 2012;19(Suppl 3):S665–74.
122. O'Reilly DR. Use of baculovirus expression vectors. Methods Mol. Biol. 1997;62:235–46.
123. Kost TA, Condreay JP. Recombinant baculoviruses as mammalian cell gene-delivery vectors. Trends Biotechnol. 2002;20:173–80.
124. Lehtolainen P, Tyynelä K, Kannasto J, et al. Baculoviruses exhibit restricted cell type specificity in rat brain: comparison of baculovirus- and adenovirus-mediated intracerebral gene transfer in vivo. Gene Ther. 2002;9:1693–9.
125. Paul A, Jardin BA, Kulamarva A, et al. Recombinant baculovirus as a highly potent vector for gene therapy of human colorectal carcinoma: molecular cloning, expression and in vitro characterization. Mol. Biotechnol. 2010;45:129–39.
126. Luo WY, Shih YS, Lo WH, et al. Baculovirus virus vectors for antiangiogenesis-based cancer gene therapy. Cancer Gene Ther. 2011;18:637–45.
127. Swift SL, Rivera GC, Dussupt V, et al. Evaluating baculovirus as a vector for human prostate cancer therapy. PLoS ONE 2013;8:e65557.
128. Zhao Y, Lam DH, Yang J, et al. Targeted suicide gene therapy for glioma using human embryonic stem cell-derived neural stem cells genetically modified by baculoviral vectors. Gene Ther. 2012;19:189–200.
129. Lundstrom K. Past, present and future of nutrigenomics and its influence on drug development. Curr. Drug Discov. Technol. 2013;10:35–46.
130. Virani S, Colacino JA, Kim JH, et al. Cancer epigenetics: a brief review. ILAR J. 2012;53:359–69.
131. Duarte JD. Epigenetics primer: why the clinician should care about epigenetics. Pharmacotherapy 2013;33(12):1362–8.
132. Timp W, Feinberg AP. Cancer as a dysregulated epigenome allowing cellular growth advantage at the expense of the host. Nat. Rev. Cancer 2013;13:497–510.
133. Liu SV, Fabbri M, Gritlitz BJ, et al. Epigenetic therapy in lung cancer. Front. Oncol. 2013;3:135.
134. Vendetti FP, Rudin CM. Epigenetic therapy in non-small-cell lung cancer: targeting DNA methyltransferases and histone acetylases. Expert Opin. Biol. Ther. 2013;19:1273–85.
135. Saha K, Hornyak TJ, Eckert RL. Epigenetic cancer prevention mechanisms in skin cancer. AAPS J. 2013;15(4):1064–71.
136. Supic G, Jagodic M, Magic Z. Epigenetics: a new link between nutrition and cancer. Nutr. Cancer 2013;65:781–92.
137. Pan Y, He B, Lirong Z, et al. Gene therapy for cancer through adenovirus vector-mediated expression of the Ad5 early region gene 1A based on loss of IGF2 imprinting. Oncol. Rep. 2013;30:1814–22.
138. Yamagata Y, Parietti V, Stockholm D, et al. Lentiviral transduction of CD34(+) cells induces genome-wide epigenetic modifications. PLoS ONE 2012;7:e48943.
139. Ginn SL, Alexander IE, Edelstein ML, et al. Gene therapy clinical trials worldwide 2012—an update. J. Gene Med. 2013;15:65–77.
140. Anon. Gene therapy clinical trials. J. Gene Med., www.abedia.com/wiley/countries.php.
141. Manilla P, Rebello T, Afable C, et al. Regulatory considerations for novel gene therapy products: a review for the process leading to the first clinical lentiviral vector. Hum. Gene Ther. 2005;16:17–25.

I. NOVEL THERAPEUTIC APPROACHES

Advances in Nanotechnology-Based Drug Delivery Platforms and Novel Drug Delivery Systems

Krishna Suri[1], *Joy Wolfram*[2], *Haifa Shen*[3], *Mauro Ferrari*[4]

[1]Houston Methodist Research Institute, Houston, TX, USA

[2]Houston Methodist Research Institute, Houston, TX, USA; National Center for Nanoscience and Technology of China, Beijing, China

[3]Department of Nanomedicine, Houston Methodist Research Institute, Houston, TX, USA; Weill Cornell Medical College, New York, NY, USA

[4]Houston Methodist Research Institute, Houston, TX, USA; Weill Cornell Medical College, New York, NY, USA

O U T L I N E

INTRODUCTION TO NANOMEDICINE

Since its inception, the term "nanotechnology" has seen considerable growth in popularity and has quickly made its way into the public domain. Nanotechnological devices can be broadly defined as synthetic material with dimensions in the nanoparticle range.[1] Within the field of medicine, nanotechnology can be utilized in a variety of ways, ranging from the

Novel Approaches and Strategies for Biologics, Vaccines and Cancer Therapies. DOI: 10.1016/B978-0-12-416603-5.00003-1

targeted delivery of drugs to the activation of nanoparticles through external stimuli once localized at the targeted site. The major characteristic of nanotherapeutics is the ability to improve the transport properties of a drug. Small-molecule drugs tend to have inadequately low accumulation at the target site, in addition to the capability to deposit in healthy tissue due to nonspecific biodistribution in the body. Nanotechnology provides a mean to overcome such disadvantages through altering and improving the biodistribution profile of drugs.

Moreover, nanotherapeutic delivery systems are highly versatile, resulting in differential patterns of localization in the body. The major mechanism that controls the accumulation of nanoparticles is selective transport across biological compartments.[1] In order to reach the target location, nanoparticles must overcome several barriers, some of which are inherently designed to be restrictive against foreign material (see Figure 3.1). These barriers include enzymatic degradation, the vascular endothelium, hemodynamics, hydrostatic pressure, the reticuloendothelial system, stromata, the interstitium, cell membranes, subcellular organelles, ionic and molecular pumps, and various excretory pathways.[2] It is important to understand how nanoparticles interact with these biological barriers when designing delivery systems that can efficiently accumulate in the region of interest. In addition, it is

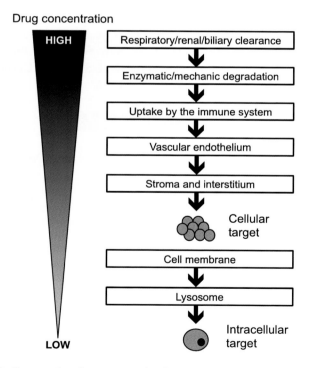

FIGURE 3.1 **Schematic diagram showing an example of the sequential biological barriers that a nanoparticle may encounter upon systemic injection.** Each barrier results in a subsequent reduction in the amount of drug that reaches the final target site.

TABLE 3.1   Strategies for Enhanced Accumulation of Nanoparticles in Tumor Tissue

Strategy	Examples of Tumor Properties Exploited	Example of Nanoparticles
Matching nanoparticle properties to the biophysical features of tumors	Vasculature with large fenestrations, altered blood flow patterns	Liposomes
Utilizing biomaterials	Enhanced uptake of certain biomaterials	Albumin-based nanoparticles
Decorating the nanoparticle surface with molecular moieties	Increased expression of certain receptors	Transferrin-targeted nanoparticles
Activating nanoparticles with external energy	Can be subjected to localized external energy	Iron oxide particles activated with a magnetic field

essential to know the long-term fate of nanoparticles. Depending on the properties of the nanoparticles, they may eventually be excreted, degraded, or permanently deposited in the body.

Accordingly, the following four strategies have been used to achieve preferential localization/activation of nanoparticles: (1) matching the properties of nanoparticles to the biophysical features of the target tissue, (2) adding molecular moieties to the surface of nanoparticles, (3) utilizing biomaterials that abundantly accumulate in tumors, and (4) using external energy sources to activate nanoparticles at a specific location (Table 3.1). All four of these strategies will be described in greater detail in this chapter. In addition to the aforementioned approaches, a next generation of multifunctional nanoparticle strategies is emerging. Among these are the multistage and time-sequential approaches, which will also be introduced in this chapter.

STRATEGIES FOR PREFERENTIAL ACCUMULATION OF NANOPARTICLES

The major goal when designing nanotherapeutics is to achieve preferential localization within the body; namely, by minimizing the drug payload that is delivered outside the target region, increased efficacy can be obtained and detrimental side effects can be averted. Therefore, it is important to understand how the differential characteristics of pathological tissue could be exploited to achieve selective localization of nanoparticles. Indeed, preclinical studies involving nanoparticles routinely include biodistribution experiments. However, biodistribution profiles can be highly variable, depending on the individual, the stage of disease, and the species. To date, four design strategies have been used in clinical and preclinical settings to obtain favorable biodistribution profiles of nanodelivery systems. These design strategies are outlined in further detail below.

Strategy I: Biophysics

The first strategy that has been used to enhance the specific accumulation of nanoparticles is known as *passive targeting*. This strategy involves identifying physical and morphological features that are unique to the pathological tissue of interest and then designing nanoparticles to take advantage of these characteristics.[2] The overall concept of passive targeting relies on the assumption that there are differences between diseased and healthy tissue. Such differences can manifest themselves in many ways, including blood flow patterns and intracellular transport. However, the term passive targeting is generally inaccurate, because designing nanoparticles based on the distinct properties of a target tissue is not a passive process but requires a thought-out approach. Hence, biophysical targeting is a more appropriate term to describe the strategy where the properties of nanoparticles are fine-tuned to be compatible with the differential biophysical features of a diseased tissue.

In essence, the exploitation of the distinct properties of diseased tissue involves the fine regulation of nanoparticle characteristics, such as size, shape, surface charge, and malleability. For example, the size of nanoparticles greatly impacts the site of accumulation in the body. It has previously been shown that particles larger than 100 nm are more likely to end up in the liver, due to recognition by macrophages, while particles smaller than 5.5 nm are excreted by the kidneys.[3,4] Likewise, particles larger than 50 nm can not gain access to pancreatic tumors, because of the distinct features of the vasculature.[3]

Consequently, a precondition for determining how particle properties affect biodistribution is the ability to synthesize nanoparticles with precisely controlled characteristics. If one wants to observe how size affects nanoparticle deposition, for example, then other parameters such as surface characteristics, shape, and deformability must be kept constant. As an example, poly(amidoamine) (PAMAM) dendrimers are highly tunable nanoparticles that can be used to evaluate how design parameters affect particle localization.[5] However, it is also important to consider how nanoparticle characteristics may change in an *in vivo* environment, as it has been shown that the size and charge of certain nanoparticles may dramatically change in the presence of serum proteins.[6]

Moreover, in order to determine the optimal characteristics of a nanotherapeutic, the transport of matter in healthy and diseased tissue should be compared. Within the field of cancer research, the governing term developed for the study of the defining features of transport in tumor tissue is *transport oncophysics*.[7,8] This field covers several aspects of transport, ranging from the movement of molecules to the movement of cells. Furthermore, transport phenomena are studied on different scales, including the blood circulation, microenvironment, and cell interior. In the section below, two distinct features of tumor tissue that have previously been utilized for biophysical targeting are discussed.

Enhanced Permeation and Retention

A commonly used application of biophysical targeting involves taking advantage of the differences in structure between the vasculature of tumor and healthy tissue. As a tumor grows, it generates a new vascular network in order to supply oxygen and nutrients to the increasing population of cancer cells, a process termed *angiogenesis*. Angiogenesis involves the formation of immature blood vessels that have an increased amount of fenestrations due to the presence of fewer pericytes and tight junctions. Such fenestrations, generally smaller than 600 nm in magnitude, allow for increased permeability of particles that are within this size range.[9] This phenomenon is more commonly referred to as the *enhanced permeation and retention* (EPR) effect. As the name suggests, tumor vasculature causes increased retention of nanoparticles. It has been proposed that this increase is due to nonspecific interactions between nanoparticles and the perivascular space.[10] However, such nonspecific binding also limits the dissemination of therapies into neighboring tissue and interstitium, highlighting the paradoxical role of retention for optimal delivery of nanotherapeutics.[11] In addition, enhanced retention is thought to arise from a lack of lymphatic drainage in tumors, which prevents macromolecules and nanoparticles from returning to the circulation, hence causing their build-up in tumor tissue.

Liposomes are an example of nanoparticles that primarily utilize the EPR effect, although this phenomenon is beneficial for all nanoparticles. Liposomes are self-assembling vesicles composed of either natural or synthetic amphipathic lipid molecules. The size of these nanoparticles can easily be fine-tuned to match the size of the fenestrations in the target tissue, thus taking advantage of the EPR effect. Liposomes can also provide several distinct advantages over their free-drug counterparts, including shielding from enzymatic and mechanical degradation, reduced renal clearance, and decreased uptake by the immune system.[12]

Indeed, decreased recognition by macrophages is usually achieved by coating the nanoparticle surface with polyethylene glycol (PEG), which serves as a steric barrier.[13] PEG hinders the binding of opsonins to the nanodelivery system. These plasma proteins serve as signals for the immune system, triggering immunological activation and phagocytosis. Although pegylation clearly helps in avoiding the initial immune surveillance, there is evidence to suggest that PEG antibodies may eventually arise.[14] The first liposome to enter the market was Doxil®, which received clinical approval in 1995 for the treatment of acquired immune deficiency syndrome (AIDS)-related Kaposi's sarcoma.[15] Since then, liposomes have been used extensively for the delivery of both hydrophilic and hydrophobic compounds. In particular, these nanoparticles can mitigate the challenges involved with the delivery of poorly water-soluble drugs.[16] Currently, 13 liposomal drugs have been approved in the United States, Europe, and elsewhere, and many more are enrolled in clinical trials.[15,17]

Utilization of the EPR effect, however, is not strictly limited to oncology. The presence of fenestrations is a characteristic of several diseases; therefore, the EPR phenomenon may be exploited in other instances to achieve high accumulation of nanoparticles in diseased tissue. Specifically in the realm of cardiovascular disease, the blood vessels of damaged tissue exhibit features similar to those of cancerous vasculature.[18,19]

Flow Patterns

In addition to particle size, other properties, such as particle shape,[20,21] surface charge,[22] and deformability,[23] also play an important role in achieving high accumulation in tumors. For example, in the preclinical setting the shapes of particles have been optimized to take advantage of the distinct blood flow patterns in tumor vasculature.[24] Interestingly, spherical nanoparticles have demonstrated low tumor accumulation, while disk-like particles have shown high accumulation in the tumor microenvironment.[24] Disk-like particles display margination along the tumor vasculature, adhesion to endothelial cells, and intravasation across the endothelial wall.[25-27] The strategy of using discoidal particles to obtain preferential tumor localization is inspired from platelets, which have a disk-like structure. This shape allows the platelets to adhere to the surface of abnormal or inflamed vasculature. Because tumor vasculature closely resembles the architecture of inflamed vessels, discoidal particles naturally accumulate along tumor blood vessels.[25]

Strategy II: Biomaterials

The second strategy to increase the localization of therapeutics in the target tissue involves the utilization of biological materials that have enhanced deposition in tumors.[2] An example of this principle is the use of albumin as a therapeutic delivery system. Serum albumin is the most abundant protein in human blood, and it serves as a endogenous chaperone for hydrophobic molecules.[28] Cancers have shown a tendency to uptake albumin in high amounts, thereby facilitating enhanced accumulation of albumin-associated lipophilic molecules in the tumor.[29] The elevated uptake of albumin in the tumor microenvironment is thought to be a consequence of the EPR effect as well as receptor-mediated endothelial transcytosis.[29] Hence, the natural transport properties of albumin, coupled with its preferential accumulation in cancers, render this protein an effective delivery vehicle for therapeutic agents. Indeed, the first clinically approved albumin-based therapeutic, Abraxane®, made it to the market in 2005. Abraxane consists of paclitaxel that is reversibly bound to albumin. Preclinical studies have demonstrated a 33% higher tumor uptake of paclitaxel when administered as Abraxane in comparison to chremophor-based paclitaxel.[30]

In essence, the exploitation of the inherent transport properties of biomaterials has several advantages. In addition to increasing tumor accumulation, this approach is also a way to mitigate toxicity associated with the intake of hydrophobic chemotherapeutics. Poorly water-soluble compounds are usually mixed with toxic solubilizing agents in order to enable drug administration. For example, paclitaxel is formulated with polyethoxylated castor oil (Cremophor® EL) and dehydrated ethanol, while docetaxel is dissolved in polysorbate 80 (Tween® 80).[31] These solvents can have adverse side effects, and many patients are required to take corticosteroids and antihistamines to avoid these reactions.[32] The reduction of toxicity achieved with the use of biomaterials also widens the therapeutic window by enabling the administration of larger and more frequent drug doses. Indeed, in a Phase III metastatic breast cancer study, the dose of paclitaxel was 49% higher when administered with albumin, in comparison to solvent-based paclitaxel.[33]

Strategy III: Molecular Moieties

The third strategy used in nanomedicine to achieve enhanced accumulation of nanoparticles within tumors is termed *active targeting*.[2] This approach involves coating the surface of nanoparticles with molecular moieties that can bind specifically to known biomarkers present in the target tissue.[34,35] The utilization of molecular moieties for drug targeting was first proposed by Paul Ehrlich, who termed this concept the "magic bullet."[36] Enrich is an early pioneer of the notion of selective delivery of drugs to a target tissue through molecular recognition. Active targeting is a misleading term, though, as nanoparticles do not actively seek out their target. Indeed, nanodelivery systems do not possess a motor to propel their movement but rely solely on the blood flow for transportation throughout the body. Nevertheless, molecular moieties can serve to increase the retention of nanoparticles once they have extravasated into the tumor microenvironment. This enhanced retention occurs due to binding between attuned moieties on the nanoparticle surface and the target tissue, such as ligand–receptor binding. In addition, molecular recognition can enhance the intracellular uptake of nanoparticles; for example, ligand–receptor binding can trigger cellular internalization of nanoparticles.[37]

The use of surface moieties can change the biophysical characteristics of nanoparticles.[38] For example, decorating the surface of nanoparticles with targeting molecules may increase the size of the delivery vehicle, in turn further complicating the penetration across biological barriers. Such alterations to the biophysical features of nanodelivery systems could undermine the benefits achieved from surface conjugation. Indeed, targeting moieties can make nanoparticles more prone to immune surveillance, more chemically reactive, less likely to extravasate, and less suitable for diffusion across the vasculature.[38,39] As a result, the utilization of surface targeting could actually hinder the successful accumulation of nanoparticles in tumor tissue. Furthermore, nanotherapeutics administered through systemic injections are subjected to plasma proteins, which form an encompassing biomolecular corona.[40] Targeting molecules on the surface of nanodelivery systems could easily be masked by a layer of proteins, thus preventing molecular recognition. Indeed, it has been shown that nanoparticles with surface ligands can lose their targeting capabilities upon entering blood circulation.[41,42] Therefore, the protein corona may be the determining factor for the biodistribution of nanoparticles.[42,43] One could potentially tailor the surface properties of nanoparticles to attract plasma proteins that have enhanced uptake in tumors.[40,44] To date, there are no clinically approved molecular targeting nanoparticles, although several such drug candidates are currently undergoing clinical trials.[45]

Molecular Targeting of Cancer Cells

Many of the targeted nanotherapeutics under development are directed toward molecules on the surface of cancer cells. This approach allows for the implementation of personalized medicine, where surface moieties can be chosen based on the characteristics of individual tumors. For example, a transferrin-coated polymer, designed for the delivery of small interfering RNA (siRNA) to tumor tissue, is a promising platform for clinical applications.[46] Indeed, the expression of the transferrin membrane receptor is increased in several tumors, making this molecule an attractive target for cancer therapy.[47] Another targeted nanoparticle that holds great promise is a polymeric vehicle decorated with a ligand against a prostate membrane antigen.[48] This nanoparticle is designed for the localized delivery of chemotherapeutics to prostate cancer cells.

Molecular Targeting of Tumor Vasculature

An alternative approach to targeting the surface of cancer cells is the utilization of distinct molecular expression patterns on tumor vasculature.[2] The cataloguing of such proteins may yield comprehensive vascular profiles, allowing for the efficient delivery of a therapeutic payload to tumor tissue.[49] The application of this concept was pioneered by David Cheresh and his research laboratory.[50] Through the identification of an angiogenic integrin $\alpha_v\beta_3$, Cheresh et al. postulated that the utilization of this key receptor pathway, previously found to be involved in the internalization of multiple viruses, could allow for greater efficacy of nanotherapeutic gene transfer. Indeed, nanoparticles conjugated to a peptide specific for $\alpha_v\beta_3$ did effectively deliver a therapeutic gene, causing apoptosis of tumor endothelium and subsequent repression of tumor growth.[51]

Moreover, the application of phage peptide libraries to the endothelium of angiogenic vasculature yields large swaths of data that can more colloquially be termed "vascular zip codes."[51] The conjugation of therapeutics to peptides that are specific for motifs identified from such zip codes can enable enhanced efficacy at the target site and reduced nonspecific cytotoxicity. In a recent study, an E-selectin thioaptamer ligand was used to target bone marrow endothelium.[52] This aptamer was conjugated to the surface of a porous silicon microparticle, which was loaded with paclitaxel-encapsulated liposomes. The results from this study reveal a dramatic increase in the accumulation of liposomes in the bone marrow when using the E-selectin-targeted delivery vehicle in comparison to a non-targeted porous silicon carrier. Vascular targeting may prove advantageous over cancer cell targeting, because it causes retention of nanoparticles at an earlier stage (i.e., before the nanoparticles come in contact with the cancer cells).

Strategy IV: External Energy

The fourth approach for designing nanotherapeutics relies on the use of external energy sources that destroy tumor tissue in the presence of nanoparticles.[2] In this setting, nanoparticles are triggered to have a therapeutic effect when subjected to external energy. This strategy relies on the notion that one is able to selectively expose a target region to therapy through the preferential accumulation of nanoparticles and/or by applying an energy source locally. The therapeutic effect of this strategy is usually achieved through the heating of nanoparticles and the subsequent thermal ablation of cells. Several different energy sources can be used to increase the temperature of nanoparticles. For example, gold particles of various shapes can be heated by infrared light or radiofrequency waves.[53,54] The use of gold nanoshells in conjunction with near-infrared radiation has proven useful for thermal cancer therapy.[55,56]

Another mechanism to achieve thermal ablation of tumor tissue involves the use of magnetic energy. Certain nanoparticles can be heated by subjecting them to an alternating magnetic field. Preclinical studies have shown that intratumoral injection of magnetic fluids combined with external energy causes tumor temperatures to reach over 70°C, resulting in a favorable therapeutic outcome.[57] Moreover, the local infusion of iron oxide particles into the brain, followed by exposure to a magnetic field, recently gained clinical approval in Europe for the treatment of glioblastoma multiforme. The Phase III clinical trial that preceded the approval of this therapy demonstrated an improvement of overall survival accompanied with only moderate side effects.[58]

In addition to metal-based particles, carbon nanotubes have also been used along with an external energy source to achieve localized hyperthermia.[59,60] Carbon nanotubes have the capability to absorb infrared radiation and subsequently release the stored energy in the form of heat.[61] Moreover, the chemical properties and structure of carbon nanotubes, such as the ability to incorporate numerous functional groups and their hollow nature, make them suitable carriers for therapeutic agents. However, the majority of strategies utilizing external energy rely on localized injection of nanoparticles rather than systemic administration. Systemically administered nanoparticles rarely accumulate in high enough concentrations inside the tumor to achieve thermal ablation, making this approach challenging.[54,62] Because 90% of cancer deaths are due to metastatic lesions that are difficult to reach by localized infusion, it is unlikely that the direct injection of nanoparticles into the tumor would prove beneficial for late-stage disease.

In addition to using heat generated from nanoparticles for thermal ablation purposes, elevated temperatures can serve as a means for increasing intratumoral permeability. The administration of drugs or nanotherapeutics, for example, can be preceded by the injection of heat-generating nanoparticles, which render the tumor vasculature more permeable.[63]

NEXT-GENERATION DRUG DELIVERY PLATFORMS

Obtaining a desirable biodistribution of drugs following systemic administration remains challenging. In the case of monoclonal antibodies, only 0.001 to 0.01% of the injected dose binds to the target upon intravenous injection.[64] In this regard, nanoparticles perform slightly better, although accumulation at the target site rarely exceeds 5% of the administered dose.[65] As previously discussed, the major reason for low accumulation of therapeutics in the target region is the presence of biological barriers. By manipulating the characteristics of nanoparticles, such barriers can be overcome. However, most current strategies designed to obtain preferential accumulation of nanotherapeutics focus only on overcoming a few obstacles within the body.

Thus, a multifaceted approach is required to develop a truly successful drug delivery system where nanoparticles bypass various barriers in a sequential manner. It is likely that successful implementation of this approach will require the use of nanovehicles consisting of several materials. Indeed, different materials can be sequentially exposed to the surrounding environment and their unique properties consecutively utilized to overcome biological barriers; for example, layer-by-layer assembly of polyelectrolytes is a useful method for synthesizing delivery vehicles that contain several layers of various nanomaterials.[66]

Time-Sequential Drug Delivery

An example of a next-generation drug delivery platform is the nanocell, developed by Ram Sasisekharan and coworkers. This nanodelivery vehicle was designed to sequentially release an antiangiogenic agent and a chemotherapeutic drug.[67,68] The delivery system was compartmentalized for optimal release and function. The outer compartment consisted of a pegylated lipid envelope encapsulating the antiangiogenic agent combretastain, while the inner compartment contained doxorubicin (a standard anthracycline chemotherapeutic) conjugated to poly-(lactic-co-glycolic) acid (PLGA). PLGA is a biodegradable polymer that can reduce the rate of drug release.[69] The idea behind this multi-component nanotherapeutic system was that the antiangiogenic agent would decrease vascular permeability, thereby trapping the slow-released chemotherapeutic drug in the tumor interstitium.[67,70]

Another example of a multimodal drug delivery system is the multistage vector (MSV). The MSV consists of three stages with different functions (see Figure 3.2).[71,72] The first stage is composed of a porous silicon microparticle, which acts as a mothership for the other two stages. Silicon is a well-characterized material that has previously been used for scaffolds, implants, and drug delivery systems.[73,74] The material is nontoxic and biodegradable, thus representing a promising carrier for biological applications.[74] The silicon particles are designed to take advantage of distinct blood flow patterns and morphological characteristics of tumor neovasculature. By using mathematical modeling, Paolo Decuzzi and his group have identified parameters that increase the vasculature adhesion of particles.[27] Indeed, discoidal particles were predicted to be superior compared to spherical particles with regard

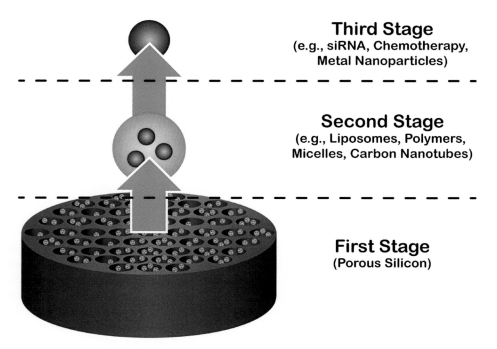

FIGURE 3.2   Schematic illustration showing the three stages of the multistage vector (MSV). The first stage consists of a discoidal porous silicon microparticle. The second stage consists of nanoparticles that are loaded inside the pores of the silicon particle. The nanoparticles, in turn, encapsulate a third stage, which consists of therapeutic or imaging agents.

to accumulation in tumor vasculature.[24] This theory was later confirmed in an *in vivo* mouse model.[25] Thus, the silicon microparticles are manufactured as disk-shaped structures for optimal interaction with tumor blood vessels, resulting in the formation of intravascular depots.[75]

In addition, the surface of silicone particles can be functionalized for the successful loading and delivery of a therapeutic payload. Moreover, by modifying the surface, different rates of degradation can be achieved. As the first stage of the MSV slowly degrades, the second-stage nanoparticles gradually exit from the pores of the silicon microparticle, subsequently entering the tumor interstitium. The nanoparticles then release the encapsulated third-stage compound consisting of a drug or imaging agent. This design makes the MSV highly versatile, as different nanoparticles and therapeutic agents can be used in various combinations. For example, siRNA-containing liposomes,[76] polymer micelles with chemotherapy,[77] and carbon nanotubes with gadolinium[78] have all been loaded into the MSV and successfully used for medical applications.

Amplifying Drug Delivery

Another emerging strategy to achieve sufficient deposition of a therapeutic agent in a target tissue involves the use of an amplifying cascade. Sangeeta Bhatia and coworkers developed a two-component drug delivery system, where a first set of nanoparticles that were deposited in the tumor attracted a second set of nanoparticles.[79] This approach was inspired from biology, as many endogenous signaling pathways rely on the activation of molecular cascades. This multifunctional platform was developed to take advantage of the coagulation cascade, due to its powerful capability for signal amplification and its prevalence in the blood. The first set of nanoparticles was engineered to activate the clotting cascade, while the second set was designed to adhere to clotting factors.

Specifically, photothermally activated gold nanorods or engineered tumor-targeted tissue factor proteins acted as the primary nanoparticles, due to their capability of tumor accumulation and initiation of coagulation. The secondary nanoparticles consisted of a chemotherapeutic liposome or an iron oxide imaging agent, both of which had been conjugated to peptides targeting the coagulation pathway. The utilization of this strategy resulted in a 40-fold increase in the accumulation of the secondary particles in the tumor tissue. With the multitude of nanoparticles under development and the vast number of endogenous signaling pathways that could potentially be exploited, the amplifying drug delivery strategy offers endless opportunities for improving preferential accumulation of therapeutics.

Biomimetic Drug Delivery

Through billions of years of evolution, natural selection has ensured that the most efficient forms of transport throughout the body are developed. On a continuous basis the body manages the transport of multiple molecules and cells. At any given moment, for example, the movement of oxygen, signaling molecules, waste products, and blood cells is precisely controlled. Any deviation in the transport of these components would most likely result in immediate death. Nevertheless, biological elements are not immune to transport barriers; rather, they have developed effective mechanisms to overcome them.

Furthermore, even pathogens, which are foreign to our bodies, have employed efficient ways of evading physiological obstacles. Intriguingly, most viruses and bacteria only cause symptoms in a select group of tissues, suggesting the preferential accumulation or activation of these pathogens. Moreover, viruses have the capability to incorporate genetic material into the host genome, thus overcoming the nuclear membrane barrier. Taken together, these phenomena suggest that the study of natural transport may prove very useful for the design of nanodelivery systems. This new realm of nanoparticles is termed *biomimetic therapies* and can be categorized on the basis of the biological features that are imitated.

An example of a biomimetic nanoplatform was already introduced in the discussion on amplifying drug delivery. In addition to utilizing endogenous signaling cascades, several other forms of biomimicry have inspired the development of innovative nanodelivery systems. Certain bacteria, such as *Clostridium beijerinckii* and *Bifidobacterium bifidum*, that display specificity toward tumor cells have served as models for the development of molecular targeting agents.[80,81]

Furthermore, integrative therapies incorporating both attenuated bacterial cells and nanoparticles have been used for cancer therapy. *Listeria monocytogenes* bacteria were conjugated to polysterene nanoparticles encapsulated with plasmid DNA to form a delivery vehicle termed *microbot*.[82] The biomimetic microbot was able to produce therapeutic proteins through utilization of the host machinery. The combined use of weakened pathogens and nanomaterials is a promising approach for the improved bypassing of biological barriers. The application of this technique across a panel of attenuated pathogens resulted in minimal non-specific toxicity.[82] However, intrinsic immune responses against pathogen delivery systems have yet to be elucidated and may pose a challenge for clinical implementation.

Similarly to bacterial pathogens, viruses offer many advantageous delivery characteristics. Viruses have through evolutionary selection become primed for self-replication and the delivery of genetic material. The field of nanomedicine has recently displayed interest in the elucidation and incorporation of viral mechanisms in the synthesis of nanoparticle systems. As an example, liposomes have been designed to mimic viral structures through the formation of a multilamellar structure and by coating the membrane with transferrin.[83] This strategy proved to be beneficial for the enhanced delivery of genetic material to the target lesion in an *in vivo* prostate cancer model.[83]

Another platform that has been used for biomimicry purposes is nanogels, which are complex nanoscale networks of hydrophilic polymer chains that can uptake biologically active molecules through various molecular interactions (e.g., hydrogen bonds, hydrophobic interactions, salt bonds).[84] Moreover, nanogels have superior loading capacity due to their ability to interact with a vast array of molecules.[84] Recently, nanogels have incorporated virus mimicking (VM) structures to improve the pharmacokinetic properties and increase the therapeutic efficacy of the delivery vehicle.[85] In order to imitate the viral capsid coat, VM nanogels contain a hydrophobic core surrounded by two hydrophilic regions conjugated with tumor-specific ligands, PEG, and bovine-serum albumin. The anticancer drug doxorubicin was encapsulated in the hydrophobic region of the carrier. Therapeutic action was invoked through a pH-sensitive mechanism, causing swelling of the carrier upon exposure to a slightly acidic endosomal environment. The swelling resulted in endosomal escape and promoted the release of doxorubicin, which had a harmful effect on the targeted cells. Subsequently, the VM nanogels proceeded to move to an adjacent cell, repeating the cytotoxic process. These virus-inspired carriers acted in remarkably similar ways to those of their virus counterparts. Although such pathogenic approaches offer new solutions for problems with drug delivery, the technology is still in its infancy and requires extensive preclinical and clinical testing.

In particular, biomimetic approaches are utilized to overcome specific problems with the transport of drug delivery vehicles. An especially pressing issue is the preferential localization of nanodelivery systems in the liver. The major reason for this phenomenon is the immune clearance of nanoparticles by macrophages that are part of the reticular connective tissue of the liver. Thus, one of the most important barriers to overcome for efficient systemic delivery of nanoparticle carriers is the RES system. By exploiting the morphological features of endogenous cells the immune system may be avoided. Leukocytes, which are components of the immune system that are involved in both specific and nonspecific immunogenicity, are an example of endogenous cells that possess superior transport characteristics.

Intriguingly, Ennio Tasciotti and colleagues have demonstrated that by coating particles with leukocyte membranes the delivery systems can impart a "Trojan-horse" effect upon systemic administration.[86] The immune system gets fooled by the endogenous appearance of the carrier and does not initiate an immune response. Tasciotti et al. used an integrative approach, where the MSV was coated with a membrane from a leukocyte, creating the "leuko-like" delivery system. *In vivo* experiments using this carrier demonstrate improved circulation times and enhanced tumor accumulation.[86] Moreover, *in vitro* transendothelial migration studies show that the leukocyte coating causes improved extravasation across an inflamed endothelial monolayer.[86]

IMPLANTS

An ideal system for drug delivery should display drug release at the target site for the duration of treatment. Although systemically administered nanoparticles display therapeutic efficacy, the primary limitation for such carriers is the requirement of repeated injections. The average life expectancy has increased, and chronic illnesses that require lifelong treatment regimens are becoming more common. Thus, implantable platforms that offer sustained drug release over long periods of time (weeks to years) can improve the quality of life by minimizing visits to healthcare providers.

In addition, an implantable system can potentially reduce overall toxicity by decreasing the drug dose per unit time while simultaneously increasing therapeutic activity.[87] Importantly, by using implants the drug concentration in the body can be maintained at a constant level, whereas the use of administered therapeutics results in peak and trough drug concentrations. Consequently, high drug concentrations may induce nonspecific toxicity, while the absence of drug may promote drug resistance.[88] Therefore, the development of implantable devices capable of controlled drug release in the time frame of months to years is needed.

When designing an implantable drug delivery system it is important to consider the biocompatibility of the device, route of implantation, drug dosage, and cost with respect to conventional dosing practice. Because implants are housed within the body for extended periods of time, it is crucial to evaluate the long-term biocompatibility. The system must be mechanically stable and not adversely affect the surrounding physiological environment.[87,89] Ideally, the drug dosage should also be precisely controlled.[90,91]

With regard to the route of administration, implants have traditionally been classified as drug implants and implantable pumps.[87] Pumps differ from drug implants in their mechanism of delivery. Pumps rely on pressure differences, and many of them utilize complex moving components to promote the release of a therapeutic agent. Implantable pumps include infusion pumps, peristaltic pumps, osmotic pumps, positive-displacement pumps, and controlled-release micropumps.

In contrast, drug implants mediate drug release by utilizing polymers and polymer membranes. The polymeric implants can further be broken down into biodegradable and nondegradable systems. The nonbiodegradable drug implants rely on drug diffusion using a polymer matrix with a homogeneously dispersed drug or a reservoir system with a drug core surrounded by a permeable membrane. The disadvantage of these systems is the need for surgical removal of the device following the cessation of treatment. In contrast, biodegradable systems rely on degradable polymers that are ultimately absorbed or excreted by the body. The rate of drug release is dependent on drug diffusion for reservoir implants and on polymer degradation kinetics for matrix implants. A disadvantage of polymeric implants is that they usually present a significant decay in the drug release profile over time.

On the whole, new innovative strategies are necessary to improve the performance of implantable drug platforms; for example, an emerging technology for such devices is the use of nanochannel membranes.[92] Nanochannel drug delivery systems enable drug release through the dense packing of dimensionally distinct nanochannels in a nanofluidic membrane. Consistent delivery of therapeutic agents occurs through molecule–surface interactions, which determine the release profile.[93] In addition, the techniques used to synthesize nanochannels provide precise control over important characteristics such as channel size and surface properties, which in turn enable the design of specific drug release regimens.[94] Alessandro Grattoni and his group constructed an implantable uniform nanochannel membrane for drug delivery,[93] and *in vitro* and *in vivo* studies have demonstrated that this nanochannel device displayed zero-order release kinetics for a prolonged period of time. In addition, the nanochannel system did not show any signs of cytotoxicity in human cells. In conclusion, implants based on nanochannels represent a promising tool for the sustained release of drugs.

References

1. Ferrari M. Cancer nanotechnology: opportunities and challenges. Nat. Rev. Cancer 2005;5:161–71.
2. Ferrari, M. Clinical Cancer Nanotherapeutics, submitted.
3. Cabral H, Matsumoto Y, Mizuno K, Chen Q, Murakami M, Kimura M, Terada Y, Kano MR, Miyazono K, Uesaka M, Nishiyama N, Kataoaka K. Accumulation of sub-100 nm polymeric micelles in poorly permeable tumours depends on size. Nat. Nanotechnol. 2011;6:815–23.
4. Choi HS, Liu W, Misra P, Tanaka E, Zimmer JP, Ipe BI, Bawendi MG, Frangioni JV. Renal clearance of quantum dots. Nat. Biotechnol. 2007;25:1165–70.
5. Menjoge AR, Kannan RM, Tomalia DA. Dendrimer-based drug and imaging conjugates: design considerations for nanomedical applications. Drug Discov. Today 2010;15:171–85.
6. Wolfram J, Suri K, Celia C, Yang Y, Shen J, Fresta M, Zhao Y, Shen H, Ferrari M. Shrinkage of pegylated and non-pegylated liposomes in serum. Colloids Surf. B Biointerfaces 2014;114:294–300.
7. Michor F, Liphardt J, Ferrari M, Widom J. What does physics have to do with cancer? Nat. Rev. Cancer 2011;11:657–70.
8. Ferrari M. Frontiers in cancer nanomedicine: directing mass transport through biological barriers. Trends Biotechnol. 2010;28:181–8.
9. Yuan F, Dellian M, Fukumura D, Leunig M, Berk DA, Torchilin VP, Jain RK. Vascular permeability in a human tumor xenograft: molecular size dependence and cutoff size. Cancer Res. 1995;55:3752–6.
10. Maeda H, Wu J, Sawa T, Matsumura Y, Hori K. Tumor vascular permeability and the EPR effect in macromolecular therapeutics: a review. J. Control. Release 2000;65:271–84.
11. Yuan F, Leunig M, Huang SK, Berk DA, Papahadjopoulos D, Jain RK. Microvascular permeability and interstitial penetration of sterically stabilized (stealth) liposomes in a human tumor xenograft. Cancer Res. 1994;54: 3352–6.
12. Gentile E, Cilurzo F, Di Marzio L, Carafa M, Ventura CA, Wolfram J, Paolino D, Celia C. Liposomal chemotherapeutics. Future Oncol. 2013;912:1849–59.
13. Li S-D, Huang L. Stealth nanoparticles: high density but sheddable PEG is a key for tumor targeting. J. Control. Release 2010;145:178–81.
14. Knop K, Hoogenboom R, Fischer D, Schubert US. Poly(ethylene glycol) in drug delivery: pros and cons as well as potential alternatives. Angew. Chem. Int. Ed. Engl. 2010;49:6288–308.
15. Chang H-I, Yeh M-K. Clinical development of liposome-based drugs: formulation, characterization, and therapeutic efficacy. Int. J. Nanomed. 2012;7:49–60.
16. Celia C, Trapasso E, Locatelli M, Navarra M, Ventura CA, Wolfram J, Carafa M, Morittu VM, Britti D, Di Marzio L, Paolino D. Anticancer activity of liposomal bergamot essential oil (BEO) on human neuroblastoma cells. Colloids Surf. B Biointerfaces 2013;112:548–53.
17. Koudelka S, Turánek J. Liposomal paclitaxel formulations. J. Control. Release 2012;163:322–34.
18. Menon C, Ghartey A, Canter R, Feldman M, Fraker DL. Tumor necrosis factor-alpha damages tumor blood vessel integrity by targeting VE-cadherin. Ann. Surg. 2006;244:781–91.
19. Weis SM. Vascular permeability in cardiovascular disease and cancer. Curr. Opin. Hematol. 2008;15:243–9.

20. Decuzzi P, Pasqualini R, Arap W, Ferrari M. Intravascular delivery of particulate systems: does geometry really matter? Pharm. Res. 2009;26:235–43.

21. Longmire MR, Ogawa M, Choyke PL, Kobayashi H. Biologically optimized nanosized molecules and particles: more than just size. Bioconjugate Chem. 2011;22:993–1000.

22. Xiao K, Li Y, Luo J, Lee J, Xiao W, Gonik A, Agarwal R, Lam K. The effect of surface charge on *in vivo* biodistribution of PEG–oligocholic acid based micellar nanoparticles. Biomaterials 2011;32:3435–46.

23. Chen H, Zhu H, Hu J, Zhao Y, Wang Q, Wan J, Yang Y, Xu H, Yang X. Highly compressed assembly of deformable nanogels into nanoscale suprastructures and their application in nanomedicine. ACS Nano 2011;5:2671–80.

24. Decuzzi P, Godin B, Tanaka T, Lee S-Y, Chiappini C, Liu X, Ferrari M. Size and shape effects in the biodistribution of intravascularly injected particles. J. Control. Release 2010;141:320–7.

25. Van de Ven AL, Kim P, Haley O, Fakhoury J, Adriani G, Schmulen J, Moloney P, Hussain F, Ferrari M, Liu X, Yun S-H, Decuzzi P. Rapid tumoritropic accumulation of systemically injected plateloid particles and their biodistribution. J. Control. Release 2012;158:148–55.

26. Adriani G, de Tullio MD, Ferrari M, Hussain F, Pascazio G, Liu X, Decuzzi P. The preferential targeting of the diseased microvasculature by disk-like particles. Biomaterials 2012;33:5504–13.

27. Decuzzi P, Ferrari M. Design maps for nanoparticles targeting the diseased microvasculature. Biomaterials 2008;29:377–84.

28. Conlin AK, Seidman AD, Bach A, Lake D, Dickler M, D'Andrea G, Traina T, Danso M, Brufsky A, Saleh M, Clawson A, Hudis C. Phase II trial of weekly nanoparticle albumin-bound paclitaxel with carboplatin and trastuzumab as first-line therapy for women with HER2-overexpressing metastatic breast cancer. Clin. Breast Cancer 2010;10:281–7.

29. Hawkins MJ, Soon-Shiong P, Desai N. Protein nanoparticles as drug carriers in clinical medicine. Adv. Drug Deliv. Rev. 2008;60:876–85.

30. Desai N, Trieu V, Yao Z, Louie L, Ci S, Yang A, Tao C, De T, Beals B, Dykes D, Noker P, Yao R, Labao E, Hawkins M, Soon-Shiong P. Increased antitumor activity, intratumor paclitaxel concentrations, and endothelial cell transport of cremophor-free, albumin-bound paclitaxel, ABI-007, compared with cremophor-based paclitaxel. Clin. Cancer Res. 2006;12:1317–24.

31. Ten Tije AJ, Verweij J, Loos WJ, Sparreboom A. Pharmacological effects of formulation vehicles: implications for cancer chemotherapy. Clin. Pharmacokinet. 2003;42:665–85.

32. Yardley DA. nab-Paclitaxel mechanisms of action and delivery. J. Control. Release 2013;170:365–72.

33. Gradishar WJ. Phase III trial of nanoparticle albumin-bound paclitaxel compared with polyethylated castor oil-based paclitaxel in women with breast cancer. J. Clin. Oncol. 2005;23:7794–803.

34. Ruoslahti E. Peptides as targeting elements and tissue penetration devices for nanoparticles. Adv. Mater. 2012;24:3747–56.

35. Cardoso MM, Peça IN, Roque ACA. Antibody-conjugated nanoparticles for therapeutic applications. Curr. Med. Chem. 2012;19:3103–27.

36. Strebhardt K, Ullrich A. Paul Ehrlich's magic bullet concept: 100 years of progress. Nat. Rev. Cancer 2008;8:473–80.

37. Pollinger K, Hennig R, Ohlmann A, Fuchshofer R, Wenzel R, Breunig M, Tessmar J, Tamm ER, Goepferich A. Ligand-functionalized nanoparticles target endothelial cells in retinal capillaries after systemic application. Proc. Natl. Acad. Sci. USA 2013;110:6115–20.

38. Sperling RA, Parak WJ. Surface modification, functionalization and bioconjugation of colloidal inorganic nanoparticles. Philos. Trans. A Math Phys. Eng. Sci. 2010;368:1333–83.

39. Wang AZ, Gu F, Zhang L, Chan J, Radovic-Moreno A, Shaikh M, Farokhzad O. Biofunctionalized targeted nanoparticles for therapeutic applications. Expert Opin. Biol. Ther. 2008;8:1063–70.

40. Lundqvist M, Stigler J, Elia G, Lynch I, Cedervall T, Dawson KA. Nanoparticle size and surface properties determine the protein corona with possible implications for biological impacts. Proc. Natl. Acad. Sci. U.S.A. 2008;105:14265–70.

41. Salvati A, Pitek AS, Monopoli MP, Prapainop K, Bombelli F, Hristov D, Kelly P, Aberg C, Mahon E, Dawson K. Transferrin-functionalized nanoparticles lose their targeting capabilities when a biomolecule corona adsorbs on the surface. Nat. Nanotechnol. 2013;8:137–43.

42. Gaspar R. Nanoparticles: pushed off target with proteins. Nat. Nanotechnol. 2013;8:79–80.

43. Monopoli MP, Aberg C, Salvati A, Dawson KA. Biomolecular coronas provide the biological identity of nanosized materials. Nat. Nanotechnol. 2012;7:779–86.

I. NOVEL THERAPEUTIC APPROACHES

44. Mahon E, Salvati A, Baldelli Bombelli F, Lynch I, Dawson KA. Designing the nanoparticle-biomolecule interface for "targeting and therapeutic delivery". J. Control. Release 2012;161:164–74.

45. Davis ME, Chen Z, Shin DM. Nanoparticle therapeutics: an emerging treatment modality for cancer. Nat. Rev. Drug Discov. 2008;7:771–82.

46. Davis ME, Zuckerman JE, Choi CHJ, Seligson D, Tolcher A, Alabi C, Yen Y, Heidel J, Ribas A. Evidence of RNAi in humans from systemically administered siRNA via targeted nanoparticles. Nature 2010;464:1067–70.

47. Daniels TR, Bernabeu E, Rodríguez JA, Patel S, Kozman M, Chiappetta D, Holler E, Ljubimova JY, Helguera G, Penichet M. The transferrin receptor and the targeted delivery of therapeutic agents against cancer. Biochim. Biophys. Acta 2012;1820:291–317.

48. Hrkach J, Von Hoff D, Ali MM, Andrianova E, Auer J, et al. Preclinical development and clinical translation of a PSMA-targeted docetaxel nanoparticle with a differentiated pharmacological profile. Sci. Transl. Med. 2012;4:128ra39.

49. Arap W. Cancer treatment by targeted drug delivery to tumor vasculature in a mouse model. Science 1998;279:377–80.

50. Hood JD. Tumor regression by targeted gene delivery to the neovasculature. Science 2002;296:2404–7.

51. Dias-Neto E, Nunes DN, Giordano RJ, Sun J, Botz G, Yang K, Setubal JC, Pasqualini R, Arap W, Ho PL. Next-generation phage display: integrating and comparing available molecular tools to enable cost-effective high-throughput analysis. PLoS ONE 2009;4:e8338.

52. Mann AP, Tanaka T, Somasunderam A, Liu X, Gorenstein DG, Ferrari M. E-selectin-targeted porous silicon particle for nanoparticle delivery to the bone marrow. Adv. Mater. 2011;23:H278–282.

53. Glazer ES, Zhu C, Massey KL, Thompson CS, Kaluarachchi WD, Hamir AN, Curley SA. Noninvasive radiofrequency field destruction of pancreatic adenocarcinoma xenografts treated with targeted gold nanoparticles. Clin. Cancer Res. 2010;16:5712–21.

54. Shen H, You J, Zhang G, Ziemys A, Li Q, Bai L, Deng X, Erm DR, Liu X, Li C, Ferrari M. Cooperative, nanoparticle-enabled thermal therapy of breast cancer. Adv. Healthcare Mater. 2012;1:84–9.

55. Hirsch LR, Stafford RJ, Bankson JA, Sershen SR, Rivera B, Price RE, Hazle JD, Halas NJ, West JL. Nanoshell-mediated near-infrared thermal therapy of tumors under magnetic resonance guidance. Proc. Natl. Acad. Sci. U.S.A. 2003;100:13549–54.

56. Gobin AM, Lee MH, Halas NJ, James WD, Drezek RA, West JL. Near-infrared resonant nanoshells for combined optical imaging and photothermal cancer therapy. Nano Lett. 2007;7:1929–34.

57. Johannsen M, Thiesen B, Jordan A, Taymoorian K, Gnevecknow U, Waldofner N, Scholz R, Koch M, Lein M, Jung K, Loening SA. Magnetic fluid hyperthermia (MFH) reduces prostate cancer growth in the orthotopic Dunning R3327 rat model. Prostate 2005;64:283–92.

58. Maier-Hauff K, Ulrich F, Nestler D, Niehoff H, Wust P, Thiesen B, Orawa H, Budach V, Jordan A. Efficacy and safety of intratumoral thermotherapy using magnetic iron-oxide nanoparticles combined with external beam radiotherapy on patients with recurrent glioblastoma multiforme. J. Neuro-Oncol. 2010;103:317–24.

59. Chakravarty P, Marches R, Zimmerman NS, Swafford ADE, Bajaj P, Musselman IH, Pantano P, Draper RK, Vitetta ES. Thermal ablation of tumor cells with antibody-functionalized single-walled carbon nanotubes. Proc. Natl. Acad. Sci. U.S.A. 2008;105:8697–702.

60. Ghosh S, Dutta S, Gomes E, Carroll D, D'Agostino R, Olson J, Guthold M, Gmeiner WH. Increased heating efficiency and selective thermal ablation of malignant tissue with DNA-encased multiwalled carbon nanotubes. ACS Nano 2009;3:2667–73.

61. Sharma A, Jain N, Sareen R. Nanocarriers for diagnosis and targeting of breast cancer. BioMed Res. Int. 2013;2013:1–10.

62. Cervadoro A, Giverso C, Pande R, Sarangi S, Preziosi L, Wosik J, Brazdeikis A, Decuzzi P. Design maps for the hyperthermic treatment of tumors with superparamagnetic nanoparticles. PLoS ONE 2013;8:e57332.

63. Li L, ten Hagen TLM, Bolkestein M, Gasselhuber A, Yatvin J, van Rhoon GC, Eggermont AMM, Haemmerich D, Koning GA. Improved intratumoral nanoparticle extravasation and penetration by mild hyperthermia. J. Control. Release 2013;167:130–7.

64. Li KCP, Pandit SD, Guccione S, Bednarski MD. Molecular imaging applications in nanomedicine. Biomed. Microdevices 2004;6:113–6.

65. Bae YH, Park K. Targeted drug delivery to tumors: myths, reality and possibility. J. Control. Release 2011;153:198–205.

66. Elbakry A, Wurster E-C, Zaky A, Liebl R, Schindler E, Bauer-Kriesel P, Blunk T, Rachel R, Goepferich A, Breunig M. Layer-by-layer coated gold nanoparticles: size-dependent delivery of DNA into cells. Small 2012;8:3847–56.
67. Sengupta S, Eavarone D, Capila I, Zhao G, Watson N, Kiziltepe T, Sasisekharan R. Temporal targeting of tumour cells and neovasculature with a nanoscale delivery system. Nature 2005;436:568–72.
68. Kerbel RS, Kamen BA. The anti-angiogenic basis of metronomic chemotherapy. Nat. Rev. Cancer 2004;4:423–36.
69. Danhier F, Ansorena E, Silva JM, Coco R, Le Breton A, Préat V. PLGA-based nanoparticles: an overview of biomedical applications. J. Control. Release 2012;161:505–22.
70. Kerbel R, Folkman J. Clinical translation of angiogenesis inhibitors. Nat. Rev. Cancer 2002;2:727–39.
71. Wong C, Stylianopoulos T, Cui J, Martin J, Chauhan VP, Jiang W, Popovic Z, Jain RK, Bawendi MG, Fukumura D. Multistage nanoparticle delivery system for deep penetration into tumor tissue. Proc. Natl. Acad. Sci. U.S.A. 2011;108:2426–31.
72. Tanaka T, Decuzzi P, Cristofanilli M, Sakamoto JH, Tasciotti E, Robertson FM, Ferrari M. Nanotechnology for breast cancer therapy. Biomed. Microdevices 2009;11:49–63.
73. Godin B, Gu J, Serda RE, Bhavane R, Tasciotti E, Chiappini C, Liu X, Tanaka T, Decuzzi P, Ferrari M. Tailoring the degradation kinetics of mesoporous silicon structures through PEGylation. J. Biomed. Mater. Res. A 2010;94:1236–43.
74. Anglin EJ, Cheng L, Freeman WR, Sailor MJ. Porous silicon in drug delivery devices and materials. Adv. Drug Deliv. Rev. 2008;60:1266–77.
75. Godin B, Tasciotti E, Liu X, Serda RE, Ferrari M. Multistage nanovectors: from concept to novel imaging contrast agents and therapeutics. Acc. Chem. Res. 2011;44:979–89.
76. Xu R, Huang Y, Mai J, Zhang G, Guo X, Xia X, Koay EJ, Qin G, Erm DR, Li Q, Liu X, Ferrari M, Shen H. Multistage vectored siRNA targeting ataxia-telangiectasia mutated for breast cancer therapy. Small 2013;9:1799–808.
77. Blanco E, Sangai T, Hsiao A, Ferrati S, Bai L, Liu X, Meric-Bernstam F, Ferrari M. Multistage delivery of chemotherapeutic nanoparticles for breast cancer treatment. Cancer Lett. 2013;334:245–52.
78. Ananta JS, Godin B, Sethi R, Moriggi L, Liu X, Serda RE, Krishnamurthy R, Muthupillai R, Bolskar R, Helm L, Ferrari M, Wilson LJ, Decuzzi P. Geometrical confinement of gadolinium-based contrast agents in nanoporous particles enhances T_1 contrast. Nat. Nanotechnol. 2010;5:815–21.
79. Von Maltzahn G, Park J-H, Lin KY, Singh N, Schwoppe C, Mesters R, Berdel WE, Ruoslahti E, Sailor MJ, Bhatia SN. Nanoparticles that communicate *in vivo* to amplify tumour targeting. Nat. Mater. 2011;10:545–52.
80. Pawelek JM, Low KB, Bermudes D. Bacteria as tumour-targeting vectors. Lancet Oncol. 2003;4:548–56.
81. Yoo J-W, Irvine DJ, Discher DE, Mitragotri S. Bio-inspired, bioengineered and biomimetic drug delivery carriers. Nat. Rev. Drug Discov. 2011;10:521–35.
82. Akin D, Sturgis J, Ragheb K, Sherman D, Burkholder K, Robinson JP, Bhunia AK, Mohammed S, Bashir R. Bacteria-mediated delivery of nanoparticles and cargo into cells. Nat. Nanotechnol. 2007;2:441–9.
83. Xu L, Frederik P, Pirollo KF, Tang W-H, Rait A, Xiang L-M, Huang W, Cruz I, Yin Y, Chang EH. Self-assembly of a virus-mimicking nanostructure system for efficient tumor-targeted gene delivery. Hum. Gene Ther. 2002;13:469–81.
84. Kabanov AV, Vinogradov SV. Nanogels as pharmaceutical carriers: finite networks of infinite capabilities. Angew. Chem. Int. Ed. 2009;48:5418–54129.
85. Lee ES, Kim D, Youn YS, Oh KT, Bae YH. A virus-mimetic nanogel vehicle. Angew. Chem. Int. Ed. 2008;47:2418–21.
86. Parodi A, Quattrocchi N, van de Ven AL, Chiappini C, Evangelopoulos M, Martinez JO, Brown BS, Khaled SZ, Yazdi IK, Enzo MV, Isenhart L, Ferrari M, Tasciotti E. Synthetic nanoparticles functionalized with biomimetic leukocyte membranes possess cell-like functions. Nat. Nanotechnol. 2013;8:61–8.
87. Dash AK, Cudworth GC 2nd. Therapeutic applications of implantable drug delivery systems. J. Pharmacol. Toxicol. Meth. 1998;40:1–12.
88. Liang X-J, Chen C, Zhao Y, Wang PC. Circumventing tumor resistance to chemotherapy by nanotechnology. In: Zhou J, editor. Multi-Drug Resistance in Cancer. Totowa, NJ: Humana Press; 2010. p. 467–88.
89. Park H, Park K. Biocompatibility issues of implantable drug delivery systems. Pharm. Res. 1996;13:1770–6.
90. Danckwerts M, Fassihi A. Implantable controlled release drug delivery systems: a review. Drug Dev. Ind. Pharm. 1991;17:1465–502.
91. Staples M, Daniel K, Cima MJ, Langer R. Application of micro- and nano-electromechanical devices to drug delivery. Pharm. Res. 2006;23:847–63.

I. NOVEL THERAPEUTIC APPROACHES

92. Grattoni A, Shen H, Fine D, Ziemys A, Gill JS, Hudson L, Hosali S, Goodall R, Liu X, Ferrari M. Nanochannel technology for constant delivery of chemotherapeutics: beyond metronomic administration. Pharm. Res. 2011;28:292–300.
93. Sih J, Bansal SS, Filippini S, Filippini S, Ferrati S, Raghuwansi K, Zabre E, Nicolov E, Fine D, Ferrari M, Palapattu G, Grattoni A. Characterization of nanochannel delivery membrane systems for the sustained release of resveratrol and atorvastatin: new perspectives on promoting heart health. Anal. Bioanal. Chem. 2013;405:1547–57.
94. Fine D, Grattoni A, Hosali S, Ziemys A, De Rosa E, Gill J, Medema R, Hudson L, Kojic M, Molosevic M, Brousseau IL, Goodall R, Ferrari M, Liu X. A robust nanofluidic membrane with tunable zero-order release for implantable dose specific drug delivery. Lab Chip 2010;10:3074–83.

Novel Approaches for the Delivery of Biologics to the Central Nervous System

Pankaj Karande[1], John Philip Trasatti[2], Divya Chandra[1]

[1]Howard P. Isermann Department of Chemical and Biological Engineering, Rensselaer Polytechnic Institute, Troy, NY, USA

[2]Chemistry and Chemical Biology, Rensselaer Polytechnic Institute, Troy, NY, USA

OUTLINE

Novel Approaches and Strategies for Biologics, Vaccines and Cancer Therapies. DOI: 10.1016/B978-0-12-416603-5.00004-3

THE RISING GLOBAL BURDEN OF CENTRAL NERVOUS SYSTEM DISORDERS

World Population and Demographics

The world population is increasing steadily. In the past six decades the total world population has increased by almost 300% and is estimated to reach ~10 billion by 2050 (Figure 4.1). This in itself is a trivial observation. What is notable and interesting is the increase in life expectancy that has accompanied this steady growth in population. The average life expectancies for a female and male in 1950 were recorded to be approximately 48 and 45 years, respectively. It is estimated that these numbers will have increased to approximately 77 years and 72 years for an average female and an average male, respectively, by 2050, indicating a 60% increase in the overall life expectancy.[1,2] Underlying these figures are the rapid and tremendous advances in healthcare sciences and medical technologies that have brought life-saving drugs that allow us to live longer. Vaccines and antibiotics, for example, have single handedly reduced the incidence rates of epidemics and infectious diseases across the globe that were long associated with widespread human morbidity. Improvements in prenatal and neonatal care have significantly reduced infant mortality rates across most parts of the world. Advances in genomics have elucidated the basic biological origins and pathologies of diseases coupled with highly effective therapies, both curative and preventative, derived from proteomics, metabolomics, and other "omic" sciences. The promise of providing longer lives has largely been delivered by the new age of science and technology. It has, unfortunately, also left us susceptible to "late-in-life" diseases. An interesting but challenging paradox of this new century will be increased longevity with increased susceptibility to newer diseases.

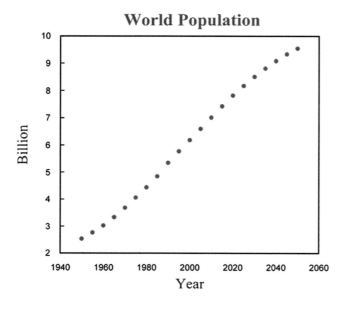

FIGURE 4.1   World Health Organization census data on world population. The world population has been increasing linearly for the past 60 years. It is expected to continue to increase and reach ~10 billion by 2050.

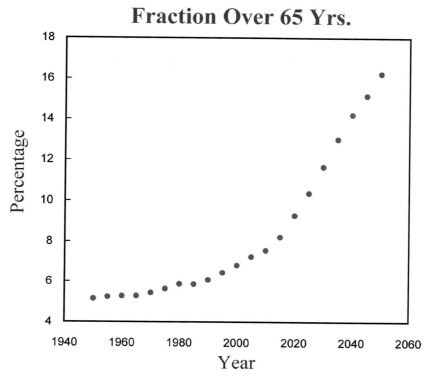

FIGURE 4.2   Fraction of the population above the age of 65. Exponential growth is projected to occur within this age group over the next 40 years. By 2050, one in five people are expected to be over the age of 65.

The so-called late-in-life diseases present an interesting challenge unlike others in the history of human evolution. A steady increase in the world population along with a steady increase in life expectancies has biased the age demographic distribution. In the 100-year period from 1950 to 2050, as the world population grows almost linearly, the fraction of the population above the age of 65 years is expected to increase exponentially, as shown in Figure 4.2.[1,2] By 2050, approximately 16% of the population, or almost 1 in 6 people, are estimated to be above the age of 65 years. This represents a critical milestone signaling a sharp increase in healthcare needs and expenditures. The burden of neurological diseases and disorders, a major contributor to late-in-life diseases, is expected to increase disproportionately.

The Rising Incidence Rates of Neurological Diseases

The World Health Organization (WHO) quantifies the impact or burden of disease on human life via disability-adjusted life years (DALYs).[1,2] DALYs for a disease or health condition are, by WHO definition, calculated as the sum of the years of life lost (YLL) due to premature mortality in the population and the years lost due to disability (YLD) for people living with the health condition or its consequences. One DALY typically represents one year of healthy life lost to disease. The sum of these DALYs across the population, or the burden of disease, can be thought of as a measurement of the gap between current health status and an ideal health situation where the entire population lives to an advanced age, free of disease and disability. The use of DALYs in lieu of mortality rates is especially critical for neurological and neurodegenerative diseases where they can significantly reduce the quality of life without inducing direct or immediate death. The 1990 Global Burden of Disease (GBD) Report particularly highlighted neuropsychiatric diseases, and injuries are major contributors to DALYs but severely underestimated when measured in terms of mortality alone.[1,2] Neurological disorders are generally defined to include two broadly defined categories:

1. Neuropsychiatric disorders covering migraine; Parkinson's, Alzheimer's, and other dementias; epilepsy; and multiple sclerosis
2. Disorders or injuries with neurological sequelae covering cerebrovascular disease, poliomyelitis, tetanus, meningitis, and Japanese encephalitis.

In 2005, neurological disorders contributed to 6.3% of the GBD, far ahead of tuberculosis, HIV/AIDS, malignant neoplasms, ischemic heart disease, respiratory disease, and digestive diseases. This number is expected to rise steadily to 6.4% by 2015 and 6.8% by 2030.

Socio-Economic Impacts of Neurological Diseases

An estimated 1 in every 17 Americans today suffers from a mental illness.[1] Every year approximately 1.5 million Americans sustain traumatic brain injuries requiring hospitalization and possibly long-term care.[2] Parkinson's disease currently affects over 1 million Americans and is one of the most common debilitating diseases in the country. It is estimated that one in 200 persons will develop Parkinson's during their lifetime. An estimated 5 million people in the United States suffer from Alzheimer's, surpassing diabetes as the sixth leading cause of deaths. In the United States, stroke is currently the third leading cause of deaths, and an estimated 150,000 people die from stroke every year. Among survivors, stroke can lead to significant disabilities, including paralysis and speech problems. Approximately 2.5 million people suffer from epilepsy in the United States. It is estimated that 10% of Americans will have experienced a seizure in their lifetimes, and of this group 3% will be diagnosed with epilepsy by the age of 80. At the current rate, more than a sixth of the population in the United States will be over the age of 65 by 2050.[3] A substantial increase in the need for drugs that act on the brain is predicted as the shift in the age demographic is expected to result in a proportional increase in brain related diseases.[3] Even otherwise healthy individuals tend to develop a range of neurological problems, from brain tumors to neurodegenerative diseases, as they grow older. The number of people living long enough to experience these conditions continues to grow, and it is estimated that this group will lose up to 25% of their healthy life to brain-related illnesses. The yearly cost of disability benefits and health care costs in the United States is nearly $125 billon, and the cost in annual lost earnings is over $190 billon.[4] Mental health related disorders represent a growing economical and societal concern, and effective therapeutic interventions are therefore imminently needed to address this concern.

CHALLENGES IN CNS DRUG DEVELOPMENT

Current and Rising Market Share of Drugs for CNS Indications

It is anticipated that over the next five years the global pharmaceutical industry will see dramatic changes. The global spending on drugs is anticipated to increase to $1.2 trillion by 2016, an increase of $70 billion from 2012 spending.[3] Yet, hidden within this global increase is a predicted decline in spending in developed markets (United States, Europe, Japan) to 57% of the global total, down from 73% only a decade prior.[3] Such a decline is due to the expiration of a significant number of key patents between 2012 and 2014, yielding a rise in generic drugs.[3,4] Furthermore, from 2007 to 2011, the total number of globally launched new molecular entities (NMEs) was less than 30, except in 2009. However, the number of globally launched NMEs is expected to rebound to 32 to 37 NMEs per year through 2016, yielding new, innovative therapies. Such NMEs are anticipated for Alzheimer's, autoimmune diseases, diabetes, cancer, heart and respiratory conditions, and other infectious and orphan diseases.[3] Additionally, by 2016, there will be a 100-fold increase in the share of spending on biologics compared to 2006 spending due to several advances in clinical research.[3] The development of biologics plays a particularly important role in the treatment of neurological diseases, as many promising biotherapeutics (proteins, peptides, gene therapies) for neurodegenerative diseases and neurological disorders are in late-stage research development and/or clinical trials.

Currently, central nervous system (CNS) drugs make up a large portion of the global pharmaceutical market share, 17% in 2008 as reported in 2009 by Lundbeck.[5] However, upon disease-specific fractionation of the CNS market share, it is apparent that the majority share is represented by drugs for the treatment of psychotic disorders, depression, and pain, while only ~10% of drugs aim to treat Alzheimer's and Parkinson's disease.[5] Yet, it is for these neurological and neurodegenerative diseases that new and effective therapeutics are urgently needed to address their growing burden within the aging population. Further, for the majority of CNS diseases, the drugs on the market aim at treating symptoms rather than being curative therapeutics. Although poor safety, low efficacy, and lack of *in vitro/* physiological models all contribute to a significant attrition of CNS drugs in Phase I and II clinical trials, the most significant contributor to this disparity is quite unequivocally the formidable blood–brain barrier that limits the penetration of actives and excipients into the brain.[6]

Approximately 98% of all small molecules and nearly all large molecules, including biotherapeutics, are excluded from penetrating into the CNS. There exist so-called "rules" which, while empirical, define attributes that CNS active drugs must adhere to in order to reach their target within the brain. For example, a molecular weight of less than 400 to 500 Daltons, formation of no more than eight to ten hydrogen bonds, and a high lipid solubility are a few that characteristically define many CNS drugs in the market today.[7] In the past 30 years, both the number of hydrogen bonding characteristics and molecular weights of developed CNS drugs have steadily increased, yet they remain a strong limiting factor in the CNS drug discovery process. The first CNS-permeating small molecules explored and developed were antipsychotics and anxiolytics.[8] Small molecules, such as these, permit structure refinement and redesign yielding generations of drugs. As an example from the antipsychotic drugs class, Thorazine® led to the development of three second-generation molecules (Clozaril®, Risperdal®, and Roxiam®), which ultimately refined into the third-generation drug Abilify®.[8] The majority of small-molecule drugs that do penetrate the CNS treat only certain neurologic disorders, including epilepsy, affective disorders, and chronic pain.[7] However, many of the neurological diseases that affect millions of patients worldwide, such as Alzheimer's, Parkinson's, and stroke, remain without effective clinical treatments. As discussed before, these are also the ailments that are likely to be the key challenges of this century. In recent years, significant successes have been made in the area of brain drug discovery, affording many new therapeutics; however, the ultimate success of these therapeutics in a clinical setting is limited by poor CNS penetration.

The Blood–Brain Barrier: A Dual Barrier

The CNS permeability of a drug is determined by the drug's ability to cross the blood–brain barrier (BBB). The BBB is a selective barrier composed of endothelial cells of the cerebral vasculature. This vasculature is a dense capillary network with a total length of 600 km in humans and average surface area of approximately 20 m².[9] Within this dense network no neuron or glial cell is more than 8 to 20 µm from a neighboring capillary.[9,10] Despite having a single endothelial cell barrier and a total intercellular brain capillary volume of 5 mL, the BBB is actually one of the most restrictive barriers found within the body.[10] The BBB's restrictive properties are achieved via a two-pronged barrier approach, acting as both a physical and metabolic barrier (Figure 4.3). The combination of these allows the BBB to maintain homeostasis and protect the surrounding brain tissue. There exist a variety of pathways by which molecules, nutrients, and ions are transported into the brain via endogenous transcellular processes, to be discussed in detail later in this chapter.

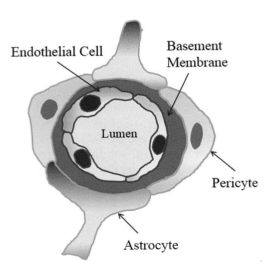

FIGURE 4.3 Cross-section of a brain microcapillary. The endothelial cells that form the capillaries make up the BBB and govern the transport of molecules from the blood into the brain tissue.

The physical barrier properties of the BBB are formed primarily by protein tight junction complexes, which restrict the paracellular permeability of molecules. The tight junction proteins found within the BBB come from a variety of families, including claudins, occludins, and junction adhesion molecules (JAMs). These tight junction complexes are transmembrane proteins expressed on the surface of endothelial cells. Adjacent endothelial cells are linked through the interaction of these tight junction proteins, causing a tight sealing of the paracellular aqueous pathway.[9] Occludin; claudins-1, -3, -5, and -12; and JAMS-A, -B, and -C are all expressed within the BBB.[9] However, the tight junction protein claudin-5 has been demonstrated *in vivo* to be one of the major protein contributors to the BBB's barrier properties.[11] Tight junctions generally restrict both large hydrophilic molecules (proteins) and ions (Na^+ and Cl^-) from crossing the BBB via the paracellular aqueous pathway. Tight junction complexes permit the BBB to exclude both blood serum proteins and restrict the movement of ions across the barrier. The penetration of serum proteins can potentially cause damage to the nervous tissue, whereas ionic fluctuations occurring within the blood can potentially disrupt neuronal signaling.[12]

The second restrictive property of the BBB is its metabolic barrier function. This metabolic barrier is achieved through the expression of efflux pumps on the surface of the endothelial cells. The most well known efflux pump, P-glycoprotein (Pgp), is located on the apical membrane of the BBB endothelial cells. Pgp is a transmembrane protein with high affinity for a variety of cationic and lipophilic compounds.[13] Another class of efflux pumps is the multidrug resistance-associated protein (MRP) family; specifically, MRP 1, 2, 5, and 6 are found on the surface of the endothelial cells of the BBB. MRPs mainly transport anionic compounds out of BBB endothelial cells.[13] Both Pgp and MRPs aim to protect the brain via the efflux of potentially harmful compounds, yet this protective mechanism also prevents many CNS drugs from reaching their targets across the BBB.[13]

Clinical Performance of CNS Drugs

Although the restrictive attributes of the BBB offer protection against xenobiotics, they also pose challenges in the development of CNS drugs. It is therefore not surprising that CNS drug discovery is a costly and risky venture costing $0.8 to 1.7 billion and taking between 10 and 16 years to bring a drug to the market. On average, this is at least 2 to 4 years longer than the development life span of a typical drug and represents the time penalty of lost opportunities for revenues. This is also the primary reason for the highest failure rates of CNS drugs in Phase I and II clinical trials (93 to 98%).[6] Effective strategies to overcome the restrictions of the BBB must therefore be developed in order to reduce the failure rate of CNS targeting drugs.

Table 4.1 lists drugs approved by the U.S. Food and Drug Administration (FDA) over the past 15 years for the treatment of CNS diseases. The majority of the drugs are small molecules that treat symptoms associated with these diseases. As can be seen from the table, several drugs have FDA approval for seizures, epilepsy, stroke, attention deficit hyperactivity disorder (ADHD), migraines, depression, multiple sclerosis, and bipolar disorder. For brain tumors, temozolomide (TMZ) and carmustine (*bis*-chloroethylnitrosourea, BCNU) are the only two drugs that are approved for therapy.[14] As mentioned by Seigal in a 2013 *NeuroOncology* review, TMZ meets all five clinical expectations of a drug:[14] effectiveness, limited systemic

TABLE 4.1   Market Survey of FDA-Approved Drugs in Clinical Use for CNS Diseases

Drug Name	Brand Name	Company	Year	Disease	Action
tPA[15]	Activase®	Genentech	1996	Ischemic brain strokes	Thrombolytic agent that breaks clots
Donepezil[16]	Aricept®	Pfizer	1996	All stages of Alzheimer's disease (AD)	Cholinesterase inhibitor that slows down disease activity that breaks down a key neurotransmitter
Galantamine hydrobromide[17]	Reminyl™	Janssen Pharmaceuticals	2001	Mild to moderate dementia of AD	Cholinesterase inhibitor
Rivastigmine[16]	Exelon®	Novartis	2000	Mild to moderate AD	Cholinesterase inhibitor, also approved in 2007 for AD and PD-related dementia
Memantine[16]	Namenda™	Forest Laboratories	2003	Moderate to severe AD	NMDA (N-methyl-D-aspartate) receptor antagonist that regulates activity of glutamate, which is important for learning and memory; protects brain from excess glutamate
Tacrine[16]	Cognex®	—	1993	Mild to moderate AD	Cholinesterase inhibitor
Gablofen (baclofen injection)[18]	—	CNS Therapeutics	2010	Severe spasticity	Anti-epileptic drug that also reduces severe spasticity due to MS, cerebral palsy, spinal cord injury, brain trauma, and stroke
Terifluonomide[19]	Aubagio®	Sanofi Aventis	2012	Multiple sclerosis	—
Perampanel[19]	Fycompa™	Eisai	2012	Epilepsy	Selective AMPA-type glutamate receptor antagonist
Levomilnacipran[17]	Fetzima™	Forest Laboratories	2013	Major depressive disorder	Selective norepinephrine and serotonin reuptake inhibitor; exact mechanism unknown
Nimodipine[17]	Nymalize™	Arbor Pharmaceuticals	2013	Ischemia/subarachnoid hemorrhage	Dihydropyridine calcium channel blocker that reduces incidence and severity of ischemic deficits
Apixaban[17]	Eliquis®	Bristol-Myers Squibb	2012	Stroke prevention	Factor Xa antagonist

TABLE 4.1   Market Survey of FDA-Approved Drugs in Clinical Use for CNS Diseases *(cont.)*

Drug Name	Brand Name	Company	Year	Disease	Action
Oxcarbazepine extended release[17]	Oxtellar XR™	Supernus Pharmaceuticals	2012	Partial seizures in adults and children (6–17 years)	Anti-epileptic drug that blocks voltage-sensitive sodium channels, stabilizes hyper-excited neural membranes, and prevents spread of seizure in the brain
Methylphenidate hydrochloride[17]	Quillivant XR™	NextWave Pharmaceuticals	2012	Attention deficit hyperactivity disorder (ADHD)	Central nervous stimulant
Ezogabine[17]	Potiga®	Valeant Pharmaceuticals	2011	Partial-onset seizures	Potassium channel agent; mechanism not fully known
Vilazodone hydrochloride[17]	Viibryd®	Clinical Data	2011	Major depressive disorder	Antidepressant; selective serotonin reuptake inhibitor and 5HT1A receptor partial agonist
Dalfampridine[17]	Ampyra®	Acorda	2010	Multiple sclerosis	Potassium channel blocker that enhances conduction in damaged nerves and improves walking in MS patients
Onabotulinumtoxin A[17]	Botox®	Allergan	2010	Chronic migraine	Binds acceptor sites on motor or sympathetic nerves and blocks transmission; inhibits the release of acetylcholine
Clonidine hydrochloride[17]	Kapvay®	Shionogi	2010	ADHD	Centrally acting alpha2-adrenergic agonist
Rifaximin[17]	Xifaxan®	Salix Pharmaceuticals	2010	Hepatic encephalopathy	Antimicrobial agent that inhibits bacterial RNA synthesis
Caprylidene[17]	Axona®	Accera	2009	Age-associated memory impairment (AAMI) and AD	Replaces depleted glucose levels in the brain
Diclofenac potassium[17]	Cambia®	Kowa Pharmaceuticals	2009	Migraine attacks	Nonsteroidal antiinflammatory drug

(Continued)

I. NOVEL THERAPEUTIC APPROACHES

TABLE 4.1   Market Survey of FDA-Approved Drugs in Clinical Use for CNS Diseases *(cont.)*

Drug Name	Brand Name	Company	Year	Disease	Action
Interferon beta-1b[17]	Extavia®	Novartis	2009	Relapsing multiple sclerosis	Modulation of immune system to reduce inflammatory damage
Guanfacine extended-release[17]	Intuniv®	Shire Pharmaceuticals	2009	ADHD in children and adolescents	Selective alpha2A-adrenergic receptor agonist; not a CNS stimulant
Vigabatrin[17]	Sabril®	Lundbeck	2009	Infantile spasms and complex partial seizures	Selective, irreversible enzyme-activated GABA transaminase inhibitor (GABA inhibits the release of dopamine)
Valproic acid delayed release[17]	Stavzor®	Banner Pharmacaps	2008	Bipolar manic disorders, seizures, and migraine headaches	Affects GABA function
Lacosamide[17]	Vimpat®	Schwarz Pharma	2008	Partial-onset seizures with adult epilepsy	Orally available anticonvulsant that selectively enhances slow inactivation of sodium channels
Tetrabenazine[17]	Xenazine®	Prestwick Pharmaceuticals	2008	Chorea due to Huntington's disease	Monoamine depletory for oral administration
Rotigotine[17]	Neupro®	Schwarz Pharma	2007	Parkinson's disease	Transdermal drug delivery system that provides non-ergolinic dopamine agonist continuously for 24 hours
Lisdexamfetamine dimesylate[17]	Vyvnase®	New River	2007	ADHD	Prodrug of dextroamphetamine that induces the release of dopamine and norephinephrine from the nerve terminals
Paliperidone[17]	Invega®	Janssen Pharmaceuticals	2006	Schizophrenia	Blocks dopamine type 2, serotonin type 2, and alpha 2 adrenergic receptors, which are implicated in schizophrenia

TABLE 4.1 Market Survey of FDA-Approved Drugs in Clinical Use for CNS Diseases *(cont.)*

Drug Name	Brand Name	Company	Year	Disease	Action
Naltrexone[17]	Vivitrol®	Alkermes	2006	Alcohol dependence	Opioid antagonist with high affinity for μ-opioid receptor
Natalizumab[17]	Tysabri®	Elan Pharmaceuticals	2006	Multiple sclerosis	Recombinant humanized IgG4k mAb
Apomorphine hydrochloride[17]	Apokyn®	Mylan Laboratories	2004	Parkinson's disease	Non-ergoline dopamine agonist
Interferon beta-1a[17]	Rebif®	Serono Laboratories	2002	Multiple sclerosis	Decreases frequency of clinical exacerbations
Eletriptan hydrobromide[17]	Relpax®	Pfizer	2002	Migraine headaches	Relieves pain in nerve endings and symptoms caused by migraine
Atomoxetine HCl[17]	Strattera®	Eli Lilly	2002	ADHD	Selective norephinephrine reuptake inhibitor
Zolmitriptan[17]	Zomig®	AstraZeneca	2001	Migraine	—
Metadate CD[17]	—	Celltech Pharmaceuticals	2001	ADHD	Capsules deliver methylphenidate in two phases
Frovatriptan succinate[17]	Frova®	Elan Pharmaceuticals	2001	Migraine attacks	Binds to stimulated serotonin (5-HT) receptors
Dexmethylphenidate HCl[17]	Focalin®	Celgene	2001	ADHD	Refined form of Ritalin®
Carbidopa-levodopa[20]	Sinemet®, Sinemet® CR	Merck Canada	1988	Parkinson's disease	Increases concentration of dopamine in the brain and improves nerve conduction
	Parcopa®	Schwarz Pharma			

and neurotoxicity, ease of introduction into the clinic, feasibility of repeated and continuous administration, and usefulness of drug/strategy to any tumor size.[14] BCNU is known to cross the BBB and has also been used in Gliadel™ wafers. For Parkinson's disease, L-dopa is still the gold standard for therapy even though various chemical modifications to this basic form have been made. To date, six drugs have been approved for Alzheimer's disease. Of those six, it has been reported that drugs two to six in Table 4.1 are only effective for 6 to 12 months in 50% of the patients who are prescribed to them. Of all the drugs approved by the FDA every year, drugs for CNS disorders form a very small fraction. For example, in 2012, the FDA approved 39 new molecular entities (NMEs) as drugs, out of which only two (Fycompa® and Aubagio®) were for CNS disorders. Thus, there is a clear need to focus on novel drug delivery strategies for brain disorders.

I. NOVEL THERAPEUTIC APPROACHES

CLINICAL STRATEGIES IN CNS DELIVERY FOR OVERCOMING THE BLOOD–BRAIN BARRIER

Here we will review existing clinical strategies for treating brain diseases that will provide further perspectives on the current status and challenges in CNS drug discovery, development, and, equally important, delivery. This section provides an overview of therapeutic strategies and devices that are FDA approved and currently in the clinic for treatment of CNS disorders.

Physical Methods

Physical methods to overcome the BBB and treat CNS disorders typically use invasive neurosurgical approaches and intracranial drug delivery systems. These include techniques such as intracerebroventricular (directly into the cerebral ventricles of the brain), intracerebral (into the cerebrum), and intrathecal (into the cerebrospinal fluid, CSF) administration of drugs, intracerebral drug implants, convection-enhanced diffusion (into a specific cavity in the brain), and the use of catheters and other devices. Intracerebral, intraventricular, intrathecal, and intracerebroventricular routes enable the direct administration or infusion of the drug into the appropriate brain cavity or the spinal cord. Typically, a majority of physical methods use catheter or catheter-based systems. Table 4.2 provides a summary of all FDA-approved catheter-based devices in clinical use for the treatment of various brain diseases such as stroke, cerebral ischemia, aneurysm, and astrocytoma.

Intracerebroventricular Drug Infusion

Intracerebroventricular (ICV) infusion helps bypass the BBB by permitting high concentrations of a drug to directly reach the central compartment of the brain.[21] For ICV drug infusion, a plastic drug reservoir can also be implanted subcutaneously in the scalp. A catheter is then used to connect the reservoir to the ventricular space in the brain. For example, the GliaSite™ radiation therapy system (RTS) from Cytyc Corporation uses an intracavitary balloon catheter to deliver radiation therapy to a surgical cavity created post-surgery and for tumor removal in various grades of fibrillary astrocytomas. In a study reported in 2006 and conducted on 95 patients with recurrent grade 3 or 4 gliomas who had previously undergone resection, GliaSite RTS was administered with lotrex at a depth of 1 cm with a median dose rate of 52.3 Gy/hr.[22] The estimated one-year survival of the patients, from the date of administration of GliaSite, was 31.1%. It was concluded from the study that GliaSite RTS after resection provided modest survival benefits as compared to surgery alone.[22] Several factors such as osmolarity, pH, volume, and diluents present in the drug can affect the efficacy of ICV drug administration.[21]

Intrathecal Drug Administration

Intrathecal delivery minimizes the drug-related side effects associated with high doses of oral medication of drugs such as baclofen, morphine, and ziconotide. Because the drug can bypass the BBB with an intrathecal injection, the resulting concentration in the CSF is higher.[23] As a result, lesser amounts of the drug can produce the desired response. Patients with different forms of spasticity and intolerable pain are typically administered drugs via the intrathecal route.

TABLE 4.2 Market Survey of FDA-Approved Catheters and Catheter-Based Systems and Therapies for CNS Diseases

Product	Company	Year Approved	Disease	Usage, Outcome, Other Information
LICOX® tunneling catheter[38]	Integra Lifesciences	2002	Prognostic and diagnostic value for several brain disorders	Brain tissue oxygen monitoring system continuously monitors dissolved oxygen and temperature in cerebral tissues.
GliaSite® Radiation Therapy System[39]	IsoRay, Inc.	2011	Diffuse fibrillary astrocytoma	Intracavitary, inflatable balloon catheter is placed in surgical cavity, and craniotomy for a resection is closed. Radiation source placed in the balloon, exposes brain tissue to radiation, continuously or at intervals.
Onyx® Liquid Embolic System (Onyx® HD-500)[39]	Ev3 Neurovascular	2007	Brain aneurysms	Onyx polymer is injected as a viscous liquid into the aneurysm via a tiny catheter. When the polymer hardens, blood circulates safely past the aneurysm.
Cordis Enterprise™ Vascular Reconstruction Device and Delivery System[39]	Cordis Neovascular, Inc.	2007	Brain aneurysm	Self-expanding stent and delivery system is composed of an introducer and delivery wire; the delivery system delivers the stent to the treatment site.
Pipeline™ Embolization Device (PED)[39]	Chestnut Medical Technologies	2011	Wide-neck brain aneurysm	Less open (yet invasive) treatment is performed with the use of a catheter placed inside blood vessel. Blood flow is redirected away from an aneurysm, causing the remaining blood in the aneurysm to clot.
cPAX Aneurysm Treatment System[39]	NeuroVasx, Inc.	2011	Wide-neck large cerebral aneurysms	Implant material is delivered through a catheter in a blood vessel up into the brain aneurysm. The implant material stops blood flow through the aneurysm and reduces the likelihood of rupture and increase in size of aneurysm.
Wingspan™ Stent System with Gateway™ PTA Balloon Catheter[39]	Boston Scientific	2005	Used to open blocked arteries in the brain	Balloon catheter opens the blocked artery, and the stent prevents recurrent blockage. It is used after clot-dissolving drugs have been used.
NeuroFlo™ catheter[39]	CoAxia, Inc.	2005	Cerebral ischemia	Long flexible tube with two small balloons is used to block blood flow in large blood vessels (lower part of body) and increase blood flow to the upper part of the body (brain). Cerebral ischemia occurs when the brain does not receive enough blood to maintain normal neurologic function (speech, movement, understanding).

Convection-Enhanced Diffusion

Convection-enhanced diffusion (CED) and delivery are an approach whereby drugs are delivered continuously to a cavity in the brain under positive pressure. Such an approach achieves better distribution of the drug as compared to simple diffusion or passive transport, which are usually performed by local intracerebral delivery of stereotactic injections. CED achieves diffusion (due to concentration gradients) and convection (due to pressure gradients). It is performed via a catheter once the proper placement site has been identified. CED, however, is a complex process where several parameters need to be identified and set, other than just the coordinates of the site of administration. Yet, foremost is the correct catheter placement to prevent backflow or leakage as this can lead to drug spreading in undesired regions of the brain and cause neurological damage, toxicity, and side effects. Another factor that determines catheter placement is the volume of distribution (V_d). Injections to the gray matter due to its relatively isotropic structure have better V_d values as compared to injections made via the white matter of the brain. Catheter size and an optimum rate of infusion also affect CED, where the optimum rate is that which enables maximum delivery over the least time. Other factors that impact CED are catheter design, volume and nature of the drug infused, dilatation of brain extracellular matrix, heart rate enhancement, and the specific regions of the brain where a drug is administered via CED. Allard et al.[24] have published a comprehensive review discussing each of these factors in detail. Even though CED has a promising scientific rationale, due to several practical challenges in the parameters described above it has not seen success over standard therapy in two large randomized clinical trials (PRECISE, TransMID).

Intracerebral Implants

Intracerebral implants make use of drug-impregnated polymers that allow controlled release of the drug at the desired site in the brain over an extended period of time.[25] Encapsulation of the drug has the added benefit of protecting it from degradation and minimizing the unwanted effects associated with an un-encapsulated drug on normal cells. Brain tumors as well as neurodegenerative diseases can especially benefit from such controlled release systems. The first, and currently considered the standard of care for patients with recurrent gliomas at the time of resection, is the implantable polymer system Gliadel® wafer. This FDA-approved product is a disc-shaped wafer that consists of PCPP:SA (poly[bis(p-carboxyphenoxyl)] propane-sebacic acid) polymer loaded with BCNU (1,3-bis (2-chloroethyl)-1-nitrosourea; carmustine), an anticancer agent for the treatment of glioblastoma multiforme (GBM).[26] Based on a similar idea, the groups of Benoit and Menei have designed PLGA (poly(lactic-co-glycolic) acid) microparticles loaded with 5-fluorouracil (5-FU).[27] Although these microparticles can be implanted at the site of the tumor, they have the added advantage that they can be administered stereotactically using a syringe.[28] Thus, tumors that can or cannot be accessed surgically can both be treated. Factors that affect the distribution of the drug from the implant to the brain are the rate of diffusive and convective drug transport, rate of elimination and degradation of the drug from the brain, and rate of binding or internalization.[29] Although several patents (e.g., US 4883666, US 20046803052, US 5601835) have been published in the area of drug-releasing implantable polymer devices for brain diseases, only one, by Brem et al.[29] (US 5651986) and marketed as the Gliadel®

wafer, has received FDA approval (1996). However, it should be noted that the Gliadel wafers have shown only limited improvement in patient survival, typically two months.[26] Also, the drug has to diffuse from the wafer to the tissue, and because tissue penetration is only up to ~1 mm, it further limits efficacy.[30] The only other implantable polymer (but not loaded with a drug) having FDA approval is the cPAX aneurysm treatment system for cerebral aneurysms (the ballooning of a cerebral artery or vein due to a weakened blood vessel wall). Rupturing of the blood vessel can lead to hemorrhage, stroke, and permanent nerve damage. Consequently, the ideal implantable drug delivery system still remains to be introduced into the clinic.

Other Physical Strategies

Other physical strategies for targeting disorders of the CNS include craniotomy, whole brain radiation therapy, radiosurgery, and deep brain stimulation. *Craniotomy*, or brain surgery, is employed for treating brain tumors and is usually carried out to cut open the brain and physically remove the tumor, metastatic growth, and a small amount of surrounding tissue. With advances in imaging technologies the precise location for the surgery can be determined in order to avoid damage to areas that are key to speech, coordination, memory, and other functions. Although craniotomy is unavoidable in severe cases of brain tumors, other techniques along with chemotherapy are used to complement the surgical procedure to avoid resurgence of tumors.

Whole brain radiation therapy (WBRT) is carried out on patients with intracranial brain metastases and rapidly progressing metastatic diseases of the brain.[31,32] The increase in medial survival of patients undergoing WBRT has been four to six months.[32] WBRT has several short-term side effects (e.g., memory loss particularly verbal memory, extreme fatigue, temporary baldness, skin rash, inflammation of outer ear, hearing loss) and long-term side effects (e.g., memory loss, confusion, lack of coordination and bladder control, dementia).[31]

Radiosurgery, also referred to as *stereotactic radiosurgery* (SRS), is considered effective in delivering very high radiation doses focused directly at the site of brain metastasis(es). This form of administering radiation is minimally invasive as it can be provided without having to actually cut the skull and can be delivered deep within the brain, thus minimizing potential side effects.[33] However, it is not a substitute for whole-brain radiation or surgery, as it cannot be administered for more than three metastases at a time or for tumors that are larger than 3 cm.[31]

Deep brain stimulation (DBS) has been used for brain disorders and motor fluctuations and dyskinesia that are long-term complications of levodopa therapy in Parkinson's disease.[34] These stimulators, implanted in the brain, deliver steady electric currents to certain structures of the brain and have been shown to suppress symptoms of severe tremor in Parkinson's disease.[35] DBS has recently been approved by the FDA for obsessive–compulsive disorders that are medication resistant. Another FDA-approved, deep brain stimulation therapy is the Activa® Parkinson's Control Therapy from Medtronic, Inc., for blocking tremors associated with Parkinson's disease (PD). Table 4.3 lists all implants and devices for CNS disorders that are currently in the market. DBS can enhance memory and learning and has the potential to be used in other diseases such as Alzheimer's disease, temporal lobe epilepsy, and injuries.[36]

TABLE 4.3   Market Survey of FDA-Approved Implants and Devices in Clinical Use for CNS Diseases

Product	Company	Year Approved	Disease	Usage and Other Information
NovoTTF™ Therapy; Novocure™ TTFields™[39]	Novocure, Ltd.	2011	Brain tumor, recurrent glioblastoma multiforme in adults	Wearable, portable device that delivers electric fields to a patient. An alternative to chemotherapy, the device inhibits mitosis and slows down and reverses tumor growth.
Reclaim™ DBS™ Therapy[39]	Medtronic Neuromodulation	2009	Chronic, treatment for resistant adult obsessive–compulsive disorder (OCD)	An implanted pulse generator (IPG) placed under the skin sends electrical stimulation pulses to the brain. The IPG is connected to a lead with four electrodes that contact a specific structure of the brain. The totally implanted brain stimulator suppresses OCD symptoms.
Medtronic Activa® Dystonia Therapy[39]	Medtronic, Inc.	2003	Management of long-term primary dystonia not responsive to drug therapy	An implanted pulse generator (IPG) placed under the skin sends electrical stimulation pulses to the brain. The IPG is connected to a lead with four electrodes that contact a specific structure of the brain. It improves symptoms associated with primary dystonia.
Activa® Parkinson's Control Therapy[39]	Medtronic, Inc.	2002	Parkinson's disease (PD)	A pulse generator placed under the skin of abdomen or collar bone sends constant tiny electrical pulses to select brain areas and blocks tremors associated with PD; may improve some symptoms associated with PD.
Gliadel[39]	Guilford Pharmaceuticals	2003	Glioblastoma multiforme	BCNU-impregnated wafers are used for intracranial implantation.
Prometra® Programmable Infusion Pump System[39]	Medasys, Inc.	2012	Chronic pain	A battery-operated pump is implanted under the abdominal skin and an infusion catheter is implanted near the spine for intrathecal delivery of controlled amounts of Infumorph®, a morphine sulfate sterile solution, into the fluid around the spinal cord (intrathecal space).

Limitations of Physical Methods

The above-mentioned physical methods have several disadvantages and limitations other than being highly invasive. Intracerebral implantation relies on diffusion of drug from the depot site to reach the target site. Diffusion scales inversely with the square of distance and drops rapidly, by as much as 90% over a few hundred microns. Consequently, therapeutically insufficient amounts (less than 1% of the administered dose) of drug reach the target site. Secretion of interstitial fluid, even though slow, from the brain microvessels generates a net flow toward the cerebrospinal fluid and works against diffusion and penetration of the drug. The renewal of CSF every five to six hours causes a continuous clearance of the drug from the brain. CED is a technique where bulk flow is forced through the brain to enhance the availability of the drug in the brain parenchyma; however, because the brain lacks a lymphatic system, intraparenchymal volume flow is limited.[37] Intracerebral implants and catheters also lead to pain and nausea and can have serious adverse side effects on the nervous system. Furthermore, seizure, bleeding, and encephalitis can be caused by improper placement of the needle or catheter in the brain. Intrathecal injections, although affording sustained delivery of agents for treatment of brain cancers, infections, pain, and inflammation, do not penetrate deeply into the brain, are frequently ineffective, and are potentially very risky. Uneven, slow, and incomplete distributions of the drug in the brain further limit intrathecal delivery. Disorders requiring chronic therapy such as Alzheimer's or Parkinson's do not stand to benefit from such approaches because recurrent brain surgery is not practical, is traumatic, and leads to several neurological side effects such as cognitive defects in the long term. Although surgery is unavoidable for removing brain tumors, a sustained drug delivery strategy is still needed for treating cases of metastatic recurring glioblastomas and astrocytomas as well as neurodegenerative diseases where chronic drug therapy is necessary. In summary, an ideal strategy is one that is minimally invasive, is clinically effective, and can be administered systemically to deliver drugs across the BBB in a patient-compliant and therapeutically effective manner.

Chemical Methods

Typically, only low-molecular-weight lipid-soluble molecules, a few peptides, and nutrients can cross the BBB via passive transmembrane diffusion or endogenous transport mechanisms. Concentration-dependent transmembrane diffusion is favored by low molecular weight and high lipid solubility, but these two factors alone do not govern BBB permeability. In fact, several low-molecular-weight (400 to 500 Da) compounds do not cross the BBB. The majority of them are substrates for P-glycoprotein efflux pumps; for example, nitrosoureas, which are small molecular weight drugs, do not reach the brain due to their short half-life, rapid clearance by hepatic metabolism, and renal excretion. On the other hand, high lipid solubility is also not a rule of thumb, as it lowers the amount of drug that reaches the BBB because it can be taken up by other tissues. Other factors that affect drug transport are charge, tertiary structure, and degree of protein binding. Therefore, additional drug optimization and formulation strategies must be employed in order to make the drugs BBB permeable.

Prodrug Approach

Prodrug approaches include chemical modifications of drugs to improve their charge and lipophilicity in favor of BBB permeability. Lipophilic prodrug agents have been used to increase brain delivery of hydrophilic molecules.[40] However, such an approach requires the process of lipidation to be reversible and the prodrug to be converted to the active agent by a chemical or an enzyme found in the brain. Several attempts to convert many anticancer drugs to prodrugs have not been successful because doing so adversely affects the pharmacokinetic profile of the drug. Nevertheless, a successful example of the prodrug approach is L-dopa in Parkinson's therapy. L-Dopa can cross the BBB and convert into the active therapeutic dopamine, which itself cannot cross the BBB. Another successful prodrug example is temozolomide (TMZ), which converts to the active agent dacarbazine under physiological pH. Chemical modification via linkage of a prodrug to a biologically active compound (e.g., coupling of phenylethylamine to nicotinic acid) has also been proven efficient by Bodor et al.[41] Other modifications include derivatization of compounds to centrally acting amines, enclosing compounds in cyclodextrin caged complexes, and covalent attachment of complexes to cationic carriers or membrane-permeable peptides.

Chemically Mediated Barrier Disruption

Another strategy for promoting entry of therapeutics across the BBB is transient disruption of the barrier using chemical agents. BBB disruption can be carried out through the use of hyperosmolar vasoactive agents, alkylating agents, immune adjuvants, or cytokines by means of intracarotid arterial infusion. By temporarily disrupting the BBB, these agents enhance passive diffusion of large and small molecule drugs. Although chemical agents are a biochemical way of achieving BBB disruption, other approaches include osmotic or ultrasound-mediated disruption. Of these, osmotic disruption using a mannitol solution is the only FDA-approved procedure to date. Hyperosmolar mannitol is rapidly infused intraarterially after transfemoral catheterization of the desired arterial region. This procedure is performed over two days by a team of experts and is repeated monthly. BBB integrity is regained after more than six hours after osmotic disruption in human subjects. A hydrophilic drug, methotrexate (MTX), has been shown to be delivered to the brain via passive transport after osmotic disruption of the BBB. In a large, multicenter study with patients with primary CNS lymphoma, BBB disruption was carried out in conjunction with chemotherapy; however, the results of the study did not demonstrate better treatment outcomes as compared to conventional chemotherapy alone. BBB disruption using biochemical agents relies on molecules such as leukotrienes, histamine, and vasoactive peptides that are capable of mediating an inflammatory response and causing temporary leakage as well increased permeability of BBB blood vessels. As an example, bradykinin agonist RMP-7 can permeabilize the BBB; however, the method requires an invasive procedure. For the treatment of malignant brain tumors, intraarterial RMP-7, in combination with carboplatin, has been evaluated in a multinational trial; however, the trial was suspended due to high toxicity. Overall, BBB disruption is associated with severe vasculopathy, neuropathologic changes, and increased risk of complications such as seizures or fatal brain edema. During the period that the BBB remains open, there is increased and unwanted uptake of plasma material into the brain, a majority of which is severely toxic for the brain. Also, the use of such solvents and agents must be evaluated for possible systemic side effects on the brain before they can be used for chronic drug administration. Many biological and biochemical processes that mediate transport across the BBB also mediate transport across other tissue barriers, including the hepatic, renal, gastrointestinal, and vascular systems in other compartments of the body. Despite the transient nature of these osmotic and biochemical BBB disruption strategies, they have not been accepted clinically, as they have not shown additional benefits over existing strategies and have been ineffective in treating large tumors and different CNS locations. The critical challenge in achieving success with these strategies is achieving the specific and reversible disruption of the BBB.

NEW DIRECTIONS IN CNS DELIVERY

Thus far, we have reviewed and discussed the key needs and challenges in the areas of CNS drug development and delivery. There are many hurdles to be overcome and critical concerns to be addressed. The challenges of BBB drug delivery are still far from being fully understood and addressed, and the goal of developing efficient CNS delivery systems is far from being achieved. Nevertheless, there is much promising work in this field that has taken advantage of new physical, chemical, and biological approaches to bring us closer to achieving this goal. Here we review and highlight novel strategies and active areas of research that are being pursued for CNS delivery.

Natural Transport Pathways

Several endogenous pathways exist in the BBB that can be used for the transport of drugs or drug carriers across the BBB. These include paracellular (aqueous) diffusion, transcellular (lipophilic), diffusion, adsorptive-mediated transcytosis (AMT), carrier-mediated transcytosis, active-efflux transport, and receptor-mediated transcytosis. There are several advantages of systemic administration of a drug via these endogenous transport pathways, primarily because they do not require invasive approaches and surgery.

Paracellular (Aqueous) Diffusion

Paracellular (aqueous) diffusion is a nonsaturable and noncompetitive transport mechanism for diffusion of substances between the cells. Due to the presence of tight junctions, this does not occur very readily in the brain except for small water-soluble molecules that can diffuse through the BBB. Transient opening of the BBB to allow for paracellular transport of drugs has been an actively pursued strategy for overcoming the BBB. For example, siRNAs that target claudin-5, a tight junction protein of the BBB, were injected in mice and a decrease in claudin-5 mRNA levels was observed for 24 to 48 hours after injection.[42] The BBB of mice injected with siRNAs showed enhanced uptake of molecules of up to 742 Da, but not 4400 Da. A 360-Da small neuropeptide thyrotropin-releasing hormone (TRH), when administered using this strategy, showed significant modifications in behavior in mice.[42] Other agents that have been studied for transient BBB opening in recent years are alkylglycerol,[43] sodium caprate,[44] and focused ultrasound using microbubbles.[45,46]

Transcellular (Lipophilic) Diffusion

Transcellular (lipophilic) diffusion is also a nonsaturable and noncompetitive mechanism; however, the higher the lipophilicity, the higher the diffusion, as long as the molecular weight of the substance is less than 450 Da. Hydrogen bonding is another factor that affects transcellular diffusion. This is essentially similar to the prodrug approach, of which there are clinically approved examples that have been reviewed earlier in this chapter. A recent example of success using this strategy in ongoing research is naproxen for the prevention and treatment of Alzheimer's disease. Naproxen has seen only limited clinical success due to poor brain distribution. Zhang et al.[47] reported a study in 2012 where they explored various prodrug designs with different chemical linkages (ester or amido bond) for naproxen. The release of naproxen from the prodrug was studied *in vitro* as well as *in vivo*. The *in vivo* results in rats demonstrated that prodrugs with ester bonds had higher brain concentrations (28.81 and 24.51% higher than control) than those with amide bonds (15.54% higher than control).

Adsorptive-Mediated Transcytosis

Adsorptive-mediated transcytosis (AMT) is the result of electrostatic, charge-based interactions between a positively charged substance (e.g., a peptide) and the negatively charged plasma membrane.[48] AMT allows for uptake of charged molecules at the apical side of the BBB and release at the basolateral side. Factors that mainly influence adsorptive-mediated transport are particle size and surface charge. One of the initial vectors used for delivery across the BBB was cationized albumin via the AMT pathway. Cationized proteins and cell-penetrating peptides (CPPs), such as Tat-derived peptides and Syn-B vectors, have been demonstrated to cross the BBB via the AMT pathway.[49] Recently, Liu and coworkers[50] successfully conjugated tanshinone IIA PEGylated nanoparticles to cationic bovine serum albumin and evaluated their efficacy in a rat model of cerebral ischemia. Tanshinone IIA is a classic example of a drug that is a potential candidate for a brain disease (in this case, cerebral ischemia) but has poor BBB penetration and a short half-life. The formulation significantly increases the half-life of the drug, showed better brain distribution and uptake, and had neuroprotective effects. However, AMT is a low-affinity interaction and does not constitute a specific interaction for transport; rather, it relies on general electrostatic interactions. In addition to that, toxicity, immunogenicity, and the relative instability of CPPs in biological fluids is another limitation of this strategy.[49] Further, the process of cationization (e.g., via conversion of carboxyls on a protein to primary amino groups) can adversely affect the bioactivity and binding affinity of large therapeutics such as antibodies.[51]

Carrier-Mediated Transcytosis

The carrier-mediated transcytosis (CMT) pathway is utilized by small molecules such as lactic acid, neutral amino acids (phenylalanine), basic amino acids (arginine), quaternary ammonium molecules (choline), and purine nucleosides (adenosine).[52] Other CMT genes help in the transport of water-soluble vitamins, thyroid hormones, and other compounds. All transporters in the CMT system are highly stereospecific and require specific structures for transporter affinity. L-Dopa is an example of a prodrug that crosses the BBB via CMT. However, to design drugs that mimic the structure of a pseudo-nutrient and can undergo transport across the BBB via CMT is quite a challenge. Prodrugs that exploit the CMT process are currently being actively pursued by Xenoport, a company that designs small molecule drugs and markets them as transported prodrugs. These prodrugs target members of the solute carrier (SLC) transporter family in the BBB and intestine; however, all Xenoport drugs currently in various clinical stages are meant for intestinal transport.

Active Efflux Transport

Active efflux transport is comprised of active efflux transporters at the BBB such as P-glycoproteins (Pgps), multidrug resistance protein (MRP), and breast cancer resistance protein 1 (Bcrp1) transporters that are involved in the efflux of molecules from brain to blood direction. A majority of drugs end up as substrates for these efflux pumps and hence cannot cross the BBB. Inhibition or modulation of active efflux transporters has been a strategy that has been explored for BBB delivery.[53] For example, Minocha et al.[54] have demonstrated the enhanced brain uptake (up to an approximately fivefold increase) of pazopanib when administered with the Pgp and Bcrp1 inhibitor elacridar. Pazopanib by itself is a substrate for both Pgp and Bcrp1.

Receptor-Mediated Transcytosis

Receptor-mediated transcytosis (RMT) is another pathway for delivery of nutrients to the brain, whereby serum proteins in systemic circulation such as transferrin, insulin, leptin, LRP1, and LRP2 bind specifically to their receptors present on the endothelial cell surface of brain microcapillary vasculature to enter the brain. This pathway has gained much attention for BBB delivery, and a longer discussion is warranted because novel RMT drug delivery strategies that are currently under development have shown immense promise. Generally, a systemically administered drug distributes evenly throughout all tissues of the body, lacks site specificity for the target, and has toxic side effects in several cases. An even biodistribution across the entire body reduces the efficacy of the drug at the target site, requiring higher dosages that can be potentially toxic or induce side effects. In an attempt to circumvent these challenges, researchers have demonstrated that target- and site-specific strategies such as receptor-mediated, polymer- and liposome-based delivery of drugs can be targeted toward specific receptors or cells, thereby enhancing the therapeutic efficacy of these drugs while minimizing the side effects on healthy cells. In the context of the BBB, proteins that are overexpressed on the endothelial cells of the brain could form potential targets for such a strategy. The use of naturally occurring proteins as drug delivery mediators or carriers is steadily increasing because the biodegradability, toxicity, and immunogenicity of these proteins are not an issue as compared to other polymer and particle based systems.[5]

One of the earliest works targeting endogenous receptor-mediated pathways for drug delivery to the brain was performed by designing molecular Trojan horses (MTHs). MTHs are peptide or protein ligands or monoclonal antibodies (mAbs) that target RMT systems.[55] When fused with a BBB-impermeable neurotherapeutic, MTHs enable the neurotherapeutic to overcome the BBB. Monoclonal antibodies (mAbs) have been designed against endothelial cell surface receptors such as the transferrin receptor or insulin receptor. OX26, a murine mAb to the rat transferrin receptor (TfR), has been used to deliver peptides, antisense pharmaceutical agents, and PEGylated liposomes to the brain.[6] OX26 has shown fourfold greater BBB permeability as compared to cationized albumin. Various conjugates of OX26 such as biotinylated basic fibroblast growth factor (bFGF) and peptide nucleic acids (PNAs) have also been shown to enter the brain.[7,8] Another mAb that has been actively pursued for RMT is 83-14 murine mAb to the human insulin receptor (HIR).[9] Coloma et al.[9,10] have genetically engineered it to form a chimeric antibody and replace the immunogenic murine sequences with human antibody sequence. When injected in rhesus monkey, this humanized antibody shows robust uptake after 2 hours in the living primate brain. Liu et al. have worked on designing a 30-amino-acid peptide (leptin30) that is derived from the hormone leptin and can enter the brain via binding to leptin receptors expressed on brain capillary endothelial cells. Dendigraft poly-L-lysine (DGL), comprised of dendrons of polylysine, was complexed to leptin30 in this study and used as a nonviral gene vector that showed cellular uptake due to leptin30-mediated receptor endocytosis.[11] Similarly, Tamaru and coworkers[56] have shown that a leptin-derived peptide (Lep70-89) acts as a ligand for mouse brain-derived endothelial cells and causes increased cellular uptake of PEG liposomes (PEG-LPs) conjugated to Lep70-89 as compared to unmodified PEG-LPs. This provides further evidence for the strategy that specific receptor-mediated transport mechanisms do in fact increase uptake of conjugated drugs and liposomes into the brain.[12]

Several MTHs have entered various phases of clinical trials. AGT-120 is a lead product from Armagen in the pre-investigational new drug (IND) stage and is being developed for treatment of stroke and neurodegenerative diseases. AGT-120 is a fusion between a brain-derived neurotrophic factor and a mAb against the human transferrin receptor. Another product from Armagen is AGT-181, which is a fusion of the IDUA (α-L-iduronidase) enzyme and a mAb against human insulin receptor. AGT-181 is meant as a therapeutic for the lysosomal storage disease Hurler's syndrome. The therapeutic 2B3-101, against Japanese encephalitis virus (JEV), is currently being developed by to-BBB and is based on CRM197, a nontoxic mimic of the diphtheria toxin. It binds to the diphtheria toxin receptor (DTR) expressed on brain capillaries, neurons, and glial cells in the brain. Yet another example of a MTH is the CORVUS peptide for delivery of siRNAs to the brain is currently in the research stage at the Immune Disease Institute of Harvard Medical School. It is a fusion between a 29-amino-acid peptide from rabies virus glycoprotein and the 9-amino-acid repeat unit of D-arginine, where the latter binds negatively charged siRNAs. Angiochem is developing peptide vectors for various brain diseases. An example of such a peptide vector is ANG4043, conjugated to anti-HER2 antibody, for the treatment of brain tumors. ANG4043 has been shown to reach the brain and target HER2-positive tumors, induce brain tumor shrinkage, and increase survival in mice that have undergone implantation with HER2-positive tumor cells. Another example is ANG1005 (in Phase I clinical trials), which makes use of the low-density lipoprotein receptor-related protein pathway for the delivery of taxane to brain tumors. A third product, ANG2002, a conjugate of Angipep-2 peptide and neurotensin, is currently being tested for its analgesic potential in preclinical studies.

In general, conjugation and fusion of neuroprotective agents and drugs to mAbs, proteins, and peptides against cell surface receptors have been an actively pursued idea. There are many review articles focusing specifically on each of the endogenous transport pathways for BBB delivery, especially the RMT pathway (due to its target specificity). Yu et al.[57] have developed monoclonal antibodies against the TfR and demonstrated that reducing the affinity of the mAb for TfR leads to their increased TfR-mediated transcytosis and brain uptake.

Other Strategies

Further discussion in this section will focus on some very recent progress made over the past few years in the general area of BBB drug delivery through some specific examples. Recently, Haqqani et al.[58] evaluated single-domain antibodies (VHHs), FC5 and FC44, for their BBB permeability. FC5 and FC44, due to their enhanced transport (50- to 100-fold) across *in vitro* rat brain endothelium as compared to control VHHs, can be used as carriers for drug delivery across the BBB. Fu et al.[59] have demonstrated the potential of a 39-amino-acid rabies virus glycoprotein-derived peptide as a carrier for delivery of three proteins of different molecular weights and pI: β-galactosidase, luciferase, and brain-derived neurotrophic factor (BDNF). Peptide vectors have long been shown to have immense potential in improving drug delivery across the BBB. To this end, Li et al.[60] carried out *in vivo* phage display to identify peptide sequences that bind to specifically to brain vascular receptors. Mice brain parenchyma was administered with a 7-mer peptide phage library intravenously. Thereafter, phages recovered from the brain parenchyma were isolated and sequenced. A particular peptide PepC7 with a cyclic conformation showed 41-fold higher brain localization as compared to native M13 phage.

Vector-Mediated Delivery

Viral Vectors

Central nervous system-targeted gene therapy aims at delivering genetic material (encoding proteins or siRNA/shRNA) into cells within the brain, with the potential for long-term treatment effects. Such genes are typically excluded from crossing the BBB via transcellular and paracellular transport due to being hydrophilic, charged, and of large molecular size. However, genes offer the benefit of a long-term therapeutic benefit following a single administration, as has been demonstrated in animal models.[13] The delivery of genes into the brain has been facilitated through the development of specialized viruses. Viruses have been employed as a biological vector system to shuttle genetic material into brain cells. The most common viral vectors employed are adeno-associated viral vectors and lentiviral vectors.[13] On their own, viruses are not readily able to cross the BBB after intravenous infusion and therefore must be injected directly into the brain. Once in the brain, viral vectors vary in their cell tropism or the affinity toward various brain cells. Such variation is crucial for the transduction of diseased tissue with minimal cross-induction of non-diseased tissues, as many neurological diseases result in the malfunction of a specific CNS compartment or tissue. Additionally, there exists a variety of brain-selective promoters, including the myelin basic protein (MBP) promoter, neuron-specific enolase (NSE) promoter, platelet-derived growth factor-β (PDGB-β) promoter, glial fibrillary acid protein (GFAP) promoter, and a number of synthetic promoters permitting selectivity within the gene itself.[13] The combination of the varied brain tissue tropism with brain-selective promoters affords increased control of the gene expression.[13]

Adeno-associated virus (AAV) is a member of the genus *Dependovirus*. Such viruses are non-autonomous, requiring a coinfected helper virus in order to replicate, and are non-pathogenic.[61] Such properties of AAV greatly reduce the risk for side effects, including immune response. The AAV virion consists of a protein shell known as a capsid which contains the viral genomic payload, is ~20 nm in size, and is restricted to contain a gene vector no greater than 4.7 kb in size.[61] Proteins of the capsid facilitate the binding of the virus to cell surface receptors. These proteins vary in their expression among the different serotypes of the virus. The predominant serotype employed in clinical applications is AAV2, which targets heparin sulfate as its primary receptor. The serotypes of AAV transduce a variety of cell types within the CNS. The majority of serotypes transduce neurons with high efficiency, where as a subset of them are able to selectively transduce astrocytes, glial, and ependymal cells. One capsid of

AAV serotype 9 (AAV9) has shown the ability to cross the BBB and transduce neurons.[61] In murine models, AAV has been shown to persist for greater than 6 months.[61] Of the ~35 AVV vectors, AAV2 is the predominant vector used to target neurological diseases. As of 2011, AAV2 accounted for 76% of therapy trials in the CNS aimed at treating Alzheimer's disease, Parkinson's disease, amyotrophic lateral sclerosis (ALS), epilepsy, and Batten disease. Currently, work is being done to expand this list to include other CNS diseases through the use of synthetic vectors having increased transduction efficiency and specificity coupled with unique tissue tropism.[61] AAV remains the preferred viral vector system for shuttling genetic material into the CNS as it is able to effectively provide a long-term, efficient gene transfer with low immunogenicity and pathogenicity.

A major downside to viral vectors is their limited ability for global brain transduction. Because viral vectors enter cells through receptor-mediated endocytosis, transduction mainly occurs at the site of injection or infusion. Such a global transduction is desired to treat diseases that arise from single gene mutations, such as lysosomal storage disorders and leukodystrophies. Strategies to enhance global neurotropism include the incorporation of peptides that mimic binding domains for cytoplasmic dynein or N-methyl-D-aspartate (NMDA) receptors into the viral vectors. Additional vector strategies are aimed at expressing brain-derived neurotrophic factor (BNDF) and glial cell-derived neurotrophic factor (GNDF) as capsid proteins to broaden the vector's transduction and increase its tissue specificity.[13]

In addition to AAV, various other viral vector therapies are also in development for CNS treatment, including a retrovirus currently being developed for use with Huntington's disease and lysosomal storage disease and a herpesvirus for Parkinson's disease and potentially anti-cancer therapy.

Stem Cells

Cell-Transplantation/Injection-Based Therapies

Cell-based therapies have shown significant promises for a variety of diseases in animal models, including Parkinson's disease, epilepsy, stroke, and spinal cord injury.[62] Administration of cells into the CNS, however, remains a major obstacle. The current widely employed delivery strategy for cell transplantation into the CNS is through the use of a stereotactically inserted straight cannula.[62] Such procedures have been successfully demonstrated in small rodent models, but the human brain is approximately 2000 times larger than the brain of a mouse. Such differences in scale raise significant issues in cell transplantation via single straight cannula injection. To overcome low volume limitations due to a single injection, a multiple injection array template was developed by which multiple injections were made along the template. However, such a strategy poses the issue of penetrating the brain parenchyma multiple times, increasing the risk of intracranial hemorrhage. Other attempts, such as increasing the number of cells delivered at a single injection site, significantly decrease cell graft viability due to the limited nutrient and oxygen diffusion into the large cell mass. In addition to the negative effects the injection causes on the implanted cells, there is also damage caused to the tissue localized around the injection site. With larger injected volumes these is also the increased risk of reflux of the infusate up the penetration tract.

A strategy developed by Potts and colleagues[62] overcomes many of these issues by using a modular cannula coupled with radially branched deployable (RBD) catheters. Their RBD device is able to transplant cells in a 4-cm^3 volume from the site of penetration. For delivery of cells to a large volumetric space within the brain, such as the putamen, transplant via the RBD system has proven to be an excellent option over single cannula delivery. An additional benefit of the RBD device is that no complications of hemorrhage were noted during injection into swine brains. It is important to note that, although the RBD device does make significant improvements over conventional straight cannula injection, there are still improvements that must be made for the large-scale transplanted cell distributions to recreate those exhibited in animal models.

Intranasal Stem Cell Delivery

Adult neural stem cells (aNSCs) are multipotent stem cells located in the ependymal cell layers of the adult brain. aNSCs have demonstrated efficacy for a variety of neuro-degenerative diseases in animal models. For example, aNSCs differentiated into olgio-dendrocytes have been shown to repair injured myelin tissue and reduce inflammatory lesions in experimental autoimmune encephalomyelitis (EAE) mice. Another example of the benefits of stems cells comes from a clinical trial of patients with secondary progressive multiple sclerosis (MS) and impaired visual pathways. The patients showed improvement after being treated with post-mesenchymal stem cells (MSCs).[63] Although the precise mechanism behind NSC therapy has yet to be understood, the benefits are evident in a variety of diseases.

Intracranial delivery of aNSCs is frequently used in animal studies, but a less invasive strategy is preferred for clinical applications. Intravenous delivery of aNSCs yields widespread systemic distribution, as well as retention of NSCs in lungs, liver, and spleen. Additionally, intravenous injection of aNSCs does not permit CNS penetration due to BBB restriction. Intranasal delivery of NSCs overcomes the restrictions of the BBB, while affording a more non-invasive delivery into the CNS than intracranial injection.[63] Additionally, intranasal delivery typically does not manifest systemic immune response outside of the CNS. Intranasal delivery of NSCs in mice models demonstrated localization of fluorescently labeled aNSCs in the olfactory bulb, cortex, and spinal cord. Intranasal delivery also yielded earlier functional recovery, as well as anti-inflammatory and remyleination as compared to intravenously injected NSCs in EAE mice.[63] Although the route that the cells take into the CNS during nasal delivery has not been fully elucidated, intranasal delivery of stems cells affords a non-invasive transplantation of stems cells, with the potential to treat a variety of neurological disorders.

CNS Targeting Using Nanomaterials

Nanocarriers provide an attractive platform for developing drug-delivery strategies for brain disorders, especially, in developing formulations of drugs that cannot themselves cross the BBB. These are typically 1 to 300 nm in size and loaded with a therapeutically active agent.[64] Examples of different types of nanocarriers are polymeric or solid lipid nanoparticles, lipid or albumin nanocapsules, liposomes and micelles, dendrimers, nanovesicles, nanogels, nano-emulsions, and nanosuspensions.[14,65] Several materials, such as polymers, lipids, ceramics, and carbon nanotubes, have been explored for nanocarrier synthesis. Typically, nanocarriers are made out of biocompatible polymers because these provide the most favorable characteristics for BBB delivery such as safety, high stability, ability to load many therapeutic agents, control of release kinetics, and ease of chemical modifications.[64] Several mechanisms have been proposed for the uptake of nanoparticles at the BBB. These include caveolae-mediated endocytosis, clathrin-mediated endocytosis, and clathrin- and caveolin-independent endocytosis.[65]

Recent literature is replete with examples of novel research conducted in the area of nanocarriers for BBB delivery. There are several excellent review articles focusing on the role of nanotechnology in overcoming the BBB and enabling CNS drug delivery.[66–71] Wohlfart et al.[71] recently published a review on BBB transport of drugs using nanoparticles. The drugs reported in the literature to cross the BBB using nanoparticles include aclarubicin, campthotecin, dalargin, dexamethasone, doxorubicin, etoposide, gemcitabine, kyotorphin, loperamide, methotrexate, NGF, obidoxime, riluzole, rivastigimine, saquinavir, sulpride, tacrine, temozolomide, tubocurarine, valproic acid, vasoactive intestinal peptide, and vascular endothelial growth factor (VEGF) antisense oligonucleotide.[71] Of these, several (such as doxorubicin) are unable to cross the BBB on their own. Nazem and Mansoori[72] have published a review of nanotechnological interventions, diagnostic as well as therapeutic, specifically for Alzheimer's disease.

Nanocarriers can also be combined with approaches such as CED to further enhance their brain uptake.[24] When combined with CED, nanocarriers can not only effectively deliver a therapeutic agent loaded onto them but also serve as tracers to continuously monitor the progress of infusion via CED.[24] Allard et al.[24] reviewed nanocarrier labeling, physicochemical properties, and survival studies from clinical trials involving nanocarriers and CED. Several CED nanocarriers involving liposomes, dendrimers, and nanoparticles are currently in preclinical and clinical studies. Mark Saltzman's group at Yale University has developed brain-penetrating nanoparticles loaded with FDA-approved agents that inhibit self-renewal and proliferation of brain cancer stem cells (BCSCs) for the treatment of glioblastoma multiforme. These particles were administered via CED to large intracranial volumes in rats and pigs. Specifically, dithiazanine iodide-loaded particles significantly increased survival in rats bearing BCSC-derived xenografts.[30] Mark E. Davis' group[73] recently demonstrated that BBB delivery of nanoparticles decorated with transferrin (Tf) can be aided by modulating avidity of nanoparticles to the transferrin receptor (TfR). Their results show that nanoparticles with large amounts of Tf remain attached to brain endothelial cells, whereas those with relatively lesser Tf can detach and transcytose from blood to the brain side of the BBB. NanoDel, a German company, is currently developing nanoparticles for targeting the brain, retina, and spinal cord.[74]

Central nervous system nanomedicine is still in its very early stages, and several technical issues need to be addressed before it can translate to a clinical setting.[14] For success in BBB delivery, nanocarriers must be less than 100 nm in size, nontoxic, biodegradable, blood stable, and noninflammatory; they must have prolonged circulation time and a low propensity for inducing platelet aggregation; they must be able to carry small molecules, peptides, proteins, and nucleic acids; and they must offer controlled release delivery.[14]

CONCLUSION

The discussion above reviews the needs, challenges, and opportunities in pharmaceutical development in the central nervous system area. As noted, many promising strategies both for drug development and drug delivery are under development. The clinical success of these strategies will be decided by the balance between their efficacy and safety in humans. Success in developing efficient and clinically relevant drug delivery strategies have the potential to provide a new lease on drugs that have been dropped from further clinical development due to poor brain penetration. Whether this materializes or not, it is clear that there needs to be a better emphasis on drug delivery challenges earlier in the CNS drug development process, making drug development and delivery a parallel challenge rather than a sequential challenge as is the norm. An orthogonal development, not explicitly discussed in this review, entails the design of representative *in vitro/vivo* models to test the preclinical validity of these various approaches. This in itself is an exciting field that is fueled by an improved understanding of the genetic and molecular understanding of the etiology and pathogenesis of the neurological diseases. We close with acknowledging the confluence of many multifaceted, creative, and impactful advances in this field that will undoubtedly prepare us to address the rising challenges of neurological disorders and neurodegenerative diseases unique to our generation.

References

1. WHO. *Global Burden of Diseases*. Geneva, Switzerland: World Health Organisation; 2008.
2. WHO. *Global Burden of Neurological Disorders: Estimates and Projections*. Geneva, Switzerland: World Health Organisation; 2006.
3. IMS. *The Global Use of Medicines: Outlook Through 2016*. Danbury, CT: IMS Institute for Healthcare Informatics; 2012. pp. 1–36 (www.theimsinstitute.org).
4. Paul SM, Mytelka DS, Dunwiddie CT, Persinger CC, Munos BH, Lindborg SR, Schacht AL. How to improve R&D productivity: the pharmaceutical industry's grand challenge. Nat. Rev. Drug Discov. 2010;9:203–14.
5. Lundbeck. *Annual Report 2009*. Valby, Denmark: H. Lundbeck A/S; 2010. pp. 1–116 (www.lundbeck.com).
6. Kola I, Landis J. Opinion: can the pharmaceutical industry reduce attrition rates? Nat. Rev. Drug Discov. 2004;3:711–6.
7. Pardridge WM. The blood–brain barrier: bottleneck in brain drug development. NeuroRx 2005;2:3–14.
8. Alavijeh MS, Chishty M, Qaiser MZ, Palmer AM. Drug metabolism and pharmacokinetics, the blood–brain barrier, and central nervous system drug discovery. NeuroRx 2005;2:554.
9. Abbott NJ, Rönnbäck L, Hansson E. Astrocyte-endothelial interactions at the blood–brain barrier. Nat. Rev. Neurosci. 2006;7:41–53.
10. Pardridge WM. Drug and gene delivery to the brain: the vascular route. Neuron 2002;36:555–8.
11. Nitta T, Hata M, Gotoh S, Seo Y, Sasaki H, Hashimoto N, Furuse M, Tsukita S. Size-selective loosening of the blood–brain barrier in claudin-5-deficient mice. J. Cell Biol. 2003;161:653–60.
12. Abbott NJ, Patabendige AK, Dolman DEM, Yusof SR, Begley DJ. Structure and function of the blood–brain barrier. Neurobiol. Dis. 2010;37:13–25.
13. De Boer AG, Gaillard PJ. Drug targeting to the brain. Annu. Rev. Pharmacol. Toxicol. 2007;47:323–55.
14. Siegal T. Which drug or drug delivery system can change clinical practice for brain tumor therapy? Neuro. Oncol. 2013;15:656–69.
15. INI. *Ischemic Stroke Treatment*. Peoria: Illinois Neurological Institute; 2014. (http://www.ini.org/services/stroke/treatments/ischemic-stroke.html).
16. Alzheimer's Association. *What We Know Today About Alzheimer's Disease*. Chicago, IL: Alzheimer's Association; 2014. (http://www.alz.org/research/science/alzheimers_disease_treatments.asp).

17. www.centerwatch.com.
18. Anon. *FDA Approves Gablofen*. Drugs.com, 2012. (http://www.drugs.com/newdrugs/fda-approves-movement-disorder-cns-therapeutics-gablofen-baclofen-severe-spasticity-2435.html).
19. Datamonitor Healthcare. *CNS Catalysts in 2013* (white paper), February 12, 2013 (http://www.datamonitor healthcare.com/cns-catalysts-in-2013/).
20. MedicineNet.com. *Levodopa-Carbidopa, Sinemet, Sinemet CR, Parc*opa, 2014 (http://www.medicinenet.com/levodopa-carbidopa/article.htm).
21. Cook AM, Mieure KD, Owen RD, Pesaturo AB, Hatton J. Intracerebroventricular administration of drugs. Pharmacotherapy 2009;29:832–45.
22. Gabayan AJ, et al. GliaSite brachytherapy for treatment of recurrent malignant gliomas: a retrospective multi-institutional analysis. Neurosurgery 2006;58:701–9.
23. Hayek SM, Deer TR, Pope JE, Panchal SJ, Patel VB. Intrathecal therapy for cancer and non-cancer pain. Pain Physician 2011;14:219–48.
24. Allard E, Passirani C, Benoit J-P. Convection-enhanced delivery of nanocarriers for the treatment of brain tumors. Biomaterials 2009;30:2302–18.
25. Brem H, Gabikian P. Biodegradable polymer implants to treat brain tumors. J. Control. Release 2001;74:63–7.
26. Brem H, Plantadosi S, Burger PC, Walker M, Selker R, Vick NA, Black K, Sisti M, Brem S, Mohr G, et al. Placebo-controlled trial of safety and efficacy of intraoperative controlled delivery by biodegradable polymers of chemo-therapy for recurrent gliomas. The Polymer-brain Tumor Treatment Group. Lancet 1995;345:1008–12.
27. Benoit JP, Faisant N, Venier-Julienne MC, Menei P. Development of microspheres for neurological disorders: from basics to clinical applications. J. Control. Release 2000;65:285–96.
28. Roullin VG, Deverre JR, Lemaire L, Hindré F, Venier-Julienne MC, Vienet R, Benoit JP. Anti-cancer drug diffusion within living rat brain tissue: an experimental study using [^{3}H](6)-5-fluorouracil-loaded PLGA microspheres. Eur. J. Pharm. Biopharm. 2002;53:293–9.
29. Pathan SA, Iqbal Z, Zeidi SM, Talegaonkar S, Vohra D, Jain GK, Azeem A, Jain N, Lalani JR, Khar RK, Ahmad FJ. CNS drug delivery systems: novel approaches. Recent Pat. Drug Deliv. Formul. 2009;3:71–89.
30. Zhou J, Patel TR, Sirianni RW, Strohbehn G, Zheng M-Q, et al. Highly penetrative, drug-loaded nanocarriers improve treatment of glioblastoma. Proc. Natl. Acad. Sci. U.S.A. 2013;110:11751–6.
31. BrainMetsBC.org. *Current Treatments for Brain Metasta*ses, 2014 (http://www.brainmetsbc.org/content/current-treatments-brain-metastases).
32. Khan AJ, Dicker AP. On the merits and limitations of whole-brain radiation therapy. J. Clin. Oncol. 2013;31:11–3.
33. Kondziolka D, Flickinger JC, Lunsford LD. Radiosurgery for brain metastases. Prog. Neurol. Surg. 2012;25:115–22.
34. Volkmann J. Deep brain stimulation for the treatment of Parkinson's disease. J. Clin. Neurophysiol. 2004;21:6–17.
35. Duke Medicine. The Brain Electric: Deep Brain Stimulation for Neurologic Disorders. Durham, NC: Duke University Health System; 2014. (http://www.dukehealth.org/health_library/health_articles/the-brain-electric).
36. Suthana N, Fried I. Deep brain stimulation for enhancement of learning and memory. Neuroimage 2013; 85(Pt. 3):996–1002.
37. Bidros DS, Liu JK, Vogelbaum MA. Future of convection-enhanced delivery in the treatment of brain tumors. Future Oncol. 2010;6:117–25.
38. Integra. Integra NeuroSciences announces FDA clearance to market a tunneled catheter for the LICOX brain tissue oxygen monitoring system; product launch to begin in second quarter (press release), April 9, 2002 (http://investor.integralife.com/releasedetail.cfm?ReleaseID=235074).
39. U.S. Food and Drug Administration, www.fda.gov.
40. Pavan B, Dalpiaz A. Prodrugs and endogenous transporters: are they suitable tools for drug targeting into the central nervous system? Curr. Pharm. Des. 2011;17:3560–76.
41. Bodor, N.S. Brain-Specific Drug Delivery, U.S. Patent No. 4540564, 1985 (http://www.patentstorm.us/patents/4540564.html).
42. Campbell M, Klang AS, Kenna PF, Kerskens C, Blau C, O'Dwyer L, Tivnan A, Kelly JA, Brankin B, Farrar GJ, Humphries P. RNAi-mediated reversible opening of the blood–brain barrier. J. Gene Med. 2008;10:930–47.
43. Erdlenbruch B, Alipour M, Fricker G, Miller DS, Kugler W, Eibl H, Lakomek M. Alkylglycerol opening of the blood–brain barrier to small and large fluorescence markers in normal and C6 glioma-bearing rats and isolated rat brain capillaries. Br. J. Pharmacol. 2003;140:1201–10.

44. Preston E, Slinn J, Vinokourov I, Stanimirovic D. Graded reversible opening of the rat blood–brain barrier by intracarotid infusion of sodium caprate. J. Neurosci. Methods 2008;168:443–9.

45. Sheikov N, McDannold N, Vykhodtseva N, Jolesz F, Hynynen K. Cellular mechanisms of the blood–brain barrier opening induced by ultrasound in presence of microbubbles. Ultrasound Med. Biol. 2004;30: 979–89.

46. Wang F, Cheng Y, Mei J, Song Y, Yang YQ, Liu Y, Wang Z. Focused ultrasound microbubble destruction-mediated changes in blood–brain barrier permeability assessed by contrast-enhanced magnetic resonance imaging. J. Ultrasound Med. 2009;28:1501–9.

47. Zhang Q, Liang Z, Chen LY, Sun X, Gong T, Zhang ZR. Novel brain targeting prodrugs of naproxen based on dimethylamino group with various linkages. Arzneimittelforschung 2012;62:261–6.

48. Lu W. Adsorptive-mediated brain delivery systems. Curr. Pharm. Biotechnol. 2012;13:2340–8.

49. Hervé F, Ghinea N, Scherrmann J-M. CNS delivery via adsorptive transcytosis. AAPS J. 2008;10:455–72.

50. Liu X, An C, Jin P, Liu X, Wang L. Protective effects of cationic bovine serum albumin-conjugated PEGylated tanshinone IIA nanoparticles on cerebral ischemia. Biomaterials 2013;34:817–30.

51. Hervé F, Ouzilou-Girod J, Scherrmann JM. Cationization, a process for the delivery of antibodies to the central nervous system. Problems encountered in its application for immunotherapy strategies such as those for clostridial poisoning. J. Soc. Biol. 2001;195:201–27.

52. Tsuji A, Tamai I. Carrier-mediated or specialized transport of drugs across the blood–brain barrier. Adv. Drug Deliv. Rev. 1999;36:277–90.

53. Minocha M, Khurana V, Qin B, Pal D, Mitra AK. Co-administration strategy to enhance brain accumulation of vandetanib by modulating P-glycoprotein (P-gp/Abcb1) and breast cancer resistance protein (Bcrp1/Abcg2) mediated efflux with m-TOR inhibitors. Int. J. Pharm. 2012;434:306–14.

54. Minocha M, Khurana V, Qin B, Pal D, Mitra AK. Enhanced brain accumulation of pazopanib by modulating P-gp and Bcrp1 mediated efflux with canertinib or erlotinib. Int. J. Pharm. 2012;436:127–34.

55. Pardridge WM, Boado RJ. Reengineering biopharmaceuticals for targeted delivery across the blood–brain barrier. Methods Enzymol. 2012;503:269–92.

56. Tamaru M, Akita H, Fujiwara T, Kajimoto K, Harashima H. Leptin-derived peptide, a targeting ligand for mouse brain-derived endothelial cells via macropinocytosis. Biochem. Biophys. Res. Commun. 2010;394(3): 587–592.

57. Yu YJ, Zhang Y, Kenrick M, Hoyte K, Luk W, Lu Y, Atwal J, Elliott JM, Prabhu S, Watts JJ, Dennis MS. Boosting brain uptake of a therapeutic antibody by reducing its affinity for a transcytosis target. Sci. Transl. Med. 2011;3:84ra44.

58. Haqqani AS, Caram-Salas N, Ding W, Brunette E, Delaney CE, Baumann E, Boileau E, Stanimirovic D. Multiplexed evaluation of serum and CSF pharmacokinetics of brain-targeting single-domain antibodies using a NanoLC-SRM-ILIS method. Mol. Pharm. 2013;10:1542–56.

59. Fu A, Wang Y, Zhan L, Zhou R. Targeted delivery of proteins into the central nervous system mediated by rabies virus glycoprotein-derived peptide. Pharm. Res. 2012;29:1562–9.

70. Li J, Zhang Q, Pang Z, Wang Y, Liu Q, Guo L, Liang X. Identification of peptide sequences that target to the brain using in vivo phage display. Amino Acids 2012;2:2373–81.

61. Lentz TB, Gray SJ, Samulski RJ. Viral vectors for gene delivery to the central nervous system. Neurobiol. Dis. 2012;48:179–88.

62. Potts MB, Silvestrini MT, Lim DA. Devices for cell transplantation into the central nervous system: design considerations and emerging technologies. Surg. Neurol. Int. 2013;4:S22–30.

63. Wu S, Li K, Yan Y, Gran B, Han Y, Zhou F, Guan YT, Rostami A, Zhang GX. Intranasal delivery of neural stem cells: a CNS-specific, non-invasive cell-based therapy for experimental autoimmune encephalomyelitis. J. Clin. Cell. Immunol. 2013;4(3).

64. Patel T, Zhou J, Piepmeier JM, Saltzman WM. Polymeric nanoparticles for drug delivery to the central nervous system. Adv. Drug Deliv. Rev. 2012;64:701–5.

65. Fernandes C, Soni U, Patravale V. Nano-interventions for neurodegenerative disorders. Pharmacol. Res. 2010;62:166–78.

66. Biddlestone-Thorpe L, Marchi N, Guo K, Ghosh C, Janigro D, Valerie K, Yang H. Nanomaterial-mediated CNS delivery of diagnostic and therapeutic agents. Adv. Drug Deliv. Rev. 2012;64:605–13.

67. Tosi G, Bortot B, Ruozi B, Dolcetta D, Vandelli MA, Forni F, Severini GM. Potential use of polymeric nanoparticles for drug delivery across the blood–brain barrier. Curr. Med. Chem. 2013;20:2212–25.

I. NOVEL THERAPEUTIC APPROACHES

68. Caraglia M, De Rosa G, Salzano G, Santini D, Lamberti M, Sperlongano P, Lombardi A, Abbruzzese A, Addeo R. Nanotech revolution for the anti-cancer drug delivery through blood–brain barrier. Curr. Cancer Drug Targets 2012;12:186–96.

69. De Rosa G, Salzano G, Caraglia M, Abbruzzese A. Nanotechnologies: a strategy to overcome blood–brain barrier. Curr. Drug Metab. 2012;13:61–9.

70. Kanwar JR, Sun X, Punj V, Sriramoju B, Mohan RR, et al. Nanoparticles in the treatment and diagnosis of neurological disorders: untamed dragon with fire power to heal. Nanomedicine 2012;8:399–414.

71. Wohlfart S, Gelperina S, Kreuter J. Transport of drugs across the blood–brain barrier by nanoparticles. J. Control. Release 2012;161:264–73.

72. Nazem A, Mansoori GA. Nanotechnology solutions for Alzheimer's disease: advances in research tools, diagnostic methods and therapeutic agents. J. Alzheimers Dis. 2008;13:199–223.

73. Wiley DT, Webster P, Gale A, Davis ME. Transcytosis and brain uptake of transferrin-containing nanoparticles by tuning avidity to transferrin receptor. Proc. Natl. Acad. Sci. U.S.A. 2013;110:8662–7.

74. Karanth H, Murthy RSR. Nanotechnology in brain targeting. Int. J. Pharm. Sci. Nanotechnol. 2008;1:9–24.

Trends in Nonparenteral Delivery of Biologics, Vaccines and Cancer Therapies

Martin J. D'Souza[1], Rikhav P. Gala[1], Ruhi V. Ubale[1],
Bernadette D'Souza[2], Trinh Phuong Vo[1], Ashwin C. Parenky[1],
Nihal S. Mulla[1], Sucheta D'Sa[1], Marissa D'Souza[1,4],
Kim Braz-Gomes[1], Nigel D'Souza[1], Maurizio Chiriva-Internati[3]

[1]Mercer University, College of Pharmacy, Vaccine Nanotechnology Laboratory, Atlanta, GA, USA
[2]Department of Pharmaceutical Sciences, McWhorter School of Pharmacy, Social and
Administrative Sciences, Samford University, Birmingham, AL, USA
[3]Texas Tech University, Health Science Center, Lubbock, TX, USA
[4]Georgia Institute of Technology, Biomedical Engineering Program, Atlanta, GA, USA

OUTLINE

(continued)

Novel Approaches and Strategies for Biologics, Vaccines and Cancer Therapies. DOI: 10.1016/B978-0-12-416603-5.00005-5

INTRODUCTION

Although more than 200 years have passed since Edward Jenner conducted the first human clinical trial of smallpox vaccine in 1796, the vaccination routes remain unchanged; subcutaneous and intramuscular remain the two main routes of vaccinations worldwide.[1] These administration routes are one of the factors that render vaccines unaffordable and unavailable in Third-World countries. The hurdles encountered include refrigeration, transport, and the need for health professionals to administer the vaccine, all which have led to higher cost. All of the shortcomings of traditional vaccinations have become a deterrent in our effort to improve world health standards. In order to ameliorate these problems, alternative vaccination routes such as oral, nasal, or buccal offer new hope. Among the alternative routes, the oral route is preferred as a result of its advantages over the other routes.

The concept of oral vaccines has been explored by numerous researchers, and oral vaccines have begun to emerge in the market, including the Polio Sabin™ oral vaccine, and Dukoral™ oral vaccine for traveler's diarrhea and cholera. The advantages of oral vaccines include improved patient compliance, ease of administration, and lower cost of production and transportation. They also serve as an alternative to the needle phobic, including young children and the elderly. More importantly, oral vaccines are capable of inducing both mucosal and systemic immunity. Recent studies have suggested that in order to produce a more effective vaccine, both systemic and mucosal immunity has to be induced.[2] Nevertheless, the oral delivery of proteins and vaccines faces major physiological barriers such as the acidic environment in the stomach and the enzymatic environment throughout the intestine, as well as formulation challenges such as stability and targeting issues.

Despite these challenges, significant levels of success are being witnessed in the veterinary field for oral delivery of *Mycobacterium pneumonia* vaccines.[3] Most biologics or vaccines generally consist of a large molecule consisting of a peptide, protein, or a conjugate. Unlike the delivery of small molecules, these products have special considerations that make it a challenge to deliver them to the site of action or its receptor. The most important consideration is the stability of the active protein or peptide in the formulation and maintaining its basic structure and its tertiary structure to obtain optimal effect. The ideal delivery system would protect the protein, peptide, or antigen from the physiological conditions encountered during administration and allow it to retain its structure (both primary and tertiary) until it reaches its site of action.

In an attempt to deliver biologics and vaccines orally, numerous strategies have been carried out by scientists around the world using various vehicles such as microparticles, liposomes, virus-like particles (VLPs), lectins, and immune stimulating complexes (ISCOMs).[4] In this chapter, we discuss various nonparenteral routes that have been employed for the delivery of these products. Nonparenteral routes offer ease of administration of the biologic formulation in nonprofessional settings and promise greater patient compliance.

FORMULATION ASPECTS OF BIOLOGICS AND VACCINES

Protein Structure

The formulation of biologics including proteins is difficult without an understanding of their structures and physicochemical properties. Proteins and peptides are formed by binding of various amino acids. There are 20 naturally occurring amino acids, and they differ only in their side chains. Proteins contain more than 50 amino acids, whereas peptides contain fewer than 20 amino acids. The four levels of protein structures are primary, secondary, tertiary, and quaternary. The primary structure includes the sequence of covalently bonded amino acids, and it is dictated by the sequence of deoxyribonucleic acid (DNA). Secondary structures consist of α-helixes, β-sheets, random coils, β-bends, and small loops of the polypeptide chain. The tertiary structure of proteins includes the overall packing in space of various elements of secondary structures, and quaternary structures represent the specific associations of separate protein chains that form a well-defined structure.[5] The primary structure of protein dictates its folding process. Generally, the overall shape is spherical with polar groups on the surface and hydrophobic groups buried in the interior. The fold structure of proteins is stabilized by both noncovalent and covalent forces. These forces include disulfide bridges between cysteine residues, hydrogen bonding, salt bridges between ionic groups, and hydrophobic interactions between side chains of amino acid residues.

Formulation of Biologics

It is evident from the above discussion that proteins have very intricate structures, which make the formulation of proteins a challenging task. In order to successfully formulate a protein, its stability and bioactivity must be maintained over its shelf life (1.5 to 2 years) and until it reaches the intended target. Any subtle changes in the secondary, tertiary, or quaternary structure will lead to physical instabilities such as denaturation, aggregation, precipitation, and adsorption. In addition, hydrolysis, deamidation, oxidation, disulfide exchange, β-elimination, and racemization will lead to chemical instability of proteins. Hence, all of these degradation pathways need to be avoided during the formulation process, and a strategy to minimize the probability of their induction should be in place. These strategies include reducing thermal stress by using the lowest temperature possible while spray drying and storing the protein at 4°C at pH 5.0 to 7.0. Harsh chemicals such as strong acids, bases, and organic solvents will disrupt the higher order structure of proteins, so their use should be avoided or minimized during the formulation process. Aqueous systems should be used rather than organic solvents. Additionally, any energy input such as shaking, vortexing, sonication, temperature increase, radiation, or ultrasound or changes in pH, ionic strength, salt concentration, buffer type, and solvent composition should be minimized to prevent the development of aggregation and eventually other degradation pathways.

Sluzky et al.[6] found significantly higher aggregations of insulin solutions in vials with overhead space and with the addition of Teflon® beads compared to aggregations of insulin in fully filled vials. This is due to the creation of air–water interphase in the partially filled vial, and Teflon beads create hydrophobic surfaces that induce aggregation.[6] Also, it has been demonstrated that vortexing causes aggregation of human growth hormone.[2] Another stress that proteins undergo during the manufacturing process is lyophilization. In lyophilization, the proteins will be exposed to moisture and elevated temperatures. Optimal moisture content actually is essential for protein stability; however, when moisture content increases above the monolayer level, other reactants at the vicinity will be mobilized, leading to aggregation, especially at elevated temperature during lyophilization.[2] For this reason, cryoprotectants such as trehalose and sucrose and lyoprotectants such as polyethylene glycol (PEG) are commonly used to stabilize the protein during lyophilization. Cryoprotectants are preferentially excluded from the protein, whereas lyoprotectants act as a water substitute and hence stabilize the folded structure of proteins. Surfactants such as Polysorbate 20, 40, 60, and 80 stabilize protein by preferential adsorption at the interphase, whereas preservatives such as phenol, m-cresol, chlorobutanol, and parabens reduce microbial contamination.

Precaution should also be taken in the selection of vials and any container for proteins because untreated surface will induce adsorption of the proteins. Siliconized and type I glass vials should be used in preference to untreated plastic vials to avoid the leaching of chemicals from the wall of the vials and induction of adsorption.

Microparticles

Among the many vehicles for successful delivery of biologics are microparticles. Microparticles are bead-like particles with a diameter greater than 1.0 μm, and they are mostly spherical in shape. Microparticulate delivery systems have been used for a wide range of drugs, including neoplastic agents, vaccines, inactivated bacteria, proteins, and peptides.[7–9]

The matrix of microparticles can be categorized into two classes; monolithic and reservoir. In the monolithic matrix the active agent is dispersed homogeneously within the polymer matrix, whereas in the reservoir matrix the drug is surrounded by the polymer matrix in the mononuclear or polynuclear state (core). The monolithic matrix has the advantage of avoiding the risk of dose dumping due to the rupture of the membrane of the reservoir matrix. Drug release from a monolithic matrix may depend on the solubility of the drug in the matrix, as well as on the porosity and tortuosity of the polymer network.[10]

The microparticulate delivery system offers the ability and flexibility to allow it to be formulated into sustained or controlled-release systems with organ or tissue targeting capability. Microparticles have been shown to selectively target drugs to an organ or diseased site.[11,12] Microparticles also possess the ability to sustain or control the release of various drugs.[13] Additionally, microparticles act as immunological adjuvants in light of the fact that they are particulate in nature.[14] Furthermore, stealth microparticles can be produced with the addition of polyethylene glycol (PEG), thus enabling the chemical attachment of PEG chains to a broad range of substances. This pegylation process increases the half-life of circulation, improves drug solubility and stability, and reduces immunogenicity.[8]

Conventional chemotherapy in cancer treatment has been widely used in the clinic but it is associated with significant systemic toxicity and the bigger problem of reoccurrence of the tumor. Immunotherapies have been recently developed to boost the immune system to detect cancer and prevent its reoccurrence, thus improving the patient's quality of life. This chapter talks about a few immunological strategies and cancer vaccines that have been researched and could be potential therapies in the future.

We will first discuss the various nonparenteral routes of administration of these therapies, the associated immunological structures in each of these routes, and the mechanistic pathways by which they act. Later in the chapter we provide specific examples.

ROUTES FOR ADMINISTRATION OF BIOLOGICS, VACCINES, AND CANCER THERAPIES

Oral Route

The oral route of administration is an attractive mode of immunization because of its ease of administration, low manufacturing cost, and high patient compliance. Intestinal Peyer's patches are the predominant sites for oral administration.[15] In the case of particles, the uptake depends on various factors such as size, charge, and hydrophobicity.[16,17] For oral delivery, it has been reported that particles of size less than 5 μm with positive charge and a hydrophobic nature can preferentially enter the Peyer's patch of the small intestine.[18] Orally delivered vaccines, especially particulate antigens, are recognized and sampled by microfold (M) cells in Peyer's patches. This is followed by transport of the particles to underlying follicles and to professional antigen-presenting cells (APCs), such as dendritic cells and macrophages. These APCs can phagocytose the particles, process them, and present them on both major histocompatibility complex (MHC) class I (through cross priming) and MHC class II molecules; as a result, both T and B cells can be triggered, as shown in Figure 5.1.[19,20]

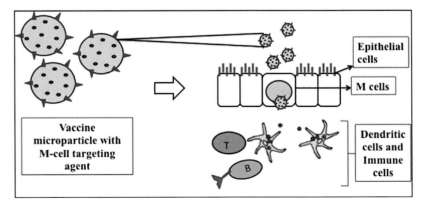

FIGURE 5.1   Schematic of vaccine microparticle uptake by microfold (M) cells of Peyer's patches in small intestine.

The major hurdle in oral delivery is protecting the active biological entity from acidic and enzymatic degradation in the gastrointestinal tract. Another obstacle to be considered while designing an oral vaccine or biologic is the probability of oral tolerance.[21] Low particle uptake and gastric degradation products of antigens can cause oral tolerance. One of the ways to avoid these issues is to formulate microparticles with enteric coating polymers.

Various studies have been reported describing the use of enteric coating polymers such as Eudragit® L 100, S 100, and L 100-55; cellulose acetate phthalate; and hydroxylpropyl methyl-cellulose phthalate/acetate succinate as polymers for particulate delivery vehicles.[22] These polymers are soluble at pH 5.5 and above and thus can render protection to antigens or active in gastric media. Oral delivery of vaccine antigens or biologics using such polymeric micro-particles offers remarkable advantages over others such as induction of mucosal as well as systemic immune response, protection of antigen from gastric degradation, prolonged presentation of antigen to the immune system, and obviation of the need of vaccine adjuvants because microparticles themselves can act as self-adjuvants.[3,14]

Strategically designed particulate delivery systems incorporate enteric polymers to protect the biological entity from harsh gastric conditions and to target ligands to enhance its uptake from M cells of the Peyer's patches in the small intestine. M cells, or microfold cells, act as sampling ports for any foreign entities encountered in the small intestine. These M cells house various dendritic cells and immune cells. For oral vaccines, particles are sampled by M cells, processed by dendritic cells or antigen-presenting cells, and presented on MHC class I or class II molecules. The antigens are further recognized by the immune cells in the vicinity, leading to the cascade of an immune response as shown in Figure 5.1. The immune response also includes a humoral response by plasma B cells that leads to production of antibodies and their class switching. The role of B cells has been debatable in the past, but a recent study by Mahmoud et al.[23] showed that humoral immunity is important in addition to cell-mediated immunity in the prognosis of cancer. Thus, this route can trigger both humoral and cell-mediated immune responses to various cancer vaccines or biologics. The use of microparticles for cancer therapies and the delivery of biologics via the oral route are discussed further later in this chapter.

Buccal Route

The oral route of drug delivery is the most preferred route by both the patient and clinician; however, there are drawbacks associated with it such as hepatic first-pass metabolism and enzymatic degradation in the gastrointestinal tract. For these reasons, other mucosal sites are being considered as alternatives to the oral route. These alternative mucosal routes of drug delivery (e.g., nasal, rectal, vaginal, ocular, buccal, sublingual) offer advantages over the peroral route with respect to bypassing first-pass metabolism and enzymatic degradation in the gastrointestinal tract.

The nasal route of drug administration has been studied[24–29] and has reached commercial status with drugs such as luteinizing hormone-releasing hormone (LHRH)[30,31] and calcitonin.[32–34] However, disadvantages such as irritation to nasal mucosa and damage to the ciliary action of the nasal cavity due to chronic use of nasal dosage forms limit the use of these drug delivery systems. Large intra- and intersubject variability can also affect drug absorption from this site. Similarly, the rectal, vaginal, and ocular sites offer advantages over the oral route but at the same time have poor patient compliance. The oral cavity, on the other hand, is much more accepted by patients; it is permeable with a rich blood supply and is robust, and it recovers quickly after stress or damage. Buccal or sublingual delivery can help to avoid first-pass metabolism and presystemic elimination in the gastrointestinal tract.

Overview of Oral Mucosa

The oral mucosa consists of an outermost layer of stratified squamous epithelium below which lies a basement membrane and a lamina propria (Figure 5.2). This is similar to stratified squamous epithelia found elsewhere in the body as it has a basal cell layer and a number of differentiating intermediate layers. The epithelial layers increase in size and become flatter as they travel from basal to superficial layers.[3]

The turnover time for the buccal epithelium has been estimated at five to six days,[35] which is probably representative of the oral mucosa as a whole. The oral mucosal thickness varies depending on the site. The buccal mucosa measures at 500 to 800 μm, whereas the mucosal thickness of the hard and soft palates, the floor of the mouth, the ventral tongue, and the gingivae measures at about 100 to 200 μm. The composition of the epithelium also varies depending on the site in the oral cavity. The mucosae of areas subject to mechanical stress (the gingivae and hard palate) are keratinized similar to the epidermis. The mucosae of the soft palate, sublingual, and buccal regions, however, are not keratinized.[35] The keratinized epithelia are relatively impermeable to water. In contrast, non-keratinized epithelia, such as

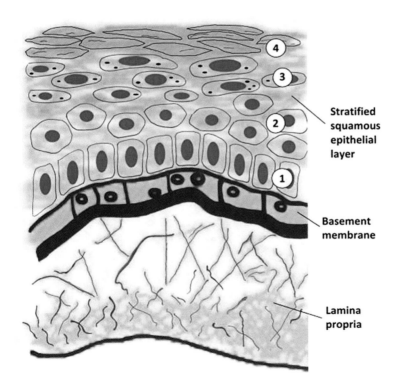

FIGURE 5.2 Structure of oral mucosa.

Stratified squamous epithelial layer

Basement membrane

Lamina propria

the floor of the mouth and the buccal epithelia, do not contain acylceramides and only have small amounts of ceramide.[36,37] They also contain small amounts of neutral but polar lipids, mainly cholesterol sulfate and glucosyl ceramides. These epithelia have been found to be considerably more permeable to water than keratinized epithelia.[35–37]

Immunology of the Buccal Cavity

It is important for a vaccine against bacterial or viral pathogens to elicit mucosal immunity, as these pathogens primarily attack the mucosal surfaces of the body. Also, the administration of a vaccine by any of the mucosal sites—oral, nasal, vaginal, or rectal—has proven to be effective and patient compliant. However, there is still a lack of vaccines that can be delivered by these routes, probably due to the challenges associated with development of an effective and stable vaccine that can be delivered by these routes. One of the mucosal routes of drug delivery that has been largely neglected for vaccine delivery is the buccal route

The mucosal surface of the oral cavity can be an ideal site for vaccination because of its easy accessibility and good antigen presentation. The buccal cavity is rich with dendritic cells similar to Langerhans cells which are a type of antigen-presenting cell. Also, a high density of T lymphocytes and mucosal-associated lymphoid tissue such as tonsils, salivary glands, Waldeyer's ring, and pharyngeal lymphoid tissue is present in the buccal mucosa. Hence, buccal immunization can help to elicit both mucosal and systemic immunity.[38,39]

Etchart et al.[40] reported that immunization with DNA injected into the buccal mucosa of mice induced a measles virus hemagglutinin-specific cytotoxic lymphocyte response in the spleen. It was also seen by Lundholm et al.[41] that pDNA administered to the oral cheek of mice using a jet injection induced production of immunoglobulin A (IgA), signifying a mucosal immune response. Wang et al.[42] reported that mucosal delivery of a melanoma vaccine in a hamster model helped treat oral melanoma and distant skin lesions. All of these studies demonstrated that buccal immunization is possible and can be very effective at the same time.

After having established the efficacy of buccal vaccination, the next step is to develop a robust and effective delivery system. Only liquid formulations containing the vaccine and adjuvant have been studied in animals so far. Hence, there is a need to develop a delivery system with prolonged residence on the buccal mucosa coupled with retention of the efficacy and stability of the vaccine antigen and adjuvant.

Pulmonary Route

Pulmonary delivery has been around for a long time and has its origins in the early civilizations; however, it has become increasingly popular and is being increasingly explored as an alternative means for the systemic delivery of drugs, including a large number of proteins and peptides. Since the latter part of the 20th century, pulmonary delivery has been used for the local delivery of drugs for diseases such as asthma and chronic obstructive pulmonary disease (COPD), but more recently it is also being considered as a viable alternative for the systemic delivery of both small and large molecules.[43]

Biologics are most certainly replacing conventional small molecule drugs as the therapy for the future. Their potency and specificity give them an edge, making them more popular with pharmaceutical and biotechnological industries. However, there are challenges associated with their delivery because of their inherent properties such as high molecular weight, hydrophilicity, and instability, which is why they are predominantly administered by parenteral routes so as to ensure their direct entry into systemic circulation. In order to improve their patient compliance, many non-invasive routes of delivery are being explored, and pulmonary delivery is one of them.[44]

Pulmonary delivery has emerged as a promising alternative because of the unique anatomical features of the lungs. The lungs provide a large absorptive surface area (up to 100 m^2), an extremely thin (0.1 to 0.2 μm) absorptive mucosal membrane, and excellent vascularization, but it is challenging to incorporate the drug in a formulation that will deliver it to such a depth in the lungs that will permit permeation of the drug into blood circulation. The respiratory system is equipped with a series of filters designed to protect the lungs from undesirable environmental material and to keep the lungs clean. This factor must be taken into consideration for a particular therapy to be sufficiently effective. Low efficiency and a large variability have been the major factors that have prevented this route of administration from gaining complete acceptance. Some of the factors that affect the deposition of the drug in the alveolar regions of the lung are uptake by alveolar macrophages and proteolytic degradation.

A number of formulation parameters are unique to pulmonary delivery, such as the aerodynamic particle behavior (particle size, density, hygroscopicity, shape, and surface charge), breathing pattern of the patient (flow rate, ventilation volume), airway anatomy, and morphometry of the patient. Irrespective of the type of drug being delivered (small molecule or large molecule), the above factors have to be considered when preparing a formulation for pulmonary delivery.[45]

Metered dose inhalers (MDIs) and dry powder inhalers (DPIs) have been traditionally used for the delivery of measured doses to the lung and are commonly used to deliver drugs to the lung for the treatment of diseases such as asthma or COPD. Another commercially available system, the AERx® Pulmonary Delivery System by Aradigm uses a bolus of aerosol particles that can be delivered at a certain time during inspiration. The bolus is produced by a piston that empties a small liquid reservoir into the inhalation air. Other devices, including the AKITA® inhalation system (Activaero) and the ProDose™ system (Profile Therapeutics), also use the bolus inhalation technique to deposit particles in the lungs. The bolus delivery technique can help to increase particle deposition in the lungs. Nectar Therapeutics, along with Pfizer, came up with Exubera® for the inhalable delivery of insulin for the treatment of diabetes. This form of insulin was expected to replace all forms of injected insulin but the product lasted on the market for only little over a year after being introduced in September 2006. It was soon recalled, as it was cost ineffective and provided the same efficacy as injected insulin. Since then, a number of other companies (e.g., MannKind Corporation, Aerogen, Dance Biopharm) have been attempting to develop a form of inhalable insulin that is less expensive to produce than Exubera.

Besides insulin, other proteins or peptides whose delivery is being attempted by the pulmonary route are hormones (e.g., insulin, calcitonin, growth hormone, somatostatin, thyroid-stimulating hormone, follicle-stimulating hormone), growth factors (e.g., granulocyte–monocyte colony-stimulating factor, granulocyte colony-stimulating factor), various interleukins, and heparin. Many of the problems associated with the stability and absorption of macromolecules are now being resolved, and these products are currently showing promise in clinical studies. This proves that, in spite of the large number of challenges that pulmonary delivery of biologics faced at the start, progress has been made in leaps and bounds, thus proving its potential.[46]

Transdermal Route

The concept of immunization evolves with knowledge of the working of the body's defense system. Vaccines are traditionally made by using live, attenuated or fragments of pathogens. The transdermal route has been explored to deliver vaccines non-invasively through the skin, thus offering a number of benefits of needle-free delivery.

Transdermal vaccine delivery (TVD) is achieved by directly applying the vaccine antigen topically. The antigen-presenting cells in the epidermis and dermis, better known as Langerhans cells, interact with the antigen to initiate an adaptive immune response by migrating from the skin to the draining lymph nodes, where they activate naïve T cells and B cells.[47] This technology, however, is limited due to the fact that vaccines are large-molecular-weight antigens which, in many instances, find it difficult to cross the outer barrier of the skin: the stratum corneum. Moreover, topically applied macromolecules may get lodged in the hair follicles and sweat ducts, preventing the vaccine from reaching an effective concentration in the skin.

Numerous methods have been successfully used to bypass the stratum corneum such as chemical enhancers, electroporation, ultrasound, iontophoresis, and the use of microneedles. These methods have the potential to increase skin permeability to a large number of therapeutic substances including macromolecules such as insulin and vaccines.[48] Such methods increase transdermal transport through the use of (1) chemical enhancers, which increase drug solubility; (2) increased diffusion coefficients (chemical enhancers, ultrasound, electroporation); and (3) external driving forces (ultrasound, iontophoresis, electroporation).[49] The stratum corneum is the outermost layer of the skin, with a thickness of 10 to 20 μm; it protects against microbes, fluids, and foreign materials. It is also the most significant barrier for transdermal delivery of many compounds, including vaccines.[50]

Much research has been carried out in the field of transdermal vaccine delivery in recent years. Bhowmik et al.[51] formulated a microparticulate whole cell lysate vaccine composed of melanoma cell line antigens, in a biodegradable matrix of bovine serum albumin (BSA) and other sustained-release polymers. The particles ranged in size from 0.165 to 1.5 μm. This formulation was delivered transdermally by creating microchannels in the skin of four- to six-week-old DBA-2/J mice, using the DermaRoller®, a device that uses microneedle technology. *In vivo* studies showed that the vaccine produced an increase in immune response. A significant increase in the IgG antibody titers was observed which may have been the result of uptake and presentation of antigen by the Langerhans cells in the skin. Also, the vaccinated mice showed no palpable tumor even when observed for 35 days after tumor induction. Thus, transdermal microparticle delivery of vaccines opens up new avenues for vaccine administration with the use of rather non-invasive methodologies that require further modifications and testing in a clinical setting.

Ongoing research is exploring drug delivery systems such as organic nanoparticles and hydrogels, polymer-based particles, solid–lipid nanoparticles, and liposomes, as well as other lipid-based vesicles for transcutaneous vaccine delivery.[48] Nanoparticles were shown to be a promising carrier for transcutaneous vaccine. These are advantageous because their small size allows them to penetrate through the hair follicles and cause the vaccine antigens to target the antigen-presenting cells and augment the immune response. Additionally, their interaction with skin lipids results in the generation of transient and reversible openings of the stratum corneum.[52] Polymers such as polylactic acid, polylactic-*co*-glycolic acid, and chitosan have shown promise in transdermal immunization by eliciting strong immune responses.[53,54] Liposomes are other exciting carrier system for delivery of vaccines via the transdermal route. The lipid-based vesicles of liposomes, especially elastic liposome, may change the bioactive permeation kinetics due to an impaired barrier function of the stratum corneum, helpful for the skin penetration.[55] Liposomes are generally composed of phosphatidylcholine and a surfactant and contain a lipid bilayer enveloping an aqueous compartment, which has a large capacity for loading drugs or vaccines. Mishra et al.[56] have demonstrated enhanced immunity against antigen using elastic liposomes loaded with hepatitis B surface antigen (HBsAg).

Research in the area of developing novel nanosized formulations may be helpful with regard to stabilizing the antigen and protecting it from disrupting lipids in the stratum corneum. These properties are of primary importance for the delivery of vaccines through the skin. However, the development of such novel nanoscale systems is limited by their low efficiency in eliciting a robust immune response. Clinical trials for transcutaneous immunization usually rely on microneedles or needle-free skin patches. Research and clinical trials are concentrated on transdermal vaccines for infectious diseases such as influenza, with cancer immunization taking a back seat. The development of future vaccine delivery strategies requires further investigation into the transdermal route because research work published thus far has shown great promise.

CHEMOTHERAPY VERSUS IMMUNOTHERAPY

Chemotherapy

Chemotherapy, the most common treatment for cancer, uses anticancer drugs to kill cancerous tissue. In chemotherapy, a single drug or a combination of drugs can be used for a particular cancer or along with treatments such as surgery and radiation. Chemotherapy may be used to achieve total remission, prevent reoccurrence of the cancer, or slow down metastasis.

Because chemotherapeutic drugs are generally given orally or as injections, not only could these drugs exert their cytotoxic effect on the cancer cells and the healthy cells around the cancer, but they could also reach other parts of the body and cause mild to devastating side effects. Side effects of chemotherapeutic drugs can range from mild symptoms such as fatigue and loss of appetite to severe effects such as vomiting or neutropenia, leading to a poor quality of life. Moreover, drugs administered by the intravenous route could cause such serious effects as extravasation. Although much progress has been made in alleviating the side effects caused by chemotherapy, there is a need for improved therapies that are less damaging to the patient.

Immunotherapy

Cancer immunotherapy is designed to modify the host's immune system or utilize the components of the immune system as cancer treatment. Immunotherapy may be preferred over the traditional chemotherapy because the treatment offers less severe side effects and sometimes may be targeted therapy. Immunological products that have received regulatory approval are either single anticancer agents or in combination with chemotherapy. These products include cytokines such as interferon-α and interleukin-2; the monoclonal antibodies trastuzumab, bevacizumab, and ipilimumab; and others such as the anticancer cell-based therapy sipuleucel-T.

When cell-mediated immune response is enhanced against tumor cells it offers various advantages over targeted therapies, particularly the generation of a long-term-memory lymphocyte population patrolling the body to attack metastases before they become visible by traditional imaging modalities.[57]

A significant interest in the development of therapeutic cancer vaccines over the last decade has led to an improvement in overall survival of cancer patients in several clinical trials. As a result, two active immunotherapy agents, sipuleucel-T and ipilimumab, have been approved by the U.S. Food and Drug Administration (FDA) for the treatment of prostate cancer and melanoma, respectively. GVAX® cellular vaccine (Cell Genesys, Inc.) is another active immunotherapy agent that targets prostate cancer and has been well studied in various clinical trials. van den Eertwegh et al.[58] studied the combination of two active immunotherapy approaches (GVAX and ipilimumab) for the treatment of metastatic castration-resistant prostate cancer. Whereas GVAX is designed to amplify the antitumor response specific to prostate cancer cells, ipilimumab contributes to T-cell activation. Thus, the authors presented the possibility of augmenting antitumor T-cell activity in two different ways.

The immunotherapeutic agent ipilimumab has helped address a significant unmet need in the treatment of advanced melanoma. Ipilimumab is a fully human monoclonal antibody that targets cytotoxic T-lymphocyte antigen-4 (CTLA-4), thereby augmenting antitumor immune responses. Ipilimumab (at a dose of 10 mg per kilogram) in combination with dacarbazine, as compared with dacarbazine plus placebo, improved overall survival in patients with previously untreated metastatic melanoma. Ipilimumab was recently approved by the FDA for the treatment of metastatic melanoma.[59]

In a pivotal Phase III trial, treatment with sipuleucel-T (provenge, dendreon), an autologous cellular vaccine consisting of activated antigen-presenting cells loaded with prostatic acid phosphatase (PAP), gave a median overall survival of 25.8 months compared with 21.7 months for placebo-treated patients, resulting in a 22% relative reduction in the risk of death.[60]

Classification of Cancer Immunotherapy

Cancer immunotherapy can be classified as two types: active and passive. Active immunotherapies that can stimulate the immune system can be further subdivided into specific immunotherapy including prophylactic or therapeutic vaccines. Nonspecific immunotherapy consists of components of the immune system such as cytokines and immune adjuvants. Passive immunotherapies are not used to boost the immune system. The passive transfers of monoclonal antibodies can increase antitumor immunity by either inhibition of immune check points or augmentation of stimulatory signals. Adoptive cell therapy involves infusion of tumor-reactive cells that are autologous tumor-infiltrating lymphocytes, T-cell receptor gene-modified lymphocytes, or chimeric antigen receptors that are recombinant receptors providing antigen-binding and T-cell activation functions.[61]

Vaccines and Active Specific Immunotherapy

Prevention or treatment with a cancer vaccine, or active specific immunotherapy, is a very attractive therapeutic option because the mechanism of action is eventually an enhanced endogenous immune response against the host's malignancy.

CURRENT IMMUNE THERAPIES

Monoclonal Antibodies

Antibodies provide protection to the immune system from microorganisms, and therapy with monoclonal antibodies targeted specifically to tumors has proven to be one of the successful forms of immune therapy in cancer. Antibodies exert their role by binding to their targets, through several effector mechanisms, including steric inhibition and neutralization, complement activation, and activation of cell-mediated cytotoxicity.

Monoclonal antibody therapy is relatively nontoxic with lesser side effects than chemotherapy when the antibodies are bound to the tumor cells.[62–64] Nine monoclonal antibodies, targeting six tumor-associated proteins, are clinically approved for the treatment of cancer. For example, rituximab, the most widely used monoclonal antibody, is now used in combination with cyclophosphamide, doxorubicin, vincristine, and prednisone for non-Hodgkin's lymphoma and has shown complete remission in patients compared with chemotherapy alone.[65–66] Monoclonal antibodies (ibritumomab tiuxetan and 131I tositumomab) have been used to target tumors directly by conjugating them to radioactive isotypes or toxic chemicals as in the case of gemcitumab.[65,67]

Cytokines

Cytokines, proteins secreted by the immune cells when stimulated by antigen, may be given systemically in certain cancers. IL-2 is a potent mediator in antiviral therapy and is used in advanced melanoma and renal cell carcinoma, both cancers that are resistant to chemotherapy alone.[68–70] Tumor necrosis factor α (TNF-α) is another cytokine used for the treatment of soft tissue carcinomas of the limb and melanoma.[71]

Cancer Vaccines

The purpose of cancer vaccines is to initiate an active immune response toward a tumor. There are several types of cancer vaccines in development: adenoviral, dendritic cell, tumor cell, adoptive T-cell transfer, and peptide.[72] Antigens from tumors and antigen-presenting cells may be used as potential vaccine approaches to enhance a preexisting antitumor immune response, or, perhaps in some cases, to induce an antitumor immune response that did not exist earlier. There are many potential sources of tumor antigens, including purified or synthesized tumor cell surface molecules, which may be peptides or proteins, cells or lysates derived from fresh or cryopreserved autologous tumor samples (actually a mixture of normal and malignant cells), and cells or lysates of allogeneic or autologous tumor cell lines. There are a variety of methods by which tumor antigens can be presented including as purified antigen, via heat shock proteins, in viruses or DNA, by antigen-presenting cells (APCs) such as dendritic cells, or as the idiotypes of monoclonal antibodies (mAbs) that have been selected by their tumor antigen recognition. There are numerous molecules that might be useful as adjuvants to enhance the immunogenicity of a vaccine. Cancer vaccines may be given by different routes: subcutaneous, intradermal, intramuscular, or intravenous.

Although the oral route is the most acceptable route of administration among patients, the formulation of an oral vaccine faces a number of challenges. Still, many researchers are focused on the aspect of formulating vaccines using novel delivery systems such as microparticles and nanoparticles. This chapter touches upon some of the research carried out in our laboratory on oral microparticulate vaccine or biologics delivery. It had long been assumed that if cancer vaccines could elicit a strong enough immune response they could overcome tumor-induced immune suppression, but after poor clinical results for so many promising vaccines it is now being realized that immunogenicity is not enough. In addition to a strong vaccine, tumor-induced immunosuppression must be actively reduced, and this may be achieved through combination with the arsenal of chemotherapy agents already in use.[73] In a Phase III trial for sipileucel-T (Provenge®, Dendreon Corporation), the first autologous vaccine consisted of activated dendritic cells comprised of granulocyte–macrophage colony-stimulating factor (GM-CSF) and prostatic acid phosphatase (PAP) approved by the FDA for treatment of advanced prostate cancer. This vaccine included a large proportion of antigen-presenting cells, which were infused back into the patient to stimulate antitumor T-cell responses.[74] The results showed higher median overall survival compared to placebo-treated patients, resulting in a 22% relative reduction in the risk of death, but it failed to show benefit in progression-free survival, and tumor regressions were rare.[60,61] This is an example of a personalized vaccine.

COMBINATION OF IMMUNOTHERAPY AND CHEMOTHERAPY

Chemotherapies can help improve the efficacy of cancer vaccines by exerting various effects on the immune system; however, there are several pitfalls to consider. Chemotherapeutic regimens are different for different cancers, stage of cancer, and patient characteristics. Adding cancer vaccines into the program introduces another layer of complexity. Indeed, several studies looking at vaccine chemotherapy combinations highlighted the fact that chemotherapies must be carefully dosed and delivered at particular times in relation to the vaccine for optimal effect.[75,76] Although substantial research has combined chemotherapies and vaccines in mouse models, information from human studies is rare.

Due to the active role the immune system plays in tumor clearance, it is likely that the benefits of cancer vaccines will be best observed in patients with early, untreated disease.[73] Gemcitabine, cyclophosphamide, and dacarbazine (or temozolomide, which is metabolized to dacarbazine *in vivo*[77]) in particular have been used. So far, no studies report the safety risks associate with chemotherapy and immunotherapy.

Recent clinical studies on combination treatments have proven chemotherapy given after vaccination is a better treatment strategy than chemotherapy pretreatment or simultaneous administration. A clinical study published by Antonia et al.[78] showed results that indicated that patients with extensive stage small cell lung cancer were essentially more responsive to second-line chemotherapy treatment after vaccination with dendritic cells transduced p53 via adenoviral vector.

In a Phase II study, a personalized peptide vaccine when combined with the anticancer drug gemcitabine to treat advanced pancreatic cancer, produced a response rate of 67% for both cellular and humoral responses.[79]

MELITAC is a peptide cancer vaccine administered after cyclophosphamide in a resected stage IIB to IV melanoma Phase I/II study, which showed that cyclophosphamide provided no detectable improvement in CD4 or CD8 T-cell responses or in clinical outcome.[67]

In addition to chemotherapy, other studies have been attempted wherein the vaccine response was improved by inactivating Treg cells through the specific targeting of the T-cell CTLA-4 receptor with a monoclonal antibody such as ipilimumab (Yervoy®, Bristol-Myers Squibb). Preliminary clinical trials suggest that administering a therapeutic vaccine followed by ipilimumab enhances immune responses and tumor reduction in prostate and ovarian cancers as well as melanoma.[80]

Similarly, in the transgenic murine prostate cancer model, a tumor shrinkage effect was observed with combination therapy of whole cell GM-CSF-secreting vaccine (GVAX) and low-dose cyclophosphamide one to two days before immunization with vaccine alone. This effect was associated with a reduced Treg population in the tumor and its lymph nodes, as well as stimulation of dendritic cell activity.[81]

Apart from chemotherapy and vaccine combinations, novel antibodies targeting certain cancers may also be used in conjunction with certain cancer vaccines and anticancer drugs. For example, anti-CTLA-4 antibody administered before a cell-based, GM-CSF-secreting vaccine (GVAX) showed a remarkable increase in the effector CD8 T-cell response.

Hence, it is possible to boost the therapeutic advantage of vaccines in combination with chemotherapy as seen in some of the cases mentioned above. However, research in this area many pose a problem as far as the chemotherapeutic aspect is concerned because the dose and the time of administration differ with different chemotherapeutic regimens for various cancers. Traditionally, patients in the last stages of cancer having limited therapeutic alternatives have been tested with experimental therapies. In these cases, such patients deteriorate with the disease and previous chemotherapies may be less likely to mount strong responses to a vaccine, thus they may not be ideal candidates.[80] Many questions remain unanswered and require further investigation. Many experimental strategies will have yet to be tried out to determine an effective combination that results in maximum therapeutic benefit with minimum side effects.

In our lab we have used particulate-based delivery systems in both the micrometer range and nanometer range delivered via the above discussed routes of administration. The particulate delivery system in general offers many advantages compared to traditional methods of drug delivery. Some of them include:

- Small and large molecules accommodated
- Multidrug therapy using one particle
- Stable delivery system for bioactive molecules
- Easy manufacturing and scale-up
- Elimination of cold-chain requirements.

MICROPARTICLE-BASED DELIVERY SYSTEMS FOR NONPARENTERAL DELIVERY OF BACTERIAL (MENINGOCOCCAL) VACCINES

Need for Micro/Nanoparticulate Meningococcal Vaccines

Neisseria meningitidis is a leading cause of bacterial meningitis and sepsis in young children and young adults in the United States and is associated with a high mortality rate.[82,83] Childhood vaccination has been shown to induce a herd immunity effect by reducing nasopharyngeal carriage.[84–86] The current available polysaccharide-based meningococcal vaccines are licensed for use in adolescents and adults but are expensive. Therefore, utilizing micro-/ nanotechnology to explore novel meningococcal vaccine formulations that boost innate and adaptive immunity and offer protection is very important. Another important aspect to be noted is that micro-/nanoparticles could facilitate the oral, transdermal, nasal, or buccal delivery of vaccines. This could prove to be an incredible boon when dealing with epidemics in Sub-Saharan African countries where the need for trained medical personnel could be effectively avoided. Needle-free vaccination has gained importance when dealing with countries where human immunodeficiency virus (HIV) is a significant concern and has improved the safety of vaccination.

Microparticle Vaccines for Polysaccharide Based Meningococcal Antigens

Capsular polysaccharides (CPS) are a major virulence factor in meningococcal infections and form the basis for serogroup designation and protective vaccines. CPS is anchored in the outer membrane through a 1,2-diacylglycerol moiety[87] and functions to protect the bacteria from complement-mediated killing while also inhibiting phagocytosis by professional phagocytes.[88,89]

Ubale et al.[90] attempted to formulate a microparticulate meningococcal vaccine to serve as a sustained-release system administered by the oral/buccal route. The vaccine formulation consisted of meningococcal CPS polymers (Serogroup A) and/or adjuvant (kdtA) encapsulated in albumin-based biodegradable matrix microparticles that mimic the chemical conjugation process of CPS to a protein carrier, thus enhancing antigen uptake via albumin receptors and eliciting a T-cell-dependent immune response.[8,12]

The ability of the CPS-loaded microparticles to induce cytokine and chemokine release from macrophages was investigated in an *in vitro* cell culture model of THP-1 human macrophage-like cells. Dose-dependent release of TNF-α (Figure 5.3) from THP-1cells exposed to meningococcal CPS-loaded microparticles, but not empty microparticles, was observed. The cytokine release reflects the recognition and immunostimulatory activity of the polysaccharide antigen in the microparticle matrix. Taken together, the data suggested that CPS-loaded microparticles are recognized by macrophages and the encapsulation in BSA matrix did not hamper the immunostimulatory activity of CPS.

Autophagy, an ancient homeostasis mechanism for macromolecule degradation, recently has been recognized to play a role in host defense and antigen presentation.[91] It was seen that CPS-loaded microparticles but not the empty microparticles strongly induced autophagic vacuoles in a dose-dependent manner (Figure 5.4). The innate immune recognition of these

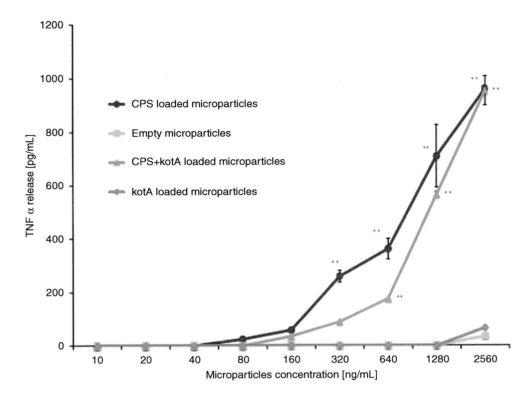

FIGURE 5.3 TNF-α release induced by microparticulate meningococcal vaccine from THP-1 cells.

vaccine-loaded microparticles is the first step and prerequisite for eliciting adaptive immune responses.

Conclusions

This case study briefly describes the use of micro-/nanoparticles as an effective alternative to the nonparenteral delivery of bacterial vaccines. This paves the way for more research and improvement in this field of vaccine delivery.

INFLUENZA VACCINE

Influenza viruses cause a highly contagious disease in the human respiratory tract, such as the nose, lungs, and throat. Symptoms of influenza infection are fever, sore throat, headache, cough, and fatigue.[92] During the influenza epidemic of 1918 the deadly virus killed approximately 50 million people globally.[93] In 2009, a new strain of influenza virus (H1N1) emerged and spread quickly throughout the world, causing the first influenza pandemic of the 21st century.

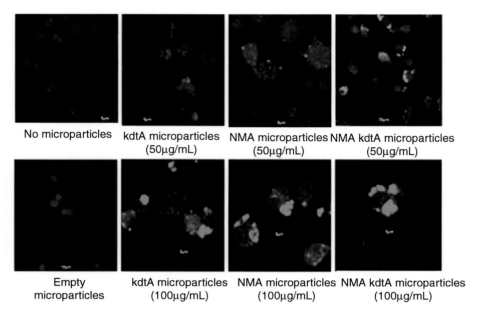

| No microparticles | kdtA microparticles (50μg/mL) | NMA microparticles (50μg/mL) | NMA kdtA microparticles (50μg/mL) |

| Empty microparticles | kdtA microparticles (100μg/mL) | NMA microparticles (100μg/mL) | NMA kdtA microparticles (100μg/mL) |

FIGURE 5.4   Autophagy induction by microparticulate meningococcal vaccine from RAW cells.

There are two types of influenza vaccines: the "flu shot" and the nasal-spray flu vaccine.[92] Flu shots contain inactivated influenza virus, while the nasal-spray flu vaccine (FluMist®) is made with live attenuated flu viruses. Oral administration is a potential route for vaccination because there is no need for trained medical personnel for administration, thus leading to increased coverage of vaccination, as seen in case of oral polio vaccination.[94] Development of a novel influenza oral vaccine will have a significant impact on improving public health.[95] In one case study, microparticulate vaccine was developed by using inactivated influenza (A/PR/34/8 H1N1) virus as an antigen, which was incorporated into a polymer matrix (Eudragit® S).[96] For *in vivo* testing, BALB/c mice were immunized with two doses within a three-week interval. Serum samples was analyzed and proved that microparticulate vaccine enhanced antigen-specific antibodies (Figure 5.5). Also, these mice were challenged with heterologous influenza viruses, and the results showed a significant induction level of protection via this technology.[96]

Another trend of developing influenza vaccine is to minimize the number of doses. One innovative approach is to broaden protective efficacy by using the extracellular domain of matrix protein 2 (M2e) antigen, which is common among influenza A viruses.[97] This group replaced the hyperimmunogenic region of *Salmonella enterica* serovar *typhimurium* flagellin (FliC) with four repeats of M2e (4.M2e-tFliC) and fused it to a membrane anchor from influenza virus hemagglutinin to establish a membrane-anchored fusion protein. The fusion protein was then integrated into influenza M1 virus-like particles. The *in vivo* studies showed a strong antigen-specific antibody in case of intramuscular and intranasal administrations.[97]

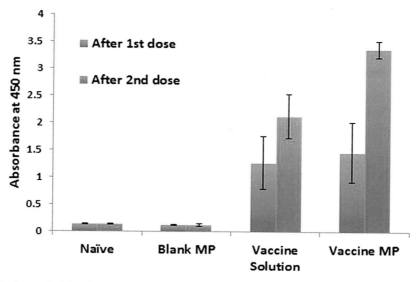

FIGURE 5.5 Serum IgG levels in BALB/c mice. Mice ($n = 6$) were vaccinated with prime followed by booster doses at 0 and 5th week, respectively. Serum samples (1:100 dilution) were analyzed at the third and seventh week. Statistical significance was calculated by two-way ANOVA comparing the results between different groups at different time points ($p < 0.0001$).

Developing influenza vaccine via the transdermal route has been investigated using microneedle technology. Influenza virus-like particles delivered through microchannels under skin showed an induction of protection against influenza infection and proved a long-tem protective efficacy.[98] In this study, influenza virus-specific total IgG and hemagglutination inhibition titers were maintained at high levels for over one year after vaccination. In addition, the levels of lung IgG and IgA antibody responses were higher compared to intramuscular administration.

Overall, many innovative technologies have been applied to develop enhanced influenza vaccines. Diverse antigens (inactivated viruses, live attenuated viruses, proteins and virus-like particles) have been studied along with various routes of administrations (transdermal, intranasal, intramuscular, and oral). These novel approaches would be promising influenza vaccines for better protection against influenza viruses and could substantially reduce the burden for public health in the future.

HUMAN PAPILLOMAVIRUS VACCINE

Human papillomavirus (HPV) is a sexually transmitted virus that causes genital warts and leads to cancer of the cervix, vulva, vagina, penis, oropharynx, and throat.[99] Approximately 600,000 women were diagnosed with cervical cancer in 2010, and that number could rise to 700,000 new cases annually by 2020 in the absence of intervention.[100] There are at least

100 distinct types of HPV, including more than 30 HPV types that can develop infection in humans. Therefore, HPV vaccination is strongly recommended for females and males, especially for girls ages 9 to 26.

Currently, two prophylactic HPV vaccines have been commercialized worldwide: the bivalent vaccines Cervarix® (GlaxoSmithKline) and Gardasil® (Merck).[101,102] However, both of these vaccines have to be injected and are very expensive (approximately $450 for a course of three doses); consequently, they are not affordable for people from developing countries.

There are numerous novel approaches to HPV vaccination with regard to different routes of administration (intranasal, oral, or transdermal) and types of antigen (virus-liked particles, DNA, or proteins). In one study, a protein-based HPV prophylactic cancer vaccine was tested in C57BL/6 mice; it was administered intranasally with a combination of E6/E7 antigens and Toll-like receptor 5 (FlaB).[103] The results showed that this combination elicited a very strong antigen-specific cytotoxic T-lymphocyte activity and antigen-specific interferon production from spleenocytes and cervical lymph node cells.[103] Such a novel approach could prove to be a very effective prophylactic HPV vaccine in the future.

DNA-based vaccines are another excellent alternative for targeting HPV infection and cervical cancer. For example, pcDNA3.1-HPV16E7 recombinant vector was used as an antigen, which passed through microchannels under skin by using microneedle arrays.[104] In this study, after BALB/c mice were immunized with one prime followed by two boosters every two weeks, serum and lymphocytes were collected to detect the functions of humoral and cellular immunities. The results proved the DNA vaccine is a promising platform for transdermal delivery via microneedles to induce specific antibodies for *in vitro* and *in vivo* studies.[104]

Recently, a nine-valent vaccine in HPV (HPV 6/11/16/18/31/33/45/52/58) has been proposed for better protection against HPV infection and cervical cancer.[105] If the nine-valent vaccine induces immunity as strong as that of Gardasil® or Cervarix®, world incidence rates could be dramatically reduced.[105]

In summary, many novel approaches for alternatives of HPV vaccines have been proposed to improve efficacy and reduce costs. Various routes of administration have been tested along with different types of antigen including protein, peptide, DNA, and virus-liked particles. A variety of adjuvants was incorporated with antigen to stimulate both humoral and cellular immune responses against HPV infection and cervical cancer.

CANCER VACCINE CASE STUDIES

Prostate Cancer Vaccines

The prostate gland is part of the male reproductive system located below the bladder and in front of the rectum. The National Cancer Institute (NCI) reported approximately 238,000 cases of prostate cancer in 2013 alone. It is the second leading cause of cancer-related deaths in America and Europe.[106] The primary goal of cancer immunotherapy is destruction of tumors by the immune system. There are several strategies to elicit an effective antitumor response, including designing vaccines that target specific tumor epitopes and modulating the activity of regulatory T cells that dampen any underlying immune response.[107] Many prostate-specific antigens are known to be immunogenic; one such antigen is the prostate-specific antigen (PSA), which also serves as a marker for disease progression.

Oral Particulate Prostate Cancer Vaccines

Nanoparticles and microparticles have been at the forefront of drug delivery. In recent years, investigators have focused on using these platforms to improve several aspects of vaccine delivery. Particulate vaccines offer a distinct advantage over antigen solutions themselves. They protect the antigen from the *in vivo* environment, improve uptake of the antigen, reduce the number of doses for primary immunization, and can be used to target specific cell populations for enhanced efficacy.[108] Several studies in our laboratory have proved the efficacy of oral microparticulate systems to elicit immune response against tumors.[109–111] The mechanism of immune system activation by the oral route is explained in the earlier section of this chapter. Our laboratory has also explored several targeting ligands that target M cells in order to enhance site-specific uptake of microparticles. Microparticles are formulated using the spray-drying technology with enteric polymers that fall under the Generally Regarded as Safe (GRAS) category classified by the FDA. Preliminary studies in our laboratory evaluated the efficacy of a microparticulate whole cell lysate vaccine of TRAMP-C2 prostate cancer cells as a prophylactic cancer vaccine therapy. It was observed that tumor growth was significantly retarded in vaccinated mice compared to the control group.[111] Recently, Chiriva-Internati et al.[112] isolated and tested AKAP-4 as a target for prostate cancer-specific immunotherapy. Our lab is currently exploring the efficacy of therapeutic oral microparticulate vaccines for prostate cancer. Preliminary studies indicate that AKAP-4 along with a whole cell lysate microparticulate vaccine system could efficiently induce antitumor immune responses, leading to a significant reduction in tumor growth *in vivo*.

Transdermal Delivery of Particulate Prostate Cancer Vaccines

The use of transdermal drug delivery for the delivery of oligonucleotides, proteins, peptides, and inactivated viruses is growing steadily. Microneedles are micron-sized needles with lengths up to 1 µm. Microneedles pierce the upper layer of skin for local or systemic delivery of small molecule drugs or biologics.[113] Delivery of vaccines to skin has been established as a promising target to elicit an immune response.[114] Our laboratory studied the efficacy of whole cell lysate vaccine microparticles with murine prostate cancer cells (TRAMP C2) on C57BL/6 mice. Vaccination was performed by the transdermal route. Mice were challenged with live murine prostate cancer cells following immunization and tumor growth was monitored for 8 weeks. Results from the study proved that mice vaccinated by the transdermal route elicited delayed tumor growth that was significant compared to control groups (Figure 5.6). Mechanistic studies revealed an increase in CD4[+] T cells and B cells in vaccinated mice compared to control. Thus, it was observed that both innate and adaptive immune responses were activated following transdermal vaccination which delayed tumor growth for vaccinated mice.

Breast Cancer Vaccine

Breast cancer is one of the most common type of cancer in females all over the world. According to the Centers for Disease Control and Prevention (CDC), about 211,731 cases were reported in 2009 and about 40,676 women died because of breast cancer.[115] In the past decade, there has been exponential growth in the research being conducted on immunotherapy.

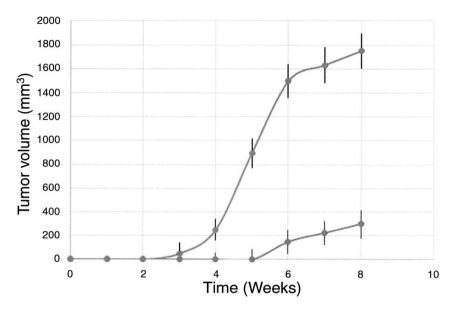

FIGURE 5.6   This graph compares the mean tumor volume of vaccinated group via the transdermal route and the naïve group following 10-week vaccination regimen. C57BL/6 mice were challenged with live 5×10^6 prostate cancer cells subcutaneously and the tumor growth was monitored for 8 weeks. Significant delay in tumor growth was observed in the vaccinated group compared to the naive ($p < 0.05$). Blue line, vaccinated group; orange line, control group.

Immunotherapy works by inducing or enhancing the body's immune system to identify and reject tumor. Several breast cancer antigens such as human epidermal growth factor receptor 2 (HER2), mucin 1 (MUC1), human telomerase reverse transcriptase (hTERT), tumor protein 53 (p53), and cancer embryonic antigen (CEA) have been used to prepare these vaccines where these tumor-associated antigens (TAAs) were represented by whole cell extracts/dendritic cells or DNA motifs.[116]

Oral and Transdermal Breast Cancer Vaccine

Whole cell vaccine was formulated into microparticles using enteric coating polymers. The microparticle formulation is optimized by using a different combination and concentration of polymers. These microparticles were administered both orally and transdermally. *In vitro* and *in vivo* studies were carried out to evaluate the humoral and cellular response against the vaccine loaded microparticles.

In vitro experiments showed that spray-dried microparticles provided protection against gastric conditions and controlled the release for about six hours. Vaccine-loaded particles were nontoxic to normal cells. The majority of the particles were in the size range of 1 to 5 μm. *In vivo* studies proved that both oral and transdermal groups were able to prevent and delay tumor growth compared to the control groups receiving blank microparticles. Flow cytometry results for the immune organs revealed that animals receiving the vaccine showed higher CD4+ T cells, CD4+, CD161+, and CD8+ levels than the control groups. A

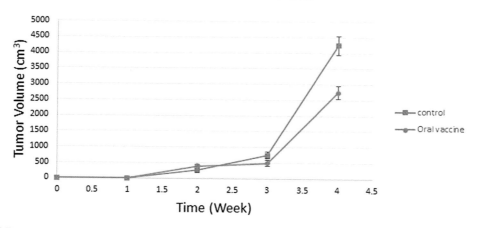

FIGURE 5.7 This graph compares the mean tumor volume of vaccinated group via oral route and the control group following a 10-week vaccination regimen. BALB/c mice were challenged with live breast cancer cells subcutaneously and the tumor growth was monitored for four weeks. Significant delay in tumor growth was observed in the vaccinated group compared to the control group ($p < 0.05$).

higher expression of these markers shows that the vaccine particles were able to induce a better immune response to fight against the cancer cells. Efficacy of vaccine microparticles could be seen with the tumor volume data (Figure 5.7).[109] Therapeutic applications of vaccine microparticles are currently being evaluated. The therapeutic efficacy of these vaccine microparticles is reportedly enhanced when given in combination with cytotoxic drug and adjuvants.

Melanoma Cancer Vaccine

Melanoma is a dangerous form of skin cancer characterized by malignant proliferation of the melanocytes. It is one of the leading causes of death and its rate of occurrence in the world is progressively increasing as people are exposed to larger amounts of damaging ultraviolet rays due to the vanishing ozone layer. The early stages of melanoma are localized and treatable to a large extent, but with time the tumor metastasizes to the visceral organs, making it more difficult to treat.

In a recent study carried out by the American Cancer Society for melanoma located near where it started, the five-year survival rate is 98%. The five-year survival rates for melanoma that has spread to the nearby lymph nodes or to other parts of the body are 62% and 15%, respectively. Melanoma accounts for only about 5% of skin cancer cases, but it is the cause of more than 75% skin cancer deaths.

The standard and approved treatments for melanoma include surgery, targeted therapy, radiation, chemotherapy and treatment with biologics. The current treatment approved by the FDA includes IFN-α and dacarbazine and requires supplementation with other treatment options such as surgery and radiation. In an extensive study conducted by the Mayo Clinic for determining the efficiency of chemotherapeutic agents, only 10 of 503 melanoma cancer patients achieved complete remission.[117]

Patients who have undergone surgery to completely remove tumors and who are at a high risk for relapse are systemically given high doses of pegylated IFN-α-2b, which is approved for the adjuvant treatment. Prospective, randomized, controlled trials with both agents have not shown an increase in overall survival when compared with observation.[118,119]

The novel monoclonal antibodies ipilimumab and vemurafenib were approved by the FDA in 2011, as they demonstrated an improvement in overall survival in international, randomized trials in patients with advanced melanoma.[120] These single agents are rarely curative; however, clinical trials that incorporate these agents are testing combinations in an attempt to prevent development of drug resistance. Vemurafenib is a selective BRAF V600E kinase inhibitor, and its indication is limited to patients with a demonstrated *BRAF* V600E mutation by an FDA-approved test.[121] Interleukin-2 (IL-2) was approved by the FDA in 1998 on the basis of durable complete response (CR) rates in a minority of patients (0 to 8%) with previously treated metastatic melanoma in eight Phase I and II studies.[122–124]

The National Cancer Institute mentions interferon and interleukin-2 as types of biologic therapy used to treat melanoma. Interferon slows tumor progression by affecting the division of cancer cells. IL-2 improves the growth and activity of many immune cells, especially lymphocytes. Lymphocytes can attack and kill cancer cells. Tumor necrosis factor (TNF) therapy is another type of biologic therapy used in conjunction with other treatments for melanoma. TNF is a cytokine released by white blood cells in response to an antigen or infection.

The success of prophylactic vaccines against infectious diseases has increased interest of researchers to explore the feasibility of using vaccines against cancer. The John Wayne Cancer Institute (Santa Clara, CA) developed a vaccination regimen in the form of a living whole cell melanoma vaccine called CancerVax. This vaccine includes a mixture of irradiated melanoma associated antigens (MAA) derived from allogenic tumor cell lines to treat melanoma.[125] Results from this vaccination study showed that the median survival rate of melanoma patients was significantly higher when compared to patients receiving other forms of treatment. This in turn has led to interest in the development of a vaccine that would trigger the immune system to stimulate the cytotoxic cells and inhibit the tumor growth.[126]

In recent years, research has been focused on developing novel vaccines such as whole cell vaccines, dendritic cell vaccines, peptide vaccines, DNA vaccines, viral vaccines, and ganglioside vaccines for either the prevention or treatment of melanoma. Melanoma vaccines that have been tested have shown poor clinical responses, thus no effective vaccine has been developed to date.[127] All of the vaccines tested, however, are given by the parenteral route.

Oral vaccines are currently being investigated for their efficacy in stimulating the mucosal as well as systemic immunity. The mucosal route of entry and initiation of primary immune response is well established where pathogens and other invasive microbes enter the host system via regions in the small intestine. Bernadette et al.[128] described a study wherein they formulated a novel prophylactic oral microparticulate vaccine composed of whole cell lysate for melanoma using the spray-drying technique. Surface morphology of microparticles evaluated by scanning electron microscopy (SEM) showed that the particles had a spherical surface with a size distribution of around 1 to 2 μm (Figure 5.8). They used an M-cell targeting ligand called aleuria aurantia lectin (ALL) that improved the uptake into the Peyer's patches of the small intestine. The results suggested that melanoma antigen microparticles were able to significantly increase the antibody titers in the mice for groups containing the lectin ligand in comparison to the other groups involved in the study. The serum IgG response of orally immunized mice with AAL ligand in the vaccine was compared with the oral group without

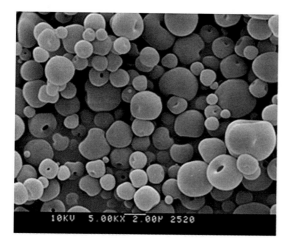

FIGURE 5.8   Surface morphology of microparticles showed that the particles had a spherical surface with a size distribution of around 1.2 ± 0.5 μm.

AAL and showed a significant increase in serum IgG titer. The results of the tumor challenge study showed that the group vaccinated with AAL-associated microparticles showed the highest level of protection against tumor development. Thus, in the future, when designing oral particulate vaccines, AAL may be incorporated in the formulation as the targeting ligand.

The major challenge in designing a successful vaccine is the delivery of antigens to the part of the immune system where maximum stimulation and proliferation of the professional immunopotent cells can be achieved. In a previous study with model antigens, it was shown that microparticles are capable of exhibiting potent serum antibody responses to entrapped antigens following oral administration.[129]

Figure 5.9 represents the cytotoxic evaluation of the melanoma-antigen microparticles in an *in vitro* cell culture model. The data show more than 80% cell viability measured as an

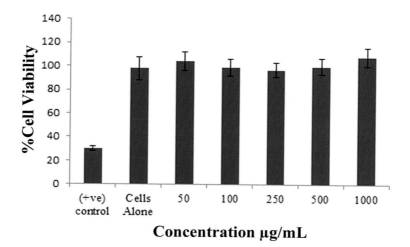

FIGURE 5.9   *In vitro* cytotoxicity assay of melanoma vaccine loaded microparticles.

average of $n = 3$ (+ SE) after 24 hours of incubation with the microparticles. The microparticle formulations were added at doses of 0.05, 0.1, 0.25, 0.5, and 1 mg/mL in 0.2 mL of complete cell culture media. Cells alone in media was used as the negative control, and atropine sulfate (cytotoxic agent) was the positive control, which resulted in cell death.

Studies are currently aimed at combining chemotherapy and novel immunotherapies, including vaccines, cytokines, and anti-CTLA4 antibodies. Hundreds of combination therapies are currently undergoing clinical trials. Vaccine therapy still remains an experimental therapy in patients with metastatic melanoma.

The vaccine delivery by the formulation demonstrated in the investigation described here opens up new avenues for vaccine administration by more patient-convenient routes for cancer therapy. Further research is needed, although a future therapy for advanced melanoma is probably a multimodal approach including vaccines, adjuvants, and negative costimulatory blockade.

Ovarian Cancer Vaccine

Among the gynecological cancers, ovarian cancer is the most lethal and the fifth leading cause of cancer-related deaths in women globally and more specifically in the United States. According to the data from the CDC, each year around 20,000 women in the US are diagnosed with ovarian cancer and 15,000 women sadly die each year due to ovarian cancer. The major reason for high mortality is that in more than 70% of women with ovarian cancer are diagnosed with advanced disease.[130]

Many vaccines have made it to the clinical trials but most of them have not progressed beyond Phase I/II studies. Although antigen-specific responses are obtained using various approaches of immunization, there is a lack of consistency in the benefits.[131,132] Here, we discuss an oral vaccination with microparticles containing the ovarian cancer antigens that can prevent or retard ovarian cancer growth. A murine ovarian cancer cell line, ID8, was used as a source of antigens as it correlates closely to human ovarian cancer cell lines in signaling pathways and results in development of tumor in mice models similar to human ovarian cancer.[133] Whole cell lysate, which is a very promising approach, provides a pool of tumor-associated antigens (TAAs) which include both CD8+ and CD4+ T cells. It also overcomes the drawbacks associated with using a single antigen or epitope vaccine.

Like other studies, to protect the antigen from the gastric conditions, enteric polymers such as methacrylic copolymers FS 30D and hydroxyl methylcellulose succinate (HPMCAS) were used to make the microparticles along with AAL for its M-cell targeting property using the spray-dryer method (Figure 5.10). In addition, inclusion of immunostimulatory molecules such as IL-2 and IL-12 was evaluated in order to enhance the overall potency of the formulated vaccines.[134,135] Characterization of the vaccine particles was done. The immunogenicity of the microparticulate vaccine was evaluated using C57BL/6 female mice model. Three different formulations such as placebo, vaccine, and vaccine with interleukins were evaluated for their efficacy. A tumor challenge study was carried out in which one week after the last vaccine was administered the mice were challenged with 1×10^7 live ID8 cells subcutaneously. Tumor volume was checked and a reduction in tumor volume was indicative of the success of the vaccine formulation.[136,137]

The morphological characterization of the particles showed that the particles were crumbled, collapsed, and irregular in shape within a micrometer size range having a net positive

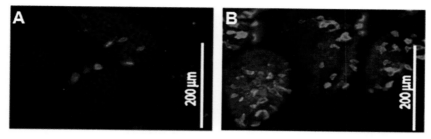

FIGURE 5.10   Increased uptake of particles by M cells (SEM images) in Peyer's patches using AAL. (A) Particles without AAL; (B) particles with AAL.

charge. The immunization studies showed that in the group of mice with the placebo particles the tumor growth was very rapid. In the vaccinated group, there was a sixfold tumor suppression as compared to the placebo. However, there was not much difference between the vaccine group and the group with interleukins, which could possibly be due to low concentrations of the interleukins.

To access the humoral immune response (B-cell mediated) the serum samples were collected before each dose and were analyzed by enzyme-linked immunosorbent assay (ELISA) for the IgG subtypes IgG_1 and IgG_{2a}. The results from the ELISA showed increased IgG titer in vaccinated mice as opposed to nonvaccinated mice. Thus, both the subtypes of IgGs indicate that a mixed Th1 and Th2 type response was generated in the vaccine-only group. But, a Th2 type response was triggered among the interleukin group. This difference could be attributed to the effect of interleukins on the Peyer's patches which has been previously reported as a strategy for increasing the immune response for oral vaccine. Similar studies were carried out by Marinaro et al.[135] where IL-12 was given orally to mice immunized with oral tetanus toxoid and cholera toxin. Their studies showed that oral IL-12 resulted in a TH2 response to the oral vaccine, and a TH1 response occurred when IL-12 was given via the intraperitoneal route.

To check for T-cell populations, lymphatic organs such as the spleen and the lymph nodes were collected. $CD4^+$ and $CD8^+$ levels were elevated in vaccinated mice as compared to the placebo group. The $CD4^+$ T-cell population was found to be elevated in the spleen cells of the vaccine + interleukin group when compared to the spleen cells of the vaccine-alone group. The B-cell population was determined in the spleen, lymph nodes, and bone marrow. For B-cell populations in spleen cells, there were elevated levels in the vaccine + interleukin group when compared to placebo and vaccine alone. B cells in bone marrow were found to be elevated in the vaccine + interleukin group compared to the placebo or vaccine-alone groups.[110]

In summary, the B-cell population was found to be more elevated in the bone marrow and spleen cells of the vaccine + interleukin group compared to the vaccine-alone group. It was higher in the lymph nodes of the vaccine-alone group as well as the vaccine + interleukin group when compared to placebo. It was found that $CD8^+$ and $CD4^+$ T cells were expanded in mice treated with vaccine with and without interleukins when compared to non-vaccinated mice (Figure 5.11). However, when a comparison was made between the vaccine-along group and the vaccine + interleukin groups, the B-cell populations in bone marrow and spleen along with $CD4^+$ T cells in spleen were found to be elevated in the vaccine + interleukin group.[110]

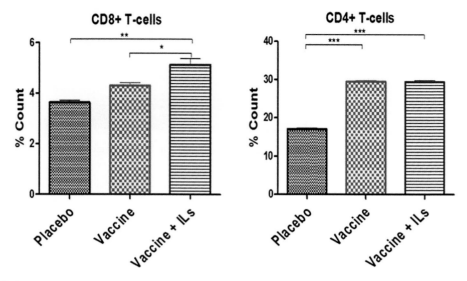

FIGURE 5.11   CD8+ T cells and CD4+ T cells in spleen and lymph nodes ($n = 6$). $*p < 0.05$, $**p < 0.01$, $***p < 0.001$.

Thus, there was overall stimulation of the humoral and cellular response upon administration of the vaccine, indicating the success of the vaccine. These results also correlate with the tumor volume reduction in the mice. Thus, this study demonstrated the efficacy of the microparticulate vaccine containing the whole cell lysate. Oral vaccine delivery could be an effective and attractive mode of immunization because of its ease of administration, low cost of manufacturing, and most importantly patient compliance.

OVERALL SUMMARY AND CONCLUSIONS

Today, there are still increasing numbers of new vaccines being developed to prevent different evolving diseases, including H5N1 bird flu, acquired immunodeficiency syndrome (AIDS), severe acute respiratory syndrome (SARS), and others. Nevertheless, the main vaccination routes are still the subcutaneous and intramuscular routes. These administration methods render vaccination unaffordable in many areas of Third-World countries. The use of a spray dryer and the formulation and development processes performed demonstrated the feasibility for scale-up and manufacture.

One of the hurdles of oral proteins or vaccines delivery is the harsh acidic environment in the stomach. To overcome this obstacle, enteric coating polymers and various combinational matrices have been used to protect the proteins. Such protection should be sufficient to ensure successful delivery of the encapsulated biologics or vaccines. Another feature of the formulations developed is their sustained- or controlled-release properties achieved by employing different combinations of polymers. This feature can be tailored to achieve desired release profiles by adjusting the compositions of the polymers used.

In light of the fact that proteins are very sensitive to any subtle changes in their microenvironment, therefore, the stability of encapsulated proteins must be evaluated. To achieve that, the physicochemical characteristics of the formulations developed were analyzed using bioactivity assays, Fourier transform infrared (FTIR) spectroscopy, differential scanning calorimetry (DSC), particle sizes analyzers, and the Zetasizer. Additionally, FTIR and DSC studies performed before and after microencapsulation showed no major changes in their native structures. These results suggest that the formulation developed can be used as an effective vehicle for delivery of proteins and vaccine.

References

1. Hilleman MR, Carlson AJ Jr, McLean AA, Vella PP, Weibel RE, Woodhour AF. *Streptococcus pneumoniae* polysaccharide vaccine: age and dose responses, safety, persistence of antibody, revaccination, and simultaneous administration of pneumococcal and influenza vaccines. Rev. Infect. Dis. 1981;3(Suppl.):S31–42.
2. Katakam M, Bell LN, Banga AK. Effect of surfactants on the physical stability of recombinant human growth hormone. J. Pharm. Sci. 1995;84(6):713–6.
3. Li C, Bhatt PP, Johnston TP. Evaluation of a mucoadhesive buccal patch for delivery of peptides: in vitro screening of bioadhesion. Drug Dev. Ind. Pharm. 1998;24(10):919–26.
4. O'Hagan DT, Palin K, Davis SS, Artursson P, Sjöholm I. Microparticles as potentially orally active immunological adjuvants. Vaccine 1989;7(5):421–4.
5. Katakam M, Banga AK. Use of poloxamer polymers to stabilize recombinant human growth hormone against various processing stresses. Pharm. Dev. Technol. 1997;2(2):143–9.
6. Sluzky V, Tamada JA, Klibanov AM, Langer R. Kinetics of insulin aggregation in aqueous solutions upon agitation in the presence of hydrophobic surfaces. Proc. Natl. Acad. Sci. U.S.A. 1991;88(21):9377–81.
7. De Rosa G, Quaglia F, La Rotonda M, Besnard M, Fattal E. Biodegradable microparticles for the controlled delivery of oligonucleotides. Int. J. Pharm. 2002;242(1-2):225–8.
8. Diwan M, Elamanchili P, Lane H, Gainer A, Samuel J. Biodegradable nanoparticle mediated antigen delivery to human cord blood derived dendritic cells for induction of primary T cell responses. J. Drug Target. 2003;11(8):495–507.
9. Lim DW, Park TG. Stereocomplex formation between enantiomeric PLA–PEG–PLA triblock copolymers: characterization and use as protein-delivery microparticulate carriers. J. Appl Polym Sci. 2000;75(13):1615–23.
10. Singh M, Kazzaz J, Chesko J, Soenawan E, Ugozzoli M, Giuliani M, et al. Anionic microparticles are a potent delivery system for recombinant antigens from *Neisseria meningitidis* serotype B. J. Pharm. Sci. 2004;93(2):273–82.
11. Lai YH, D'Souza MJ. Formulation and evaluation of an oral melanoma vaccine. J. Microencapsul. 2007;24(3):235–52.
12. Yeboah KG, D'Souza MJ. Evaluation of albumin microspheres as oral delivery system for *Mycobacterium tuberculosis* vaccines. J. Microencapsul. 2009;26(2):166–79.
13. Martin ME, Dewar JB, Newman JF. Polymerized serum albumin beads possessing slow release properties for use in vaccines. Vaccine 1988;6(1):33–8.
14. O'Hagan DT, Singh M. Microparticles as vaccine adjuvants and delivery systems. Expert Rev Vaccines 2003;2(2):269–83.
15. Lai YH, D'Souza MJ. Microparticle transport in the human intestinal M cell model. J. Drug Target. 2008;16(1):36–42.
16. Andrianov P. Polymeric carriers for oral uptake of microparticulates. Adv. Drug Deliv. Rev. 1998;34(2-3):155–70.
17. Vyas SP, Gupta PN. Implication of nanoparticles/microparticles in mucosal vaccine delivery. Expert Rev. Vaccines 2007;6(3):401–18.
18. Xiang SD, Scholzen A, Minigo G, David C, Apostolopoulos V, Mottram PL, et al. Pathogen recognition and development of particulate vaccines: does size matter? Methods San Diego Calif. 2006;40(1):1–9.
19. Men Y, Audran R, Thomasin C, Eberl G, Demotz S, Merkle HP, et al. MHC class I- and class II-restricted processing and presentation of microencapsulated antigens. Vaccine 1999;17(9-10):1047–56.
20. Shen H, Ackerman AL, Cody V, Giodini A, Hinson ER, Cresswell P, et al. Enhanced and prolonged cross-presentation following endosomal escape of exogenous antigens encapsulated in biodegradable nanoparticles. Immunology 2006;117(1):78–88.
21. Zho F, Neutra MR. Antigen delivery to mucosa-associated lymphoid tissues using liposomes as a carrier. Biosci. Rep. 2002;22(2):355–69.

22. Hori M, Onishi H, Machida Y. Evaluation of Eudragit-coated chitosan microparticles as an oral immune delivery system. Int. J. Pharm. 2005;297(1-2):223–34.

23. Mahmoud SM, Lee AH, Paish EC, Macmillan RD, Ellis IO, Green AR. The prognostic significance of B lymphocytes in invasive carcinoma of the breast. Breast Cancer Res Treat. 2012 Apr;132(2):545–53.

24. Aungst BJ, Rogers NJ. Site dependence of absorption-promoting actions of laureth-9, Na salicylate, Na$_2$EDTA., and aprotinin on rectal, nasal, and buccal insulin delivery. Pharm. Res. 1988;5(5):305–8.

25. Aungst BJ, Rogers NJ, Shefter E. Comparison of nasal, rectal, buccal, sublingual and intramuscular insulin efficacy and the effects of a bile salt absorption promoter. J. Pharmacol. Exp. Ther. 1988;244(1):23–7.

26. Tengamnuay P, Mitra AK. Bile salt-fatty acid mixed micelles as nasal absorption promoters of peptides. I. Effects of ionic strength, adjuvant composition, and lipid structure on the nasal absorption of [D-Arg2]-kyotorphin. Pharm. Res. 1990;7(2):127–33.

27. Shao Z, Mitra AK. Nasal membrane and intracellular protein and enzyme release by bile salts and bile salt-fatty acid mixed micelles: correlation with facilitated drug transport. Pharm. Res. 1992;9(9):1184–9.

28. Shao Z, Mitra AK. Bile salt-fatty acid mixed micelles as nasal absorption promoters. III. Effects on nasal transport and enzymatic degradation of acyclovir prodrugs. Pharm. Res. 1994;11(2):243–50.

29. Sayani AP, Chien YW. Systemic delivery of peptides and proteins across absorptive mucosae. Crit. Rev. Ther. Drug Carrier Syst. 1996;13(1-2):85–184.

30. Adjei A, Sundberg D, Miller J, Chun A. Bioavailability of leuprolide acetate following nasal and inhalation delivery to rats and healthy humans. Pharm. Res. 1992;9(2):244–9.

31. Shimamoto T. Pharmaceutical aspects. Nasal and depot formulations of leuprolide. J. Androl. 1987;8(1):S14–16.

32. Dal Negro R, Turco P, Pomari C, Trevisan F. Calcitonin nasal spray in patients with chronic asthma: a double-blind crossover study vs. placebo. Int. J. Clin. Pharmacol. 1991;29(4):144–6.

33. Plosker GL, McTavish D. Intranasal salcatonin (salmon calcitonin). A review of its pharmacological properties and role in the management of postmenopausal osteoporosis. Drugs Aging 1996;8(5):378–400.

34. Reginster JY, Lecart MP. Efficacy and safety of drugs for Paget's disease of bone. Bone 1995;17(5 Suppl.):485S–S488.

35. Harris D, Robinson JR. Drug delivery via the mucous membranes of the oral cavity. J. Pharm Sci. 1992;81(1):1–10.

36. Wertz PW, Squier CA. Cellular and molecular basis of barrier function in oral epithelium. Crit. Rev. Ther. Drug Carrier Syst. 1991;8(3):237–69.

37. Squier CA, Cox P, Wertz PW. Lipid content and water permeability of skin and oral mucosa. J. Invest. Dermatol. 1991;96(1):123–6.

38. Cui Z, Mumper RJ. Bilayer films for mucosal (genetic) immunization via the buccal route in rabbits. Pharm. Res. 2002;19(7):947–53.

39. Amorij J-P, Kersten GFA, Saluja V, Tonnis WF, Hinrichs WLJ, Slütter B, et al. Towards tailored vaccine delivery: needs, challenges and perspectives. J. Control. Release 2012;161(2):363–76.

40. Etchart N, Hennino A, Friede M, Dahel K, Dupouy M, Goujon-Henry C, et al. Safety and efficacy of transcutaneous vaccination using a patch with the live-attenuated measles vaccine in humans. Vaccine 2007;25(39-40):6891–9.

41. Lundholm P, Asakura Y, Hinkula J, Lucht E, Wahren B. Induction of mucosal IgA by a novel jet delivery technique for HIV-1 DNA. Vaccine 1999;17(15-16):2036–42.

42. Wang J, Murakami T, Hakamata Y, Ajiki T, Jinbu Y, Akasaka Y, et al. Gene gun-mediated oral mucosal transfer of interleukin 12 cDNA coupled with an irradiated melanoma vaccine in a hamster model: successful treatment of oral melanoma and distant skin lesion. Cancer Gene Ther. 2001;8(10):705–12.

43. Gonda I. The ascent of pulmonary drug delivery. J. Pharm Sci. 2000;89(7):940–5.

44. Chung SW, Hil-lal TA, Byun Y. Strategies for non-invasive delivery of biologics. J. Drug Target. 2012;20(6):481–501.

45. Ghilzai, N.K. *Pulmonary Drug Delivery*, 2008, http://www.drugdel.com/Pulm_review.pdf.

46. Scheuch G, Siekmeier R. Novel approaches to enhance pulmonary delivery of proteins and peptides. J. Physiol. Pharmacol. 2007;58(Suppl. 5, Pt. 2):615–25.

47. Kripke ML, Munn CG, Jeevan A, Tang JM, Bucana C. Evidence that cutaneous antigen-presenting cells migrate to regional lymph nodes during contact sensitization. J. Immunol. 1990;145(9):2833–8.

48. Lawson LB, Freytag LC, Clements JD. Use of nanocarriers for transdermal vaccine delivery. Clin. Pharmacol. Ther. 2007;82(6):641–3.

49. Mitragotri S. Breaking the skin barrier. Adv. Drug Deliv. Rev. 2004;56(5):555–6.

50. Babiuk S, Baca-Estrada M, Babiuk LA, Ewen C, Foldvari M. Cutaneous vaccination: the skin as an immunologically active tissue and the challenge of antigen delivery. J. Control. Release 2000;66(2-3):199–214.

51. Bhowmik T, D'Souza B, Shashidharamurthy R, Oettinger C, Selvaraj P, D'Souza MJ. A novel microparticulate vaccine for melanoma cancer using transdermal delivery. J. Microencapsul. 2011;28(4):294–300.

52. Kohli AK, Alpar HO. Potential use of nanoparticles for transcutaneous vaccine delivery: effect of particle size and charge. Int. J. Pharm. 2004;275(1-2):13–7.

53. Panyam J, Labhasetwar V. Biodegradable nanoparticles for drug and gene delivery to cells and tissue. Adv. Drug Deliv. Rev. 2003;55(3):329–47.

54. Lee P-W, Peng S-F, Su C-J, Mi F-L, Chen H-L, Wei M-C, et al. The use of biodegradable polymeric nanoparticles in combination with a low-pressure gene gun for transdermal DNA delivery. Biomaterials 2008;29(6):742–51.

55. Li N, Peng L-H, Chen X, Nakagawa S, Gao J-Q. Transcutaneous vaccines: novel advances in technology and delivery for overcoming the barriers. Vaccine 2011;29(37):6179–90.

56. Mishra D, Dubey V, Asthana A, Saraf DK, Jain NK. Elastic liposomes mediated transcutaneous immunization against hepatitis B. Vaccine 2006;24(22):4847–55.

57. Gao J, Bernatchez C, Sharma P, Radvanyi LG, Hwu P. Advances in the development of cancer immunotherapies. Trends Immunol. 2013;34(2):90–8.

58. Santegoets SJAM, Stam AGM, Lougheed SM, Gall H, Scholten PET, Reijm M, et al. T cell profiling reveals high CD4+CTLA-4 + T cell frequency as dominant predictor for survival after prostate GVAX/ipilimumab treatment. Cancer Immunol Immunother CII. 2013 Feb;62(2):245–56.

59. Page DB, Postow MA, Callahan MK, Wolchok JD. Checkpoint modulation in melanoma: an update on ipilimumab and future directions. Curr. Oncol. Rep. 2013;15(5):500–8.

60. Gerritsen WR. The evolving role of immunotherapy in prostate cancer. Ann. Oncol. 2012;23(Suppl. 8):viii22–7.

61. Ito F, Chang AE. Cancer immunotherapy: current status and future directions. Surg. Oncol. Clin. N. Am. 2013;22(4):765–83.

62. Byrd JC, Waselenko JK, Maneatis TJ, Murphy T, Ward FT, Monahan BP, et al. Rituximab therapy in hematologic malignancy patients with circulating blood tumor cells: association with increased infusion-related side effects and rapid blood tumor clearance. J. Clin. Oncol. 1999;17(3):791–5.

63. Hurwitz H, Fehrenbacher L, Novotny W, Cartwright T, Hainsworth J, Heim W, et al. Bevacizumab plus irinotecan, fluorouracil, and leucovorin for metastatic colorectal cancer. N. Engl. J. Med. 2004;350(23):2335–42.

64. Slamon DJ, Leyland-Jones B, Shak S, Fuchs H, Paton V, Bajamonde A, et al. Use of chemotherapy plus a monoclonal antibody against HER2 for metastatic breast cancer that overexpresses HER2. N. Engl. J. Med. 2001;344(11):783–92.

65. Coiffier B, Lepage E, Briere J, Herbrecht R, Tilly H, Bouabdallah R, et al. CHOP chemotherapy plus rituximab compared with CHOP alone in elderly patients with diffuse large-B-cell lymphoma. N. Engl. J. Med. 2002;346(4):235–42.

66. Marcus R, Hagenbeek A. The therapeutic use of rituximab in non-Hodgkin's lymphoma. Eur. J. Haematol. Suppl. 2007;(67):5–14.

67. Witzig TE, Gordon LI, Cabanillas F, Czuczman MS, Emmanouilides C, Joyce R, et al. Randomized controlled trial of yttrium-90-labeled ibritumomab tiuxetan radioimmunotherapy versus rituximab immunotherapy for patients with relapsed or refractory low-grade, follicular, or transformed B-cell non-Hodgkin's lymphoma. J. Clin Oncol. 2002;20(10):2453–63.

68. Fyfe G, Fisher RI, Rosenberg SA, Sznol M, Parkinson DR, Louie AC. Results of treatment of 255 patients with metastatic renal cell carcinoma who received high-dose recombinant interleukin-2 therapy. J. Clin. Oncol. 1995;13(3):688–96.

69. Atkins MB, Lotze MT, Dutcher JP, Fisher RI, Weiss G, Margolin K, et al. High-dose recombinant interleukin 2 therapy for patients with metastatic melanoma: analysis of 270 patients treated between 1985 and 1993. J. Clin. Oncol. 1999;17(7):2105–16.

70. Motzer RJ, Bacik J, Murphy BA, Russo P, Mazumdar M. Interferon-alfa as a comparative treatment for clinical trials of new therapies against advanced renal cell carcinoma. J. Clin. Oncol. 2002;20(1):289–96.

71. Lans TE, Grünhagen DJ, de Wilt JHW, van Geel AN, Eggermont AMM. Isolated limb perfusions with tumor necrosis factor and melphalan for locally recurrent soft tissue sarcoma in previously irradiated limbs. Ann. Surg. Oncol. 2005;12(5):406–11.

72. Jain KK. Personalized cancer vaccines. Expert Opin. Biol. Ther. 2010;10(12):1637–47.

I. NOVEL THERAPEUTIC APPROACHES

73. Weir GM, Liwski RS, Mansour M. Immune modulation by chemotherapy or immunotherapy to enhance cancer vaccines. Cancers 2011;3(3):3114–42.

74. Anassi E, Ndefo UA. Sipuleucel-T (provenge) injection: the first immunotherapy agent (vaccine) for hormone-refractory prostate cancer. Pharm. Ther. 2011;36(4):197–202.

75. Tongu M, Harashima N, Yamada T, Harada T, Harada M. Immunogenic chemotherapy with cyclophosphamide and doxorubicin against established murine carcinoma. Cancer Immunol Immunother. 2010;59(5): 769–77.

76. Emens LA, Asquith JM, Leatherman JM, Kobrin BJ, Petrik S, Laiko M, et al. Timed sequential treatment with cyclophosphamide, doxorubicin, and an allogeneic granulocyte-macrophage colony-stimulating factor-secreting breast tumor vaccine: a chemotherapy dose-ranging factorial study of safety and immune activation. J. Clin. Oncol. 2009;27(35):5911–8.

77. Kyte JA, Gaudernack G, Dueland S, Trachsel S, Julsrud L, Aamdal S. Telomerase peptide vaccination combined with temozolomide: a clinical trial in stage IV melanoma patients. Clin. Cancer Res. 2011;17(13):4568–80.

78. Antonia SJ, Mirza N, Fricke I, Chiappori A, Thompson P, Williams N, et al. Combination of p53 cancer vaccine with chemotherapy in patients with extensive stage small cell lung cancer. Clin. Cancer Res. 2006;12(3, Pt. 1):878–87.

79. Yanagimoto H, Shiomi H, Satoi S, Mine T, Toyokawa H, Yamamoto T, et al. A Phase II study of personalized peptide vaccination combined with gemcitabine for non-resectable pancreatic cancer patients. Oncol. Rep. 2010;24(3):795–801.

80. Slovin S. Chemotherapy and immunotherapy combination in advanced prostate cancer. Clin. Adv. Hematol. Oncol. 2012;10(2):90–100.

81. Wada S, Yoshimura K, Hipkiss EL, Harris TJ, Yen H-R, Goldberg MV, et al. Cyclophosphamide augments antitumor immunity: studies in an autochthonous prostate cancer model. Cancer Res. 2009;69(10):4309–18.

82. Kaplan SL, Schutze GE, Leake JAD, Barson WJ, Halasa NB, Byington CL, et al. Multicenter surveillance of invasive meningococcal infections in children. Pediatrics 2006;118(4):e979–84.

83. Shepard CW, Rosenstein NE, Fischer M. Active Bacterial Core Surveillance Team. Neonatal meningococcal disease in the United States. 1990 to 1999. Pediatr. Infect. Dis. J. 2003;22(5):418–22.

84. Chiavaroli C, Moore A. An hypothesis to link the opposing immunological effects induced by the bacterial lysate OM-89 in urinary tract infection and rheumatoid arthritis. BioDrugs Clin. Immunother. Biopharm. Gene Ther. 2006;20(3):141–9.

85. Barin JG, Baldeviano GC, Talor MV, Wu L, Ong S, Quader F, et al. Macrophages participate in IL-17-mediated inflammation. Eur. J. Immunol. 2012;42(3):726–36.

86. Peng H, Huang Y, Rose J, Erichsen D, Herek S, Fujii N, et al. Stromal cell-derived factor 1-mediated CXCR4 signaling in rat and human cortical neural progenitor cells. J. Neurosci. Res. 2004;76(1):35–50.

87. Tzeng Y-L, Datta AK, Strole CA, Lobritz MA, Carlson RW, Stephens DS. Translocation and surface expression of lipidated serogroup B capsular polysaccharide in *Neisseria meningitidis*. Infect. Immun. 2005;73(3):1491–505.

88. Choudhury B, Kahler CM, Datta A, Stephens DS, Carlson RW. The structure of the L9 immunotype lipooligosaccharide from Neisseria meningitidis NMA Z2491. Carbohydr. Res. 2008;343(17):2971–9.

89. Spinosa MR, Progida C, Talà A, Cogli L, Alifano P, Bucci C. The *Neisseria meningitidis* capsule is important for intracellular survival in human cells. Infect. Immun. 2007;75(7):3594–603.

90. Ubale RV, D'Souza MJ, Infield DT, McCarty NA, Zughaier SM. Formulation of meningococcal capsular polysaccharide vaccine-loaded microparticles with robust innate immune recognition. J Microencapsul. 2013;30(1): 28–41.

91. Levine B, Deretic V. Unveiling the roles of autophagy in innate and adaptive immunity. Nat. Rev. Immunol. 2007;7(10):767–77.

92. CDC. *Seasonal Influenza (Flu)*, 2014, http://www.cdc.gov/flu/.

93. Billings, M. *The Influenza Pandemic of 1918*, 2005, http://www.stanford.edu/group/virus/uda/.

94. Modlin JF, Onorato IM, McBean A, et al. The humoral immune response to type 1 oral poliovirus vaccine in children previously immunized with enhanced potency inactivated poliovirus vaccine or live oral poliovirus vaccine. Am. J. Dis. Child. 1990;144(4):480–4.

95. Germann TC, Kadau K, Longini IM, Macken CA. Mitigation strategies for pandemic influenza in the United States. Proc. Natl. Acad. Sci. U.S.A. 2006;103(15):5935–40.

96. Shastri PN, Kim M-C, Quan F-S, D'Souza MJ, Kang S-M. Immunogenicity and protection of oral influenza vaccines formulated into microparticles. J. Pharm. Sci. 2012;101(10):3623–35.

97. Wang B-Z, Gill HS, Kang S-M, Wang L, Wang Y-C, Vassilieva EV, et al. Enhanced influenza virus-like particle vaccines containing the extracellular domain of matrix protein 2 and a Toll-like receptor ligand. Clin. Vaccine Immunol. 2012;19(8):1119–25.

98. Quan F-S, Kim Y-C, Song J-M, Hwang HS, Compans RW, Prausnitz MR, et al. Long-term protective immunity from an influenza virus-like particle vaccine administered with a microneedle patch. Clin. Vaccine Immunol. 2013;20(9):1433–9.

99. CDC. *Genital HPV Infection—Fact Sheet*, 2014, http://www.cdc.gov/std/HPV/STDFact-HPV.htm.

100. Parkin DM, Bray F. The burden of HPV-related cancers. Vaccine 2006;24(Suppl. 3):S3/11–25.

101. GlaxoSmithKline. *Cervarix® [Human Papillomavirus Bivalent (Types 16 and 18) Vaccine, Recombinant]*, 2014, http://www.gsksource.com/gskprm/en/US/adirect/gskprm?cmd=ProductDetailPage&product_id=1262876367943&featureKey=601720.

102. European Medicines Agency. *Gardasil [Human Papillomavirus Vaccine (Types 6, 11, 16, 18) Recombinant, Absorbed]: Summary of Product Characteristics*, http://ec.europa.eu/health/documents/community-register/2011/20110801107489/anx_107489_en.pdf.

103. Nguyen CT, Hong SH, Ung TT, Verma V, Kim SY, Rhee JH, et al. Intranasal immunization with a flagellin-adjuvanted peptide anticancer vaccine prevents tumor development by enhancing specific cytotoxic T lymphocyte response in a mouse model. Clin. Exp. Vaccine Res. 2013;2(2):128–34.

104. Gao H, Pan J-C, Chen B, Xue Z-F, Li H-D. The effect of HPV16E7 DNA vaccine transdermal delivery with microneedle array. Zhonghua Yu Fang Yi Xue Za Zhi 2008;42(9):663–6.

105. Serrano B, Alemany L, Tous S, Bruni L, Clifford GM, Weiss T, et al. Potential impact of a nine-valent vaccine in human papillomavirus related cervical disease. Infect Agent Cancer 2012;7(1):38.

106. Geary SM, Salem AK. Prostate cancer vaccines. Oncoimmunology 2013;2(5):e24523. (http://www.ncbi.nlm.nih.gov/pmc/articles/PMC3667918/).

107. Gulley JL, Madan RA, Heery CR. Therapeutic vaccines and immunotherapy in castration-resistant prostate cancer. Am. Soc. Clin. Oncol. Educ. Book 2013;2013:166–70.

108. Gupta RK, Chang AC, Siber GR. Biodegradable polymer microspheres as vaccine adjuvants and delivery systems. Dev. Biol. Stand. 1998;92:63–78.

109. Chablani L, Tawde SA, Akalkotkar A, D'Souza C, Selvaraj P, D'Souza MJ. Formulation and evaluation of a particulate oral breast cancer vaccine. J. Pharm Sci. 2012;101(10):3661–71.

110. Tawde SA, Chablani L, Akalkotkar A, D'Souza C, Chiriva-Internati M, Selvaraj P, et al. Formulation and evaluation of oral microparticulate ovarian cancer vaccines. Vaccine 2012;30(38):5675–81.

111. Akalkotkar A, Tawde SA, Chablani L, D'Souza MJ. Oral delivery of particulate prostate cancer vaccine: *in vitro* and *in vivo* evaluation. J. Drug Target. 2012;20(4):338–46.

112. Chiriva-Internati M, Yu Y, Mirandola L, D'Cunha N, Hardwicke F, Cannon MJ, et al. Identification of AKAP-4 as a new cancer/testis antigen for detection and immunotherapy of prostate cancer. Prostate 2012;72(1):12–23.

113. Van der Maaden K, Jiskoot W, Bouwstra J. Microneedle technologies for (trans)dermal drug and vaccine delivery. J. Control. Release 2012;161(2):645–55.

114. Prausnitz MR, Mikszta JA, Cormier M, Andrianov AK. Microneedle-based vaccines. Curr. Top. Microbiol. Immunol. 2009;333:369–93.

115. CDC. *Breast Cancer Statistics*, 2013, http://www.cdc.gov/cancer/breast/statistics/.

116. Benavides LC, Sears AK, Gates JD, Clifton GT, Clive KS, Carmichael MG, et al. Comparison of different HER2/neu vaccines in adjuvant breast cancer trials: implications for dosing of peptide vaccines. Expert Rev Vaccines 2011;10(2):201–10.

117. Ahmann DL, Creagan ET, Hahn RG, Edmonson JH, Bisel HF, Schaid DJ. Complete responses and long-term survivals after systemic chemotherapy for patients with advanced malignant melanoma. Cancer 1989;63(2):224–7.

118. Kirkwood JM, Strawderman MH, Ernstoff MS, Smith TJ, Borden EC, Blum RH. Interferon alfa-2b adjuvant therapy of high-risk resected cutaneous melanoma: the Eastern Cooperative Oncology Group Trial EST 1684. J. Clin. Onco. 1996;14(1):7–17.

119. Eggermont AMM, Suciu S, Santinami M, Testori A, Kruit WHJ, Marsden J, et al. Adjuvant therapy with pegylated interferon alfa-2b versus observation alone in resected stage III melanoma: final results of EORTC 18991, a randomised Phase III trial. Lancet 2008;372(9633):117–26.

120. Luke JJ, Hodi FS. Ipilimumab, vemurafenib, dabrafenib, and trametinib: synergistic competitors in the clinical management of BRAF mutant malignant melanoma. Oncologist 2013;18(6):717–25.

I. NOVEL THERAPEUTIC APPROACHES

121. Su F, Viros A, Milagre C, Trunzer K, Bollag G, Spleiss O, et al. RAS mutations in cutaneous squamous-cell carcinomas in patients treated with BRAF inhibitors. N. Engl. J. Med. 2012;366(3):207–15.

122. Atkins MB, Lotze MT, Dutcher JP, Fisher RI, Weiss G, Margolin K, et al. High-dose recombinant interleukin 2 therapy for patients with metastatic melanoma: analysis of 270 patients treated between 1985 and 1993. J. Clin. Oncol. 1999;17(7):2105–16.

123. Atkins MB, Kunkel L, Sznol M, Rosenberg SA. High-dose recombinant interleukin-2 therapy in patients with metastatic melanoma: long-term survival update. Cancer J. Sci. Am. 2000;6(Suppl. 1):S11–14.

124. Lee ML, Tomsu K, Von Eschen KB. Duration of survival for disseminated malignant melanoma: results of a meta-analysis. Melanoma Res. 2000;10(1):81–92.

125. Morton DL, Barth A. Vaccine therapy for malignant melanoma. CA Cancer J. Clin. 1996;46(4):225–44.

126. Morton DL, Foshag LJ, Hoon DS, Nizze JA, Famatiga E, Wanek LA, et al. Prolongation of survival in metastatic melanoma after active specific immunotherapy with a new polyvalent melanoma vaccine. Ann. Surg. 1992;216(4):463–82.

127. Lens M. The role of vaccine therapy in the treatment of melanoma. Expert Opin. Biol. Ther. 2008;8(3):315–23.

128. D'Souza B, Bhowmik T, Shashidharamurthy R, Oettinger C, Selvaraj P, D'Souza M. Oral microparticulate vaccine for melanoma using M-cell targeting. J Drug Target. 2012 Feb;20(2):166–73.

129. O'Hagan DT. Microparticles and polymers for the mucosal delivery of vaccines. Adv. Drug Deliv. Rev. 1998;34(2-3):305–20.

130. Stuart GCE. First-line treatment regimens and the role of consolidation therapy in advanced ovarian cancer. Gynecol. Oncol. 2003;90(3, Pt. 2):S8–15.

131. Leffers N, Daemen T, Boezen HM, Melief KJM, Nijman HW. Vaccine-based clinical trials in ovarian cancer. Expert Rev Vaccines 2011;10(6):775–84.

132. Thibodeaux SR, Curiel TJ. Immune therapy for ovarian cancer: promise and pitfalls. Int. Rev. Immunol. 2011;30(2-3):102–19.

133. Pengetnze Y, Steed M, Roby KF, Terranova PF, Taylor CC. Src tyrosine kinase promotes survival and resistance to chemotherapeutics in a mouse ovarian cancer cell line. Biochem. Biophys. Res. Commun. 2003;309(2):377–83.

134. Babai I, Samira S, Barenholz Y, Zakay-Rones Z, Kedar E. A novel influenza subunit vaccine composed of liposome-encapsulated haemagglutinin/neuraminidase and IL-2 or GM-CSF. II. Induction of TH1 and TH2 responses in mice. Vaccine 1999;17(9-10):1239–50.

135. Marinaro M, Boyaka PN, Finkelman FD, Kiyono H, Jackson RJ, Jirillo E, et al. Oral but not parenteral interleukin (IL)-12 redirects T helper 2 (Th2)-type responses to an oral vaccine without altering mucosal IgA responses. J. Exp. Med. 1997;185(3):415–27.

136. Benencia F, Courrèges MC, Conejo-García JR, Mohammed-Hadley A, Coukos G. Direct vaccination with tumor cells killed with ICP4-deficient HSVd120 elicits effective antitumor immunity. Cancer Biol. Ther. 2006;5(7):867–74.

137. Sharma RK, Srivastava AK, Yolcu ES, MacLeod KJ, Schabowsky R-H, Madireddi S, et al. SA-4-1BBL as the immunomodulatory component of a HPV-16 E7 protein based vaccine shows robust therapeutic efficacy in a mouse cervical cancer model. Vaccine 2010;28(36):5794–802.

Novel Generation of Antibody-Based Therapeutics

Randall J. Brezski

Principal Scientist, Biologics Research, Janssen R&D, LLC, USA

INTRODUCTION

Monoclonal antibodies (mAbs) are one of the fastest growing biological therapeutic agents, with as many as 28 approved mAbs in the United States and the European Union.[1] Approved mAb-based therapeutics have been used in the treatment of a broad array of diseases including autoimmune disorders, coronary artery disease, tissue transplantation, infectious disease, and cancer.[1] MAb therapies have been successful based on their diversity, selectivity, stability, solubility, tolerability, and long circulating half-life. The potential of mAb-based therapies is exemplified by the fact that there are currently more than 350 mAbs in the clinical pipeline.[2]

This chapter focuses on three categories for which mAbs are employed for therapeutic effect and reviews engineering strategies intended to improve clinical efficacy. One category,

Novel Approaches and Strategies for Biologics, Vaccines and Cancer Therapies. DOI: 10.1016/B978-0-12-416603-5.00006-7

antagonistic mAbs, involves blocking receptor–ligand interactions either by neutralizing soluble factors such as cytokines or by binding directly to a cell surface receptor and blocking its ability to engage ligand. A second group, agonistic mAbs, includes mAbs that engage cell surface targets and mimic the action of endogenous ligands. The third category, cytotoxic mAbs, involves binding to a cell surface receptor followed by recruitment of immune effector functions to destroy targeted cells, such as bacteria or cancer. Whereas the ability of a mAb to function as an antagonist is largely dependent on the selectivity of the mAb for targets, the second and third categories require that multiple parts of the antibody function in concert to engage the target while at the same time recruiting components of the immune system to either amplify agonist function or kill the targeted cell. Advances in protein engineering technologies have afforded investigators the ability to design fit-for-purpose antibody-based therapeutics where the functional properties for each of the aforementioned categories can be improved based on the intended therapeutic need.

IgG STRUCTURE

The basic composition of a monomeric immunoglobulin (Ig) consists of two identical Ig light chains (LCs) attached to two identical Ig heavy chains (HCs) by both noncovalent and disulfide bonds. In humans and mice, there are two dominant LC subclasses, kappa (κ) and lambda (λ), and five HC isotypes or subclasses: IgM, IgD, IgG, IgA, and IgE. At present, all of the approved mAbs are of the IgG subclass, which are the focus for the chapter. Each IgG LC consists of a single variable domain (V_L) and a single constant domain (C_L), and each IgG HC consists of a single variable domain (V_H) and three constant domains (C_H1, C_H2, and C_H3). The structure of an IgG consists of two fragment antigen-binding (Fab) arms linked to a single fragment crystalizable (Fc) domain by a flexible hinge region (Figure 6.1A). This structural

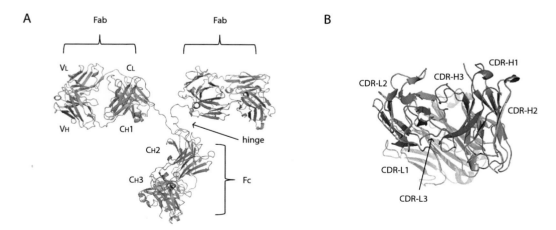

FIGURE 6.1   **Structure of an IgG.** (A) The IgG heavy chains are shown in purple and the light chains are shown in gray (PDBID: 1IGT). (B) Depiction of the antigen-binding region of an IgG within the variable region. CDR-L1, CDR-L2, and CDR-L3 are highlighted in green and CDR-H1, CDR-H2, and CDR-H3 are highlighted in magenta (PDBID: 1IGT). The figure was generated with PyMol.

organization affords IgGs the ability to engage target antigen through the Fab arms and then recruit humoral and cellular components of the immune system via the Fc region.

IgG interactions with cellular components of the immune system predominantly occur through immune cell-bearing Fc gamma receptors (FcγRs). In humans, there are three activating FcγRs: the high-affinity FcγRI, which is capable of binding to a monomeric antibody, and the lower affinity FcγRIIa and FcγRIIIa. Both human FcγRIIa and FcγRIIIa can be further divided by a lower affinity polymorphism (i.e., R131 for FcγRIIa and F158 for FcγRIIIa) and a higher affinity polymorphism (i.e., H131 for FcγRIIa and V158 for FcγRIIIa). Antibody Fc interactions with these activating receptors initiate phosphorylation of an immunoreceptor tyrosine-based activation motif (ITAM), which triggers a signaling cascade and ultimately stimulates immune effector functions such as antibody-dependent cellular cytotoxicity (ADCC) and antibody-dependent cellular phagocytosis (ADCP) (Figure 6.2A,B). Humans also have one inhibitory receptor, FcγRIIb,[3] which, in contrast to the activating receptors, contains an immunoreceptor tyrosine-based inhibitory motif (ITIM). Signaling through this receptor recruits tyrosine phosphatases, which opposes signal transduction through the activating FcγRs.[3] For the most part, IgG interactions with humoral components of the immune system are triggered by Fc binding to the C1q component of complement. This event leads to the recruitment of additional factors of the complement cascade, ultimately leading to the formation of the membrane attack complex and lysis of the targeted cell, a process often referred to as *complement-dependent cytotoxicity* (CDC) (Figure 6.2C).

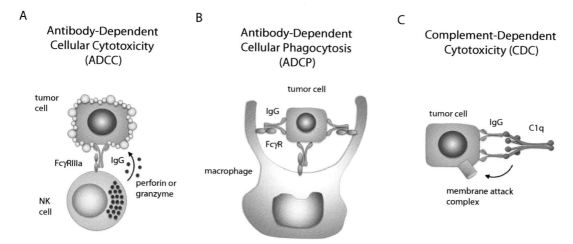

FIGURE 6.2 **Immune effector mechanisms recruited to kill mAb-targeted cells.** (A) Antibody-dependent cellular cytotoxicity (ADCC) is initiated when antibodies opsonize a tumor cell then recruit immune effectors cells through Fc interactions with FcγRs. This initiates a signal in the immune cell that causes the release of perforin and granzymes that will permeabilize the cellular membrane and induce apoptosis in the tumor cell. (B) Antibody-dependent cellular phagocytosis (ADCP) occurs when antibody-opsonized tumor cells recruit macrophages via Fc–FcγR interactions, resulting in engulfment and lysosome targeting and destruction of the tumor cell. (C) Classical complement-dependent cytotoxicity (CDC) requires antibody opsonization of a tumor cell, followed by fixation of C1q on the Fc portion of the IgG. This results in activation of a series of proteolytic events known as the complement cascade, ultimately leading to the formation of the membrane attack complex (MAC) and lysis of the tumor cell.

IgGs contain a complex carbohydrate attached to a conserved amino acid (N297) in the C_H2 domain. The core structure of this carbohydrate consists of *N*-acetylglucosamine (GlcNAc) and mannose, where additional modifications can include fucose, galactose, and sialic acid.[4] The structure of the carbohydrate can have a profound effect on Fc-dependent effector functions, and many glycoengineering efforts have been made to modulate effector function.

Amino acid residues located proximal to the C_H2/C_H3 junction can influence binding to the MHC class I-related receptor, also known as the neonatal Fc receptor (FcRn). Fc interactions with FcRn contribute to transporting IgG across the fetal/maternal barrier, in addition to protecting IgGs from catabolism, which contributes, in part, to the long circulating half-life of IgGs.[5] Numerous technologies have been employed to modulate mAb half-life.

Human IgGs are divided into four subclasses, IgG_1, IgG_2, IgG_3, and IgG_4. The nomenclature is based on the prevalence of IgGs found in human circulation, with IgG_1 having the highest amount (~60%), followed by IgG_2 (~25%), IgG_3 (~10%), and IgG_4 (~5%).[6] Currently, there are approved therapeutic mAbs that utilize the IgG_1, IgG_2, and IgG_4 subclasses, and the sequence alignments of the hinge and C_H2/C_H3 regions for these subclasses are shown in Figure 6.3A. As will be discussed, each subclass has distinct biophysical and functional properties. Further, a wealth of information about IgG structure and function has allowed investigators to engineer IgGs with unique properties in an attempt to fine-tune the mAb platform for the biology of the target.

GENERATION AND SELECTION OF ANTIBODY V-REGIONS

B cells and the antibodies they generate are integral components of the adaptive immune response. The mechanisms that regulate generation of B-cell antigen receptors (BCRs), which can subsequently be secreted as antibodies, result in an extraordinary amount of diversity in terms of the amount of antigens that antibodies can recognize. Heavy-chain diversity is initially regulated by a process known as V(D)J recombination, whereby gene segments known as the variable (V), diversity (D), and joining (J) segments are brought together to form the V_H domain. Light-chain diversity is initially regulated by VJ recombination to form the V_L domain. Further diversity occurs through contributions from somatic mechanisms such as somatic hypermutation[7] and gene conversion[8] and are concentrated within the complementarity-determining regions (CDRs). Each V_H contains three CDRs (CDR-H1, CDR-H2, and CDR-H3) and each V_L contains three CDRs (CDR-L1, CDR-L2, and CDR-L3). Each CDR is alternated with conserved regions known as framework regions (FRs). There are four regions in the V_L (FR-L1, FR-L2, FR-L3, and FR-L4) and four regions in the V_H (FR-H1, FR-H2, FR-H3, and FR-H4). These six CDRs are brought together via folding and noncovalent associations to form the antigen-binding site (Figure 6.1B) and are responsible for the specificity of antigen recognition as well as the affinity for the antigen. As shown in Figure 6.1B, CDR-L3 and CDR-H3 are located centrally in the antigen-binding site and are often considered the most critical CDRs for antigen recognition.

Hybridoma technology was a key enabling breakthrough for the field of monoclonal antibodies. This technology involves immunizing a host animal, typically a BALB/c mouse, then isolating B cells from the spleen or lymph nodes. The B cells are then fused with an immortalized myeloma cell, resulting in a cell line that can stably produce a single antibody

A

	Upper hinge												Core hinge				Lower hinge						
EU	214	215	216	217	218	219	220	221	222	223	224	225	226	227	228	229	230	231	232	233	234	235	236
IgG1	K	V	E	P	K	S	C	D	K	T	H	T	C	P	P	C	P	A	P	E	L	L	G
IgG2	T	V	E	R	K	C	C	-	V	-	E	-	C	P	P	C	P	A	P	P	V	A	
IgG4	R	V	E	S	K	Y	G	-	-	-	-	P	C	P	S	C	P	A	P	E	F	L	G

	start CH2																						
EU	237	238	239	240	241	242	243	244	245	246	247	248	249	250	251	252	253	254	255	256	257	258	259
IgG1	G	P	S	V	F	L	F	P	P	K	P	K	D	T	L	M	I	S	R	T	P	E	V
IgG2	G	P	S	V	F	L	F	P	P	K	P	K	D	T	L	M	I	S	R	T	P	E	V
IgG4	G	P	S	V	F	L	F	P	P	K	P	K	D	T	L	M	I	S	R	T	P	E	V

EU	260	261	262	263	264	265	266	267	268	269	270	271	272	273	274	275	276	277	278	279	280	281	282
IgG1	T	C	V	V	V	D	V	S	H	E	D	P	E	V	K	F	N	W	Y	V	D	G	V
IgG2	T	C	V	V	V	D	V	S	H	E	D	P	E	V	Q	F	N	W	Y	V	D	G	V
IgG4	T	C	V	V	V	D	V	S	Q	E	D	P	E	V	Q	F	N	W	Y	V	D	G	V

													N-linked glycosylation site										
EU	283	284	285	286	287	288	289	290	291	292	293	294	295	296	297	298	299	300	301	302	303	304	305
IgG1	E	V	H	N	A	K	T	K	P	R	E	E	Q	Y	N	S	T	Y	R	V	V	S	V
IgG2	E	V	H	N	A	K	T	K	P	R	E	E	Q	F	N	S	T	F	R	V	V	S	V
IgG4	E	V	H	N	A	K	T	K	P	R	E	E	Q	F	N	S	T	Y	R	V	V	S	V

EU	306	307	308	309	310	311	312	313	314	315	316	317	318	319	320	321	322	323	324	325	326	327	328
IgG1	L	T	V	L	H	Q	D	W	L	N	G	K	E	Y	K	C	K	V	S	N	K	A	L
IgG2	L	T	V	V	H	Q	D	W	L	N	G	K	E	Y	K	C	K	V	S	N	K	A	L
IgG4	L	T	V	L	H	Q	D	W	L	N	G	K	E	Y	K	C	K	V	S	N	K	G	L

												start CH3											
EU	329	330	331	332	333	334	335	336	337	338	339	340	341	342	343	344	345	346	347	348	349	350	351
IgG1	P	A	P	I	E	K	T	I	S	K	A	K	G	Q	P	R	E	P	Q	V	Y	T	L
IgG2	P	A	P	I	E	K	T	I	S	K	T	K	G	Q	P	R	E	P	Q	V	Y	T	L
IgG4	P	S	S	I	E	K	T	I	S	K	A	K	G	Q	P	R	E	P	Q	V	Y	T	L

EU	352	353	354	355	356	357	358	359	360	361	362	363	364	365	366	367	368	369	370	371	372	373	374
IgG1	P	P	S	R	D	E	L	T	K	N	Q	V	S	L	T	C	L	V	K	G	F	Y	P
IgG2	P	P	S	R	E	E	M	T	K	N	Q	V	S	L	T	C	L	V	K	G	F	Y	P
IgG4	P	P	S	Q	E	E	M	T	K	N	Q	V	S	L	T	C	L	V	K	G	F	Y	P

EU	375	376	377	378	379	380	381	382	383	384	385	386	387	388	389	390	391	392	393	394	395	396	397
IgG1	S	D	I	A	V	E	W	E	S	N	G	Q	P	E	N	N	Y	K	T	T	P	P	V
IgG2	S	D	I	S	V	E	W	E	S	N	G	Q	P	E	N	N	Y	K	T	T	P	P	V
IgG4	S	D	I	A	V	E	W	E	S	N	G	Q	P	E	N	N	Y	K	T	T	P	P	M

EU	398	399	400	401	402	403	404	405	406	407	408	409	410	411	412	413	414	415	416	417	418	419	420
IgG1	L	D	S	D	G	S	F	F	L	Y	S	K	L	T	V	D	K	S	R	W	Q	Q	G
IgG2	L	D	S	D	G	S	F	F	L	Y	S	K	L	T	V	D	K	S	R	W	Q	Q	G
IgG4	L	D	S	D	G	S	F	F	L	Y	S	R	L	T	V	D	K	S	R	W	Q	E	G

EU	421	422	423	424	425	426	427	428	429	430	431	432	433	434	435	436	437	438	439	440	441	442	443
IgG1	N	V	F	S	C	S	V	M	H	E	A	L	H	N	H	Y	T	Q	K	S	L	S	L
IgG2	N	V	F	S	C	S	V	M	H	E	A	L	H	N	H	Y	T	Q	K	S	L	S	L
IgG4	N	V	F	S	C	S	V	M	H	E	A	L	H	N	H	Y	T	Q	K	S	L	S	L

EU	444	445	446	447
IgG1	S	P	G	K
IgG2	S	P	G	K
IgG4	S	L	G	K

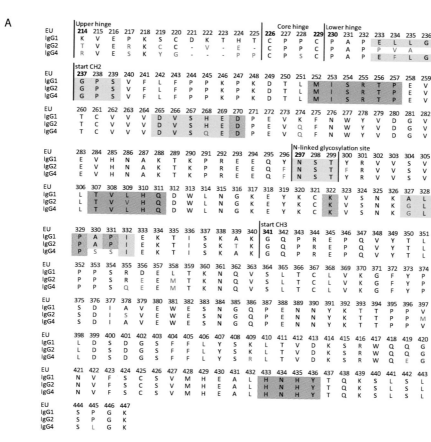

B

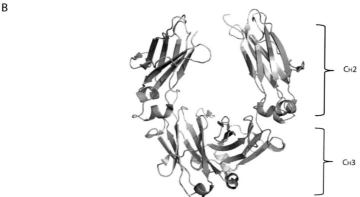

FIGURE 6.3 **Sequence alignment and critical motifs for Fc functional activity.** (A) Sequence alignment of the hinge, C$_H$2, and C$_H$3 regions of human IgG$_1$, IgG$_2$, and IgG$_4$, the three human IgG subclasses currently utilized in approved mAb therapeutics. Sequence differences of IgG$_2$ and IgG$_4$ that are distinct from IgG$_1$ are highlighted in red. Numbers correspond to the Kabat numbering system aligned to the human IgG$_1$ EU sequence.[117] Key motifs for interactions with FcγRs are highlighted in yellow, and key motifs for interactions with FcRn are highlighted in green. The four amino acids deemed critical for interactions with the C1q component of complement are highlighted in blue. This figure is adapted from the one previously published by Strohl.[118] (B) A depiction of the lower hinge, C$_H$2, and C$_H$3 regions of the human IgG$_1$ Fc is shown (PDBID: 3AVE). The same amino acids in the linear sequence as highlighted above are shown in the three-dimensional structure. Note that key recognition motifs for FcγR and C1q binding (yellow and blue, respectively) are present at the top of the C$_H$2 region, and key FcRn recognition motifs (green) are present at the interface of the C$_H$2 and C$_H$3 region. Figure 6.3B was generated with PyMol.

clone, which is advantageous for large-scale production.[9] V-region sourcing from hybridomas utilizes the endogenous BCR generation process to generate antibodies specific for a given target. This approach was used to produce the first therapeutic antibody approved for use in humans, the anti-CD3 murine IgG$_{2a}$ mAb muromonab-CD3 (OKT3). However, it was realized early on that administration of a murine antibody into humans elicited antibodies against the murine variable and constant domains, which could neutralize the function of the mAb and contribute to rapid clearance of the mAb upon successive dosing.[10–12]

Early antibody engineering efforts to reduce immunogenicity against murine components of the IgG involved a process known as *chimerization*, whereby the murine constant regions were replaced with the human counterparts.[13] This approach was successfully adopted by investigators at Centocor for the second approved therapeutic mAb, abciximab, a Fab fragment recognizing GPIIb/IIIa that contains a murine variable region and human C$_H$1 and C$_L$ regions.[14] Further engineering technologies included humanization,[15] the use of phage display technologies to screen human antibodies *in vitro*,[16] and the generation of transgenic mice that encode human variable and constant regions.[17] At present, all of these technologies are being utilized to source V-regions with the appropriate specificity and affinity as well as attempt to limit immunogenicity.[18]

ENGINEERING FIT-FOR-PURPOSE ANTIBODY-BASED THERAPEUTICS

Overview of IgG Fc Interactions with the FcγRs and Complement

Immunoglobulins are among the most well-characterized proteins studied to date, and this wealth of information has been used to modify the biochemical, biophysical, and functional aspects of IgGs.[18] Detailed analyses of the different IgG subclasses combined with mutational studies have provided a framework of knowledge from which many subsequent engineering efforts derived. A review of several early papers that defined key IgG Fc recognition motifs for both FcγR and complement binding follows. One of the first studies to implicate a consensus sequence in the lower hinge/proximal C$_H$2 region of IgGs (Figure 6.3A) was published by Woof et al.,[19] where the authors examined different human IgG subclasses and IgG subclasses from different species for their ability to bind to human monocytes or the human cell lines U937 or HL-60 (both of which are of myeloid lineage). These studies indicated that human IgG$_1$ and IgG$_4$ bound to monocytes, with IgG$_4$ having approximately tenfold less affinity. An additional observation in this study was that when the sequences of immune function capable antibodies were aligned with the sequences of non-immune activating subclasses between different species (e.g., human, mouse, rabbit, guinea pig), those antibodies capable of activating immune function had conserved sequences in the both the lower hinge and C$_H$2 region, whereas non-immune activating subclass sequences did not share these common motifs. Jefferis et al.[20] designed a series of single-point mutations in the lower hinge region of IgG$_3$, including L234A, L235A or L235E, G236A, and G237A. The authors found that the mutations L234A, L235A or L235E, and G237A all decreased rosette formation with U937 cells—a functional assessment for FcγR-binding—whereas the mutation of G236A had little effect. Canfield and Morrison[21] published a series of recombinant IgG_2/IgG_3 molecules. In this study, they performed exon shuffling experiments between IgG_2 and IgG_3 and used a four-number designation for each construct. For example, a construct designated 2-2-2-3 would have IgG_2 C_H1, IgG_2 hinge, IgG_2 C_H2, and IgG_3 C_H3. It is important to note that in this study the authors' designation of the C_H2 domain includes the lower hinge, such that the C_H2 domain of IgG_2 would start with A231, whereas currently the start of the C_H2 region more commonly begins with the amino acid stretch G237–P238–S239 (Figure 6.3A). The study indicated that the C_H3 domain of either IgG_2 or IgG_3 did not contribute to FcγRI-binding. Rather, the C_H2 domain of IgG_2 abrogated FcγRI binding, whereas the C_H2 domain of IgG_3 allowed FcγRI binding. Another interesting finding was that the construct 2-2-3-2 bound to FcγRI with an affinity of $2.8 \times 10^8 \, M^{-1}$ (compared to IgG_3 $1.2 \times 10^9 \, M^{-1}$). This finding suggested that the sequence disparity in the upper hinge of IgG_2 (T214–VERKCCV–E224 compared to K214–VEPKSCDKTH–T225 of IgG_1) does not completely block FcγRI binding, further implicating the lower hinge/proximal C_H2 as critical for interactions with FcγRs. Chappel et al.[22] published a series of recombinant IgG_1/IgG_2 hybrid molecules and showed that inclusion of the lower hinge/proximal C_H2 domain of IgG_2 (including A231–P232–P233–V234–A235 with G236 deleted) abolished FcγRI binding. Inclusion of the lower hinge/proximal C_H2 domain of IgG_1 (including A231–P232–E233–L234–L235–G236) into IgG_2 restored binding to FcγRI. They went on to perform single-point mutations of the lower hinge of IgG_1 into IgG_2 and *vice versa*. All point mutations of IgG_2 into IgG_1 (with the exception of L234V) abolished FcγRI binding of IgG_1. In contrast, point mutations of the lower hinge/proximal C_H2 of IgG_1 into IgG_2 did not restore effector function. Only the triple mutant (V234L–A235L and addition of G236) or complete substitution of the lower hinge of IgG_1 into IgG_2 (P233E–V234L–A235L and addition of G236) restored binding to FcγRI. This study specifically implicated the entire stretch of E233–L234–L235–G236–G237 as critical for FcγRI binding.

A study published by Lund et al.[23] used a series of point mutations in the lower hinge of IgG_3 to determine binding to either FcγRI or FcγRII (the study does not distinguish between activating FcγRIIa and inhibitory FcγRIIb). For FcγRI binding, the mutation of L235E resulted in a 100-fold reduction in binding, whereas the mutation of L235A only showed a 10-fold decrease as determined by competition binding to U937 cells. The G236A mutation did not affect FcγRII binding; instead, L234A and G237A reduced binding to FcγRII as determined by rosette formation with Daudi cells, which only express FcγRII. This study also indicated the importance of G237 in both FcγRI and FcγRII binding. A study published by Sarmay et al.[24] expanded on the previously reported series of single-point mutations in the lower hinge of IgG_3 to look at Fc-mediated effector function (i.e., rosette formation or cell lysis) by U937 cells, HL-60 cells, and NK cells. The results indicated that for NK-cell-mediated lysis, individual mutations of L234A, L235A, L235E, or G237A all decreased lysis, whereas the mutation G236A had little effect on lysis. This study concluded that the lower hinge of IgGs contributed to interactions with all three FcγRs, but the individual binding sites are not necessarily equivalent. Parren and colleagues[25] modified the lower hinge of IgG_1 with L234A–L235A and demonstrated both a loss in FcγR function as well as complement activation.

The importance of the lower hinge/proximal C_H2 region is perhaps further exemplified by the observation that many physiologically relevant proteases secreted by pathogenic bacteria and invasive cancers specifically cleave IgGs within this region, which results in a profound loss of Fc-dependent cell-killing functions.[26] Several groups have demonstrated that cleavage of amino acids within the E233–G237 stretch of amino acids in human IgG$_1$ by physiologically relevant proteases occurs in a two-step process, where the first heavy-chain lesion generates a singly-cleaved intermediate.[27-30] Cleavage of the opposing heavy chain results in the complete dissociation of the Fc fragment from the F(ab′)$_2$ fragment. The singly-cleaved intermediate displays a loss of ADCC and CDC activity *in vitro* and a loss of cell-killing functions *in vivo*.[27,31] Investigators at Centocor demonstrated that the singly-cleaved intermediate accumulates on the surface of mAb-opsonized cancer cells in the presence of an IgG-cleaving protease.[27] Von Pawel-Rammingen and colleagues[32] recently demonstrated that during *in vitro* proteolysis reactions nearly all of the IgG is converted to the singly-cleaved intermediate before cleavage of the second heavy chain is observed. Interestingly, the singly-cleaved intermediate maintains antigen-binding capabilities as well as the long circulating half-life of intact IgGs.[27] As such, several groups have suggested that cleavage of IgGs may function as an immune evasion mechanism to subvert host immune responses by specifically disabling a critical recognition motif for Fc-dependent cell-killing functions.[26,33]

Taken together, these studies indicated that the lower hinge/proximal C$_H$2 region of IgG spanning residues from Kabat 233 to 237 are critical for interactions with FcγRs and complement; as will be discussed, some of the earliest attempts to engineer fit-for-purpose mAbs for therapeutic intervention focused on modifying this region.

Detailed studies of each human IgG subclass have also provided many insights later used to engineer fit-for-purpose mAbs including both modifications to render the Fc silent or to enhance Fc effector functions. Human IgG$_1$ and IgG$_3$ are traditionally considered the most immune function activating subclasses due to potent ADCC and CDC, whereas human IgG$_2$ and IgG$_4$ were considered silent due to their inability to elicit either ADCC or CDC.[34] However, although IgG$_2$ and IgG$_4$ are silent in terms of ADCC and CDC, both are capable of eliciting ADCP. Although IgG$_2$ has markedly reduced binding to FcγRI and FcγRIIIa, IgG$_2$ demonstrates binding to FcγRIIa H131[35] and is capable of eliciting immune effector functions from myeloid cell-bearing FcγRIIa.[36,37] Additionally, IgG$_2$s can form covalent dimers with other IgG$_2$s, which may augment agonist activity.[38] IgG$_2$ can also undergo disulfide isomerism in the upper hinge, which has been linked to a decrease in potency.[39,40] Although human IgG$_4$ has reduced binding to FcγRIIa and FcγRIIIa, it only has about a tenfold decrease in binding to FcγRI compared to IgG$_1$.[19] Monocytes and macrophages can express FcγRI, and numerous studies have demonstrated that IgG$_4$ is capable of eliciting monocyte/macrophage-mediated cell killing,[41,42] and IgG$_4$-mediated depletion of target cells has been demonstrated in humans.[43] Native IgG$_4$ can also undergo a process known as Fab arm exchange both *in vitro* and *in vivo*, where the Fab-Fc half of one IgG$_4$ exchanges with the Fab-Fc of another IgG$_4$, resulting in a bispecific molecule and functional monovalency.[44,45] There are two factors which contribute to Fab-arm exchange, one deriving from an instability of the intra-heavy-chain disulfide bonds in the core hinge region due to the presence of a S228 (Figure 6.3A), and the second involves weak noncovalent associations in the C$_H$3 region of IgG$_4$ compared to other isotypes.[45,46] Taken together, although these studies have provided many insights into both the silent and immune-activating aspects of human IgG$_2$ and IgG$_4$, they also demonstrate that unmodified versions of these subclasses contain individual idiosyncrasies that make them unsuitable as truly silent Fc platforms.

Antibody Engineering for Reduced or Silent Effector Function

In cases where the intended mechanism of action of a mAb is to engage a receptor on the surface of a cell but not to deplete the target cell population, it may be desirable to engineer out immune effector function.[47] Other indications where binding to FcγRs would be unwanted include the use of antibody–drug conjugates (ADCs), where unintended binding to FcγRs on immune cells could lead to off-target cytotoxicity (e.g., leukopenia). Additionally, FcγR interactions with a mAb bound to a cell surface receptor can lead to crosslinking of the targeted receptor. In some cases, unintentional crosslinking can convert an antagonist mAb into an agonist.[47] Crosslinking has also led to immune cell activation and cytokine storm, a situation that has led to adverse events in the clinical setting. Therefore, efforts to silence interactions with both FcγRs and complement have been underway for over 20 years.

There are several examples where unwanted interactions with FcγRs have led to adverse events in the clinical setting. The first approved mAb for treatment in humans was the anti-CD3 epsilon mAb muromonab-CD3 (also known as OKT3), which was a murine IgG$_{2a}$. The therapeutic intent for OKT3 was to prevent T-cell responses in cases where patients received tissue transplants, including a donor heart, lung, or kidney.[48] However, in many cases, treatment with OKT3 led to adverse events ascribed in part to increased levels of proinflammatory cytokines,[49] which were attributed to OKT3 Fc interactions with FcγRs.[50–52] This induction of cytokines contributed to the removal of murine IgG$_{2a}$ OKT3 from the clinic. Unintended agonist activity with the IgG$_4$ anti-CD28 mAb, TGN1412, elicited cytokine storm and multiorgan failure in a Phase I clinical trial.[53] Several groups have speculated that residual binding to FcγRs, particularly FcγRI, may have contributed to the catastrophic adverse events associated with the administration of TGN1412 in humans.[6,54] These observations argue for the importance of engineering silent platforms for use in the clinical setting.

Some of the earliest attempts to generate silent mAbs involved complete removal of the glycan at N297, which was historically accomplished by mutation of the N-linked glycosylation site with either N297A or N297Q[55,56] or more recently N297G.[57] Aglycosylated IgGs demonstrated low to undetectable binding to FcγRs and complement under monomeric conditions. However, it was noted early on that aglycosylated IgGs maintain detectable levels of FcγR binding under conditions that take into account the sum of multimeric interactions between antigen-engaged IgGs and FcγRs, a situation known as avidity-based binding.[55] More recently, Nesspor et al.[41] compared aglycosylated IgG binding under both monomeric and avidity-based conditions. As expected, under monomeric conditions, binding to FcγRs on immune cells was not detected. In contrast, when aglycosylated IgGs were tested under avidity-based conditions, not only was binding detected, but also the aglycosylated IgG was capable of driving macrophage-based ADCP comparable to an IgG$_1$ WT in the absence of any competing IgG. The inclusion of 10% competing serum abrogated the ability of the aglycosylated IgG to elicit ADCP, suggesting that aglycosylated therapeutic IgG would remain silent in human circulation, where the level of IgGs in serum can range from 10 to 20 mg/mL.

As was reviewed above, the lower hinge/proximal C$_H$2 region is typically considered critical to elicit immune function. Several early attempts to render IgGs silent by mutating the lower hinge/proximal C$_H$2 were intended to reduce or eliminate the cytokine storm elicited by OKT3. Bluestone and colleagues[52] generated variants including the IgG$_4$ mutations of either L235E or F234A-L235A[50,51] and the human IgG$_1$ variant L234A-L235A. All of these variants demonstrated decreased binding to FcγRs and, in turn, lower induction of cytokines.

More recent attempts to engineer IgG-based mAbs devoid of Fc effector functions have included substituting amino acids from different subclasses to generate novel silent platforms. The approved anticomplement protein C5 mAb eculizumab is used to inhibit the complement cascade in patients with paroxysmal nocturnal hemoglobinuria, which causes the depletion of red blood cells.[58] The investigators desired a silent Fc platform and achieved this by shuffling the domains of IgG$_2$ and IgG$_4$,[58] two subclasses with limited effector functions relative to IgG$_1$. Eculizumab contains the Kabat sequences stretching from 118 to 260 of IgG$_2$ and 261 to 447 of IgG$_4$ (see Figure 6.3A) and as such does not elicit immune effector function.[59] The successful use of eculizumab in humans provides proof-of-concept that silenced Fc platforms can be incorporated in fit-for-purpose therapeutic strategies.

A study by Williamson and colleagues[61] introduced the IgG$_2$ residues P233–V234–A235 and deletion of G236 in place of the IgG$_1$ residues E233–L234–L235–G236,[60] which decreased binding to FcγRs. The authors used the domain swap approach because they reasoned that exchanging residues between two different IgG subclasses would decrease the chance of immunogenicity compared to incorporating novel amino acid substitutions. A later refinement of this strategy by the same group involved mutating multiple amino acid residues in an active subclass (e.g., IgG$_1$) to corresponding residues in a more silent subclass (e.g., IgG$_2$, IgG$_4$). The authors generated the variant K214T–E233P–L234V–L235A–(G236-deleted)–A327G–A330S–P331S–D356E–L358M for reduced FcγR-binding and complement activation. Investigators at Merck engineered a variant of IgG$_2$, termed IgG$_2$m4, containing the mutations H268Q–V309L–A330S–P331S, which had reduced Fc functionality but maintained comparable half-life in rhesus monkeys compared to IgG$_1$.[62] This finding was perhaps not unexpected, as the recognition motifs for FcγR/C1q interactions are distal from FcRn recognition motifs (see Figure 6.3B). Leabman et al.[57] further assessed whether silencing mutations (e.g., N297A, N297G, L234–L235A) affects half-life by performing a comprehensive half-life analysis in cynomolgus monkeys. They demonstrated comparable half-lives for all tested variants tested compared to IgG$_1$ WT controls. These results indicated that engineering approaches could be utilized to reduce Fc effector function without adversely affecting half-life.

Investigators at Janssen Research & Development recently engineered a silent platform based on the IgG$_2$ subclass, termed IgG$_{2\sigma}$ (V234A–G237A–P238S–H268A–V309L–A330S–P331S), with the intent to abrogate all immune effector functions as assessed by both monomeric and avidity-based binding assays.[54] This variant demonstrated the highest reduction in Fc effector functions compared to other silent platforms such as an aglycosylated IgG$_1$, IgG$_2$m4,[62] or an IgG$_4$ variant with F234A–L235A.[51] Additionally, the three-dimensional structure of the Fc of IgG$_{2\sigma}$ was solved, and modeling studies were performed to assess how the mutations may have affected binding to FcγRs and complement activation. The results demonstrated that conformational changes at position P329 potentially abrogate binding to FcγRs, and structural changes at both positions D270 and P329 could negatively impact binding to the C1q component of complement.

As was mentioned previously, there are some cases when mAb-mediated crosslinking of a receptor can initiate a signaling cascade through the receptor, which would confound the mechanism of action if the mAb is intended as an antagonist. For example, bivalent antibodies targeting the receptor tyrosine kinase cMET can often trigger tyrosine phosphorylation and at times augment motility and invasive growth of tumor cells expressing cMET.[63] Fab fragments would not elicit receptor crosslinking and have been previously approved for use as human therapeutics (e.g., abciximab, ranibizumab, certolizumab pegol);[1] however, Fab fragments have a very short *in vivo* half-life due to the lack of Fc interactions with FcRn. In order to generate an antibody devoid of receptor crosslinking activity that maintains normal half-life, researchers at Genentech engineered a monovalent mAb platform. This was accomplished using a knobs-into-holes technology[64] whereby a single heavy-chain/light-chain heterodimer containing a "hole" (T366S–L368A–Y407V) could pair with a hinge–C_H1–C_H2 Fc fragment containing a "knob" (T366W), resulting in a single Fab arm linked to an Fc.[65] Additionally, the monovalent mAb construct was produced in *Escherichia coli* and was not glycosylated, further limiting the ability of FcγR-mediated clustering. This technology incorporates two silencing engineering strategies into a single molecular entity (i.e., non-crosslinking monovalency and reduced Fc effector function due to aglycosylation), representing a new class of silent Fc platform. At the time of the writing of this chapter, Genentech's MetMAb (anti-MET monovalent monoclonal antibody), onartuzumab, was entered into clinical trials for the treatment of glioblastoma, liver cancer, gastric cancer, non-small-cell lung cancer, colorectal cancer, and breast cancer (see http://clinicaltrials.gov).

Antibody Engineering for Enhanced Effector Function

The mechanism of action for many anticancer therapeutic antibodies is thought to rely, in part, on the ability of the Fc region of the mAb to interact with cellular and serum components of the immune system. Additionally, in some cases, clinical studies suggested that individuals expressing higher affinity FcγR polymorphisms (i.e., FcγRIIa H131 and FcγRIIIa V158) had increased progression-free survival compared to patients expressing lower affinity polymorphisms (i.e., FcγRIIa R131 and FcγRIIIa F158).[66–68] Therefore, many initial attempts to enhance effector function were often designed to augment the ability of antibodies to bind to activating FcγRs, thereby increasing the ability of the mAb to facilitate ADCC or ADCP. Augmenting FcγR-dependent binding has been accomplished by modifying the glycan attached to N297 or by altering the sequence of the Fc region. Other attempts have been made to increase the ability of a mAb to interact with the C1q component of complement, thereby increasing CDC. However, as will be discussed later in this section, recent evidence has suggested that increasing the ability of a mAb to bind to the inhibitory FcγRIIb can augment mAb-mediated agonist activity, particularly in the case for agonistic mAb's targeting tumor necrosis factor alpha (TNFα) superfamily members.[69]

Glycoengineering for Altered Effector Function

Because the Fc glycan can have a profound effect on modulating interactions with FcγRs and complement, many investigators have modified the content of the glycan in an attempt to augment Fc effector functions. Umana and colleagues[70] utilized a Chinese hamster ovary (CHO) cell line expressing β(1,4)-N-acetylglucosaminyltransferase III to glycoengineer mAbs to express bisected oligosaccharides and demonstrated increased ADCC activity relative to controls. Genentech researchers later used an engineered CHO cell line to produce mAbs that were devoid of fucose content and showed that afucosylation alone was sufficient to augment

ADCC activity up to 50-fold.[71] Shinkawa et al.[72] later demonstrated that the lack of fucose on the Fc glycan had a greater impact on improving ADCC function compared to the presence of bisected oligosaccharides. These initial studies focused on glycoengineering human IgG_1 mAbs for improved ADCC activity. However, Niwa et al.[73] demonstrated that augmented ADCC with afucosylated mAbs was not limited to the IgG_1 subclass alone. In particular, they demonstrated that afucosylation of both human IgG_2 and IgG_4 resulted in detectable ADCC activity, whereas the normal fucose parental mAbs did not have detectable ADCC. Additionally, lowering the overall fucose content can augment $Fc\gamma RIIIa$ binding and Fc functional activity,[74,75] demonstrating that absolute afucosylation is not required to generate mAbs with enhanced ADCC. There are now many different platforms to lower or remove fucose content on IgGs, including Kyowa Hakko Kirin's Potelligent® technology,[76] Merck-GlycoFi's yeast technology,[77] and Roche-Glycart's GlycoMAb® technology.[78]

There are several perceived benefits for using glycoengineering technologies to lower the fucose content on IgGs. Shields et al.[71] demonstrated that afucosylated mAbs generated from their glycoengineered Chinese hamster ovary (CHO) cells had oligosaccharides comparable to other mAbs produced in normal CHO cells as well as oligosaccharides found on IgGs from human serum. Therefore, because normal human serum (NHS) had comparable oligosaccharide patterns, and afucosylated IgGs are present in NHS, it is suggested that the absence of fucose would not induce immunogenicity. Lower fucosylated IgGs can also increase NK cell ADCC activity with peripheral blood mononuclear cell (PBMC) donors that express the low-affinity polymorphism of $Fc\gamma RIIIa$, F158.[79] Ferrara et al.[80,81] have demonstrated the putative mechanism responsible for improved binding of afucosylated IgGs to $Fc\gamma RIIIa$. Human $Fc\gamma RIIIa$ contains a glycan at N162, and the lack of fucose allows carbohydrate/carbohydrate interactions between the Fc and $Fc\gamma RIIIa$, increasing the strength of binding. The presence of fucose weakens these interactions. The increased affinity for $Fc\gamma RIIIa$ is thought to play a key role in eliciting ADCC in the presence of competing serum. Preither et al.[82] determined that very high concentrations of mAb are required to drive ADCC in the presence of competing IgG compared to ADCC assays performed in the absence of competing IgG. Several groups have now shown that mAbs with decreased fucose content can facilitate ADCC in the presence of competing IgGs, whereas mAbs containing normal fucose levels have weak to undetectable ADCC activity.[83,84]

Two recent cases where glycoengineered technologies to reduce fucosylation have made an impact during clinical trials include the anti-CCR4 mogamulizumab and the anti-CD20 obinutuzumab. Mogamulizumab is indicated for the treatment of relapsed or refractory CCR4-positive T-cell leukemia-lymphoma and represents the first approved glycoengineered mAb (received approval in Japan in 2012). Mogamulizumab was generated using Kyowa Hakko Kirin's Potelligent® technology.[85] Obinutuzumab (also known as GA101) is produced by Roche-Glycart's GlycoMAb® technology to reduce fucosylation[84] and was granted the breakthrough therapy designation by the U.S. Food and Drug Administration (FDA) in 2013.[2] Obinutuzumab utilizes two engineering approaches to improve efficacy. One approach includes reduced fucosylation in the Fc, and the other involves an alteration in the elbow hinge region, an area that can impact the flexibility of the Fab domains.[84] Obinutuzumab was humanized from a parental murine anti-CD20, B-ly1, and during the humanization process a leucine present in the FR-1 of the murine mAb was converted to a valine. This modification resulted in a change in the elbow hinge angle, which the authors suggested increased the direct cell death induction elicited by this type II anti-CD20 mAb.[84] The successful use of mogamulizumab and breakthrough designation for obinutuzumab demonstrate that enhanced effector function Fc platforms can be incorporated in fit-for-purpose therapeutic strategies.

Investigators are now adopting additional glycoengineering approaches to improve the efficacy of mAbs. One example involves rendering the glycan resistant to endoglycosidase activity. The *Streptococcus pyogenes* endoglycosidase S (EndoS) hydrolyzes the glycan on native IgG,[86] which has been demonstrated to block the activity of pathogenic antibodies *in vivo*,[87] presumably due to decreased ability of the glycan-hydrolyzed IgGs to elicit immune effector functions. Based on the glycan-hydrolyzing efficiency of EndoS, investigators have suggested that treatment with a therapeutic preparation of EndoS may be a means to ameliorate autoimmune conditions associated with pathogenic autoantibodies.[87] Baruah et al.[88] developed an approach where they engineered the IgG glycan to be resistant to EndoS activity. By coadministering EndoS and a therapeutic mAb containing an EndoS-resistant glycan into human serum, the investigators were able to significantly increase the FcγRIIIa-binding capacity of their glycoengineered mAb. These studies demonstrate the potential utility of glycoengineering beyond merely modulating the fucose content.

Amino Acid Modifications to Enhance Fc Effector Function

Numerous methodologies have been employed to augment FcγR binding by modifying the amino acid sequence, including domain exchange among human IgG subclasses, alanine scanning, random mutagenesis, computational structure-based analysis, and molecular evolution strategies employed in both bacteria and yeast.[34] Researchers at Genentech performed an alanine scan of almost all of the solvent-exposed residues in the C_H2/C_H3 region of IgG_1 to identify single amino acid residues that influence binding to FcγRs.[89] By combining multiple mutations that augmented FcγR-binding, they were able to generate combinatorial variants with improved ADCC activity (e.g., S298A–E333A–K334A). Investigators at Xencor utilized computational three-dimensional modeling and high-throughput screening to identify variants with increased binding to FcγRs.[90] The variants S239D–I332E and S239D–A330L–I332E had increased ADCC activity. The main difference among the two variants was that the addition of A330L ablated CDC activity, affording the ability to fine-tune effector functions. The crystal structure of an Fc fragment containing the S239D–A330L–I332E mutations was solved, and modeling studies suggested that the enhanced ADCC activity may be due to additional hydrogen bonds, hydrophobic contacts, and/or electrostatic interactions.[91] Xencor investigators also engineered a variant with improved binding to FcγRIIa (G236A–S239D–I332E), which demonstrated increased ADCP activity.[92] As of the writing of this chapter, an anti-CD19 mAb with one of Xencor's augmented FcγR-binding variants (S239D–I332E)[93] is currently being utilized by MorphoSys AG in Phase II clinical trials for the treatment of B-cell acute lymphoblastic leukemia (B-ALL) and non-Hodgkin lymphoma (NHL) (see http://clinicaltrials.gov). Researchers at Macrogenics employed a yeast surface display technology to screen a library of Fc variants and identified a number of constructs (e.g., F243L–R292P–Y300L–V305I–P396L) with increased binding to FcγRs and enhanced ADCC.[94] A Macrogenics anti-HER2 mAb, MGAH22 or margetuximab, with enhanced ADCC activity[95] is currently in Phase II clinical trials for the treatment of metastatic breast cancer (see http://clinicaltrials.gov).

Several groups have modified the sequence of the Fc to improve binding to the C1q component of complement with the intent to augment CDC function. Genentech researchers demonstrated that the mutations of K326W–E333S confer CDC activity to human IgG_2, a subclass that is otherwise devoid of classical CDC. The authors suggested that mutations at these two positions influence structural associations between C1q and the Fc.[96] An Fc variant engineered by investigators at Kyowa Hakko Kirin that mixed the C_H1 and hinge region of IgG_1 with the C_H2 and C_H3 regions of IgG_3 (termed 1133) demonstrated augmented CDC activity relative to an IgG_1. Key differences among IgG_1 and IgG_3 reside in the C_H2 domain (e.g., K274Q–N276K–Y300F) proximal to the residues D270–K322–P329–P331, which have been deemed critical for C1q interactions with human IgG.[97,98] However, since the 1133 variant also demonstrated increased CDC activity relative to parental IgG_3, additional contributions from the domain exchange may have influenced the increased CDC activity. The authors further demonstrated that afucosylation of the IgG_1/IgG_3 hybrids maintained not only the increased CDC activity but also the enhanced ADCC activity, indicating that combining amino acid mutations with Fc glycan engineering can simultaneously augment independent Fc effector functions.[99] Xencor investigators engineered a series of variants with increased CDC activity, with the IgG_1 variant S267E–H268F–S324T demonstrating the greatest increase in CDC.[100] The authors identified that S267E was the most potent single amino acid substitution, and they argued that this mutation alters the charge of the C_H2 region, which in turn could augment ionic interactions with the C1q subunit B. Together, these studies indicated that mutations within the C_H2 region, particularly those that modulate the charge of the C_H2 region, can strongly influence CDC activity.

New fit-for-purpose technologies are emerging based on specific insights into particular disease microenvironments. As was previously mentioned, physiologically relevant proteases can cleave IgGs in the lower hinge/proximal C_H2 region, rendering them silent. In order to overcome the potential of protease-mediated immune evasion, researchers at Janssen have engineered a protease-resistant platform.[36] The engineering strategy was based on knowledge that human IgG_2 is resistant to cleavage in the lower hinge/proximal C_H2 by a number of physiologically relevant proteases.[101] The mutations of E233P–L234V–L235A with G236 deleted conferred protease resistance but also resulted in a profound loss of Fc effector function. However, this loss of function could be compensated for by the addition of point mutations in the C_H2 (e.g., K326A–E333A restored CDC and S239D and/or I332E restored or enhanced ADCC). Insights into which mutations restored either ADCC/ADCP activity or CDC activity afforded the ability to engineer protease-resistant mAbs with selective cell-killing functions.

The above-mentioned amino acid modifications have all been geared toward increasing interactions with activating FcγRs or the C1q component of complement; however, several variants have been engineered with the intent to increase interactions with FcγRIIb, the sole inhibitory FcγR. FcγRIIb is the most broadly expressed FcγR and is present on almost all leukocytes with the exception of neutrophils, NK cells, and T cells.[3] Historically, engagement of FcγRIIb has been attributed to (1) opposing activating signals generated through activating FcγRs and (2) modulating B-cell responses and maintaining tolerance.[3] However, recent evidence in the literature has suggested that selective engagement of FcγRIIb could potentially be advantageous for numerous therapeutic settings beyond its role in inhibiting immune responses.

Researchers at Genentech demonstrated that mAbs directed against death-domain-containing tumor necrosis factor receptor (TNFR) superfamily members (e.g., DR4, DR5) have increased pro-apoptotic agonist activity when FcγRs are engaged, and it was determined that either activating FcγRs or FcγRIIb could induce apoptotic activity.[102] The authors suggested that FcγRs could serve as a crosslinking scaffold to drive mAb-dependent, pro-apoptotic signals. Li and Ravetch[103] demonstrated that selective engagement of FcγRIIb with mAbs directed against immunostimulatory TNFR superfamily members (e.g., CD40) elicited an immune adjuvant effect that helped enable cross-presentation of dendritic cell-targeted antigen to effector T cells. White et al.[104] showed that the agonist activity of an anti-mouse CD40 mAb was dependent on binding to FcγRIIb, such that agonist activity was lost in FcγRIIb$^{-/-}$ mice. However, the authors did note that in *in vitro* studies, both activating FcγRs and FcγRIIb could augment agonist activity and concluded that the *in vivo* dependence on interactions with FcγRIIb was most likely a result of FcγRIIb-bearing cells being in closer proximity to CD40-expressing cells, thereby providing more crosslinking activity. Based on these observations, Li and Ravetch[69] have suggested that selective engagement of FcγRIIb for mAbs targeting TNFR superfamily members may be a general requirement. One purported advantage of selectively engaging the inhibitory FcγRIIb in the absence of engaging activating FcγRs is that FcγRIIb can serve as a crosslinking scaffold to drive agonist signals without engaging immune effector mechanisms that would result in depletion of the targeted cell.[105] One caveat for these preclinical studies is that they were carried out in mice. Many of the current Fc engineering approaches being employed to augment binding to FcγRIIb either simultaneously increase binding to activating FcγRIIa R131 (e.g., Xencor's S267E-L328F mutations[106]) or maintain normal binding to FcγRIIa R131 (e.g., Chugai's E233D–G237D–H268D–P271G–A330R mutations).[107] Several studies have shown that engagement of FcγRIIa on macrophages is sufficient to drive antibody-dependent cellular phagocytosis (ADCP) and kill mAb-targeted cells.[37,92] Further, both of these variants may engage complement-dependent cytotoxicity (CDC), leading to destruction of the targeted cell. Because the preclinical studies were carried out in mice, neither ADCP nor CDC would have been detected because mice do not express FcγRIIa,[3] and human IgGs often fail to elicit CDC with mouse serum.[99] Therefore, because several existing Fc engineering strategies to selectively engage FcγIIb also engage FcγRIIa and may retain (or have enhanced) CDC activity, it will be important to determine if increased agonist affects can be balanced against the potential to deplete targeted cells.

Antibody Engineering for Altered Half-Life

Increasing antibody half-life can confer a number of favorable properties to mAb-based therapeutics, including decreased costs of goods, increased bioavailability, decreased or extended dosing schedules, and the potential reduction of toxicity associated with high doses.[5] For the most part, the long circulating half-life of IgGs (estimated between 7 and 21 days[108]) is regulated by interactions of amino acid motifs proximal to the C_H2/C_H3 interface of IgG Fc with FcRn (see Figure 6.3B). The structure of FcRn is comprised of a transmembrane α-chain noncovalently associated with $β_2$-microglobulin ($β_2$m). IgG/FcRn interactions are highly pH dependent, such that the Fc binds to FcRn with high affinity at low pH (e.g., <6.5) but much lower affinity at physiologic pH (e.g., pH 7.4, the pH of blood). Upon pinocytosis, IgG can bind to FcRn within acidified endosomes as a result of histidine protonation, which protects the IgG from degradation. Two histidines at positions 310 and 435 have been deemed critical for pH dependent binding,[109] whereas I253, H433, and Y436 are also thought to contribute to binding.[110] If the endosome reassociates with the cell surface, the pH will be neutralized, and the IgG can release from FcRn and reenter circulation. IgGs that do not associate with FcRn within acidified endosomes are thought to be directed toward lysosomes, resulting in IgG degradation. β_2m knockout mice have a reduced IgG half-life, which supports the dependence on Fc/FcRn interactions for maintaining a long half-life;[111] therefore, many investigators have attempted to increase interactions with FcRn in order to augment IgG half-life.

Several molecular evolution or computational approaches have been employed to modify the amino acid sequence of IgGs in order to increase half-life. Researchers at MedImmune employed phage display to generate Fc variants and screened for increased binding to FcRn at low pH.[112] In particular, the authors identified the variant M252Y–S254T–T256E, termed "YTE," which demonstrated an 11-fold increased binding to FcRn at pH 6.0 compared to IgG$_1$. MedImmune researchers later demonstrated that the YTE variant had a fourfold increased half-life in cynomolgus monkeys compared to IgG$_1$.[113] The YTE variant also demonstrated decreased ADCC activity relative to IgG$_1$, but the addition of S239D–I332E on the YTE variant restored ADCC.[113] Investigators at Protein Design Labs utilized a molecular modeling approach and mutagenesis to identify variants with increased binding to FcRn. The variant T250Q–M428L displayed a 28-fold increased binding to FcRn at low pH and a 2.5-fold increase in half-life in rhesus monkeys.[114,115] Xencor investigators engineered a variant, M428L–N434S, that displayed an 11-fold increased binding to FcRn at pH 6.0 and a 3.2-fold increased half-life in cynomolgus monkeys compared to IgG$_1$.[116] These examples indicate that a number of amino acid modifications can be employed to improve interactions with FcRn and increase mAb half-life.

CONCLUSIONS

With more than 350 mAb-based therapeutics in the clinical pipeline, the need for differentiation from competitors is becoming increasingly imperative. A deep understanding of the molecular events that regulate antibody interactions with the immune system has resulted in a number of engineering strategies to modulate mAb effector functions. Further, as investigators uncover additional insights into the mechanisms of action for mAb-based drugs, researchers now have the ability to select or fine-tune mAb platforms for disease-specific microenvironments. The recent approval of a glycoengineered mAb for the treatment of cancer has provided proof-of-concept that next generation mAbs with enhanced effector functions can have a clinical impact. The next few years should prove to be an exciting time for mAb-based therapies as more novel engineered platforms progress through clinical trials.

References

1. Reichert JM. Marketed therapeutic antibodies compendium. MAbs. 2012;4:413–5.
2. Reichert JM. Which are the antibodies to watch in 2013? MAbs. 2013;5:1–4.
3. Nimmerjahn F, Ravetch JV. Fcgamma receptors as regulators of immune responses. Nat. Rev. Immunol. 2008;8:34–47.

4. Raju TS. Terminal sugars of Fc glycans influence antibody effector functions of IgGs. Curr. Opin. Immunol. 2008;20:471–8.
5. Roopenian DC, Akilesh S. FcRn: the neonatal Fc receptor comes of age. Nat. Rev. Immunol. 2007;7:715–25.
6. Jefferis R. Antibody therapeutics: isotype and glycoform selection. Expert Opin. Biol. Ther. 2007;7:1401–13.
7. Neuberger MS. Antibody diversification by somatic mutation: from Burnet onwards. Immunol. Cell Biol. 2008;86:124–32.
8. Mage RG, Lanning D, Knight KL. B cell and antibody repertoire development in rabbits: the requirement of gut–associated lymphoid tissues. Dev. Comp. Immunol. 2006;30:137–53.
9. Kohler G, Milstein C. Continuous cultures of fused cells secreting antibody of predefined specificity. Nature 1975;256:495–7.
10. Legendre C, Kreis H, Bach JF, Chatenoud L. Prediction of successful allograft rejection retreatment with OKT3. Transplantation 1992;53:87–90.
11. Norman DJ, Shield CF 3rd, Henell KR, Kimball J, Barry JM, Bennett WM, Leone M. Effectiveness of a second course of OKT3 monoclonal anti-T cell antibody for treatment of renal allograft rejection. Transplantation 1988;46:523–9.
12. Woodle ES, Thistlethwaite JR, Jolliffe LK, Fucello AJ, Stuart FP, Bluestone JA. Anti-CD3 monoclonal antibody therapy. An approach toward optimization by in vitro analysis of new anti-CD3 antibodies. Transplantation 1991;52:361–8.
13. Morrison SL, Johnson MJ, Herzenberg LA, Oi VT. Chimeric human antibody molecules: mouse antigen-binding domains with human constant region domains. Proc. Natl. Acad. Sci. U.S.A. 1984;81:6851–5.
14. Knight DM, Wagner C, Jordan R, McAleer MF, DeRita R, Fass DN, Coller BS, Weisman HF, Ghrayeb J. The immunogenicity of the 7E3 murine monoclonal Fab antibody fragment variable region is dramatically reduced in humans by substitution of human for murine constant regions. Mol. Immunol. 1995;32:1271–81.
15. Jones PT, Dear PH, Foote J, Neuberger MS, Winter G. Replacing the complementarity-determining regions in a human antibody with those from a mouse. Nature 1986;321:522–5.
16. McCafferty J, Griffiths AD, Winter G, Chiswell DJ. Phage antibodies: filamentous phage displaying antibody variable domains. Nature 1990;348:552–4.
17. Lonberg N, Taylor LD, Harding FA, Trounstine M, Higgins KM, Schramm SR, Kuo CC, Mashayekh R, Wymore K, McCabe JG, et al. Antigen-specific human antibodies from mice comprising four distinct genetic modifications. Nature 1994;368:856–9.
18. Strohl WR, Strohl LM. Therapeutic Antibody Engineering: Current and Future Advances Driving the Strongest Growth Area in the Pharmaceutical Industry. Cambridge, U.K: Woodhead Publishing; 2012.
19. Woof JM, Partridge LJ, Jefferis R, Burton DR. Localisation of the monocyte–binding region on human immunoglobulin G. Mol. Immunol. 1986;23:319–30.
20. Jefferis R, Lund J, Pound J. Molecular definition of interaction sites on human IgG for Fc receptors (huFc gamma R). Mol. Immunol. 1990;27:1237–40.
21. Canfield SM, Morrison SL. The binding affinity of human IgG for its high affinity Fc receptor is determined by multiple amino acids in the C_H2 domain and is modulated by the hinge region. J. Exp. Med. 1991;173:1483–91.
22. Chappel MS, Isenman DE, Everett M, Xu YY, Dorrington KJ, Klein MH. Identification of the Fc gamma receptor class I binding site in human IgG through the use of recombinant IgG_1/IgG_2 hybrid and point-mutated antibodies. Proc. Natl. Acad. Sci. U.S.A. 1991;88:9036–40.
23. Lund J, Winter G, Jones PT, Pound JD, Tanaka T, Walker MR, Artymiuk PJ, Arata Y, Burton DR, Jefferis R, et al. Human Fc gamma RI and Fc gamma RII interact with distinct but overlapping sites on human IgG. J. Immunol. 1991;147:2657–62.
24. Sarmay G, Lund J, Rozsnyay Z, Gergely J, Jefferis R. Mapping and comparison of the interaction sites on the Fc region of IgG responsible for triggering antibody dependent cellular cytotoxicity (ADCC) through different types of human Fc gamma receptor. Mol. Immunol. 1992;29:633–9.
25. Hezareh M, Hessell AJ, Jensen RC, van de Winkel JG, Parren PW. Effector function activities of a panel of mutants of a broadly neutralizing antibody against human immunodeficiency virus type 1. J. Virol. 2001;75:12161–8.
26. Brezski RJ, Jordan RE. Cleavage of IgGs by proteases associated with invasive diseases: an evasion tactic against host immunity? MAbs. 2010;2:212–20.
27. Brezski RJ, Vafa O, Petrone D, Tam SH, Powers G, Ryan MH, Luongo JL, Oberholtzer A, Knight DM, Jordan RE. Tumor-associated and microbial proteases compromise host IgG effector functions by a single cleavage proximal to the hinge. Proc. Natl. Acad. Sci. U.S.A. 2009;106:17864–9.

28. Gearing AJ, Thorpe SJ, Miller K, Mangan M, Varley PG, Dudgeon T, Ward G, Turner C, Thorpe R. Selective cleavage of human IgG by the matrix metalloproteinases, matrilysin and stromelysin. Immunol. Lett. 2002;81: 41–8.

29. Ryan MH, Petrone D, Nemeth JF, Barnathan E, Bjorck L, Jordan RE. Proteolysis of purified IgGs by human and bacterial enzymes *in vitro* and the detection of specific proteolytic fragments of endogenous IgG in rheumatoid synovial fluid. Mol. Immunol. 2008;45:1837–46.

30. Vincents B, von Pawel-Rammingen U, Björck L, Abrahamson M. Enzymatic characterization of the streptococcal endopeptidase, IdeS, reveals that it is a cysteine protease with strict specificity for IgG cleavage due to exosite binding. Biochemistry 2004;43:15540–9.

31. Fan X, Brezski RJ, Fa M, Deng H, Oberholtzer A, Gonzalez A, Dubinsky WP, Strohl WR, Jordan RE, Zhang N, An Z. A single proteolytic cleavage within the lower hinge of trastuzumab reduces immune effector function and *in vivo* efficacy. Breast Cancer Res. 2012;14:R116.

32. Vindebro R, Spoerry C, von Pawel-Rammingen U. Rapid IgG heavy chain cleavage by the streptococcal IgG endopeptidase IdeS is mediated by IdeS monomers and is not due to enzyme dimerization. FEBS Lett. 2013;587:1818–22.

33. von Pawel-Rammingen U. Streptococcal IdeS and its impact on immune response and inflammation. J. Innate Immun. 2012;4:132–40.

34. Brezski RJ, Almagro JC. Application of antibody engineering in the development of next generation antibody-based therapuetics. In: Tabrizi MA, Bornstein GG, Klakamp SL, editors. Development of Antibody-Based Therapeutics: Translational Considerations. New York: Springer; 2012. p. 65–93.

35. Bruhns P, Iannascoli B, England P, Mancardi DA, Fernandez N, Jorieux S, Daeron M. Specificity and affinity of human Fcgamma receptors and their polymorphic variants for human IgG subclasses. Blood 2009;113: 3716–25.

36. Kinder M, Greenplate AR, Grugan KD, Soring KL, Heeringa KA, McCarthy SG, Bannish G, Perpetua M, Lynch F, Jordan RE, Strohl WR, Brezski RJ. Engineered protease-resistant antibodies with selectable cell–killing functions. J. Biol. Chem. 2013;288:30843–54.

37. Schneider-Merck T, Lammerts van Bueren JJ, Berger S, Rossen K, van Berkel PH, Derer S, Beyer T, Lohse S, Bleeker WK, Peipp M, Parren PW, van de Winkel JG, Valerius T, Dechant M. Human IgG_2 antibodies against epidermal growth factor receptor effectively trigger antibody-dependent cellular cytotoxicity but, in contrast to IgG_1, only by cells of myeloid lineage. J. Immunol. 2009;184:512–20.

38. Yoo EM, Wims LA, Chan LA, Morrison SL. Human IgG_2 can form covalent dimers. J. Immunol. 2003;170: 3134–8.

39. Dillon TM, Ricci MS, Vezina C, Flynn GC, Liu YD, Rehder DS, Plant M, Henkle B, Li Y, Deechongkit S, Varnum B, Wypych J, Balland A, Bondarenko PV. Structural and functional characterization of disulfide isoforms of the human IgG_2 subclass. J. Biol. Chem. 2008;283:16206–15.

40. Wypych J, Li M, Guo A, Zhang Z, Martinez T, Allen MJ, Fodor S, Kelner DN, Flynn GC, Liu YD, Bondarenko PV, Ricci MS, Dillon TM, Balland A. Human IgG_2 antibodies display disulfide-mediated structural isoforms. J. Biol. Chem. 2008;283:16194–205.

41. Nesspor TC, Raju TS, Chin CN, Vafa O, Brezski RJ. Avidity confers FcgammaR binding and immune effector function to aglycosylated immunoglobulin G_1. J. Mol. Recognit. 2012;25:147–54.

42. Steplewski Z, Sun LK, Shearman CW, Ghrayeb J, Daddona P, Koprowski H. Biological activity of human–mouse IgG_1, IgG_2, IgG_3, and IgG_4 chimeric monoclonal antibodies with antitumor specificity. Proc. Natl. Acad. Sci. U.S.A. 1988;85:4852–6.

43. Isaacs JD, Wing MG, Greenwood JD, Hazleman BL, Hale G, Waldmann H. A therapeutic human IgG_4 monoclonal antibody that depletes target cells in humans. Clin. Exp. Immunol. 1996;106:427–33.

44. Schuurman J, Van Ree R, Perdok GJ, Van Doorn HR, Tan KY, Aalberse RC. Normal human immunoglobulin G_4 is bispecific: it has two different antigen-combining sites. Immunology 1999;97:693–8.

45. van der Neut Kolfschoten M, Schuurman J, Losen M, Bleeker WK, Martinez-Martinez P, Vermeulen E, den Bleker TH, Wiegman L, Vink T, Aarden LA, De Baets MH, van de Winkel JG, Aalberse RC, Parren PW. Anti-inflammatory activity of human IgG_4 antibodies by dynamic Fab arm exchange. Science 2007;317:1554–7.

46. Dall'Acqua W, Simon AL, Mulkerrin MG, Carter P. Contribution of domain interface residues to the stability of antibody CH3 domain homodimers. Biochemistry 1998;37:9266–73.

47. Labrijn AF, Aalberse RC, Schuurman J. When binding is enough: nonactivating antibody formats. Curr. Opin. Immunol. 2008;20:479–85.

48. Chatenoud L, Bluestone JA. CD3-specific antibodies: a portal to the treatment of autoimmunity. Nat. Rev. Immunol. 2007;7:622–32.

49. Chatenoud L, Ferran C, Legendre C, Thouard I, Merite S, Reuter A, Gevaert Y, Kreis H, Franchimont P, Bach JF. *In vivo* cell activation following OKT3 administration. Systemic cytokine release and modulation by corticosteroids. Transplantation 1990;49:697–702.

50. Alegre M-L, Collins AM, Pulito VL, Brosius RA, Olson WC, Zivin RA, Knowles R, Thistlethwaite JR, Jolliffe LK, Bluestone JA. Effect of a single amino acid mutation on the activating and immunosuppressive properties of a "humanized" OKT3 monoclonal antibody. J. Immunol. 1992;148:3461–8.

51. Alegre M-L, Peterson LJ, Xu D, Sattar HA, Jeyarajah DR, Kowalkowski K, Thistlethwaite JR, Zivin RA, Jolliffe L, Bluestone JA. A non-activating "humanized" anti-CD3 monoclonal antibody retains immunosuppressive properties *in vivo*. Transplantation 1994;57:1537–43.

52. Xu D, Alegre ML, Varga SS, Rothermel AL, Collins AM, Pulito VL, Hanna LS, Dolan KP, Parren PW, Bluestone JA, Jolliffe LK, Zivin RA. *In vitro* characterization of five humanized OKT3 effector function variant antibodies. Cell Immunol. 2000;200:16–26.

53. Suntharalingam G, Perry MR, Ward S, Brett SJ, Castello-Cortes A, Brunner MD, Panoskaltsis N. Cytokine storm in a phase 1 trial of the anti-CD28 monoclonal antibody TGN1412. N. Engl. J. Med. 2006;355:1018–28.

54. Vafa O, Gilliland GL, Brezski RJ, Strake B, Wilkinson T, Lacy ER, Scallon B, Teplyakov A, Malia TJ, Strohl WR. An engineered Fc variant of an IgG eliminates all immune effector functions via structural perturbations. Methods 2013;65:114–26.

55. Bolt S, Routledge E, Lloyd I, Chatenoud L, Pope H, Gorman SD, Clark M, Waldmann H. The generation of a humanized, non–mitogenic CD3 monoclonal antibody which retains *in vitro* immunosuppressive properties. Eur J. Immunol. 1993;23:403–11.

56. Walker MR, Lund J, Thompson KM, Jefferis R. Aglycosylation of human IgG_1 and IgG_3 monoclonal antibodies can eliminate recognition by human cells expressing Fc gamma RI and/or Fc gamma RII receptors. Biochem. J. 1989;259:347–53.

57. Leabman MK, Gloria Meng Y, Kelley RF, DeForge LE, Cowan KJ, Iyer S. Effects of altered FcgR binding on antibody pharmacokinetics in cynomolgus monkeys. MAbs. 2013;5:894–901.

58. Rother RP, Rollins SA, Mojcik CF, Brodsky RA, Bell L. Discovery and development of the complement inhibitor eculizumab for the treatment of paroxysmal nocturnal hemoglobinuria. Nat. Biotechnol. 2007;25:1256–64.

59. Mueller JP, Giannoni MA, Hartman SL, Elliott EA, Squinto SP, Matis LA, Evans MJ. Humanized porcine VCAM–specific monoclonal antibodies with chimeric IgG_2/G_4 constant regions block human leukocyte binding to porcine endothelial cells. Mol. Immunol. 1997;34:441–52.

60. Armour KL, Clark MR, Hadley AG, Williamson LM. Recombinant human IgG molecules lacking Fcγ receptor I binding and monocyte triggering activities. Eur. J. Immunol. 1999;29:2613–24.

61. Ghevaert C, Wilcox DA, Fang J, Armour KL, Clark MR, Ouwehand WH, Williamson LM. Developing recombinant HPA–1a–specific antibodies with abrogated Fcgamma receptor binding for the treatment of fetomaternal alloimmune thrombocytopenia. J. Clin. Invest. 2008;118:2929–38.

62. An Z, Forrest G, Moore R, Cukan M, Haytko P, Huang L, Vitelli S, Zhao JZ, Lu P, Hua J, Gibson CR, Harvey BR, Montgomery D, Zaller D, Wang F, Strohl W. IgG_2m4, an engineered antibody isotype with reduced Fc function. MAbs. 2009;1:572–9.

63. Prat M, Crepaldi T, Pennacchietti S, Bussolino F, Comoglio PM. Agonistic monoclonal antibodies against the Met receptor dissect the biological responses to HGF. Journal of cell science 1998;111(Pt. 2):237–47.

64. Ridgway JB, Presta LG, Carter P. Knobs-into-holes" engineering of antibody CH3 domains for heavy chain heterodimerization. Protein Eng. 1996;9:617–21.

65. Merchant M, Ma X, Maun HR, Zheng Z, Peng J, Romero M, Huang A, Yang NY, Nishimura M, Greve J, et al. Monovalent antibody design and mechanism of action of onartuzumab, a MET antagonist with anti-tumor activity as a therapeutic agent. Proc. Natl. Acad. Sci. U.S.A. 2013;110:E2987–2996.

66. Bibeau F, Lopez–Crapez E, Di Fiore F, Thezenas S, Ychou M, Blanchard F, Lamy A, Penault-Llorca F, Frebourg T, Michel P, Sabourin JC, Boissiere–Michot F. Impact of Fc{gamma}RIIa–Fc{gamma}RIIIa polymorphisms and KRAS mutations on the clinical outcome of patients with metastatic colorectal cancer treated with cetuximab plus irinotecan. J. Clin. Oncol. 2009;27:1122–9.

67. Cartron G, Dacheux L, Salles G, Solal-Celigny P, Bardos P, Colombat P, Watier H. Therapeutic activity of humanized anti-CD20 monoclonal antibody and polymorphism in IgG Fc receptor FcgammaRIIIa gene. Blood 2002;99:754–8.

68. Musolino A, Naldi N, Bortesi B, Pezzuolo D, Capelletti M, Missale G, Laccabue D, Zerbini A, Camisa R, Bisagni G, Neri TM, Ardizzoni A. Immunoglobulin G fragment C receptor polymorphisms and clinical efficacy of trastuzumab-based therapy in patients with HER-2/neu-positive metastatic breast cancer. J. Clin. Oncol. 2008;26:1789–96.

69. Li F, Ravetch JV. A general requirement for FcγRIIB co-engagement of agonistic anti-TNFR antibodies. Cell Cycle 2012;11:3343–4.

70. Umana P, Jean-Mairet J, Moudry R, Amstutz H, Bailey JE. Engineered glycoforms of an antineuroblastoma IgG$_1$ with optimized antibody-dependent cellular cytotoxic activity. Nat. Biotechnol. 1999;17:176–80.

71. Shields RL, Lai J, Keck R, O'Connell LY, Hong K, Meng YG, Weikert SH, Presta LG. Lack of fucose on human IgG$_1$ N–linked oligosaccharide improves binding to human Fcγ RIII and antibody-dependent cellular toxicity. J. Biol. Chem. 2002;277:26733–40.

72. Shinkawa T, Nakamura K, Yamane N, Shoji–Hosaka E, Kanda Y, Sakurada M, Uchida K, Anazawa H, Satoh M, Yamasaki M, Hanai N, Shitara K. The absence of fucose but not the presence of galactose or bisecting N-acetylglucosamine of human IgG$_1$ complex-type oligosaccharides shows the critical role of enhancing antibody-dependent cellular cytotoxicity. J. Biol. Chem. 2003;278:3466–73.

73. Niwa R, Natsume A, Uehara A, Wakitani M, Iida S, Uchida K, Satoh M, Shitara K. IgG subclass-independent improvement of antibody-dependent cellular cytotoxicity by fucose removal from Asn297-linked oligosaccharides. J. Immunol. Methods 2005;306:151–60.

74. Chung S, Quarmby V, Gao X, Ying Y, Lin L, Reed C, Fong C, Lau W, Qiu ZJ, Shen A, Vanderlaan M, Song A. Quantitative evaluation of fucose reducing effects in a humanized antibody on Fcγ receptor binding and antibody-dependent cell-mediated cytotoxicity activities. MAbs. 2012;4:326–40.

75. Scallon B, McCarthy S, Radewonuk J, Cai A, Naso M, Raju TS, Capocasale R. Quantitative *in vivo* comparisons of the Fc gamma receptor-dependent agonist activities of different fucosylation variants of an immunoglobulin G antibody. Int. Immunopharmacol. 2007;7:761–72.

76. Yamane-Ohnuki N, Satoh M. Production of therapeutic antibodies with controlled fucosylation. MAbs. 2009;1:230–6.

77. Zhang N, Liu L, Dumitru CD, Cummings NR, Cukan M, Jiang Y, Li Y, Li F, Mitchell T, Mallem MR, Ou Y, Patel RN, Vo K, Wang H, Burnina I, Choi BK, Huber HE, Stadheim TA, Zha D. Glycoengineered *Pichia* produced anti-HER2 is comparable to trastuzumab in preclinical study. MAbs. 2011;3:289–98.

78. Sehn LH, Assouline SE, Stewart DA, Mangel J, Gascoyne RD, Fine G, Frances-Lasserre S, Carlile DJ, Crump M. A phase 1 study of obinutuzumab induction followed by 2 years of maintenance in patients with relapsed CD20-positive B-cell malignancies. Blood 2012;119:5118–25.

79. Niwa R, Hatanaka S, Shoji-Hosaka E, Sakurada M, Kobayashi Y, Uehara A, Yokoi H, Nakamura K, Shitara K. Enhancement of the antibody-dependent cellular cytotoxicity of low-fucose IgG$_1$ is independent of FcγRIIIa functional polymorphism. Clin. Cancer Res. 2004;10:6248–55.

80. Ferrara C, Grau S, Jager C, Sondermann P, Brunker P, Waldhauer I, Hennig M, Ruf A, Rufer AC, Stihle M, Umana P, Benz J. Unique carbohydrate–carbohydrate interactions are required for high affinity binding between FcγRIII and antibodies lacking core fucose. Proc. Natl. Acad. Sci. U.S.A. 2011;108:12669–74.

81. Ferrara C, Stuart F, Sondermann P, Brunker P, Umana P. The carbohydrate at FcγRIIIa Asn-162. An element required for high affinity binding to non-fucosylated IgG glycoforms. J. Biol. Chem. 2006;281:5032–6.

82. Preithner S, Elm S, Lippold S, Locher M, Wolf A, da Silva AJ, Baeuerle PA, Prang NS. High concentrations of therapeutic IgG$_1$ antibodies are needed to compensate for inhibition of antibody-dependent cellular cytotoxicity by excess endogenous immunoglobulin G. Mol. Immunol. 2006;43:1183–93.

83. Iida S, Misaka H, Inoue M, Shibata M, Nakano R, Yamane-Ohnuki N, Wakitani M, Yano K, Shitara K, Satoh M. Nonfucosylated therapeutic IgG$_1$ antibody can evade the inhibitory effect of serum immunoglobulin G on antibody-dependent cellular cytotoxicity through its high binding to FcγRIIIa. Clin. Cancer Res. 2006;12:2879–87.

84. Mossner E, Brunker P, Moser S, Puntener U, Schmidt C, Herter S, Grau R, Gerdes C, Nopora A, van Puijenbroek E, et al. Increasing the efficacy of CD20 antibody therapy through the engineering of a new type II anti-CD20 antibody with enhanced direct and immune effector cell-mediated B-cell cytotoxicity. Blood 2010;115:4393–402.

85. Beck A, Reichert JM. Marketing approval of mogamulizumab: a triumph for glyco-engineering. MAbs. 2012;4:419–25.

86. Collin M, Olsen A. Effect of SpeB and EndoS from *Streptococcus pyogenes* on human immunoglobulins. Infect. Immun. 2001;69:7187–9.

87. Collin M, Shannon O, Bjorck L. IgG glycan hydrolysis by a bacterial enzyme as a therapy against autoimmune conditions. Proc. Natl. Acad. Sci. U.S.A. 2008;105:4265–70.

88. Baruah K, Bowden TA, Krishna BA, Dwek RA, Crispin M, Scanlan CN. Selective deactivation of serum IgG: a general strategy for the enhancement of monoclonal antibody receptor interactions. J. Mol. Biol. 2012;420:1–7.

89. Shields RL, Namenuk AK, Hong K, Meng YG, Rae J, Briggs J, Xie D, Lai J, Stadlen A, Li B, Fox JA, Presta LG. High resolution mapping of the binding site on human IgG_1 for Fc gamma RI, Fc gamma RII, Fc gamma RIII, and FcRn and design of IgG_1 variants with improved binding to the Fc gamma R. J Biol Chem 2001;276: 6591–604.

90. Lazar GA, Dang W, Karki S, Vafa O, Peng JS, Hyun L, Chan C, Chung HS, Eivazi A, Yoder SC, Vielmetter J, Carmichael DF, Hayes RJ, Dahiyat BI. Engineered antibody Fc variants with enhanced effector function. Proc. Natl. Acad. Sci. U.S.A. 2006;103:4005–10.

91. Oganesyan V, Damschroder MM, Leach W, Wu H, Dall'Acqua WF. Structural characterization of a mutated, ADCC-enhanced human Fc fragment. Mol. Immunol. 2008;45:1872–82.

92. Richards JO, Karki S, Lazar GA, Chen H, Dang W, Desjarlais JR. Optimization of antibody binding to FcγRIIa enhances macrophage phagocytosis of tumor cells. Mol. Cancer Ther. 2008;7:2517–27.

93. Horton HM, Bernett MJ, Pong E, Peipp M, Karki S, Chu SY, Richards JO, Vostiar I, Joyce PF, Repp R, Desjarlais JR, Zhukovsky EA. Potent *in vitro* and *in vivo* activity of an Fc-engineered anti-CD19 monoclonal antibody against lymphoma and leukemia. Cancer Res 2008;68:8049–57.

94. Stavenhagen JB, Gorlatov S, Tuaillon N, Rankin CT, Li H, Burke S, Huang L, Vijh S, Johnson S, Bonvini E, Koenig S. Fc optimization of therapeutic antibodies enhances their ability to kill tumor cells *in vitro* and controls tumor expansion *in vivo* via low-affinity activating Fcγ receptors. Cancer Res. 2007;67:8882–90.

95. Nordstrom JL, Gorlatov S, Zhang W, Yang Y, Huang L, Burke S, Li H, Ciccarone V, Zhang T, Stavenhagen J, Koenig S, Stewart SJ, Moore PA, Johnson S, Bonvini E. Anti–tumor activity and toxicokinetics analysis of MGAH22, an anti-HER2 monoclonal antibody with enhanced Fcγ receptor binding properties. Breast Cancer Res. 2011;13:R123.

96. Idusogie EE, Wong PY, Presta LG, Gazzano-Santoro H, Totpal K, Ultsch M, Mulkerrin MG. Engineered antibodies with increased activity to recruit complement. J. Immunol. 2001;166:2571–5.

97. Isusogie EE, Presta LG, Gazzano–Santoro H, Totpal K, Wong PY, Ultsch M, Meng YG, Mulkerrin MG. Mapping of the C1q binding site on Rituxan, a chimeric antibody with a human IgG_1 Fc. J. Immunol. 2000;164:4178–84.

98. Thommesen JE, Michaelsen TE, Løset GA, Sandlie I, Brekke OH. Lysine 322 in the human IgG_3 C_H2 domain is crucial for antibody dependent complement activation. Mol. Immunol. 2000;37:995–1004.

99. Natsume A, In M, Takamura H, Nakagawa T, Shimizu Y, Kitajima K, Wakitani M, Ohta S, Satoh M, Shitara K, Niwa R. Engineered antibodies of IgG_1/IgG_3 mixed isotype with enhanced cytotoxic activities. Cancer Res. 2008;68:3863–72.

100. Moore GL, Chen H, Karki S, Lazar GA. Engineered Fc variant antibodies with enhanced ability to recruit complement and mediate effector functions. MAbs. 2010;2:181–9.

101. Brezski RJ, Oberholtzer A, Strake B, Jordan RE. The *in vitro* resistance of IgG_2 to proteolytic attack concurs with a comparative paucity of autoantibodies against peptide analogs of the IgG_2 hinge. MAbs. 2011;3:558–67.

102. Wilson NS, Yang B, Yang A, Loeser S, Marsters S, Lawrence D, Li Y, Pitti R, Totpal K, Yee S, et al. An Fcgamma receptor-dependent mechanism drives antibody-mediated target–receptor signaling in cancer cells. Cancer Cell 2011;19:101–13.

103. Li F, Ravetch JV. Inhibitory Fcγ receptor engagement drives adjuvant and anti-tumor activities of agonistic CD40 antibodies. Science 2011;333:1030–4.

104. White AL, Chan HT, Roghanian A, French RR, Mockridge CI, Tutt AL, Dixon SV, Ajona D, Verbeek JS, Al-Shamkhani A, et al. Interaction with FcγRIIB is critical for the agonistic activity of anti-CD40 monoclonal antibody. J. Immunol. 2011;187:1754–63.

105. Kim JM, Ashkenazi A. Fcgamma receptors enable anticancer action of proapoptotic and immune-modulatory antibodies. J. Exp. Med. 2013;210:1647–51.

106. Chu SY, Vostiar I, Karki S, Moore GL, Lazar GA, Pong E, Joyce PF, Szymkowski DE, Desjarlais JR. Inhibition of B cell receptor-mediated activation of primary human B cells by coengagement of CD19 and FcγRIIb with Fc-engineered antibodies. Mol. Immunol. 2008;45:3926–33.

107. Mimoto F, Katada H, Kadono S, Igawa T, Kuramochi T, Muraoka M, Wada Y, Haraya K, Miyazaki T, Hattori K. Engineered antibody Fc variant with selectively enhanced FcγRIIb binding over both FcγRIIaR131 and FcγRIIaH131. Protein Eng. Des. Sel. 2013;26:589–98.

108. Morell A, Terry WD, Waldmann TA. Metabolic properties of IgG subclasses in man. J. Clin. Invest. 1970;49: 673–80.

109. Martin WL, West AP Jr, Gan L, Bjorkman PJ. Crystal structure at 2.8 A of an FcRn/heterodimeric Fc complex: mechanism of pH-dependent binding. Mol. Cell 2001;7:867–77.

110. Kuo TT, Baker K, Yoshida M, Qiao SW, Aveson VG, Lencer WI, Blumberg RS. Neonatal Fc receptor: from immunity to therapeutics. J. Clin. Immunol. 2010;30:777–89.

111. Ghetie V, Hubbard JG, Kim JK, Tsen MF, Lee Y, Ward ES. Abnormally short serum half-lives of IgG in beta 2-microglobulin-deficient mice. Eur J. Immunol. 1996;26:690–6.

112. Dall'Acqua WF, Woods RM, Ward ES, Palaszynski SR, Patel NK, Brewah YA, Wu H, Kiener PA, Langermann S. Increasing the affinity of a human IgG$_1$ for the neonatal Fc receptor: biological consequences. J. Immunol. 2002;169:5171–80.

113. Dall'Acqua WF, Kiener PA, Wu H. Properties of human IgG$_1$s engineered for enhanced binding to the neonatal Fc receptor (FcRn). J. Biol. Chem. 2006;281:23514–24.

114. Hinton PR, Johlfs MG, Xiong JM, Hanestad K, Ong KC, Bullock C, Keller S, Tang MT, Tso JY, Vasquez M, Tsurushita N. Engineered human IgG antibodies with longer serum half-lives in primates. J. Biol. Chem. 2004;279:6213–6.

115. Hinton PR, Xiong JM, Johlfs MG, Tang MT, Keller S, Tsurushita N. An engineered human IgG$_1$ antibody with longer serum half-life. J. Immunol. 2006;176:346–56.

116. Zalevsky J, Chamberlain AK, Horton HM, Karki S, Leung IW, Sproule TJ, Lazar GA, Roopenian DC, Desjarlais JR. Enhanced antibody half-life improves *in vivo* activity. Nat. Biotechnol. 2010;28:157–9.

117. Edelman GM, Cunningham BA, Gall WE, Gottlieb PD, Rutishauser U, Waxdal MJ. The covalent structure of an entire gammaG immunoglobulin molecule. Proc. Natl. Acad. Sci. U.S.A. 1969;63:78–85.

118. Strohl WR. Optimization of Fc–mediated effector functions of monoclonal antibodies. Curr. Opin. Biotechnol. 2009;20:685–91.

Novel Approaches in Discovery and Design of Antibody-Based Therapeutics

Juan C. Almagro, Sreekumar Kodangattil

CTI-Boston, Pfizer, Inc., Boston, MA, USA

O U T L I N E

INTRODUCTION

Antibody-based drugs have become important medical and commercial products with application in a wide range of human diseases. Antibodies are large, multidomain, complex glycoproteins (Figure 7.1) composed of two antigen-binding fragments (Fabs) and one crystallizable fragment (Fc). Each fragment plays a role in the functioning of the molecule and thus in defining the efficacy and safety of the antibody-based therapy. The Fc is formed by pairing the constant (C) domains from the heavy chains, and it determines a variety of functions including multiple cell killing mechanisms and plasma half-life of the antibody. The Fabs contain the Fv fragments, which are assembled by heavy and light variable (V) regions. The V regions contain the antigen-binding site and thus determine the antigen-binding characteristics of the antibody, including specificity, affinity for the target, and cross-reactivity with orthologs.[1,2]

Novel Approaches and Strategies for Biologics, Vaccines and Cancer Therapies. DOI: 10.1016/B978-0-12-416603-5.00007-9

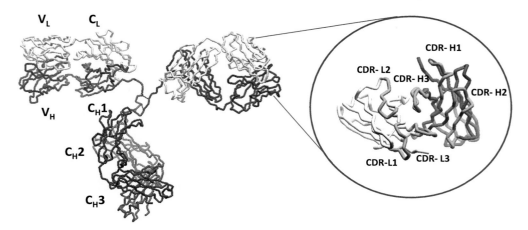

FIGURE 7.1   Structure of an IgG comprising several domains. LCs are colored in silver. HCs are colored in violet. The coordinates used to generate the figure correspond to the structure with Protein Data Bank (PDB) code 1IGT. On the left is a close-up of the Fv fragment looking from the antigen perspective. The antigen-binding site is colored in orange, following Kabat's definition of complementarity determining regions (CDRs).

In this chapter, we first review one of the new technologies impacting the antibody discovery and optimization processes: next-generation sequencing (NGS). This technology is providing the means to study whole natural and manmade repertoires in expedited ways and at relatively low cost. Having access to the complete information encoded in antibody repertoires before and after selection under a variety of selection conditions or after immunization has revealed features of the antibody repertoire that are impacting the theories addressing its origin and evolution.[3,4] NGS is also quickly becoming part of the arsenal of tools for discovery and optimization of antibodies.[5] It has been utilized to assess the quality of antibody repertoires designed to isolate molecules with potential therapeutic use and has complemented screening strategies to discover antibodies via immunization or phage display.

Second, we discuss novel sources of V regions for discovery and engineering of therapeutic antibodies, specifically species other than humans and rodents, including chickens and rabbits. These species are gaining attention as substrates for the development of therapeutic antibodies. Rabbits and chickens have been known for decades for producing high-affinity antibodies with exquisite specificity and the ability to recognize unique epitopes. Because both species are evolutionary more distant from humans than mice and rats, chickens and rabbits also have the capability of generating antibodies against epitopes conserved between rodents and humans. The development of technologies to isolate single-specificity rabbit[6] and chicken[7] antibodies and the subsequent successful humanization of their V regions have enabled development of therapeutic antibodies from these species.

Finally, we review molecular modalities beyond natural antibodies, in particular bi- and multispecific modalities. With the relatively recent approval of catumaxomab in Europe,[8] a rat/murine hybrid, trifunctional, bispecific (anti-human epithelial cell adhesion molecule

[EpCAM] × anti-CD3) monoclonal antibody, the field of bi- and multifunctional molecules has gained momentum. Currently, dozens of different molecular formats are in the early stages of validation as therapeutics and clinical trials.[9–12] Due to the proven impact on efficacy and potential new indications, these antibody-like modalities may lead to a new wave of marketed biologics in the near future, particularly in the field of oncology.

ANTIBODY DISCOVERY AND OPTIMIZATION VIA DATA MINING

Although antibody-based therapies have been used to treat diverse maladies for at least a century, the development of hybridoma technology described by Köhler and Milstein in 1975,[13] who were awarded the Nobel Prize in 1984, was the key advancement that ultimately led to the modern antibody-based therapies. Recombinant human antibody discovery using display technologies followed.[14] Display-based antibody discovery and development platforms, such as phage, bacterial, yeast, mammalian, and ribosome display, have heavily relied on enrichment and screening the large initial pool of antibody variants prior to sequencing a small set of clones of the order of a few hundreds. Similarly, screening and selection are practiced in hybridoma-based antibody discovery approaches prior to sequencing a small number of clones. These approaches have been constrained by the low throughput and high cost associated with the Sanger sequencing technology[15] that dominated the field until the development of the second-generation sequencing technologies beginning in 2005.[16]

The Roche 454 Sequencing™ platform, Illumina/Solexa platform, and Applied Biosystems' SOLiD™, which initiated the sequencing revolution, can produce thousands to billions of 25- to 800-nucleotide-long reads within days at a cost much lower than the per-base sequencing cost of the Sanger sequencing technology.[17] These new sequencing platforms have been utilized to generate sequences of antibodies at a number unimaginable until just a few years ago. Such efforts combined with data mining have been useful in analyzing the complexities of the immune repertoire in humans and model organisms, differentiating the immune repertoire under normal and pathological conditions, evaluating the quality of antibody phage libraries, following enrichment of antibody clones in phage display,[5] and identifying dominant clones and target specific binders from immunized animals.[18,19]

The premise of the antibody discovery by deep sequencing and data mining is that clones positively selected for binding to a given target in a display system or preferentially selected and retained in an immunized animal will be present at high frequency in the selection pools and the lymphoid organs, respectively. These enriched clones can be identified in an appropriate sample, based on the their high frequency in comparison to their frequency in an unselected library, in a library selected with a different target, in lymphoid organs of a naïve animal, or in the lymphoid organs of an animal immunized with a different antigen. One of the main requirements of this method is the sequencing of a large number of clones (10^4 to 10^6) from an appropriate sample, which is accomplished by employing one of the second-generation sequencing technologies. Data mining-aided antibody discovery may be applied to antibody discovery or antibody optimization from generic libraries or focused libraries without high-throughput screening and to antibody discovery from immunized animals without generating hybridomas.

Deep Sequencing of Antibody Libraries

The libraries used in conjunction with the display technologies have a diversity on the order of 10^8 to 10^{11} members. The task of identifying a small number of potential target specific binders is simplified by selectively retaining binders and amplifying them for two or three rounds, called selection, and then screening about 10^5 clones. The selection strategy is critical for the success of the panning campaign, hence multiple branches of selection under different conditions and stringency are carried out. Because of the availability of multiple selection pools and the practical limit of the number of individual clones that can be screened by high-throughput sequencing, the number of clones that are screened from each selection pool often falls below 10^5. However, it is possible to generate few hundred thousand sequences from each selection pool through the application of deep sequencing, and the clones that are over-represented in these populations can be identified by data mining. Samples from more than one selection pool tagged with distinct molecular barcodes can be combined and run on a single lane. In order to identify clones from antibody discovery libraries that are enriched after two or three rounds of selection for binding to the target, it is important to use a high throughput sequencing technology such as the Roche 454 Sequencing platform, which can provide reads of length 350 to 400 bases.

Saggy et al.[20] were successful in discovering antibodies against trinitophenyl by deep sequencing and data mining of a phage display library generated from splenocytes of mouse immunized with trinitrophenyl conjugated with bovine serum albumin (BSA). For antibody discovery from affinity maturation and lead optimization libraries, long reads generated by the Roche 454 Sequencing platform may not be required unless side-chain diversification is done over many dispersed residues. Sequencing read lengths provided by the paired-end methodology of the Illumina HiSeq™ platform (2×90 bases) may be sufficient to probe the diversity introduced into individual CDRs, as one might want to do in an affinity optimization library. Ravn et al.[5] bypassed the *in vitro* screening step in discovering anti-idiotype antibodies and anti-human interferon γ antibodies from a synthetic library with amino acid randomization limited to the CDR-L3 and CDR-H3 by applying the data-mining approach on sequence data generated by the Illumina technology. The sequencing strategy they used provided partial sequence of FW3, which was sufficient to identify the germline gene used in the synthetic library construction, and the complete sequence of CDR3, which was necessary to identify the major component of the target binding property. The choices for the most appropriate sequencing platform for a particular application will continue to evolve as the sequencing technology evolves.

Sample Preparation and Sequencing for Antibody Discovery Libraries

Sample preparation of an antibody library for NGS-based quality assessment consists of amplifying the variable domain of heavy and light chains using primers that would not introduce primer-related amplification bias. This can be accomplished by designing primers annealing to a common region on the vector flanking the light- and heavy-chain variable domain (Figure 7.2A,B). Alternatively, the vector DNA can be sheared and size fractionated before ligating molecular identification tag (MID) and sequencing adapters. Attaching MID and sequencing adapters is required when the sample is prepared by amplification as well. This can be achieved by designing fusion primers (Figure 7.2C) that consist of the

(A) Single chain

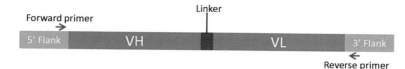

(B) Fab

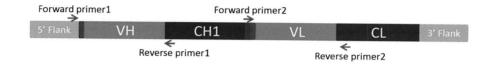

(C) Fusion primer

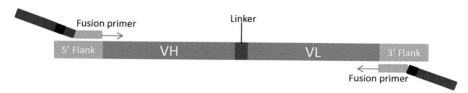

FIGURE 7.2   Primer design for the amplification of the V region from the (A) single-chain Fv library, (B) Fab library, and (C) fusion primer for Roche 454 Sequencing™. Primers are designed to anneal within the region flanking the V region. The fusion primer consists of the target-specific region (green), the molecular identifier (red), a stretch of four bases that forms the library key sequence (black), and either primer A or primer B (blue). The fusion primer set shown in the figure would generate sequences reads of the heavy-chain variable (VH) domain. A similar fusion primer set should be designed to read the light-chain variable (VL) domain.

sequencing adapter, the MID, and the target-specific sequence. In order to reduce the errors introduced during the polymerase chain reaction (PCR), the amplification is carried out for as few cycles as possible with polymerase having high fidelity at conditions such as deoxynucleotide triphosphate (dNTP) and salt concentrations that are optimal for the polymerase. The amplicon obtained with the use of fusion primers is cleaned to get rid of unincorporated nucleotides and any remaining primers and is used in the emulsion PCR. It is important to keep in mind the issues related to the pyrosequencing technology, specifically incorrect homopolymer length as well as relatively higher number of insertion and deletion errors. An estimate of the errors introduced by PCR and sequencing can be obtained by amplifying control DNA having similar sequence composition as the target DNA and spiking the control amplicon at 0.1 to 0.5% prior to the emulsion PCR. Readers are recommended to follow the manufacturers' methods for emulsion PCR, library pooling, and sequencing.

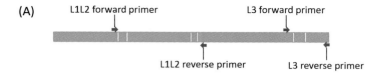

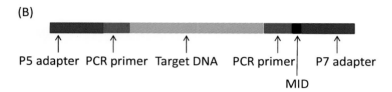

FIGURE 7.3   Primer design for the analysis of antibody optimization library. (A) An example of primer design for the analysis of an example light-chain construct where side-chain randomizations are introduced in CDRs L1, L2, and L3. (B) Schematic of the PCR amplicon after attaching the molecular identifier (MID) and adapters for Illumina sequencing. The PCR product generated by the L1L2 forward/reverse primers would be approximately 150 bp, a length appropriate for paired-end sequencing with the Illumina platform as described in the text. A sequencing library made out of this PCR product will be able to interrogate diversity spanning from CDR-L1 to CDR-L2. Similarly, the PCR product of the L3 forward/reverse primer could be 90 to 120 bp, a length sufficient to investigate the diversity in and around CDR-L3.

Sample Preparation and Sequencing for Affinity Maturation Libraries

For the samples to be sequenced on the Illumina HiSeq platform, the forward and reverse primers used for the PCR could amplify 150 to 160 bp which would give an overlap of 20 to 30 bases in the paired-end reads (Figure 7.3A). Therefore, amino acid diversification over approximately 50 residues can be evaluated by paired-end sequencing using the Illumina platform, which is sufficient to give coverage over single CDRs or, when appropriately positioned, give coverage of two CDRs. As in the case of samples for the Roche 454 Sequencing platform, it is a good practice to limit the number of PCR cycles and fine-tune the amplification conditions to limit PCR-introduced errors. An Illumina sequencing library should then be generated from the amplicons by adding the molecular identifier (MID) and sequencing adapters as shown in Figure 7.3B. Readers are recommended to follow the manufacturers' methods for cluster generation and sequencing

Sequence Analysis for Antibody Discovery

The sequence data obtained are subjected to standard Roche 454 Sequencing processing. Low-quality sequence reads such as those with homopolymers of length 8 or more and those with ambiguous base calls should be discarded from further consideration. Further, it is recommended to trim reads when the per-base quality score falls below 23 or when the average quality score of a 50-base moving window falls below 35. Reads of acceptable quality are then assigned to germline genes and translated, and CDRs are identified using IMGT®/High

V-QUEST,[21] VDJ-Fasta,[22] or other custom software. It is recommended to use a curated germline gene database that contains a comprehensive collection of functional full-length genes as annotated by IMGT. Generally, we exclude all but the *01 allele for those genes with multiple allelic forms. The analysis and annotation can be expedited by parallel processing on a compute cluster. Translated and annotated sequences are further processed to remove those with incomplete variable domains, stop codons, or frameshift mutations.

Sequence Analysis for Antibody Optimization

The bioinformatics procedure for quality assessment of focused libraries followed in our laboratory is as follows. After standard quality filtering, each pair of the paired-end reads is mapped to the target DNA, merged to give a 150- to 160-nucleotide-long sequence, and then translated using custom Perl scripts. Information from all of the pairs is used to compute amino acid diversity at each of the positions which is then used to identify the over-represented clones.

Data mining and Interpretation

To determine the representation of clones in the selection pools enriched for binders to a given target and the dynamics of enrichment under different selection conditions, the annotated sequences are classified into clonal groups. Members of a clonal group have the same variable and joining gene assignments in addition to having identical CDR3 sequences, but they may not have identical sequences. Highly populated clonal groups, which are considered to be preferentially selected, are identified by comparing the frequency of sequences having the same variable and joining genes and the CDR3 in an unselected library or in selection pools against a different target. Within a clonal group, the largest subgroup having identical sequence over the entire variable domain is usually chosen as the representative sequence. Depending on the availability of resources, representative sequences from the top 10 to 20 clonal groups are chosen for further experiments. Given the limitations on the length of reads with acceptable quality scores, it is often difficult if not impossible to determine the pairing of heavy and light chains. We combine the top heavy-chain sequences with the top light-chain sequences in a combinatorial manner in preliminary high-throughput expression experiments followed by binding assessment by enzyme-linked immunosorbent assay (ELISA). In the case of affinity maturation libraries, the sequences that are selected for further experiments should be the top clones, not clonal groups.

Pros and Cons

Antibody discovery based on data mining has its advantages as well as disadvantages. The data-mining method could be complementary to the traditional high-throughput sequencing (HTS) in that false-negative binders that do not express well in the display host could be identified based on their frequency in the population and characterized further. Not all binders identified by HTS are necessarily identified in the data-mining method, again suggesting that a two-pronged strategy of combining HTS with data mining, when resources permit, will enhance the success rate in antibody discovery campaigns. Deciphering the heavy- and light-chain pair based on data mining is often difficult, if not impossible. Depending on the display vector design and the distance between the VH and VL domains, it may be possible to design sequencing strategies to identify the over-represented VH/VL pairs from antibody libraries. If the predominant VH/VL pairs cannot be deciphered from the sequence data, it is necessary to express and screen combinations of predominant heavy and light chains to identify the potential binders.

Deep-Sequencing of cDNA from Immunized Animals

Very few B cells form successful fusions with the immortalizing cell line, hence there is a high probability that some potent binders are lost in the process. Moreover, the generation of fusions, screening, and subcloning are labor intensive and time consuming. Deep sequencing brings the prospect of sequencing nearly all of the antibodies expressed in the lymphoid organs of an immunized animal, and the high-abundance antibodies of the immunome are the ones hypothesized to be enriched due to immunization with the antigen. Antibody discovery driven by data mining opens up the possibility of developing monoclonal antibodies from organisms that lack a well-established fusion partner and protocol. One limitation inherent to this method is that the light- and heavy-chain pairing used in the immune response may not be correctly identified.

High-affinity antibodies against three antigens were identified from immunized mice through the application of high-throughput sequencing of bone marrow plasma cells and data mining.[18] Two other studies combined proteomics with high-throughput sequencing to identify antigen-specific antibodies from serum.[19,23] In both the studies, the high-throughput sequencing data were used to create a case-specific database of antibody V regions against which the protein fingerprints were searched.

Sample preparation for sequencing begins with isolation of mRNA from bone marrow, spleen, other lymphoid tissue such as lymph nodes, isolated splenocytes or isolated plasma cells of bone marrow followed by generation of cDNA. The cDNA is amplified using fusion primers containing the target-specific sequences and sequenced as described in the "Sample Preparation and Sequencing for Affinity Maturation Libraries" section earlier. Data analysis can be performed as described in "Sequence Analysis for Antibody Discovery" section, with the exception that the germline gene database used for gene assignment should include the germline genes of the organism used in the immunization. Direct sequencing antibodies from lymphoid tissue does not provide information on the pairing of heavy and light chains; thus, it is absolutely essential to experimentally determine the correct pairing by combining all selected heavy chains with all selected light chains. For many antibodies, it is the heavy chain that determines the specificity, and the light chain contributes toward affinity; therefore, it may be possible to combine a well-behaved human light-chain germline gene sequence with the heavy chains selected from the immunized animal to derive a "half-human" antigen-specific binder.[24]

SPECIES OTHER THAN HUMANS AND RODENTS AS SOURCE OF V REGIONS

Hybridoma technology was originally developed for rodents. In fact, except for the human antibodies obtained through phage display or immunization of transgenic animals, all the marketed antibodies at the time of writing this chapter were generated in mice or rats (see http://www.antibodysociety.org/news/approved_mabs.php). The success of antibody-based drugs has fueled the diversification of platforms for discovery and optimization of more efficacious, safer, and developable therapeutic antibodies,[25] including immunization of species other than rodents. Rabbits and chickens are species that are capable of generating highly potent antibodies against unique epitopes, and they offer the practical advantages of rodents with regard to obtaining, characterizing, and engineering therapeutic antibodies. In the following sections, we describe the functional and structural repertoire of rabbits and chickens and discuss engineering strategies to humanize antibodies from these species.

Rabbit Antibodies

It is well known that rabbits (*Oryctolagus cuniculus*) have the capability of generating high-affinity antibodies with exquisite specificity.[6,26] This capability, compounded with the possibility of obtaining large amounts of anti-sera relative to mice and rats, have made rabbit polyclonal antibodies attractive reagents for research and diagnostics for decades. Rabbit polyclonal antibodies have also been utilized in transplantation in the last two decades. For example, the antithymocyte globulin (ATG) purified IgG fraction of sera from rabbits has successfully been used in allogeneic stem-cell transplantation and solid-organ transplantation.[27] In the mid-1990s, development of a myeloma rabbit B-cell fusion partner[28] enabled the generation of rabbit monoclonal antibodies, expanding the interest in rabbit V genes as substrates for the development of therapeutic antibodies.

Fv Functional Repertoire

Genomic mapping of the rabbit IGH locus has revealed the existence of over 200 IGHV germline genes.[29–31] Over 50% have been found to be nonfunctional, with about 80 to 90% of the circulating antibodies derived from the IGHV1 gene and expressing the IGHVa1-3 allotypic markers. The VH chains of the remaining 10 to 20% of circulating antibodies are encoded by the IGHVn genes, which are localized at least 100 Kb upstream of IGHV1. The coding regions of the IGHJ genes from different haplotypes are also conserved,[30] and the repertoire of VDJ rearrangements is limited by the use of a small number of IGHD and IGHJ genes. Out of six IGHJ genes, IGHJ4 has been found in 80% of the VDJ gene rearrangements and IGHJ2 in the other 20%. Of the 12 IGHD gene segments, most VDJ gene rearrangements use D2a (D9), D2b (Df), D3, or D5; D4 and D6 are rarely utilized. The limited usage of IGHV, IGHD, and IGHJ genes is thought to be compensated by diversity generated at N regions. The size of the functional rabbit repertoire has not yet been estimated, and the basis for the preferential usage of the IGHV1 and IGHJ4 gene in VDJ rearrangements remains unanswered.[30]

Different from other species such as humans and rodents, where the VH domain plays a fundamental role in antigen recognition, VL seems to be a major contributor to the rabbit antibody diversity and thus specificity.[32] Estimates of the number of rabbit IGKV germline genes have suggested a repertoire greater than 50 IGKV functional genes and the preferential use of one IGKJ gene.[32–34] Importantly, the IGKV genes encode at least seven CDR-L3 lengths, resulting in a potentially larger repertoire of CDR-L3 loop lengths than its mouse or human counterparts.[33] A diverse repertoire of VK chains, together with gene conversion as a means to diversify the repertoire of antibodies,[33] seems to compensate for the limited repertoire of VH chains to build the rabbit immune response.

Using the Roche 454 deep-sequencing technology we recently explored the functional diversity of the rabbit antibody repertoire.[35] We sequenced the VH and VL repertoires of bone marrow (BM) and spleen (SP) of a naïve New Zealand white rabbit (NZW; *Oryctolagus cuniculus*) and those of lymphocytes collected from a NZW rabbit immunized (IM) with a 16-mer peptide. Consistent with a previous study,[19] two closely related IGHV genes, IGHVS140 (VH1a3) and IGHVS145 (VH4), accounted for more than 90% of the BM and SP VH sequences. Interestingly, as much as 40% of the IM sequences were assigned to the IGHV1S69 gene (VH1a1). The difference in the IGHV usage may be explained by the fact that the BM and SP samples were obtained from the same rabbit, whereas the IM sample was obtained from another rabbit. Alternatively, the distinct IGHV gene usage could be due the peptide immunization.

The IGHJ germline gene usage of BM and SP samples was also consistent with previous studies,[19] with approximately 80% of the sequences assigned to IGHJ4. A distinct IGHJ usage was observed in the IM sample. Only 54% of IM sequences were assigned to IGHJ4, whereas 26% of the sequences were assigned to IGHJ2. This difference might be due to the distinct IGHV usage; that is, IGHV1S40 and/or IGHV1S45 might recombine preferentially with IGHJ4, whereas IGHV1S69 might have a preference to recombine with IGHJ2.

Out of the 68 rabbit IGKV germline genes reported in IMGT,[36] we found[35] that 23 contributed with a frequency of 1% of more and seven contributed to the repertoire of rearranged sequences with a frequency of 5% or higher in at least one of the samples. In contrast to VH, none of the genes contributed more than 20% of the sample. Differences in the IGKV gene usage were also observed among the BM, SP, and IM samples. For example, IGKVS1 is underexpressed in IM when compared to BM and SP, whereas IGKVS52 is overexpressed in SP and IM when compared to BM. However, the bias is not as apparent as in VH.

Interestingly, the CDR-H3 length distribution was similar in the three samples, which implies that it is independent of the bias observed in IGHV and IGHJ gene usage among the BM, SP, and IM samples. The rabbit CDR-H3 lengths resembled a normal distribution with the highest frequency at 11-amino-acid loops. Human CDR-H3 loops tended to be slightly longer with an average of 13 amino acids,[37] (Kabat's definition) with a range of 1 to 35. Mice CDR-H3 loops are shorter, with an average length of 9 amino acids and a range of 1 to 21 amino acids.[37]

In addition to the length distribution, the amino acid composition of the CDR-H3 loop is of critical importance to the antibody repertoire function, and detailed characterization of the diversity encoded in this loop has aided the design of libraries for antibody discovery.[38,39] The stems of the loop (i.e., Cys 92, Ala 93, and Arg 94 at the N-terminal region of the loop) and four residues at the C-terminal, before the conserved Trp-102 (YFNI/L for IGHJ4 and NAFDP for IGHJ2), reflect the amino acid composition of the IGHV and the IGHJ genes, respectively. The apical region of the loops is rich in Gly, Ser, and Tyr, with frequencies that vary between 15% and 35%, depending on position in the loop. Loop lengths of 11 and 12 amino acids also have a high content (~30%) of Asp at position 95, which is due to recombination events between the IGHV and IGHJ genes. Overall, the rabbit CDR-H3 amino acid composition is similar to that of humans and mice,[37] with both species having a strong preference for the use of Tyr, Ser, and Gly residues.

Similar to the CDR-H3, the CDR-L3 length distribution did not differ in the BM, SP, and IM samples.[35] It followed a normal distribution with average lengths of 11 amino acids and a range of 8 lengths. Thus, the CDR-L3 of rabbits is more diverse than its human counterpart.[40]

In humans, as much as 70% of loops are seven residues in length. Few human antibodies have one deletion with respect to the seven-residue loop or one or two insertions, yielding a range of lengths of six to nine amino acids.

The composition of the CDR-L3 loops with frequencies above 10% (lengths of 10 to 13 residues) reflects the amino acid composition of the IGVK and the IGJK genes, due to their very high content (50 to 80%) of Gly, Ser, Tyr, or Asp in certain positions. Approximately 10% of the loops have Cys in position 91, regardless of the length and the sample. These antibodies may present liabilities with regard to the development of therapeutic antibodies.[41] Twelve-residue loops of IM samples are also rich (~65%) in Cys at positions 95 and 95e.

Structural Repertoire

Knowledge of the structural repertoire of antigen-binding sites of human antibodies has been crucial in library design for antibody discovery and optimization.[42] It has also contributed to knowledge-based methods for antibody three-dimensional modeling,[43] where it is used as a tool to engineer antibodies for therapeutic settings (i.e., humanization, affinity optimization, and developability enhancement).[41] An alignment of the amino-acid sequences of the most prevalent rabbit IGHV genes—IGHV1S45, IGHV1S40, and IGHV1S69—is shown in Figure 7.4A. IGHV1S40 and IGHVIS45 differ by one deletion in position 2 and five mutations, two of them in the CDR-1. In contrast, IGHV1S69s differ from IGHV1S40/45 by 13 mutations and three deletions, one in each CDR, and the third in FR-3. Therefore, antibodies derived from IGHV1S40 and IGHVIS45 genes should generate similar antigen-binding sites, whereas antibodies encoded by IGHV1S69 may result in quite different ones. Another interesting difference between IGHV1S40/45 and IGHV1S69 is the presence of two cysteine residues in the CDRs (Cys^{L35} and Cys^{L50}) of the former.

Figure 7.4B shows an alignment of the VK genes contributing >5% of functional repertoire of rabbits.[35] These genes can be clustered into two groups (Figure 7.4C) and differ by a deletion of two residues in the CDR-L1. In addition to the diversity of rabbit CDR-L3 in terms of lengths (see above), the conformation of these loops seems to be structurally less constrained than that of human CDR-L3 loops. The vast majority of the human and mouse germline loops encode Pro at position 95, restraining the loop to a definite canonical structure, type 1.[44,45] Such a constraint does not exist in rabbit antibodies, as amino acids other than Pro are found in position 95.

At the time of writing, five rabbit Fab structures were available or pending release at the Protein Data Bank (PDB). Four PDB entries—4JO1, 4JO2, 4JO3, and 4JO4—contained coordinates for two rabbit antibodies, R56 (4JO1 and 4JO2) and R20 (4JO3 and 4JO4), raised against the third variable region (V3) of HIV-1 gp120.[46] The fifth structure, 4MA3, was a direct deposit to be released by the beginning of 2014 (Gary Gilliland, pers. comm.). A comparison of the structures indicates that R56 and 4MA3 have a closely related VL, whereas R56 and R20 have similar VHs. Therefore, these structures represent two different VHs and two VLs.

The R56/R20 VHs were likely derived from IGHV1S40/45 or other closely related genes. They have eight mutations and no insertions/deletions with respect to IGHV1S40/45. When compared to IGHV1S69, R56/R20 VH have nine mutations and one deletion in FR-3. The VH of 4MA3, on other hand, only has the same CDR-H1 and H2 loop lengths as IGHV1S69, with five mutations and one deletion in the FR-3. Hence, the known rabbit structures represent the main CDR-H1 and CDR-H2 loop lengths of the prevalent rabbit VH repertoire.

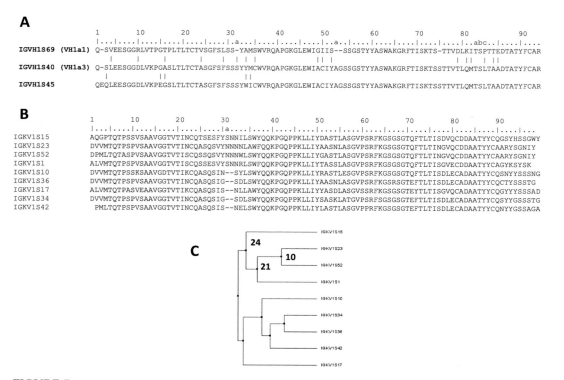

FIGURE 7.4 Most prevalent IGVH and IGVK genes. Amino-acid sequence alignment of the most prevalent (A) IGVH and (B) IGVK genes observed in the samples analyzed. (C) Dendogram showing the diversity and relationship of the IGVK genes. Residues are numbered according to Chothia convention. The VK amino-acid sequences in the dendogram were aligned and dendogram was plotted based on average distance calculated from percent identity using Jalview. The numbers close to the branches represent number of mutations.

Regarding VK, R56 and 4MA3 are 84% identical and have the same length in all the CDRs, including two Cys in positions 95 and 95e. When compared with the most prevalent IGKV germline genes, R20/4MA3 is close to the IGKVIS01 germline gene with no indels in the CDRs. R56 matches IGKVS36 with no indels. Therefore, as in VH, the known VL rabbit structures represent the main groups of CDR lengths of the most prevalent germline gene in the rabbit antibody repertoire.

Comparison with known canonical structures indicates that the CDR-L1 of R20 belongs to the group defined by North et al.[47] as L1-11, whereas the CDR-L1 of R26 and 4MA3 represents a new canonical structure. The CDR-L2 has the conserved typical canonical structure observed in most of human and mouse antibodies. The non-canonical cysteines at positions 95 and 95e in the CDR-L3 form a disulfide bond that stabilizes a conformation conserved in R20 and 4MA3. The other non-canonical Cys in FR-3 (Cys^{L80}) forms an interdomain disulfide bond with Cys^{L170} in the Cκ domain.

The CDR-H1 of R56 and R20 can be classified as H1-14 and the CDR-H1 of 4MA3 as H1-13.[47] The CDR-H2 of 4MA3 has the canonical structure defined as H2-9, while R56 and

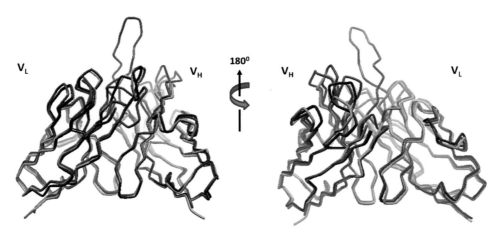

FIGURE 7.5 Molecular overlay of the three rabbit Fvs of known structure. R26 (PDB: 1JO3) in blue; 4MA3 in green; R20 (PDB: 1J01) in red.

R20 have a new conformation. It is probably stabilized by an interdomain disulfide bond formed between Cys^{H50} and Cys^{H35} in the CDR-H1. Noncanonical disulfide bonds are found with very low frequency in human and mouse CDRs but often in other species, including chickens (see below). These disulfide bonds may limit the flexibility of the Fv and the loops forming the antigen-binding site and hence help to increase the binding affinity of antibodies by reducing the entropy.

Most of the anti-protein antibodies have canonical structures determined by short CDR-L1 loops (six to eight residues).[48] This is in contrast to anti-peptide and anti-hapten antibodies, which predominantly have canonical structures made of long CDR-L1 loops (11 to 13 residues). The remaining loops show little difference in the canonical structure distribution across anti-protein, anti-peptide, and anti-hapten antibodies. The combination of short CDR1 and 2 in rabbit VH and VL generates a relative flat binding site. This topography is modified by the CDR-L3 and CDR-H3. Note in Figure 7.5, for example, the difference in R20 with respect to R56 and 4MA3 that forms a finger-like topography found in antibodies that recognize recessed epitopes[49] and the relative flat binding site of R26 and 4MA3.

Engineering Rabbit Antibodies for Therapeutic Applications

One of the main concerns when developing biologics is the potential immunogenicity of the therapeutic product.[50] Since the pioneering work by Greg Winter in the mid-1980s, several methods have been validated to humanize antibodies and therefore minimize immunogenicity.[51] For rabbit antibodies, three methods have been described thus far.

First, Rader and coworkers[52] described a method that relied on a combination of CDR grafting and FR fine-tuning by phage display selection. Selected rabbit sequences using phage display were first aligned with human IGV and IGJ germline genes. The best matches, which happened to be genes encoding well-behaved antibodies and FR frequently used in humanization campaigns (e.g., human genes from the IGHV3 and IGKV1 families), were combined with CDRs (Kabat's definition) of rabbit clones with higher expression levels. For the FR fine-tuning, residues important for stabilizing and positioning the CDRs, also known as Vernier residues,[53] at six positions in VH and four positions in Vκ are diversified. A new phage library displaying Fabs with the diversified human FRs sequence and rabbit CDRs are then selected by panning against immobilized target using highly stringent conditions. The resulting humanized antibodies were found to retain both high specificity and affinity for human A33 antigen, the target used as immunogen and known to be an antigen for the immunotherapy of colon cancer.

Recognizing that the repertoire of rabbit antibodies is relatively simple, another approach[54] developed a human scFv scaffold, termed FW1.4, designed to accommodate CDRs derived from a broad variety of rabbit V domains. Using as human FRs IGHV3 and IGKV1 genes, a motif consisting of five structurally relevant residues (T^{H23}, G^{H49}, T^{H73}, V^{H78}, and R^{H94}) that are highly conserved in rabbit variable domains was introduced into FW1.4. Grafting of CDRs from 15 different rabbit antibodies onto FW1.4 and their derivatives resulted in humanized scFvs with binding affinities in the picomolar range. In addition, the developability profile of the humanized scFvs improved significantly, including good production yields in *Escherichia coli* and the apparent melting temperature (T_m) of some antibodies reaching 80°C. By using this minimalistic approach, 15 different rabbit antibodies directed against tumor necrosis factor-α (TNF-α) or vascular endothelial growth factor (VEGF) were humanized.

The third method, called mutational lineage-guided (MLG), was developed by Epitomics.[55] It is based on comparing V-region sequences that have the same biological functions and are presumably derived from the same parental B cell during the *in vivo* antibody affinity maturation process. In brief, a number of V regions with similar binding profiles are identified from each immunized rabbit using either a cell-based or a biochemical assay. Amino-acid sequences of both VH and VL are obtained and aligned to form a phylogenetic tree. It is assumed that the sequences in each lineage likely share a common B cell ancestor and conserved sequences in a lineage-related group, thus representing important residues for the structure and function of such antibodies. Conversely, nonconserved residues are assumed to be well-tolerated mutations that do not compromise specificity and/or affinity. If these mutations occurred at the positions that are different between the rabbit and the human FRs, human residues at these positions should be well tolerated in the humanized antibody. More importantly, if such mutations are found in the CDRs, such replacements should render the antibody more human-like, without affecting the structure or binding, thereby yielding a less immunogenic molecule. The MLG humanization method has been used in more than ten engineering projects with success.[6]

Chicken Antibodies

Chickens (*Gallus gallus*) have some practical advantages compared to mammals as sources of V regions for antibody therapeutic development. Avians are phylogenetically more distant from humans than rodents (and even rabbits), which makes it possible to isolate cross-reactive antibodies against conserved epitopes in these species. Another advantage is that chicken antibodies can be collected directly from the egg yolk and the antibodies can be purified in one step in large amounts. This non-invasive collection of antibodies and their straightforward purification facilitate follow-up of immunization campaigns and easy characterization of chicken polyclonal antibodies. Furthermore, the V gene repertoire of chickens is simpler than that of mammals, enabling the identification and engineering of V regions for the development of therapeutic antibodies at low cost.

Fv Functional Repertoire

Characterization of the repertoire of chicken antibodies began with the seminal work of Reynaud and coworkers.[56,57] The equivalent to mammalian IgGs in chickens is called IgY due to the presence of this immunoglobulin in high concentration (5 to 15 mg/mL) in the egg yolk.[58] IgY is similar to IgG except that it has four Cγ domains[59] and lacks the flexible hinge region. The lack of hinge structure is also found in mammalian IgE. Hence, the IgY exhibit structural features of both mammalian IgE and IgG. The V repertoire of IgYs is integrated by a single functional VH and VL genes that recombine with unique J$_H$ and D-J$_H$ segments.[60–62] Chicken antibodies also differ in the content of λ and κ isotype[63] with respect to humans, mice, and rabbits. The functional VL genes are λ-type, thus making chicken antibodies exclusively λ-type. Human antibodies are 40:60 λ:κ, mouse is 95% κ, and rabbit is almost exclusively κ-type. Despite the limited V gene repertoire of chickens, high-affinity antibodies to a broad arrange of antigens including proteins, peptides, and haptens,[64–67] have been obtained in this species.

Chickens have in common with rabbits[68] the use of gene conversion to diversify their single VH and VL genes.[62,63] Such diversification occurs via the incorporation of segments from upstream pseudogenes that lack recombination signal sequences. Based on sequence homology between the pseudogene and the germline gene which acts as the acceptor, the process diversifies both CDRs and FRs.[69] However, recent chicken V$_H$ repertoire analysis suggests that the requirement for sequence homology between the germ line and pseudogene leads to a low level of mutagenesis in the FRs but hypervariability in the CDRs.[70] Interestingly, this was coupled with strong maintenance of common CDR structural residues that have also been observed in mammals[71] but modulation of residues that affect VH–VL interaction[72] and CDRs[53]. Thus, the chicken V$_H$ repertoire increases structural diversity by changing the CDRs residues and angle of interaction between the VH and VL domains[73].

The CDR-H3 repertoire of chickens differs substantially from that of humans and mice, in both length distribution and amino acid content. Chickens have 15 functional D segments, all of which are highly homologous; some (e.g., D9/12/13, D4/8/11) are even identical in amino-acid sequence.[61] In contrast to human, mice, and rabbits, the chicken naive repertoire is not normally distributed and favors much longer sequences. The majority (89%) of chicken CDR-H3 are between 15 and 23 residues in length. Shorter CDR-H3 lengths are found to be relatively rare.

The CDR-H3 amino-acid content in the chicken is also very different from humans, mice,[74] and rabbits. There is a bias toward small amino acids (G/S/A/C/T, but not P), while large aromatic and hydrophobic residues are strongly disfavored, including an unusually low representation of Y, the dominant residue in the repertoires of mice and humans. This observation may be important, as synthetic antibody repertoire studies have suggested that Y is a critical amino acid for target binding.[75–78] Additionally, the chicken CDR3 repertoire has a low representation of positively charged residues (K/R). This may be of practical importance, as excess positive charge in the VH CDR3 is associated with polyreactivity[79] and a poor pK profile *in vivo*[80] but can lower the pI of the antibody.

The presence of Cys residues in the CDR-H3 suggests an important functional role. Human functional CDR-H3 sequences contain pairs of cysteines;[38] however, they are found at a low frequency.[81] The high incorporation rate of C in the chicken CDR-H3 creates loops with intra-CDR disulfide bridges and insertion of single C residues in the VH CDRs 1 and 2 for inter-CDR disulfide bonding. These covalent bonds between CDRs are structurally analogous to those observed at high frequency in antibodies of other species, such as camelids,[82] sharks,[83,84] cows,[85–87] and pigs.[88] Mutagenesis studies have shown that these disulfide bonds, in either IgG or single-domain antibodies, are essential for both V-domain stability and binding function.[89–91]

Structural Repertoire and Engineering of Chicken Antibodies

Given the limited number of chicken V regions, the topography of chicken antigen-binding sites is mainly modulated by the repertoire of CDR-H3 conformations. Recently, the structure of an anti-phospho-tau chicken Fab (pT231/pS235_1) in complex with the cognate phospho-peptide was determined at 1.9 Å resolution (PDB code: 4GLR). The CDR-L2, CDR-L3, CDR-H1, and CDR-H2 can be classified within the known canonical conformations described by North et al.[47] as L2–8, L3–11, H1–13, and H2–10, respectively. The CDR-L1 is shorter by three residues than any of the known canonical structures.[47,93] The combination of the short CDR-L1 with the other loops generates a relatively flat topography, similar to rabbit antibodies (Figure 7.6, top). This basic theme can be modulated by indels in the CDRs, pairing of VH and VL, and the CDR-H3 conformation, which in turns is stabilized by disulfide bonds. For example, as described by Shih et al.,[92] pT231/pS235_1 exhibits a "bowl-like" conformation in CDR-H2 that interacts with the phospho-Thr-231 phosphate group. The CDR-H3 is 18 amino acids in length and is constrained by a disulfide bond between C^{H100B} and C^{H100Y} (Figure 7.6, bottom). It forms a surface that makes numerous interactions with the non-phosphorylated part of the epitope.

Humanization of chicken antibodies seems to be relatively straightforward. The functional VH gene has ~70% homology with members of the human IGHV3 family, whereas VL is close (~60% homology) to members of the human IGLV3 family. Using human VH and VL genes from these families as FR donors, in one approach back mutations were designed to accommodate the chicken CDRs in the human FRs.[7] In another example, libraries of residues in Vernier positions[53] were designed similar to rabbit humanization and cloned, and the optimal combination of mutations was selected by phage display.[66] In the rational approach—design of back mutations—the affinities of a humanized antibody to human and mouse IL-12 were nearly identical to those of a chicken–human chimeric. By phage display selection, most of the humanized variants also retained affinity comparable to the parental chicken antibody.

Because chickens are phylogenetically more distant from humans than rodents, it is reasonable to think that chicken antibodies are more immunogenic than murine antibodies when used in human therapy. Interestingly, as mentioned above, chicken V genes are 60 to 70% homologous to human V genes, and the CDR conformations are similar to the

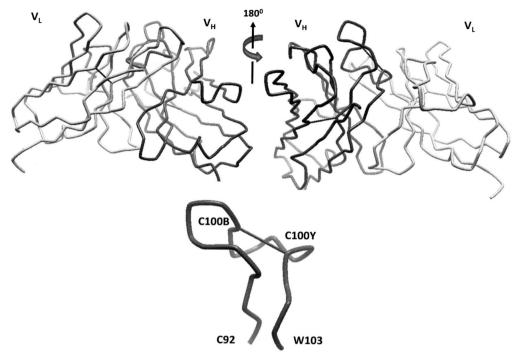

FIGURE 7.6 Chicken Fv of known structure in blue. (Top) Side views of the Fv. (Bottom) Long CDR-H3 stabilized with a disulfide bride between Cys H100b and Cys H100Y.

structure of known human and mouse antibodies. In addition, FR replacement during humanization should minimize immunogenicity in the FR, and in recent years methodologies have been developed to identify nonhuman residues and/or immunogenic spots in the CDRs and mutate them to human germline gene residues without compromising binding.[94,95] In one method,[94] the closest matching human germline sequence for the humanized antibody was identified based on sequence comparison, and all possible single substitutions that increase the sequence identity of the engineered antibody sequence to the closest human germline sequence were screened for binding. In another method, the CDRs were scanned with overlapping peptides and tested for their ability to induce proliferative responses with CD4+ T cells and dendritic cells from community donors.[95] Peptides carrying T-cell epitopes were deimmunized by modifying the amino-acid sequence of the CDRs and testing the impact of the mutations in antigen-binding assays. The engineered antibodies retained binding and were indistinguishable from or closely related to human antibodies isolated from transgenic mice or human antibody libraries. This methodology can be applied to minimize immunogenicity in chicken antibodies, and, although the immunogenicity of the chicken engineered antibodies has to be determined in the clinic, chicken therapeutic antibodies may not be that different or might be less immunogenic than rodent antibodies.

BI- AND MULTISPECIFICS INSPIRED IN THE MODULARITY OF ANTIBODIES

As Riethmüller[12] pointed out, the concept of antibody-like multifunctional molecules can be traced back to the pioneering work of Nisonoff, Wissler, and Lipman.[96] In this seminal paper, which contributed to elucidating the modular nature of antibodies, the authors suggested the possibility of making "antibodies of mixed specificity." Over 20 years later,[97] this concept was realized in the development of hybrid hybridomas. In this modality, two hybridomas generating monoclonal antibodies of distinct specificity are fused to produce a quadroma that expresses a trispecific molecule, in which each Fab arm binds two distinct targets and the Fc engages Fc receptors triggering effector functions as an intact IgG molecule (Figure 7.7A). The product of a hybrid hybridoma, catumaxomab was approved in Europe in 2009,[8] raising renewed interest in the field of multispecific modalities. Catumaxomab was developed by Fresenius Biotech and Trion Pharma and approved for the treatment of malignant ascites in patients with EpCAM-positive cancer when a standard therapy is not available.

The key assumption behind the development of bi- and multispecific molecules is that binding two or more targets simultaneously with a single molecular entity increases therapeutic efficacy over binding the individual targets. Alternative modalities to bi- and multispecifics

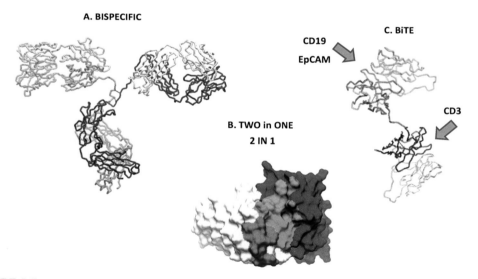

FIGURE 7.7 Three representative bispecifics. (A) Hybrid hybridomas combining the LC and HC from one antibody (yellow and orange, respectively) with LC and HC from another antibody (silver and violet, respectively) to generate a hybrid IgG molecule with each Fab arm recognizing a different target. (B) Connolly surface of the same Fv shown in Figure 7.1 now illustrating the two-in-one format. Residues determining binding to one of the targets are colored in blue. Residues determining binding to a second target are colored in red. Residues shared by the two targets are in green. (C) Tandem of scFvs that bind two different targets; in the case of BiTE, one of the targets is CD3 and the other is a target in a tumor, such as CD19 (MT103) or EpCAM (MT110). Linkers are colored in green, and blue arrows indicate the position of the binding sites. The coordinates used to generate the figure correspond to the structure with PDB code 1IN2.

such as mixtures of antibodies have also emerged in the last years.[98] Similar to bispecifics, mixtures of antibodies could recognize two or more targets or distinct epitopes on the same target and thus complement each other to combat diseases. However, linking two or more targets with a single bispecific molecule has advantages. For example, if one the targets is displayed on a cancer cell and the other target is on the surface of the immune system cells, the bispecific molecule could recruit the immune response to destroy the tumor, similar to the natural Fc killing function. In fact, bi- and multispecifics have found applications in multiple therapeutic areas,[11] including allergic and infectious diseases and inflammatory disorders, but the vast majority of indications are being validated in the oncology field.[9] Targets on the tumor cells include carcinoembryonic antigen (CEA), human epidermal growth factor receptor 2 (HER2), cluster of differentiation 19 (CD19), epithelial cell adhesion molecule (EpCAM), and B-lymphocyte antigen CD20. To recruit the immune system, targets include CD3 and CD28 on T cells, CD16 on natural killer (NK) cells, and CD46 on monocytes and neutrophils.

The main limitation in development of hybrid hybridomas has been the low yield of the bispecific entity, which makes the manufacturing process expensive or even impractical. Immunogenicity associated with nonhuman antibodies has been another major roadblock in developing hybrid hybridomas as sources of therapeutic molecules. Technologies to clone and manipulate DNA are overcoming these limitations by making humanization possible (see above) and expanding the concept of antibodies of mixed specificity to several dozen bi- and multispecificity formats with superior manufacturability. These formats include two main types: Fc-fusion proteins and Fc-less fusions.

Fc fusions are of several types: (1) combining two antibodies to generate a hybrid IgG molecule with each Fab arm recognizing a different target similar to the hybrid of hybridomas but engineering the C_H3 domain, the VH/VL interface, or the Fab to maximize the pairing of the bispecific molecule over the pairing of the monospecific antibodies;[99] (2) attaching Fabs, Fvs, or V domains at the amino- or carboxy-terminal or both ends of a known antibody or the Fc; and (3) engineering antigen-binding sites to bind more than one target[100] (Figure 7.7B). In addition to binding two or more targets, the Fc domain in these modalities can activate immune effector pathways. The hinge region of IgG and the C_H2 domain contain critical residues to interact with the Fc gamma family of receptors (FcγRs) and complement. Engagement of FcγRs triggers cellular responses such as antibody-dependent cellular cytotoxicity (ADCC) and antibody-dependent cellular phagocytosis (ADCP), whereas complement fixation leads to activation and formation of the membrane attack complex, which results in cellular lysis.

The second type of multispecific format (i.e., Fc-less molecules) includes the fusion of two Fabs, Fvs, or V domains with distinct binding profiles via a peptide or a protein linker. One of the simplest but most successful formats is BiTE® (bispecific T-cell engager) developed by Micromet, recently acquired by Amgen (Figure 7.7C). BiTE consists of linking two scFvs via a peptide. One of the scFvs is specific for a target in a tumor and the other is specific for CD3. BiTEs exhibit 10^2 to 10^4 higher efficacy in tumor cell lysis than other CD3-bispecific formats. In addition, BiTEs are nonglycosylated proteins that are stable, homogeneous, and soluble and can be manufactured in large amounts. Several BiTE programs have entered into clinical trials. The first BiTE to enter into clinical trials, blinatumomab (MT103), is specific for tumor-associated CD19 and has shown evidence of remission in acute lymphoblastic leukemia.[101] Another BiTE (MT110) specific for EpCAM is currently in clinical trials in patients with advanced solid tumors.

CONCLUSIONS

The approval of several dozen therapeutic antibodies in the last two decades, combined with the high probability of success of antibodies in clinical trials relative to small molecules, the expiration of patents of key technologies such as CDR grafting to humanize antibodies, and the lowering manufacturing costs of biologics, is leading to an acceleration in the discovery and optimization of antibody-based medicines. New technologies such as NGS are enabling this acceleration by assisting screening and complementing assays and hold the promise of simplifying the antibody discovery and optimization processes. Exploitation of new sources of V regions, including, but not limited to, rabbit and chicken V regions, can lead to new specificities and highly potent antibodies offering some advantages over rodents for engineering therapeutic antibodies. Also, validation of diverse novel formats of bi- and multispecific molecules inspired in the modularity of antibodies are leading to superior efficacy in some diseases, especially in the oncology indications. These advances in the discovery and design of antibodies, together with other novel technologies such as antibody–drug conjugates and mixtures of antibodies, are changing the landscape of antibody-based therapies.

Acknowledgments

We would like to thank William Finlay for comments and valuable discussions on the chicken antibodies.

References

1. Wu TT, Kabat EA. An analysis of the sequences of the variable regions of Bence Jones proteins and myeloma light chains and their implications for antibody complementarity. J. Exp. Med. 1970;132:211–50.
2. Davies DR, Padlan EA, Sheriff S. Antibody–antigen complexes. Annu. Rev. Biochem. 1990;59:439–73.
3. Mathonet P, Ullman C. The application of next generation sequencing to the understanding of antibody repertoires. Front. Immunol. 2013;4:1–5.
4. Weinstein J, Jiang N, White RR, Fisher D, Quake S. High-throughput sequencing of the zebrafish antibody repertoire. Science 2009;324:807–10.
5. Ravn U, Gueneau F, Baerlocher L, Osteras M, Desmurs M, Malinge P, Magistrelli G, Farinelli L, Kosco-Vilbois M, Fischer N. By-passing *in vitro* screening—next generation sequencing technologies applied to antibody display and *in silico* candidate selection. Nucleic Acids Res. 2010;38:e193.
6. Yu G, Yang X. High affinity rabbit monoclonal antibodies. Curr. Drug Discov. Technol. 2013. Oct. 30 [Epub ahead of print].
7. Tsurushita N, Park M, Pakabunto K, Ong K, Avdalovic A, Fu H, Jia A, Vásquez M, Kumar S. Humanization of a chicken anti-IL-12 monoclonal antibody. J. Immunol. Methods 2004;295:9–19.
8. Seimetz D, Lindhofer H, Bokemeyer C. Development and approval of the trifunctional antibody catumaxomab (anti-EpCAM x anti-CD3) as a targeted cancer immunotherapy. Cancer Treat. Rev. 2010;36:458–67.
9. Weidle U, Tiefenthaler G, Weiss E, Georges G, Brinkmann U. The intriguing options of multispecific antibody formats for treatment of cancer. Cancer Genomics Proteomics 2013;10:1–18.
10. Kontermann RE. Dual targeting strategies with bispecific antibodies. MAbs 2012;4:182–97.
11. Byrne H, Conroy P, Whisstock J, O'Kennedy R. A tale of two specificities: bispecific antibodies for therapeutic and diagnostic applications. Trends Biotechnol. 2013;31:621–32.
12. Riethmüller G. Symmetry breaking: bispecific antibodies, the beginnings, and 50 years on. Cancer Immun. 2012;12:1–7.
13. Köhler G, Milstein C. Continuous cultures of fused cells secreting antibody of predefined specificity. Nature 1975;256:495–7.

14. Winter G, Griffiths AD, Hawkins RE, Hoogenboom HR. Making antibodies by phage display technology. Annu. Rev. Immunol. 1994;12:433–55.

15. Sanger F, Coulson A. A rapid method for determining sequences in DNA by primed synthesis with DNA polymerase. J. Mol. Biol. 1975;94:441–8.

16. Shendure J, Ji H. Next-generation DNA sequencing. Nat. Biotechnol. 2008;26:1135–45.

17. Ozsolak F. Third-generation sequencing techniques and applications to drug discovery. Expert Opin. Drug Discov. 2012;7:231–43.

18. Reddy S, Ge X, Miklos AE, Hughes RA, Kang SH, Hoi KH, Chrysostomou C, Hunicke-Smith SP, Iverson BL, Tucker PW, Ellington AD, Georgiou G. Monoclonal antibodies isolated without screening by analyzing the variable-gene repertoire of plasma cells. Nat. Biotechnol. 2010;28:965–9.

19. Wine Y, Boutz D, Lavinder J, Miklos A, Hughes R, Hoi K, Jung S, Horton A, Murrin E, Ellington A, Marcotte E, Georgiou G. Molecular deconvolution of the monoclonal antibodies that comprise the polyclonal serum response. Proc. Natl. Acad. Sci. U.S.A. 2013;110:2993–8.

20. Saggy I, Wine Y, Shefet-Carasso L, Nahary L, Georgiou G, Benhar I. Antibody isolation from immunized animals: comparison of phage display and antibody discovery via V gene repertoire mining. Protein Eng. Des. Sel. 2012;25:539–49.

21. Alamyar E, Duroux P, Lefranc M, Giudicelli V. IMGT® tools for the nucleotide analysis of immunoglobulin (IG) and T cell receptor (TR) V-(D)-J repertoires, polymorphisms, and IG mutations: IMGT/V-QUEST and IMGT/HighV-QUEST for NGS. Methods Mol. Biol. 2012;882:569–604.

22. Glanville J, Zhai W, Berka J, Telman D, Huerta G, Mehta G, Ni I, Mei L, Sundar P, Day G, Cox D, Rajpal A, Pons J. Precise determination of the diversity of a combinatorial antibody library gives insight into the human immunoglobulin repertoire. Proc. Natl. Acad. Sci. U.S.A. 2009;106:20216–21.

23. Cheung W, Beausoleil S, Zhang X, Sato S, Schieferl S, Wieler J, Beaudet J, Ramenani R, Popova L, Comb M, Rush J, Polakiewicz R. A proteomics approach for the identification and cloning of monoclonal antibodies from serum. Nat. Biotechnol. 2012;30:447–52.

24. Rojas G, Almagro J, Acevedo B, Gavilondo J. Phage antibody fragments library combining a single human light chain variable region with immune mouse heavy chain variable regions. J. Biotechnol. 2002;94:287–98.

25. Almagro J, Strohl W. Antibody engineering: humanization, affinity maturation and selection methods. In: An Z, editor. Therapeutic Monoclonal Antibodies: From Bench to Clinic. New York: John Wiley & Sons; 2009. p. 307–27.

26. An Z, editor. Therapeutic Monoclonal Antibodies: From the Bench to the Clinic. New York: John Wiley & Sons; 2009. p. 151–69.

27. Popow I, Leitner J, Majdic O, Kovarik J, Saemann M, Zlabinger G, Steinberger P. Assessment of batch to batch variation in polyclonal antithymocyte globulin preparations. Transplantation 2012;93:32–40.

28. Spieker-Polet H, Sethupathi P, Yam P, Knight K. Rabbit monoclonal antibodies: generating a fusion partner to produce rabbit–rabbit hybridomas. Proc. Natl. Acad. Sci. U.S.A. 1995;92:9348–52.

29. Currier S, Gallarda J, Knight K. Partial molecular genetic map of the rabbit VH chromosomal region. J. Immunol. 1988;140:1651–9.

30. Mage R, Lanning D, Knight K. B cell and antibody repertoire development in rabbits: the requirement of gut-associated lymphoid tissues. Dev. Comp. Immunol. 2006;30:137–53.

31. Ros F, Puels J, Reichenberger N, Schooten WV, Buelow R, Platzer J. Sequence analysis of 0.5 Mb of the rabbit germline immunoglobulin heavy chain locus. Gene 2004;330:49–59.

32. Sehgal D, Johnson G, Wu T, Mage R. Generation of the primary antibody repertoire in rabbits: expression of a diverse set of Igk-V genes may compensate for limited combinatorial diversity at the heavy chain locus. Immunogenetics 1999;50:31–42.

33. Ros F, Reichenberger N, Dragicevic T, Schooten WV, Buelow R, Platzer J. Sequence analysis of 0.4 megabases of the rabbit germline immunoglobulin kappa1 light chain locus. Anim. Genet. 2005;36:51–7.

34. Reynaud C, Weill J. Postrearrangement diversification processes in gut-associated lymphoid tissues. Curr. Top. Microbiol. Immunol. 1996;212:7–15.

35. Kodangattil S, Huard C, Ross C, Li J, Gao H, Mascioni A, Hodawadekar S, Naik S, Visintin A, Almagro J. The functional repertoire of rabbit antibodies and antibody discovery via next-generation sequencing. mAbs 2013;6:628–36.

36. Lefranc M-P, Giudicelli V, Kaas Q, Duprat E, Jabado-Michaloud J, Scaviner D, Ginestoux C, Clement O, Chaume D, Lefranc G. IMGT®, the international ImMunoGeneTics information system. Nucleic Acids Res. 2005;33:D593–7.

37. Zemlin M, Klinger M, Link J, Zemlin C, Bauer K, Engler JA, Schroeder HW Jr, Kirkham PM. Expressed murine and human CDR-H3 intervals of equal length exhibit distinct repertoires that differ in their amino acid composition and predicted range of structures. J. Mol. Biol. 2003;334:733–49.

38. Schroeder HW Jr. Similarity and divergence in the development and expression of the mouse and human antibody repertoires. Dev. Comp. Immunol. 2006;30:119–35.

39. Schroeder HW Jr, Hillson JL, Perlmutter RM. Early restriction of the human antibody repertoire. Science 1987;238:791–3.

40. Tomlinson I, Cox J, Gherardi E, Lesk A, Chothia C. The structural repertoire of the human V kappa domain. EMBO J. 1995;14:4628–38.

41. Gilliland G, Luo J, Vafa O, Almagro J. Leveraging SBDD in protein therapeutic development: antibody engineering. Methods Mol. Biol. 2012;841:321–49.

42. Finlay W, Almagro J. Natural and man-made V-gene repertoires for antibody discovery. Front. Immunol. 2012;3:342.

43. Almagro J, Beavers M, Hernandez-Guzman F, Maier J, Shaulsky J, Butenhof K, Labute P, Thorsteinson N, Kelly K, Teplyakov T, Luo J, Sweet R, Gilliland G. Antibody modeling assessment. Proteins 2011;79: 3050–66.

44. Al-Lazikani B, Lesk AM, Chothia C. Standard conformations for the canonical structures of immunoglobulins. J. Mol. Biol. 1997;273:927–48.

45. Kuroda D, Shirai H, Kobori M, Nakamura H. Systematic classification of CDR-L3 in antibodies: implications of the light chain subtypes and the VL-VH interface. Proteins 2009;75:139–46.

46. Pan R, Sampson J, Chen Y, Vaine M, Wang S, Lu S, Kong X. Rabbit anti-HIV-1 monoclonal antibodies raised by immunization can mimic the antigen-binding modes of antibodies derived from HIV-1-infected humans. J. Virol. 2013;87:10221–31.

47. North B, Lehmann A, Dunbrack RJ. A new clustering of antibody CDR loop conformations. J. Mol. Biol. 2011;406:228–56.

48. Raghunathan G, Smart J, Williams J, Almagro J. Antigen-binding site anatomy and somatic mutations in antibodies that recognize different types of antigens. J. Mol. Recognit. 2012;25:103–13.

49. Saphire E, Parren P, Pantophlet R, Zwick M, Morris G, Rudd P, Dwek R, Stanfield R, Burton D, Wilson I. Crystal structure of a neutralizing human IGG against HIV-1: a template for vaccine design. Science 2001;293: 1155–9.

50. Schellekens H, Crommelin D, Jiskoot W. Immunogenicity of antibody therapeutics. In: Dübel S, editor. Handbook of Therapeutic Antibodies. New York: John Wiley & Sons; 2007. p. 267–76.

51. Almagro J, Fransson J. Humanization of antibodies. Front. Biosci. 2008;13:1619–33.

52. Rader C, Ritter G, Nathan S, Elia M, Gout I, Jungbluth AA, Cohen LS, Welt S, Old LJ, Barbas CF 3rd. The rabbit antibody repertoire as a novel source for the generation of therapeutic human antibodies. J. Biol. Chem. 2000;275:13668–76.

53. Foote J, Winter G. Antibody framework residues affecting the conformation of the hypervariable loops. J. Mol. Biol. 1992;224:487–99.

54. Borras L, Gunde T, Tietz J, Bauer U, Hulmann-Cottier V, Grimshaw J, Urech D. Generic approach for the generation of stable humanized single-chain Fv fragments from rabbit monoclonal antibodies. J. Biol. Chem. 2010;285:9054–66.

55. Couto J, Hendricks K, Wallace SE, Yu GL. Methods for Antibody Engineering. International Patent Application No: PCT/US2005/039930; Publication No. WO/2006/050491.

56. Reynaud C, Dahan A, Weill J. Complete sequence of a chicken lambda light chain immunoglobulin derived from the nucleotide sequence of its mRNA. Proc. Natl. Acad. Sci U.S.A. 1983;80:4099–103.

57. Reynaud C, Dahan A, Anquez V, Weill J. Somatic hyperconversion diversifies the single VH gene of the chicken with a high incidence in the D region. Cell 1989;59:171–83.

58. Spillner E, Braren I, Greunke K, Seismann H, Blank S, du Plessis D. Avian IgY antibodies and their recombinant equivalents in research, diagnostics and therapy. Biologicals 2012;40:313–22.

59. Parvari R, Avivi A, Lentner F, Ziv E, Tel-Or S, Burstein Y, Schechter I. Chicken immunoglobulin gamma-heavy chains: limited VH gene repertoire, combinatorial diversification by D gene segments and evolution of the heavy chain locus. EMBO J. 1988;7:739–44.

60. Parvari R, Ziv E, Lantner F, Heller D, Schechter I. Somatic diversification of chicken immunoglobulin light chains by point mutations. Proc. Natl. Acad. Sci. U.S.A. 1990;87:3072–6.

61. Reynaud CA, Anquez V, Weill JC. The chicken D locus and its contribution to the immunoglobulin heavy chain repertoire. Eur. J. Immunol. 1991;21:2661–70.

62. Reynaud CA, Dahan A, Anquez V, Weill JC. Somatic hyperconversion diversifies the single Vh gene of the chicken with a high incidence 2in the D region. Cell 1989;59:171–83.

63. Reynaud CA, Anquez V, Grimal H, Weill JC. A hyperconversion mechanism generates the chicken light chain preimmune repertoire. Cell 1987;48:379–88.

64. Finlay WJ, deVore NC, Dobrovolskaia EN, Gam A, Goodyear CS, Slater JE. Exploiting the avian immunoglobulin system to simplify the generation of recombinant antibodies to allergenic proteins. Clin. Exp. Allergy 2005;35:1040–8.

65. Finlay WJ, Shaw I, Reilly JP, Kane M. Generation of high-affinity chicken single-chain Fv antibody fragments for measurement of the *Pseudonitzschia pungens* toxin domoic acid. Appl. Environ. Microbiol. 2006;72:3343–9.

66. Nishibori N, Horiuchi H, Furusawa S, Matsuda H. Humanization of chicken monoclonal antibody using phage-display system. Mol. Immunol. 2006;43:634–42.

67. Yamanaka HI, Inoue T, Ikeda-Tanaka O. Chicken monoclonal antibody isolated by a phage display system. J. Immunol. 1996;157:1156–62.

68. Weill JC, Reynaud CA. Early B-cell development in chickens, sheep and rabbits. Curr. Opin. Immunol. 1992;4:177–80.

69. Ratcliffe MJ. Antibodies, immunoglobulin genes and the bursa of Fabricius in chicken B cell development. Dev. Comp. Immunol. 2006;30:101–18.

70. Wu L. Fundamental characteristics of the immunoglobulin VH repertoire of chickens in comparison to those of humans, mice and camelids. J. Immunol. 2012;188:322–33.

71. Lee CV, Liang WC, Dennis MS, Eigenbrot C, Sidhu SS, Fuh G. High-affinity human antibodies from phage-displayed synthetic Fab libraries with a single framework scaffold. J. Mol. Biol. 2004;340:1073–93.

72. Padlan EA. Anatomy of the antibody molecule. Mol. Immunol. 1994;31:169–217.

73. Abhinandan KR, Martin AC. Analysis and prediction of VH/VL packing in antibodies. Protein Eng. Des. Sel. 2010;23:689–97.

74. Wu L, Oficjalska K, Lambert M, Fennell BJ, Darmanin-Sheehan A, Ni Shuilleabhain D, Autin B, Cummins E, Tchistiakova L, Bloom L, Paulsen J, Gill D, Cunningham O, Finlay WJ. Fundamental characteristics of the immunoglobulin VH repertoire of chickens in comparison with those of humans, mice, and camelids. J. Immunol. 2011;188:322–33.

75. Fellouse FA, Barthelemy PA, Kelley RF, Sidhu SS. Tyrosine plays a dominant functional role in the paratope of a synthetic antibody derived from a four amino acid code. J. Mol. Biol. 2006;357:100–14.

76. Fellouse FA, Esaki K, Birtalan S, Raptis D, Cancasci VJ, Koide A, Jhurani P, Vasser M, Wiesmann C, Kossiakoff AA, Koide S, Sidhu SS. High-throughput generation of synthetic antibodies from highly functional minimalist phage-displayed libraries. J. Mol. Biol. 2007;373:924–40.

77. Fellouse FA, Li B, Compaan DM, Peden AA, Hymowitz SG, Sidhu SS. Molecular recognition by a binary code. J. Mol. Biol. 2005;348:1153–62.

78. Fellouse FA, Wiesmann C, Sidhu SS. Synthetic antibodies from a four-amino-acid code: a dominant role for tyrosine in antigen recognition. Proc. Natl. Acad. Sci. U.S.A. 2004;101:12467–72.

79. Li H, Jiang Y, Prak EL, Radic M, Weigert M. Editors and editing of anti-DNA receptors. Immunity 2001;15:947–57.

80. Boswell CA, Tesar DB, Mukhyala K, Theil FP, Fielder PJ, Khawli LA. Effects of charge on antibody tissue distribution and pharmacokinetics. Bioconjug. Chem. 2010;21:2153–63.

81. Raaphorst FM, Raman CS, Nall BT, Teale JM. Molecular mechanisms governing reading frame choice of immunoglobulin diversity genes. Immunol. Today 1997;18:37–43.

82. Harmsen MM, Ruuls RC, Nijman IJ, Niewold TA, Frenken LG, de Geus B. Llama heavy-chain V regions consist of at least four distinct subfamilies revealing novel sequence features. Mol. Immunol. 2000;37:579–90.

83. Dooley H, Flajnik MF, Porter AJ. Selection and characterization of naturally occurring single-domain (IgNAR) antibody fragments from immunized sharks by phage display. Mol. Immunol. 2003;40:25–33.

84. Stanfield RL, Dooley H, Flajnik MF, Wilson IA. Crystal structure of a shark single-domain antibody V region in complex with lysozyme. Science 2004;305:1770–3.

85. Aitken R, Gilchrist J, Sinclair MC. A single diversified VH gene family dominates the bovine immunoglobulin repertoire. Biochem. Soc. Trans. 1997;25:326S.

86. O'Brien PM, Aitken R, O'Neil BW, Campo MS. Generation of native bovine mAbs by phage display. Proc. Natl. Acad. Sci. U.S.A. 1999;96:640–5.

87. Sinclair MC, Gilchrist J, Aitken R. Bovine IgG repertoire is dominated by a single diversified VH gene family. J. Immunol. 1997;159:3883–9.

88. Li F, Aitken R. Cloning of porcine scFv antibodies by phage display and expression in *Escherichia coli*. Vet. Immunol. Immunopathol. 2004;97:39–51.

89. Fennell BJ, Darmanin-Sheehan A, Hufton SE, Calabro V, Wu L, Muller MR, Cao W, Gill D, Cunningham O, Finlay WJ. Dissection of the IgNAR V domain: molecular scanning and orthologue database mining define novel IgNAR hallmarks and affinity maturation mechanisms. J. Mol. Biol. 2010;400:155–70.

90. Lee CV, Hymowitz SG, Wallweber HJ, Gordon NC, Billeci KL, Tsai SP, Compaan DM, Yin J, Gong Q, Kelley RF, DeForge LE, Martin F, Starovasnik MA, Fuh G. Synthetic anti-BR3 antibodies that mimic BAFF binding and target both human and murine B cells. Blood 2006;108:3103–11.

91. Govaert J, Pellis M, Deschacht N, Vincke C, Conrath K, Muyldermans S, Saerens D. Dual beneficial effect of interloop disulfide bond for single domain antibody fragments. J. Biol. Chem. 2012;287:1970–9.

92. Shih H, Tu C, Cao W, Klein A, Ramsey R, Fennell B, Lambert M, Shúilleabháin DN, Autin B, Kouranova E, et al. An ultra-specific avian antibody to phosphorylated tau protein reveals a unique mechanism for phospho-epitope recognition. J. Biol. Chem. 2012;287:44425–34.

93. Chailyan A, Marcatili P, Cirillo D, Tramontano A. Structural repertoire of immunoglobulin λ light chains. Proteins 2011;79:1513–24.

94. Bernett MJ, Karki S, Moore GL, Leung IW, Chen H, Pong E, Nguyen DH, Jacinto J, Zalevsky J, Muchhal US, Desjarlais JR, Lazar GA. Engineering fully human monoclonal antibodies from murine variable regions. J. Mol. Biol. 2010;396:1474–90.

95. Harding FA, Stickler MM, Razo J, DuBridge RB. The immunogenicity of humanized and fully human antibodies: residual immunogenicity resides in the CDR regions. MAbs. 2010;2:256–65.

96. Nisonoff A, Wissler F, Lipman L. Properties of the major component of a peptic digest of rabbit antibody. Science 1960;132:1770–1.

97. Suresh M, Cuello A, Milstein C. Bispecific monoclonal antibodies from hybrid hybridomas. Methods Enzymol. 1986;121:210–28.

98. Raju T, Strohl W. Potential therapeutic roles for antibody mixtures. Expert Opin. Biol. Ther. 2013;13:1347–52.

99. Klein C, Sustmann C, Thomas M, Stubenrauch K, Croasdale R, Schanzer J, Brinkmann U, Kettenberger H, Regula J, Schaefer W. Progress in overcoming the chain association issue in bispecific heterodimeric IgG antibodies. MAbs. 2012;4:653–63.

100. Bostrom J, Yu S, Kan D, Appleton B, Lee C, Billeci K, Man W, Peale F, Ross S, Wiesmann C, Fuh G. Variants of the antibody herceptin that interact with HER2 and VEGF at the antigen binding site. Science 2009;323:1610–4.

101. Wickramasinghe D. Tumor and T cell engagement by BiTE. Discov. Med. 2013;16:149–52.

Novel Therapeutic Proteins and Peptides

Andrew Buchanan, Jefferson D. Revell

Antibody Discovery and Protein Engineering, MedImmune, Cambridge, UK

INTRODUCTION

Proteins and peptides have evolved to play dynamic and diverse roles in the body, signaling as ligands and receptors, acting as transporters, regulating gene expression, and catalyzing intracellular and extracellular reactions. There are over 20,000 functionally distinct proteins and peptides, and viewed from the perspective of medicines there is a tremendous opportunity to utilize and innovate with these molecules and pathways to bring benefit to patients. There have been two key revolutions in the use of therapeutic proteins and peptides. The first was recognition of their therapeutic potential, and the second was the development of methods to manufacture them at a large scale for clinical use. The use of therapeutic antibodies can be traced back to Emil von Behring's serum therapy, or antitoxins, to treat diphtheria and tetanus in the 1890s; von Behring was awarded the first Nobel Prize for Physiology or Medicine in 1901. The first non-antibody therapeutic protein was Frederick

Novel Approaches and Strategies for Biologics, Vaccines and Cancer Therapies. DOI: 10.1016/B978-0-12-416603-5.00008-0

Banting's use of insulin to treat diabetes mellitus in 1922; he was also awarded the Nobel Prize in 1923. These first proteins were purified from their native sources of immunized horse serum and ox pancreas extract. respectively. However, the breakthroughs in recombinant DNA technology (1980 Nobel Prize for Chemistry to Berg, Gilbert, and Sanger)—the "simple and ingenuous" solid-phase peptide synthesis (1984 Nobel Prize for Chemistry to Merrifield) and solution-phase peptide synthesis, or a combination of both—have revolutionized research into and the manufacture of therapeutic proteins and peptides. The first recombinant expressed medicines were the hormones somatostatin in 1977 and human insulin in 1979;[1,2] oxytocin represents the first chemical synthesis of a full peptide, which occurred in 1953.[3]

As of August 2013 there were 181 widely launched therapeutic recombinant proteins and peptides, 39 therapeutic synthetic peptides, and over 1000 proteins and peptides in clinical trials. To help appreciate their diversity, therapeutic proteins and peptides can be grouped in a number of ways. Based on their molecular types they can be divided into engineered protein scaffolds, Fc fusions, enzymes, growth hormones, interferons, interleukins, bone morphogenic proteins, blood factors, anticoagulants, and thrombolytics.[4] Alternatively, they can be classified on their pharmacological mechanism of action into five main groups: (1) replacing a protein that is deficient or abnormal; (2) augmenting an existing pathway; (3) providing a novel function or activity; (4) interfering with a molecule of organism; and (5) delivering other compounds or proteins.[5]

The advantages of proteins and peptides include their high affinity, potency, and specificity for the target, in addition to a well-defined mechanism of action that drives efficacy and leads to a reduced incidence of unexpected adverse events. Safety concerns for this class of medicines are primarily related to exaggerated pharmacology. However, proteins and peptides have several significant limitations as therapeutics. Small proteins (<50 to 60 kDa) and peptides are rapidly cleared from circulation by renal filtration, thus their efficacy is limited by a short circulating half-life. In terms of target class, they are currently limited to extracellular and cell surface targets, approximately 35% of the proteome.[6] Intracellular delivery, although possible in the laboratory, has not been demonstrated in the clinic. Because protein and peptide drugs are denatured and/or proteolyzed in the gut, they are not orally bioavailable and must be administered via subcutaneous, intravenous, or intramuscular injection. Large doses over a treatment course can result in a high cost of goods which can limit their clinical use. All protein therapeutics, including peptides, are potentially immunogenic in patients, eliciting an antidrug antibody (ADA) response that may compromise drug efficacy and patient safety. Finally, the requirements for large-scale manufacture, high-concentration liquid formulations, and long-term storage introduce additional the requirements of high stability and levels of expression. Many protein and peptide engineering strategies have been developed to optimize next-generation therapeutics to address these challenges of potency, pharmacokinetics, stability, and immunogenicity, which are outlined below. However, the most important factor in developing new medicines is defining the unmet medical need and understanding the disease biology and how target modulation can translate into clinical benefit for patients. With an increased understanding of target biology and translation to humans there is a greater potential for new breakthrough therapies as well as new and exciting challenges for protein and peptide engineering in research and development.

INNOVATION IN RECOMBINANT THERAPEUTIC PROTEINS AND PEPTIDES

Antibodies may be the most successful and best-studied therapeutic proteins, but many other types of proteins and peptide have been developed as therapeutic agents. These can be viewed as falling into two broad categories: (1) engineered scaffolds, which are used as alternatives to traditional monoclonal antibodies or antibody derivates, and (2) endogenous proteins and peptides with the prerequisite pharmacology for specific indications which are engineered to address specific limitations in pharmacokinetics, solubility, stability, and manufacturability.

Engineered Scaffolds

The original drivers for engineered scaffolds revolved around independent intellectual property and overcoming the perceived drawbacks of antibodies, such as their large size, which may limit tissue penetration and the tendency of some antibody derivates to aggregate. These limitations of antibodies are being addressed by engineering for improved stability and developments in eukaryotic, microbial, and cell free translation systems.[7–10] Nevertheless, engineered scaffolds can complement antibodies, particularly in applications requiring small multispecific agents or where Fc-mediated functions are not required.

More than 50 different classes of engineered protein scaffolds have been described, with one approved for therapy and many more progressing successfully into clinical trials. Key features of these scaffolds are that they are small, modular, monomeric, single-chain polypeptides (<200 amino acids) with a defined three-dimensional structure that tolerates insertions, deletions, and substitutions; they have high solubility and stability; they often lack disulfide bonds or glycoslyation; and they are readily expressed in microbial hosts. Scaffolds can be engineered in much the same way as antibodies. Large combinatorial synthetic libraries are generated by randomizing surface-accessible residues, which are selected on a target using ribosome/m-RNA, phage, or yeast display.[11] In this section, we briefly review the industrially advanced scaffolds, not including the single-domain or multimer formats based on Ig variable domains, and we highlight some novel scaffolds from the literature.

Industrially Advanced Scaffolds

Kunitz-type Domains

Kunitz-type domains are ubiquitous in nature, acting as both serine protease inhibitors and toxins in animal venoms. They consist of between 50 and 70 amino acids, adopting a conserved structural fold with two antiparallel β-sheets and one or two helical regions that are stabilized with three disulfide bridges (Figure 8.1A). The first Kunitz domain for therapy, developed by Dyax, was based on engineering a human lipoprotein-associated coagulation inhibitor scaffold to generate ecallantide, a specific inhibitor of plasma kallikrein that was approved for the treatment of hereditary angioedema in 2009.[12] Kunitz-type domain inhibitors have been identified to potassium channels,[13] a challenging target class for biologics, and additional proteases[14,15] and strategies to enhance stability for therapeutic use have been described.[16]

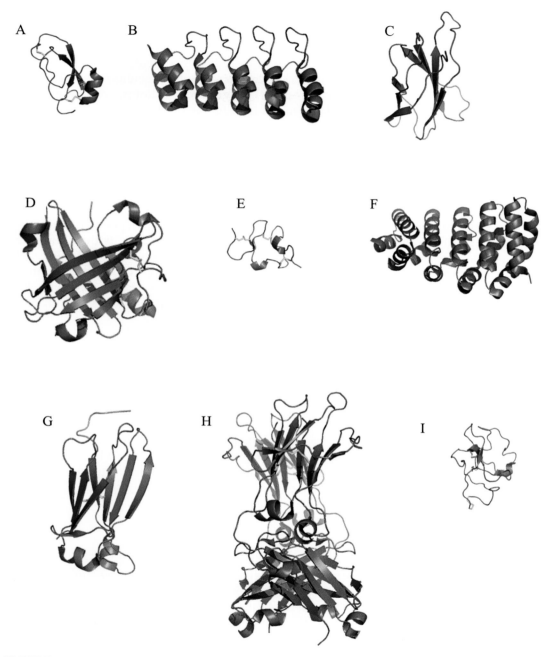

FIGURE 8.1 Structural representations of protein and peptide scaffolds. In red are residues and loops that are mutated to engineer binding specificity and affinity. In yellow are the disulfide bonds. (A) Kunitz domain (1AAP). (B) DARPin with three repeats, N and C terminal caps (2QYJ). (C) Fn3 domain (1FNF). (D) Lipocalin (3DSZ). (E) Avimer A-domain subunit (1AJJ). (F) Armadillo domain with three repeats, N and C terminal caps (4DB6). (G) CH2 domain with N-terminal deletion in orange (1HZH). (H) CH2-CH3 domain (1OQO). (I) Kringle domain (1I5K).

Ankyrin Repeat (AR) Proteins

Ankyrin repeat (AR) proteins are a prominent repeat protein family regulating protein–protein interactions. Designed AR proteins (DARPins), developed by Molecular Partners, are engineered scaffolds based on a consensus AR module of 33 amino acids which form a β-turn followed by two antiparallel α-helices with six diversified positions in the β-turn and first α-helix (Figure 8.1B). Libraries consist of two to four repeat units between N and C terminal capping repeats which protect the hydrophobic interface of the AR modules.[17] The C-terminal cap has been reengineered to increase the developability of the molecules.[18] DARPins can be selected in ribosome or phage display formats and expressed in the cytoplasm of *Escherichia coli* as soluble monomers with high thermodynamic stability. In addition they can be fused to form multivalent or multispecific molecules.[19] The most advanced DARPin is AGN-150998, an antivascular endothelial growth factor A (VEGF-A) antagonist that successfully completed a Phase I trial in age-related macular degeneration (AMD) and diabetic macular edema and is currently in a Phase II AMD study.[20]

Fibronectin Scaffolds

Multiple academic groups and biotechnology companies have worked on fibronectin type III domain (Fn3) scaffolds derived from human fibronectin or tenascin-C, abundant extracellular proteins.[21–23] The Fn3 fold is an Ig-like β sandwich of seven β-strands with three solvent accessible loops at each pole, encoded in approximately 90 amino acids with no disulfide bridges (Figure 8.1C). The earliest libraries were based on the tenth Fn3 domain and randomized two loops, BC and FG, analogous to antibody complementarity-determining region (CDR) 1 and CDR3.[24] Fn3 library design has increased in complexity and sophistication with tailored diversity in the three CDR-like loops and in the opposite-pole AB loop. Recently, a new Fn3 library was described that diversifies a single loop and the face of a β-sheet to present a concave paratope, distinct from the flat or convex paratopes of typical loop libraries.[25] This new library produced binders, termed *monobodies*, with similar efficiency to loop libraries and may offer advantages for binders to convex targets. Fn3 libraries have been selected in phage, mRNA, and yeast display and are expressed as stable proteins in *E. coli*. Adnexus (a Bristol-Myers Squibb company) led the development of Fn3 scaffolds termed Adnectins™. The most advanced Adnectin, CT-322, an anti-VEGFR-2 antagonist, has successfully completed Phase I clinical trials and is now in Phase II trails for treatment of metastatic colorectal cancer.[26] The first example of a modular bispecific Adnectin combined epidermal growth factor receptor (EGFR) and insulin-like growth factor 1 receptor (IGF-1R) monospecific Adnectins linked via a flexible linker comprising ten glycine–serine repeats. This bispecific molecule demonstrated high levels of soluble expression in *E. coli*, was >95% monomer, and was relatively stable with a T_m of 57.5°C.[27]

Lipocalins

Lipocalins are abundant in plasma and other body fluids and are involved in the transport or storage of vitamins, hormones, and metabolites. The family has a conserved cup-shaped β-barrel structure that supports four loops at the open pole, encoded in 160 to 180 amino acids with one disulfide bridge (Figure 8.1D). The loops have a high degree of structural plasticity, and libraries based on human tear lipocalin and neutrophil gelatinase-associated lipocalin, with 16 to 24 randomized residues, have been successfully used to generate potential therapeutics.[28] Pieris has led the development of lipocalins termed Anticalins®. Anticalins have selected in phage and bacterial display and are expressed as soluble monomers in *E. coli* and yeast. The most advanced Anticalin, PRS-050, a VEGF-A antagonist, was well tolerated in Phase I clinical trials.[29]

Avimers

A-domains occur as strings of multiple domains in several proteins, where each domain binds a unique target epitope, providing an avidity effect to achieve high affinity and specificity. Avimer proteins, developed by Avidia (now part of Amgen), are based on human A domains forming avidity multimers. The A-domain is comprised of approximately 40 residues, of which 12 form a conserved motif, including six cysteines (Figure 8.1E). A phage display library was generated based on a consensus of human A domains with diversity in the intercysteine loops, and avimers binders were identified to a range of targets.[30] Multimers of up to eight domains have been generated, and despite the presence of three disulfide bridges per domain they are expressed solubly in the cytoplasm of E. coli. The most advanced avimer, C326, targeting interleukin 6 (IL-6), has been in the clinic but clinical development has been halted. Recently, a novel agonist bispecific avimer, C3201, mimicking fibroblast growth factor 21 (FGF21), has been reported.[31] This molecule is a fusion of a monomeric avimer targeting FGFR1c and a dimer avimer targeting β-Klotho. C3201 requires the presence of both β-Klotho and FGFR1c to trigger signaling and unlike FGF21 does not bind other FGF receptors. This provides a novel therapeutic agent to treat diabetes and obesity.

Novel Scaffolds

Alternative Repeat Proteins

In addition to DARPins, based on human ankarin repeats, alternative scaffolds have been successfully generated from other non-human repeat proteins that have a modular architecture and are involved in protein–protein interactions. Examples include leucine-rich repeats from lamprays and hagfish, artificial alpha-helical repeat proteins based on thermophilic organisms' HEAT repeats, and armadillo repeat proteins.[32–34] Common to all of these approaches are randomized library repeat modules flanked by engineered N- and C-terminal caps that can be expressed in the cytoplasm of E. coli as stable monomeric molecules (Figure 8.1F). These new scaffolds are generally applicable to generate binding reagents, with one limitation being the potential immunogenicity in humans if used as therapeutics.[34]

Immunoglobulin Constant Domains

Recently, two academic groups have published new scaffolds based on human IgG Fc fragment. The first scaffold is based on the C_H2 domain (Figure 8.1G), with diversity introduced into loops BC and FG, analogous to CDR1 and CDR3.[35] C_H2 libraries were selected by phage or yeast display and expressed in E. coli. However, most clones generated from this library aggregated. Deletion of the seven N-terminal residues significantly improved stability and aggregation resistance of these shortened C_H2 domains.[36] The truncated C_H2 scaffold is predicted to lack binding to FcγRs and retain binding to FcRn. An alternative Fc scaffold is based on the full C_H2–C_H3 domain (Figure 8.1H) with diversity introduced into the short loops AB and EF at the C-terminal tip of C_H3,[37] now being developed by F-star as Fcab™ (Fc antigen binding). This library was selected by yeast display and clones expressed in mammalian cells. Clones from Fcab libraries had decreased thermal stability compared to wild-type Fc. Two strategies to improve stability have been employed. Introducing an additional one or two disulfide bonds into C_H3 increased the T_m by up to 19°C.[38] Directed evolution for stability did enhance stability but also reduced the affinity of the molecules.[39] Despite the low nanomolar binding affinity of the Fcabs, they do retain binding to the FcγRs, C1q, and FcRn. Therefore, Fcabs, unlike C_H2s, retain full IgG-like effector function and both are predicted to have extended half-lives *in vivo*.

Small Disulfide-Rich Domains

In addition to avimers, other cysteine-rich miniproteins have been evaluated as scaffolds, including knottins, cyclotides, and kringle domains. These encoded intramolecular disulfide bonds result in small scaffolds with extraordinary chemical and thermal stability and the potential for oral delivery. Research on these domains has been primarily in the synthetic arena, but increasingly they are being addressed by recombinant methods.[40–43] For example, the kringle domain (KD), composed of ~80 amino acids, forms a cysteine knot with seven surface-exposed loops (Figure 8.1I) that can be divided into two clusters based on the direction they face. Yeast display libraries were built on the human PgnKD2 domain, with 45 residues in the exposed loops randomized and novel functional binding proteins generated.[44] This group went on to demonstrate that the two clusters of loops can act as independent binding sites to generate bivalent and bispecific functionality in a single domain, an attribute that has not been reported in other scaffolds.[45]

Endogenous Proteins and Peptides

Scaffolds and antibodies have demonstrated clinical and commercial value but are not the universal solution for all biological therapeutics. Endogenous proteins and peptides have been successfully developed as therapeutic agents for example human insulin, which in 1982 became the first recombinant protein therapeutic for the treatment of diabetes mellitus type I and type II. Many native peptides and proteins are in clinical use, including glucagon-like peptide 1 (GLP-1), growth hormone (GH), IGF-1, interferons (IFNs), bone morphogenetic proteins (BMPs), coagulation factors, and enzymes. As we understand the mechanisms underlying complex disease pathology, natural ligands and receptors provide a valuable starting point for drug discovery as they have unique attributes. Soluble proteins and peptides may have no known binding partner but drive relevant pharmacology. Ligands and receptors are often promiscuous with complex and overlapping interactions that introduce redundant cell signaling pathways (e.g., ErbB or FGFR families). Finally, endogenous molecules can have unique epitopes on the target receptor that are crucial for activity or a specific mechanism of action, such as agonism or enzymatic degradation. These attributes can often be difficult and complex to deconvolute or mimic with specific scaffolds or antibodies and therefore provide a starting point for drug discovery and therapeutics.

Peptides

The majority of approved peptide drugs are synthesized chemically.[46] However, there are examples of clinically successful peptides that are produced recombinantly. The choice of manufacturing platform is sequence dependent, and currently recombinant platforms are particularly useful for molecules of ~50 natural amino acids or longer that require posttranslational modification for activity or half-life (e.g., glycoslyation, disulfide formation, C terminal α-amidation). Examples of recombinant therapeutic polypeptides include insulin, glucagon, and IGF-1. Human glucagon, a single-chain, 29-amino-acid peptide, is produced in *Saccharomyces cerevisiae* (Novo Nordisk) or *E. coli* (Eli Lilly) and is used to treat diabetic patients with very low blood sugar levels (hypoglycemic) who are treated with insulin.[47] IGF-1 is comprised of 70 amino acids, and two different forms are approved for growth hormone-insensitivity syndrome. One form, Increlex™, is recombinant human IGF-1 produced in *E. coli*. In order to prolong the half-life of IGF-1 a second form, iPLEX™, was produced. This is a combination of IGF-1 and IGF binding protein 3 (IGFBP-3) that is manufactured as two separate compounds, which are then combined in equimolar proportions.[48] IGF-1 and IGFBP-3 have a binding affinity of ~50 p*M* and can form a 140-kDa ternary complex in circulation with an 85-kDa protein, termed the acid-labile subunit, that reduces renal clearance and prolongs half-life. The demarcation between chemical synthesis and recombinant expression of polypeptides may well disappear as both approaches make technical progress. For example, many academic groups are reporting recombinant expression of endogenous peptides that up to now have been chemically synthesized, such as *E. coli* expression of PYY 3-36, oxyntomodulin, and GLP-1 and *Pichia pastoris* expression of GLP-1 and extendin-4.[49–52]

Insulin is important in the maintenance of blood sugar levels. It is the only therapeutic agent for type I diabetes and is increasingly used in advanced cases of type II diabetes. Insulin is a 51-amino-acid hormone comprised of an A and B chain linked by two disulfide bridges (Figure 8.2). When synthesized in pancreatic β-cells, insulin forms hexamers, which are inactive; upon release, the hexamers dissociate into active dimers and monomers. The therapeutic agent has advanced from animal pancreas purified protein in the 1920s to human insulin expressed in either *E. coli* (Humulin®, Eli Lilly) or *Saccharomyces cerevisiae* (Novolin®, Novo Nordisk) in the 1980s. More recently, insulin analogs have been engineered for either more rapid onset with short duration or prolonged duration of action. This has enabled physicians to tailor therapy to more closely mimic the natural insulin physiology of stable baseline secretion and surges following food ingestion that return to baseline within two to three hours.

Before the advent of insulin analogs the principle method of modifying insulin pharmacokinetics was via formulation. The addition of protamine or zinc stabilized the hexamer,

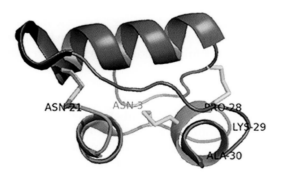

FIGURE 8.2 Structure of insulin (3I3Z) highlighting residues targeted to alter duration of action. The A chain is in green, the B chain is in blue, and the disulfide bridges are in yellow.

delayed adsorption, and resulted in a slow release of active monomers and dimers. The solution of a high-resolution crystal structure of insulin hexamer enabled the rational design of rapid-acting analogs by destabilizing the self-association interface.[53] Mutations in the B chain were identified that weaken dimer and hexamer formation while maintaining potency. Three rapid-acting insulin analogs are currently in use: lispro (Humalog®, Eli Lilly), which switches the order of two residues, P28 and K29, in the B chain; aspart (NovoLog®, Novo Nordisk), which has a B-chain mutation, P28D; and glulisin (Apidra®, Sanofi-Aventis), which has two B-chain mutations, N3K and K29E.[54] Insulin analogs with prolonged, basal action have been developed using a range of mechanisms. The most widely used is glargine (Lantus®, Sanofi-Aventis), which has one A-chain mutation, D21K, and the insertion of two Rs at the end of the B chain to switch the isoelectric point from pH 5.4 to 6.7. This molecule precipitates following injection to form a subcutaneous depot that delays absorption and prolongs its duration of action. An alternative long-acting insulin is detemir (Levemir®, Novo Nordisk), which is acylated at K29. This enhances the stability of the hexamer and enables binding to serum albumin.[55] Two other basal analogs are currently in clinical trials: insulin degludec (Novo Nordisk), which forms a dimer of hexamers linked by a novel acyl modification that delays absorption, and LY2605541 (Eli Lilly), a PEGylated derivative of lispro, which delays absorption and reduces clearance.[56,57]

Proteases

Proteases, enzymes that cleave peptide bonds to activate or inactivate proteins, have great promise as therapeutics. The catalytic mechanism of action of proteases theoretically enables smaller therapeutic doses and a lower cost of goods compared to monoclonal antibodies (mAbs) and scaffolds that have a stoichiometric mechanism of action. However, there are two significant limitations in developing proteases as therapeutics. First is a lack of specificity, as proteases have up to 100 different substrates, and second is the presence of endogenous activators and inhibitors.[58] The current approved therapeutic proteases have few substrates and include urokinase-type plasminogen activator (u-PA) and tissue-type plasminogen activator (t-PA) for thrombolysis; coagulation factors FVIIa, FIX, and thrombin for traumatic bleeding; and botulinum toxins for muscle spasms. Next-generation protease drugs are in development, with the potential to improve upon existing therapeutics, and novel native proteases are also being evaluated.[59]

The clinical utility of proteases could be greatly expanded if their substrate specificity can be improved and interactions with inhibitors minimized. The serpin superfamily represents important protease inhibitors that use suicide inhibition to inactivate both the serpin and protease by forming a covalent complex that is rapidly cleared. Engineering proteases to minimize interaction with serpin inhibitors is challenging, as inhibitors bind in close proximity to the active site. Using a rational structure-guided approach has made it possible to create t-PA variants that are resistant to the serpin PAI-1.[60] As many potential therapeutic proteases are serine proteases, like t-PA encoding the trypsin fold, such rational engineering approaches should be transferable. Engineering specificities into protease has been challenging via rational and directed evolution strategies. Early breakthroughs in swapping substrate specificity (e.g., trypsin with chemotrypsin or subtilisin with furin) has not led to the simple introduction of novel or fine-tuned specificity and activity. The use of brute force mutagenesis, high-throughput expression, and novel yeast display platforms provides innovative tools to engineer proteases and exploit their potential to deactivate valid disease targets in a unique catalytic manner that could result in significantly lower doses or an ability to address targets that are present in very high concentrations.[61,62]

Cytokines

Cytokines are a heterogeneous group of small proteins, ranging in size from ~130 to 190 amino acids, that are extremely potent and involved in every important biological process. These molecules include interleukins, interferons, growth factors, and hormones. Many cytokine molecules have been developed as approved therapies, such as erythropoietin to treat anemia, granulocyte colony-stimulating factor (G-CSF) for neutropenic patients, IL-2 for cancer, derivatives of IFN-α for viral infection and cancer, IFN-γ for cancer and osteoporosis, BMPs for bone injury repair, and leptin for the treatment for metabolic disorders such as lipodystrophy.[5] Therapy with immunomodulatory cytokines has historically been limited by their severe toxicity; for example, high doses of IL-2 are associated with vascular leak syndrome, where fluid accumulates in organs such as lung and liver. However, innovative combination therapies, alternative delivery strategies, and the design of novel engineered cytokines, or superkines, are extending the potential clinical benefits of cytokine-based therapy.

One strategy to address toxicity is to direct the cytokine to the site of action and thus limit the systemic toxicity. Selectikine (Merck) is a fusion of anti-DNA IgG$_2$ with IL-2 at the C-terminus of the Fc chain. The mAb targets the DNA–histone complex in the necrotic core of tumors, and a mutation in IL-2 potentially removes a toxin motif responsible for endothelial cell binding driving toxicity.[63] Phase I clinical trials with this molecule demonstrated no severe toxicity and prolonged disease stabilization.[64] A second strategy to potentially address cytokine toxicity involves engineering cytokine affinity for components of the receptor complex. Most cytokines trigger signaling by first binding to high-affinity receptor α and then recruiting the low-affinity receptors β and γ. The potency of the cytokine is dependent on recruitment of the β and γ receptors. Using a combination of *in vitro* evolution and rational design, Garcia's group has engineered IL-2 and IL-4 variants with high affinity for the β and γ receptors, independent of receptor α, that are potent agonists but with reduced toxicity *in vivo*.[65,66] In a similar manner, IL-15–IL-15Rα fusions have been generated to increase affinity for the β and γ receptors and also as mAb protein conjugates.[67,68] Approaches like these could improve the selectivity and reduce the toxicity of immunomodulatory cytokine therapy.

Recombinant human erythropoietin (EPO) provides an interesting example of how an innovator molecule (Epogen®, Amgen) was followed by a few next-generation molecules and then a flood of biosimilar molecules. This is a pattern that is being repeated for other successful biologic therapeutics. EPO, a 165-amino-acid, four-helix bundle, was characterized in 1985 and first approved in the European Union in 1988. The innovator molecule epoetin alfa is produced in CHO cells, as glycoslyation is critical for activity, and with a half-life of 6 to 9 hours it is dosed two to three times weekly. The next-generation EPO molecules were developed to have a longer half-life, enabling less frequent dosing. Darbepoetin alfa (Aranesp®, Amgen), approved in 2001, was engineered to introduce two additional *N*-glycans and increase the number of sialic acids from 14 to 22.[69] This resulted in greater biologic activity due to the long half-life of 25 hours which enabled weekly dosing. Methooxy-PEG-epoetin beta

(Mircera®, Roche), approved in 2007, is a chemically modified EPO incorporating a 30-KDa PEG polymer resulting in a half-life of 130 to 140 hours.[70] As the patents for epoetin alfa have expired the door has opened for biosimilars. Biosimilars are biologic agents that encode the same gene and aim to deliver similar efficacy, safety, and quality as the approved product. However, differences in the manufacturing process can result in substantial differences in the agents biological and clinical properties.[71] Currently, among the over 80 different EPOs marketed globally, only a few have been approved in the highly regulated pharmaceutical markets.[72]

Protein Engineering Strategies

Recombinant expression of proteins and peptides has delivered effective medicines. However, engineering and optimizing the attributes of these molecules represent the next major step in improving their clinical potential, as described above for insulin and EPO. Two of the major challenges for the clinical use of proteins and peptide are serum half-life and immunogenicity.[4] Being able to engineer molecules with increased half-life has the potential benefit of increasing exposure, thus driving improved efficacy as well as lower or less frequent dosing. Immunogenicity in patients is a risk for all biotherapeutics and may result in antibodies that interfere with the drugs activity or compromise patient safety.

Fc Fusion and Fc Engineering

The advent of immunoglobulin Fc fusion has been clinically successful at increasing small biologics half-life from minutes or hours to days and weeks due to pH-dependent Fc binding to the neonatal receptor (FcRn). It is interesting to note that Fc fusion proteins have a lower affinity for FcRn in comparison to IgG. One explanation for this is that the fusion partner is subtly altering the C_H2–C_H3 interface with FcRn.[73] Fc fusion can also improve expression and stability and enables conventional protein A purification, facilitating the manufacture of therapeutic molecules. Beyond conventional half-life extension, engineering of the Fc provides additional options to modulate valency, increase or decrease effector function, or further extend half-life.

Currently, there are seven approved IgG1-Fc fusion proteins and peptides, including Enbrel® (Amgen/Pfizer), Orenica® (BMS), and NPlate® (Amgen/Pfizer), the first peptide–Fc fusion. Many others are in clinical and preclinical development, including dulaglutide (Eli Lilly), a GLP-1 IgG_4–Fc fusion. In engineering these recombinant fusion molecules, careful attention must be paid to both the orientation of the active molecule and the linker. Certain proteins and peptides are more active when fused to the N- or C-terminus, depending on the structure–function relationship.[74] The direct fusion of GLP-1 to the Ig hinge dramatically reduced activity, but the addition of a 19-amino-acid Gly-Ser linker enhanced activity fourfold.[75] Fc fusion enables dimeric presentation, and additional avidity and potency can be introduced by concatemerizing the active molecule (i.e., two peptides spaced by a linker as in the case of NPlate). Alternative strategies to increase the valency have been described, including use of the 18-amino-acid tailpiece from human IgM to form hexamer Fc fusion proteins.[76]

The use of Fc fusion proteins introduces the option of modulating effector functions. The approved Fc fusions have an IgG_1–Fc, which can elicit antibody-dependent cellular cytotoxicity (ADCC) and antibody-dependent cellular phagocytosis (ADCP) via the activating FcγRs, but cannot trigger complement as they lack the Fab domain that contributes to the interaction with C1q.[77] For some specific therapeutic applications, the activation of FcγRs is best avoided. Although IgG$_2$ and IgG$_4$ have reduced effector functions relative to IgG$_1$, engineered Fcs that lack effector function have been reported. For example, the triple mutations L234F, L235E, and P331S in the lower hinge and C$_H$2 domain of human IgG$_1$ eliminated ADCC, and dula-glutide is fused to an IgG$_4$ with similar mutations in C$_H$2, F234A, and L235A that significantly reduced ADCC.[78,75] In the context of antibodies, other variant Fcs or Fc peptide mimetics have been reported with enhanced effector function by mutation or glycoengineering, altered FcγR selectivity, and monomeric Fcs that could lead to therapeutic benefits for fusion proteins in particular settings.[79–82] The pH-dependent binding of Fc to the FcRn is critical for the long half-life of antibodies. Several groups have designed Fcs that have even longer half-lives than natural IgG by enhancing Fc binding to FcRn at pH 6, thus rescuing the therapeutic from lysosomal degradation and recycling it to the cell surface.[83] The use of such Fc variants could provide significant half-life extension to next-generation Fc fusion proteins, resulting in less frequent patient administration compared to native Fc fusions.

Alternative Half-Life Extension Technologies

Most therapeutic molecules, with the exception of antibodies, are rapidly cleared from circulation by renal filtration, as they are below the 60-kDa glomerular filtration cutoff. Additional clearance mechanisms include proteolytic degradation and receptor mediated clearance, which are dependent on the biology of the individual target; for example, native GLP-1 is rapidly inactivated by enzymatic cleavage of the N-terminus, and cytokines are rapidly depleted by receptor mediated endocytosis. Many recombinant and chemical strategies have been proposed to extend the circulating half-life of proteins and peptides, in addition to Fc fusions, by addressing renal clearance. The most successful of these is PEGylation, the chemical coupling with the synthetic polymer polyethylene glycol (PEG), which has been used on over ten approved proteins and peptides[84] and will be discussed below with other synthetic solutions to increase half-life. The recombinant engineering approaches to extending half-life can be grouped into two main categories: (1) genetic fusion to albumin or albumin-binding domains, and (2) genetic fusions to long flexible polypeptides.

Albumin has an extraordinary half-life of 19 days as a result of its size and pH-dependent interaction and recycling via FcRn that protects it from catabolism. A large variety of proteins and peptides have been fused to albumin, and five are currently in clinical testing.[85] The most advanced of these is albigultide (Human Genome Sciences/GSK), which is under regulatory review. Albigultide is a protease-resistant GLP-1 fused to the N-terminus of human albumin that has been shown to increase the half-life in patients from 2 minutes to 5 days, thus enabling a once-per-week dose regime.[86] An additional benefit of protein fusion to albumin has been the improved stability reported for G-CSF, GH, and IFNα2b.[87] The molecular mechanism of albumin's pH-dependent binding to FcRn has recently been elucidated, facilitating the design of next-generation albumin fusions to modulate half-life in a manner similar to Fc:FcRn engineering.[88] In addition to direct albumin fusion, molecules that bind to albumin have been used as fusion partners to extend the half-life of therapeutics. These include the albumin-binding domain of streptococcal protein G, peptides, domain antibodies, and engineered scaffolds that have been evaluated preclinically but have not yet reached the clinic.

To address some of the drawbacks of synthetic PEG e.g., it does not biodegrade and so can accumulate in tissues such as kidney and interfere with normal function, unstructured recombinant polypeptides have recently been developed to increase the half-life of proteins and peptides in a manner similar to that of PEG. The first of these, XTEN, encodes an unstructured polypeptide designed from the natural amino acids A, E, G, P, S, and T.[89] The length of the polypeptide can be modified to tune the half-life, and the genetic fusion molecules can be expressed solubley in the *E. coli* cytoplasm. The use of XTEN fusion resulted in peptide–XTEN fusions with a half-life in cynomologus monkeys ranging from 9 to 60 hours, compared to 10 to 30 minutes for the unmodified peptides. An alternative unstructured polypeptide based on P, A, and S (PAS) has also been described with properties very similar to those of XTEN.[90] To date, the one unstructured polypeptide fusion in Phase I clinical trials (VRS-317, a GH–XTEN fusion for GH-deficient patients) indicates the safety and tolerability of these recombinant PEG-like molecules.[91]

Additional protein engineering strategies to increase half-life have been described. The glycoengineering for EPO that resulted in Aranesp was discussed above and was also successful in maintaining activity and increasing the half-life of leptin and Mpl in preclinical models.[69] The use of histidine switching to introduce pH-dependent binding into G-CSF for G-CFSR demonstrated the potential to increase half-life.[92] However, neither of these strategies has been widely adopted for therapeutic proteins and peptides. One novel approach to potentially extend half-life is genetic fusion to a short FcRn binding peptide that facilitates FcRn binding, but the impact on half-life has yet to be demonstrated.[93]

Addressing Immunogenicity

All protein and peptide therapeutics, including native sequences, are potentially immunogenic in patients and may elicit antidrug antibodies (ADAs). The ADA response is typically polyclonal and can have neutralizing and non-neutralizing effects on the therapeutic molecule, which can lead to unfavorable outcomes, such as patients having to withdraw from therapy.[94] If the therapeutic is derived from endogenous sequences, as in the case of EPO, neutralizing ADAs can cross-react with the endogenous protein, resulting in patient morbidity and mortality.[95] Factors that can drive immunogenicity include amino acid sequence, aggregation, formulation, route of administration, patient disease status, and co-medications. Recent examples of immunogenic molecules include Omontys® (Peginesatide, Takeda/Affymax), a dimeric PEGylated agonist peptide to EPO receptor, which was withdrawn in 2013 as a result of serious hypersensitivity reactions in patients, including life-threatening or fatal anaphylaxis.[96] Another example is AMG 819 (Amgen), an antagonistic anti-NGF peptide IgG$_1$–Fc fusion; in a Phase I study, 37% of patients developed ADAs, which were a major impediment to further development.[74] Protein engineering strategies can be used to potentially reduce immunogenicity by mutating sequences that can either be recognized by the naive antibody repertoire (B-cell epitopes) or bind class II major histocompatibility complex (MHC-II) molecules and elicit T-cell-dependent immune responses (T-cell epitopes).

The identification and removal of B-cell epitopes is very challenging as they are conformational epitopes that cannot currently be predicted from the diverse naive antibody repertoire *in silico*. However, there has been one recent example of the removal of human B-cell epitopes from the *Pseudomonas* exotoxin A (PE) component (encoding domain II and III of PE, known as PE38) of the recombinant immunotoxin moxetumomab pasudotx (HA22, MedImmune).

B cells were obtained from patients with ADAs to HA22 and used to identify mAbs to PE38. These mAbs were epitope mapped onto PE38 and as expected the B-cell epitopes were dispersed over the surface of the molecule. Seven mutations and a domain deletion were introduced to remove ADA binding and retain cytotoxicity.[97] The toxin variant no longer reacted with the existing patient ADA sera, but there is the potential that the mutations have introduced novel epitopes that may be recognized by the immune system.

Significant progress has been made in addressing T-cell epitopes, with academics and companies developing technologies to identify T-cell epitopes, to directly measure their impact on human T-cell activation *in vitro*, and to assess immunogenicity with novel transgenic mice and immune system transplantation models preclinically.[98] The use of *in silico* algorithms can predict peptides that bind to MHC-II with reasonable accuracy to highlight residues that could be mutated. This *in silico* approach can also be combined with structural modeling to simultaneously consider protein structure, stability, and function as in the case of the EpiSweep algorithm.[99] The major limitation common to all of the *in silico* approaches is the over-prediction of false positives, as they do not account for others factors such as protein/peptide processing, recognition by T-cell receptors, and T-cell tolerance, all of which influence the formation of T-cell epitopes. *In vitro* T-cell culture systems overcome some of these limitations, and by testing whole proteins and peptide fragments a T-cell epitope map and relative immunogenicity can be assessed preclinically. By combining *in silico* and *in vitro* methods, the immunogenicity of AMG 819 was mapped to 14 amino acids at the C-terminus of the bioactive peptide, illustrating how such immunogenicity could be assessed and eliminated in early drug development.[74] The combination of innovative protein engineering and *in vitro* T-cell assays was used to deimmunize the chemotherapeutic bacterial enzyme ELSPAR® (L-aspararginase II, Lundbeck/Recordati), to which 60% of patients generate ADAs. The mutant aspararginase contained eight amino-acid substitutions, retained catalytic activity and stability, and demonstrated reduced immunogenicity in transgenic mice.[100] Developing the next generation of safe and effective medicine for patients will involve harnessing the existing clinical data and employing cutting-edge immunobioengineering technologies.

INNOVATION IN SYNTHETIC THERAPEUTICS PEPTIDES

Despite both our ever-increasing understanding of nature's extensive use of peptides and our ability to design and manufacture them, their development as therapeutics remains challenging.[101] These challenges stem largely from renal ultrafiltration and proteolytic degradation, which invariably lead to rapid elimination and/or inactivation of small natural peptides. This section discusses some recent innovations in the development of therapeutic peptides, addressing metabolic stability, short circulatory half-life, and current trends in oral dosing of peptide drugs.

Addressing Metabolic Instability

Most small natural peptides undergo rapid and extensive proteolysis *in vivo*, resulting in a short serum half-life and a poor therapeutic window. Numerous techniques have been devised to overcome enzymatic catabolism, with simple chemical derivatization yielding promising results. These modifications usually involve changes to the primary sequence of the peptide, particularly in degradation-prone regions; examples include acetylation, lipidation, PEGylation, or glycosylation of the peptide backbone or termini. Sequence modifications have also been thoroughly explored and may include deletions, truncations, retro-inverso configuration and/or incorporation of unnatural amino acids, such as D-amino acids,[102] or homologated analogs such as β- or γ-amino acids, which are unrecognized by proteases.[103]

Naturally occurring covalent modifications that radically alter peptide secondary structure and influence biology include macrocyclization, lactamization, and inter- or intramolecular disulfide bridging. Widely observed in nature, such modifications frequently enhance ligand–receptor binding affinity, increase metabolic stability, and improve oral bioavailability. Perhaps the most inspiring example is cyclosporin A (CsA), a non-ribosomal macrocyclic peptide of fungal origin, developed as an immunosuppressant by Sandoz AG (now Novartis AG) and approved in 1983 as Sandimmune™. CsA is comprised of 11 amino acids (Figure 8.3A), seven of which are N-methylated and one of which is in the unusual D-configuration, is orally bioavailable and cell permeable, and displays a remarkable resistance to proteolysis.

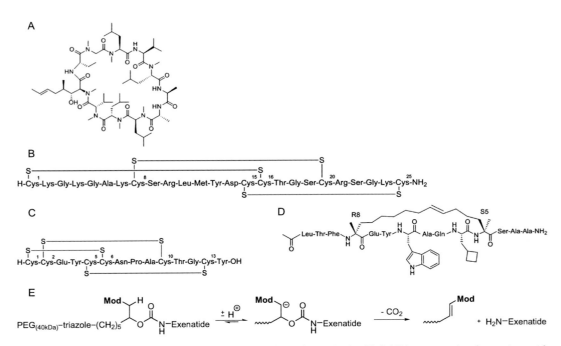

FIGURE 8.3   (A) Non-ribosomal macrocyclic peptide cyclosporin A. (B) Inhibitory cysteine knot ziconotide. (C) Orally bioavailable linaclotide. (D) Hydrocarbon-stapled peptide ATSP-7041. (E) Half-life extension with tunable release of exenatide; here, Mod = $PhSO_2^-$.

At ~1200 Da, CsA is also a well-known contradiction to Lipinski's rules, which state that molecules over ~500 Da, bearing more than five hydrogen-bond donors or ten hydrogen-bond acceptors, are likely to be poorly absorbed. The unusual physicochemical properties of CsA stem from its conformation-dependent hydrophobicity, switching of which allows membrane permeation with unexpected ease. These unusual characteristics inspired decades of intense research to deconvolute CsA to a simple template upon which other peptide drugs of interest could be grafted. The hope was that new drugs with similar oral bioavailability, *in vivo* stability, and cell permeability would ensue. Although no universal template has emerged, the quest for CsA's secret has led to technological revolution in the field brought about by new understanding and driven by a desire to innovate.[104]

Constrained Peptides

Although most small linear endogenous peptides lack a preferential conformation in solution when unbound from their native receptor, cyclic peptides derive many biological advantages from their restricted conformation. Inhibitory cysteine knots (ICKs) are a class of cyclic peptides abundant in nature, possessing a broad and well-defined pharmacology, and showing enormous potential as structural scaffolds for future drug design.[104] The ICK peptide ziconotide, approved in 2004 (Prialt™, Azur Pharma, Ltd.) for treatment of severe chronic pain is the synthetic form of natural conotoxin ω-MVIIA. Ziconotide (Figure 8.3B) is a venom component of the cone snail *Conus magus* that antagonizes centrally located N-type voltage-gated calcium channels following intrathecal injection. However, intrathecal dosing is the most expensive and invasive route of drug administration, carrying with it significant health risks, and the use of ziconotide is restricted to individuals suffering with severe chronic pain (e.g., cancer pain). Despite its restrictions, the approval of ziconotide has led to renewed interest in the development of other ICKs as therapeutics for chronic pain, notably antagonists of TTX-sensitive voltage-gated sodium channels such as Nav1.7.[105]

The hostile enzymatic environment of the gastrointestinal tract usually precludes oral dosing of unmodified proteinogenic peptides; yet, many disulfide-rich peptides (DRPs), including ICKs, feature remarkable stability toward proteolysis. Recent efforts have focused on understanding the unique nature of this stability and development of DRPs as orally available peptide therapeutics in their own right and as structural scaffolds for further drug design. The 14-residue, triple disulfide-bridged peptide linaclotide (Linzess™, Ironwood Pharmaceuticals) is a DRP that was approved in 2012 and is indicated for treatment of irritable bowel syndrome with constipation. Linaclotide (Figure 8.3C) is a potent agonist of the guanylate cyclase type-C receptor which plays a key role in regulating intestinal fluid and electrolyte homeostasis in the intestine.[106]

Combining the structural features of both classical macrocycles and ICKs, cyclotides are a class of small disulfide-rich peptides which are also head-to-tail cyclized along their peptide backbone. Otherwise known as cyclic cysteine knots (CCKs), cyclotides are predominantly found in plants and generally exhibit the greatest degree of thermal, chemical, and enzymatic stability of all classes of constrained peptides. Kalata B1 is one representative member of the cyclotide family shown to inhibit proliferation of human peripheral blood mononuclear cells, suppressing T-cell polyfunctionality and arresting proliferation of immune-competent cells by inhibiting IL-2 biology.[107] Hence, cyclotides potentially offer an orally bioavailable therapeutic platform for treatment of immune-related disorders via T-cell mediated immunosuppression.

The immense stabilizing potential of intramolecular disulfide bonds in certain naturally occurring peptide classes (e.g., venoms) highlights the value of using covalent reinforcement within the peptide backbone. Such observations have resulted in development of novel chemistries offering still more robust chemical bridges which are even less susceptible to chemical and enzymatic degradation than disulfides. Currently, the two most widely acknowledged and successfully exploited methods for bridging or "stapling" peptides intramolecularly are metathesis-mediated hydrocarbon stapling, and the classical natural use of lactams (cyclic amides).

Hydrocarbon-Stapled Peptides

Collaborating with Hoffmann-La Roche, Aileron Therapeutics is making progress in moving their novel modality of hydrocarbon-stapled α-helical peptides toward the clinic. Combining improved membrane permeability and metabolic stability, hydrocarbon stapling of small helical peptides retains a high-affinity conformation permitting modulation of protein–protein interactions out of the context of a much larger regulatory protein. Recently, ATSP-7041, a potent and selective dual inhibitor of MDM2 and MDMX, which effectively activates the human transcription factor protein p53 pathway in tumors, demonstrated growth suppression in xenograft cancer models.[108] ATSP-7041 (Figure 8.3D) exhibits more favorable tissue distribution and pharmacokinetics than small-molecule inhibitors of MDMX and MDM2 and appears potentially amenable to a once-weekly dosing regimen.

Lactamized Peptides

GLP-1 replacement therapies are promising treatments for type 2 diabetics who are insensitive to or produce inadequate GLP-1 endogenously. However, as a messenger peptide, GLP-1 is short lived, and once secreted has a blood serum half-life of only 2 minutes due mainly to the combined actions of the proteases dipeptidylpeptidase-IV (DPP-IV) and neutral endopeptidase (NEP). Consequently, decades of research have been invested into development of metabolically stable GLP-1 and glucagon variants as T2DM therapeutics. This has resulted in the identification of multiple residues amenable to chemical modification by lactamization, resulting in increased stability, potency, and *in vivo* half-life.[109]

Circulatory Half-Life Extension Strategies

In extending the circulatory half-life of a therapeutic peptide we must address both its proteolytic instabilities and the rate of renal clearance. Chemical modification strategies, as outlined above, can be used to address specific sequence liabilities through relevant enzymatic cleavage studies. The rate of clearance may be reduced significantly through site-specific conjugation of the peptide to an appropriate carrier molecule, thereby overcoming elimination via kidney ultrafiltration. Techniques include functionalization with small-molecule albumin-binding tags (e.g., lipidation), conjugation to large inert polymers (e.g., PEG), and fusion to long-lived carrier proteins such as serum albumin. These approaches have collectively driven development of therapeutics based on the incretins GLP-1, GIP, oxyntomodulin, and glucagon, all of which have enjoyed decades of innovation and refinement and today make up a significant proportion of the global market in treatments for type 2 diabetes.

Lipidation

Lipidation may improve metabolic stability, membrane permeability, and bioavailability and favorably alter both the pharmacokinetic and pharmacodynamic profile of the substrate peptide.[110] Hence, lipidation of synthetic peptides has become a common method for imparting favorable qualities to otherwise poor peptide drug candidates. Currently, liraglutide (Victoza®, Novo Nordisk), a long-acting lipidated-GLP-1 agonist indicated for treatment of type 2 diabetes, represents the gold-standard treatment for this condition despite requiring daily subcutaneous injections in order to maintain a therapeutically relevant concentration systemically. Liraglutide's palmitoyl lipid moiety allows association with serum albumin in a reversible manner, affording a circulating pool of the peptide. The combined hydrodynamic radius of the peptide–albumin complex is larger than the cut-off for renal ultrafiltration (~8 nm), hence liraglutide is not readily cleared from circulation until proteolytic cleavage either at the site of lipidation or within the backbone of the peptide occurs.[111]

PEGylation

Covalent attachment of the hydrophilic polymer polyethylene glycol (PEG) to peptides is a well-known technique for improving proteolytic resistance through steric shielding, vastly increasing the hydrodynamic radius of the resulting peptide chimera, and reducing glomerular filtration and thereby prolonging residence time in blood serum.[112] Lee and coworkers[113] applied a site-specific PEGylation strategy to GLP-1, functionalizing at a variety of basic positions in a selective manner and demonstrating that PEGylation at Lys^{34} yielded superior insulinotropic activity and proteolytic resistance. Conjugation of peptides to high-molecular-weight PEGs of around ~40 kD has already proven to afford active drugs with half-lives extending out to ~7 days in humans in several cases.

PEGylation of peptides is often accompanied by a reduction in their potency, derived from the newly imposed limited degrees of freedom within which the peptide may interact with its receptor. Hence, high potency prior to conjugation and administration of relatively high concentrations of peptide–PEG conjugates are usually necessary to achieve the required pharmacology. In addition, despite the improved metabolic stability of peptide–PEG conjugates, there remain long-standing concerns at the risk of accumulation of long-chain PEGs in the liver.

Recent innovations to peptide–PEG conjugates offering tunable pharmacologies include the development of selectively cleavable linkers positioned between peptide and PEG, offering the possibility of a releasable peptide drug cargo. Many of the earlier releasable linkers proposed resulted in unpredictable rates of peptide release, relying on unselective esterases to cleave labile ester functions formed between a PEG alcohol and the carboxylate C-terminus of the peptide. Of the many linker strategies considered for this approach, one of the most promising to date includes that proposed by Santi et al.,[114] in which a drug is functionalized through an available amino group itself masked as a carbamate moiety through which a macromolecular carrier such as PEG is tethered (Figure 8.3E).

Conjugation to a Stable Carrier Protein

The long half-life and high molecular weight of human serum albumin (hSA) make it an attractive target for the covalent attachment of peptide drugs, notably to native Cys^{34} by means of maleimide or vinylsulfone chemistry. The clinical utility of GLP-1 homolog exendin-4 (exenatide, Byetta™, Amylin/BMS/AZ) is limited by its relatively short circulating half-life; however, Los Angeles-based ConjuChem recently demonstrated homogeneous preparation of an albumin–exendin-4 conjugate, CJC-1134-PC, suitable for once-weekly dosing. The exendin-4 analog is covalently bound to a recombinantly produced hSA (Recombumin®, Novozymes), yielding a preformed albumin–peptide conjugate with much longer half-life and greater efficacy than the peptide alone. CJC-1134-PC is a highly soluble liquid formulation suitable for injection and is stable in prefilled syringes at room temperature for at least one month. CJC-1134-PC is currently in Phase II clinical trials and showing a significantly extended half-life over exendin-4.

Oral Delivery of Peptides

The relatively high cost associated with formulation for parenteral delivery of therapeutics peptides has prompted significant innovations in orally bioavailable peptides. Though still very much an emerging area, oral dosing of peptide therapeutics has already met with several notable successes. The following section details four novel strategies.

Biocon PEGalkylation

Acquired by Biocon in 2006, Nobex's technology exploits a hybrid PEGalkylation strategy that involves selective functionalization of a peptide of interest with small (<500 Da) monodisperse oligomers consisting of both a water-soluble PEG moiety and lipid-soluble alkyl chain. This approach creates a molecule with amphiphilic characteristics, facilitating passage through the manifold environments inside our bodies, including translocation over the gastric mucosa into the bloodstream. Biocon/Nobex claim that their oral insulin drug, which is currently in Phase I in the United States and Phase III in India, reproduces the first-phase spike of insulin produced by the pancreas following ingestion of a meal, something that remains a challenge for both injectable and inhaled forms of insulin.

Eligen®

In 2009, Emisphere demonstrated successful oral dosing of peptides GLP-1 and PYY_{3-36} using their proprietary Eligen® technology in an appetite suppression study. Eligen uses amphiphilic small-molecule chaperones, such as sodium N-[8-(2-hydroxybenzoyl) amino]-caprylate (SNAC), to facilitate oral delivery of drugs including peptides with known poor bioavailability and/or gastrointestinal stability. The technology has proven itself effective in achieving therapeutic levels of peptides that otherwise would not have sufficient epithelial permeability to cross the gastric mucosa prior to degradation by digestive enzymes.

Chaperones including SNAC, which received Generally Regarded As Safe (GRAS) status in 2009, are postulated to form weak noncovalent nonspecific interactions with the peptide of interest, increasing its hydrophobicity, possibly as the result of displacement of the water of hydration or by inducing a more lipophilic conformation. Additionally, the presence of these delivery agents has been shown to slow degradation of peptides in the gastrointestinal tract.[115] Novo Nordisk is making good use of a combined alkyl–PEGylation and chaperone strategy with their most recent type 2 diabetes treatment, semaglutide

(NN9535), a GLP-1 analog that entered Phase III trials in 2013 as a once-weekly injectable. Novo recently announced that when tableted with a suitable chaperone, semaglutide given orally has achieved therapeutically relevant concentrations in the bloodstream during Phase I trials.

Designed Thiomers

ThioMatrix used thiolated polymeric excipients, or designed thiomers, to further improve upon the mucoadhesion properties of well-established polymeric excipients including poly(acrylates) and chitosans. These thiolated polymers form disulfide bonds with cysteine-rich subdomains abundant on the surface of the gastric mucosa, leading to numerous pharmaceutical improvements including enhanced permeation, controlled release from the polymeric network, inhibition of enzyme, and efflux-pump activity. Thiolation of chitosan was shown to increase gastric residence time by at least 140-fold, and ThioMatrix reported a sustained 40% decrease in blood-sugar level over almost 24 hours after oral administration of a thiomer-formulated PEGylated insulin in diabetic mice.[116] Administration of an unformulated insulin derivative showed no comparable pharmacology.

Peptelligence™

Having acquired the Peptelligence™ platform and a recombinant manufacturing process for therapeutically relevant peptides from Unigene Laboratories, Enteris Biopharma has become an industry leader in oral dosage formulations. Peptelligence utilizes an enteric-tablet formulation, ensuring that the contents of the tablet are delivered to the pH-neutral environment of the small intestine. The tablet is formulated with protease inhibitors and excipients comprising two main components. The first is a surfactant-type permeation enhancer that increases solubility and loosens tight junctions in the intestinal enterocytes to improve paracellular transport. The second key component, citric acid, chelates calcium, enhances membrane permeation, and has been shown to increase absorptive flux and membrane wetting/charge dispersal. Enteris currently has several peptides in clinical trials including calcitonin (Phase II for osteopenia, Phase III for osteoporosis) and parathyroid hormone (Phase II for osteoporosis).

NOVEL OPPORTUNITIES FOR BIOLOGICS

At the start of this chapter we highlighted two key revolutions, or paradigm shifts, in the use of therapeutic proteins and peptides: the recognition of their therapeutic potential and methods to manufacture them on a large scale for clinical use. New breakthroughs in understanding disease biology and pharmacology continue to drive thinking in what is the optimal strategy to address a disease mechanism and what is the right drug format for the patient. Although there have been no new Nobel Prizes awarded in how to make proteins and peptides, there continue to be gradual improvements in recombinant and synthetic engineering approaches. Most notable among these are (1) strategies that combine recombinant and synthetic approaches, and (2) strategies to address intracellular targets.

The combination of recombinant and synthetic methods in the development of new medicines is best demonstrated with the antibody–drug conjugates (ADCs). The use of ADCs is now clinically validated for the targeted killing of cancer cells, as Adcentris® (Seattle Genetics) and Kadcyla® (ImmunoGen) have been approved in the last two years. The next generation of oncology ADCs field is focused on producing more homogeneous drug product through site-specific conjugation and delivering more potent payloads. However, this concept of combined synthetic and recombinant components can be extended beyond cell killing to drive new innovations in protein engineering and drug delivery. For example, in diabetes an ADC approach generated a long-acting antidiabetic FGF21 mimetic.[117] FGF21 has metabolically beneficial effects via mechanisms that are not completely clear. However, it has a very short half-life and the N- and C-termini are required for biological activity, thus limiting the use of genetic fusions. Introducing a free cysteine residue in the middle of FGF21 (A129C) enabled site-specific chemical conjugation to an engineered IgG$_1$, generating a molecule with extended half-life and preserving the full therapeutic functionality in preclinical models. Many labs are now combining the strengths of traditional recombinant engineering strategies and chemical synthesis to overcome technical limitations in drug discovery. The chemical macrocyclization of recombinant peptide–Fc fusions for a next generation of ADCs,[118] the use of new vectors to enable high-throughput mammalian expression of peptide–Fc fusions directly from phage display selections,[119] and the combination of bacterial display for lead isolation and optimization prior to the final chemical synthesis of small disulfide-rich domains,[120] among other approaches, can accelerate the discovery new peptides and proteins.

Proteins and peptides drugs are currently restricted to modulating soluble or plasma membrane associated targets that account for around 35% of human proteins.[6] The intracellular compartment is beyond the reach of conventional proteins and peptides and the intracellular protein–protein interactions are, by and large, not tractable by small molecules. Therefore, the potential to deliver proteins and peptides intracellularly has the potential to open up new avenues for therapeutic intervention. However, there are two main challenges to achieve this. The first step is active uptake of the molecule, typically by active receptor-mediated endocytosis. The second step is then to escape the endocytic pathway before entering the lysosome where active degradation takes place. As a result of endocytic uptake only a fraction of the active molecule enters the cell cytoplasm. Examples of successful delivery of protein payloads to the cytoplasm are rare, but one example is the recombinant immunotoxin moxetumomab pasudotox (MedImmune/NCI). In this case, specific internalization is achieved by the anti-CD22 antibody, and the lysosomal degradation of the genetically fused PE38 results in the cytoplasmic release of a toxin fragment. Various protein and peptide intracellular delivery strategies have been developed, including cell-penetrating peptides (CPPs), stapled peptides, supercharged proteins, and targeted nanoparticles.[121–124] To date, these approaches for intracellular delivery have proven to be inefficient and require further technical advances to enable efficient delivery of the protein payload to the cytoplasmic site of action.

Significant progress has been made in the development of protein and peptide therapeutics in the last 35 years and they will have an expanding role in medicine in the future. Incorporating the novel modalities and technologies from both recombinant and synthetic approaches will enable the design of new therapeutic molecules to modulate targets more effectively to bring healthcare benefits to patients.

References

1. Itakura K, Hirose T, Crea R, Riggs AD, Heyneker HL, Bolivar F, Boyer HW. Expression in *Escherichia coli* of a chemically synthesized gene for the hormone somatostatin. Science 1977;198:1056–63.
2. Goeddel DV, Kleid DG, Bolivar F, Heyneker HL, Yansura DG, Crea R, Hirose T, Krasewski A, Itakura K, Roggs AD. Expression in *Escherichia coli* of chemically synthesized genes for human insulin. Proc. Natl. Acad. Sci. U.S.A. 1979;76:106–10.
3. du Vigneaud V, Ressler C, Swan JM, Roberst CW, Katsoyannis PG, Gordon S. The synthesis of an octapeptide amide with the hormonal activity of oxytocin. J. Am. Chem. Soc. 1953;75:4879–80.
4. Carter PJ. Introduction to current and future protein therapeutics: A protein engineering perspective. Exp. Cell Res. 2011;317:1261–9.
5. Leader B, Baca QJ, Golan DE. Protein therapeutics: a summary and pharmacological classification. Nat. Rev. Drug Discov. 2008;7:21–39.
6. Rastogi S, Rost B. LocDB: experimental annotations of localization for homo sapiens and arabidopsis thaliana. Nucleic Acids Res. 2011;39:230–4.
7. Buchanan A, Clementel V, Woods R, Harn N, Bowen MA, Mo W, Popovic B, Bishop SM, Dall'Acqua W, Minter R, Jermutus L, Bedian V. Engineering a therapeutic IgG molecule to address cysteinylation, aggregation and enhance thermal stability and expression. mAbs 2013;5:255–62.
8. Buchanan A, Ferraro F, Rust S, Sridharan S, Franks R, Dean G, McCourt M, Jermutus L, Minter R. Improved drug-like properties of therapeutic proteins by directed evolution. Protein Eng. Des. Sel. 2012;25:631–8.
9. Murray CJ, Baliga R. Cell-free translation of peptides and proteins: From high throughput screening to clinical production. Curr. Opin. Chem. Biol. 2013;17:420–6.
10. Agrawal V, Bal M. Strategies for rapid production of therapeutic proteins in mammalian cells. BioProcess Int. 2012;10:32–48.
11. Binz HK, Amstutz P, Plückthun A. Engineering novel binding proteins from nonimmunoglobulin domains. Nat. Biotechnol. 2005;23:1257–68.
12. Martello JL, Woytowish MR, Chambers H. Ecallantide for treatment of acute attacks of hereditary angioedema. Am. J. Health Syst. Pharm. 2012;69:651–7.
13. Chen Z, Hu Y, Yang W, He Y, Feng J, Wang B, Zhao R, Ding J, Cao Z, Li W, Wu Y. Hg1: novel peptide inhibitor specific for Kv1.3 channels from first scorpion Kunitz-type potassium channel toxin family. J. Biol. Chem. 2012;287:13813–21.
14. Wan H, Leem KS, Kim BY, Zou FM, Yoon HJ, Je YH, Li J, Jin BR. A spider-derived Kunitz-type serine protease inhibitor that acts as a plasmin inhibitor and an elastase inhibitor. PLoS ONE 2013;8:e53343.
15. Devy L, Rabbani SA, Stochl M, Ruskowski M, Mackie I, Naa L, Toews M, Van Gool R, Chen J, Ley A, Ladner RC, Dransfield DT, Henderikx P. PEGylated DX-1000: pharmacokinetics and antineoplastic activity of a specific plasmin inhibitor. Neoplasia 2007;9:927–37.
16. Salameh MA, Soares AS, Navaneetham D, Sinha D, Walsh PN, Radisky ES. Determinants of affinity and proteolytic stability in interactions of Kunitz family protease inhibitors with mesotrypsin. J. Biol. Chem. 2010;285:36884–96.
17. Binz HK, Amstutz P, Kohl A, Stumpp MT, Briand C, Forrer P, Grütter MG, Plückthun A. High-affinity binders selected from designed ankyrin repeat protein libraries. Nat. Biotechnol. 2004;22:575–82.
18. Interlandi G, Wetzel SK, Settanni G, Plückthun A, Caflisch A. Characterization and further stabilization of designed ankyrin repeat proteins by combining molecular dynamics simulations and experiments. J. Mol. Biol. 2008;375:837–54.
19. Boersma YL, Chao G, Steiner D, Wittrup KD, Plückthun A. Bispecific designed ankyrin repeat proteins (DARPins) targeting epidermal growth factor receptor inhibit A431 cell proliferation and receptor recycling. J. Biol. Chem. 2011;286:41273–85.
20. Campochiaro PA, Channa R, Berger BB, Heier JS, Brown DM, Fiedler U, Hepp J, Stumpp MT. Treatment of diabetic macular edema with a designed ankyrin repeat protein that binds vascular endothelial growth factor: A phase I/II study. Am. J. Ophthalmol. 2013;155:697–704.
21. Lipovsek D. Adnectins: engineered target-binding protein therapeutics. Protein Eng. Des. Sel. 2011;24:3–9.
22. Jacobs SA, Diem MD, Luo J, Teplyakov A, Obmolova G, Malia T, Gilliland GL, Oneil KT. Design of novel FN3 domains with high stability by a consensus sequence approach. Protein Eng. Des. Sel. 2012;25:107–17.

23. Swers JS, Grinberg L, Wang L, Feng H, Lekstrom K, Carrasco R, Xiao Z, Inigo I, Leow CC, Wu H, Tice DA, Baca M. Multivalent scaffold proteins as superagonists of TRAIL receptor 2-induced apoptosis. Mol. Cancer Ther. 2013;12:1235–44.

24. Koide A, Bailey CW, Huang X, Koide S. The fibronectin type III domain as a scaffold for novel binding proteins. J. Mol. Biol. 1998;284:1141–51.

25. Koide A, Wojcik J, Gilbreth RN, Hoey RJ, Koide S. Teaching an old scaffold new tricks: monobodies constructed using alternative surfaces of the FN3 scaffold. J. Mol. Biol. 2012;415:393–405.

26. Tolcher AW, Sweeney CJ, Papadopoulos K, Patnaik A, Chiorean EG, Mita AC, Sankhala K, Furfine E, Gokemeijer J, Iacono L, Eaton C, Silver BA, Mita M. Phase I and pharmacokinetic study of CT-322 (BMS-844203), a targeted adnectin inhibitor of VEGFR-2 based on a domain of human fibronectin. Clin. Cancer Res. 2011;17:363–71.

27. Emanuel SL, Engle LJ, Chao G, Zhu R, Cao C, Lin Z, Yamniuk A, Hosbach J, Brown J, Fitzpatrick E, et al. A fibronectin scaffold approach to bispecific inhibitors of epidermal growth factor receptor and insulin-like growth factor-I receptor. mAbs 2011;3:38–48.

28. Gebauer M, Schiefner A, Matschiner G, Skerra A. Combinatorial design of an anticalin directed against the extra-domain B for the specific targeting of oncofetal fibronectin. J. Mol. Biol. 2013;425:780–802.

29. Mross K, Fischer R, Richly H, Scharr D, Buechert M, Stern A, Hoth D, Gille H, Audoly LP, Scheulen ME. First in human Phase I study of PRS-050 (Angiocal), a VEGF-A targeting anticalin, in patients with advanced solid tumours: results of a dose escalation study. PLoS ONE 2013;8:e83232.

30. Silverman J, Lu Q, Bakker A, To W, Duguay A, Alba BM, Smith R, Rivas A, Li P, Le H, Whitehorn E, Moore KW, Swimmer C, Perlroth V, Vogt M, Kolkman J, Stemmer WPC. Multivalent avimer proteins evolved by exon shuffling of a family of human receptor domains. Nat. Biotechnol. 2005;23:1556–61.

31. Smith R, Duguay A, Bakker A, Li P, Weiszmann J, Thomas MR, Alba BM, Wu X, Gupte J, Yang L, Stevens J, Hamburger A, Smith S, Chen J, Komorowski R, Moore KW, Veniant MM, Li Y. FGF21 can be mimicked *in vitro* and *in vivo* by a novel anti-FGFR1c/beta-Klotho bispecific protein. PLoS ONE 2013;8:e61432.

32. Lee S, Park K, Han J, Lee JJ, Kim HJ, Hong S, Heu W, Kim YJ, Ha JS, Lee SG, Cheong HK, Jeon YH, Kim D, Kim HS. Design of a binding scaffold based on variable lymphocyte receptors of jawless vertebrates by module engineering. Proc. Natl. Acad. Sci U.S.A. 2012;109:3299–304.

33. Urvoas A, Guellouz A, Valerio-Lepiniec M, Graille M, Durand D, Desravines DC, van Tilbeurgh H, Desmadril M, Minard P. Design, production and molecular structure of a new family of artificial alpha-helicoidal repeat proteins (αRep) based on thermostable HEAT-like repeats. J. Mol. Biol. 2010;404:307–27.

34. Varadamsetty G, Tremmel D, Hansen S, Parmeggiani F, Plückthun A. Designed armadillo repeat proteins: library generation, characterization and selection of peptide binders with high specificity. J. Mol. Biol. 2012;424:68–87.

35. Xiao X, Feng Y, Vu BK, Ishima R, Dimitrov DS. A large library based on a novel (CH2) scaffold: identification of HIV-1 inhibitors. Biochem. Biophys. Res. Commun. 2009;387:387–92.

36. Gong R, Wang Y, Ying T, Feng Y, Streaker E, Prabakaran P, Dimitrov DS. N-terminal truncation of an isolated human IgG$_1$ C$_H$2 domain significantly increases its stability and aggregation resistance. Mol. Pharmaceutics. 2013;10:2642–52.

37. Wozniak-Knopp G, Bartl S, Bauer A, Mostageer M, Woisetschlager M, Antes B, Ettl K, Kainer M, Weberhofer G, Wiederkum S, Himmler G, Mudde GC, Ruker F. Introducing antigen-binding sites in structural loops of immunoglobulin constant domains: Fc fragments with engineered HER2/neu-binding sites and antibody properties. Protein Eng. Des. Sel. 2010;23:289–97.

38. Wozniak-Knopp G, Stadlmann J, Ruker F. Stabilisation of the Fc fragment of human IgG$_1$ by engineered intra-domain disulfide bonds. PLoS ONE 2012;7:e30083.

39. Traxlmayr MW, Lobner E, Antes B, Kainer M, Wiederkum S, Hasenhindl C, Stadlmayr G, Ruker F, Woisetschlager M, Moulder K, Obinger C. Directed evolution of Her2/neu-binding IgG$_1$-Fc for improved stability and resistance to aggregation by using yeast surface display. Protein Eng. Des. Sel. 2013;26:255–65.

40. Kolmar H. Alternative binding proteins: biological activity and therapeutic potential of cystine-knot miniproteins. FEBS J. 2008;275:2684–90.

41. Moore SJ, Leung CL, Cochran JR. Knottins: disulphide-bonded therapeutic and diagnostic peptides. Drug Discov. Today 2013;9:e3–e11.

42. Gould A, Ji Y, Aboye TL, Camarero JA. Cyclotides, a novel ultrastable polypeptide scaffold for drug discovery. Curr. Pharm. Des. 2011;17:4294–307.

II. NOVEL APPROACHES FOR BIOLOGICS

43. Austin J, Wang W, Puttamadappa S, Shekhtman A, Camarero JA. Biosynthesis and biological screening of a genetically encoded library based on the cyclotide MCoTI-I. Chembiochem. 2009;10:2663–70.

44. Lee C, Park K, Sung E, Kim A, Choi JD, Kim JS, Kim SH, Kwon MH, Kim YS. Engineering of a human kringle domain into agonistic and antagonistic binding proteins functioning *in vitro* and *in vivo*. Proc. Natl. Acad. Sci. U.S.A. 2010;107:9567–71.

45. Lee C, Park K, Kim SJ, Kwon O, Jeong KJ, Kim A, Kim Y. Generation of bivalent and bispecific kringle single domains by loop grafting as potent agonists against death receptors 4 and 5. J. Mol. Biol. 2011;411:201–19.

46. Craik DJ, Fairlie DP, Liras S, Price D. The future of peptide-based drugs. Chem. Biol. Drug Des. 2013;81: 136–47.

47. Moody AJ, Norris F, Norris K. The secretion of glucagon by transformed yeast strains. FEBS Lett. 1987;212:302–6.

48. Williams RM, McDonald A, O'Savage M, Dunger DB. Mecasermin rinfabate: rhIGF-I/rhIGFBP-3 complex: iPLEX. Expert Opin. Drug Metab. Toxicol. 2008;4:311–24.

49. Fazen CH, Kahkoska AR, Doyle RP. Expression and purification of human PYY(3-36) in *Escherichia coli* using a His-tagged small ubiquitin-like modifier fusion. Protein Expr. Purif. 2012;85:51–9.

50. Stepanenko VN, Esipov RS, Gurevich AI, Chupova LA, Miroshnikov AI. Recombinant oxyntomodulin [in Russian]. Bioorg. Khim. 2007;33:227–32.

51. Kim S, Shin S, Park Y, Shin C, Seo J. Production and solid-phase refolding of human glucagon-like peptide-1 using recombinant *Escherichia coli*. Protein Expr. Purif. 2011;78:197–203.

52. Zhou J, Chu J, Wang Y, Wang H, Zhuang Y, Zhang S. Purification and bioactivity of exendin-4, a peptide analogue of GLP-1, expressed in *Pichia pastoris*. Biotechnol. Lett. 2008;30:651–6.

53. Baker EN, Blundell TL, Cutfield JF, Cutfield SM, Dodson EJ, Dodson GG, Hodgkin DM, Hubbard RE, Isaacs NW, Reynolds CD. The structure of 2Zn pig insulin crystals at 1.5 A resolution. Philos. Trans. R. Soc. Lond. B Biol. Sci. 1988;319:369–456.

54. Pandyarajan V, Weiss MA. Design of non-standard insulin analogs for the treatment of diabetes mellitus. Curr. Diabetes Rep. 2012;12:697–704.

55. Whittingham JL, Jonassen I, Havelund S, Roberts SM, Dodson EJ, Verma CS, Wilkinson AJ, Dodson GG. Crystallographic and solution studies of *N*-lithocholyl insulin: a new generation of prolonged-acting human insulins. Biochemistry 2004;43:5987–95.

56. Jonassen I, Havelund S, Hoeg-Jensen T, Steensgaard DB, Wahlund PO, Ribel U. Design of the novel protraction mechanism of insulin degludec, an ultra-long-acting basal insulin. Pharm. Res. 2012;29:2104–14.

57. Bergenstal RM, Rosenstock J, Arakaki RF, Prince MJ, Qu Y, Sinha VP, Howey DC, Jacober SJ. A randomized, controlled study of once-daily LY2605541, a novel long-acting basal insulin, versus insulin glargine in basal insulin-treated patients with type 2 diabetes. Diabetes Care 2012;35:2140–7.

58. Craik CS, Page MJ, Madison EL. Proteases as therapeutics. Biochem. J. 2011;435:1–16.

59. Li Q, Yi L, Marek P, Iverson BL. Commercial proteases: present and future. FEBS Lett. 2013;587:1155–63.

60. Madison EL, Goldsmith EJ, Gerard RD, Gething MH, Sambrook JF. Serpin-resistant mutants of human tissue-type plasminogen activator. Nature 1989;339:721–4.

61. Varadarajan N, Rodriguez S, Hwang B, Georgiou G, Iverson BL. Highly active and selective endopeptidases with programmed substrate specificities. Nat. Chem. Biol. 2008;4:290–4.

62. Yi L, Gebhard MC, Li Q, Taft JM, Georgiou G, Iverson BL. Engineering of TEV protease variants by yeast ER sequestration screening (YESS) of combinatorial libraries. Proc. Natl. Acad. Sci. U.S.A. 2013;110:7229–34.

63. Gillies SD, Lan Y, Hettmann T, Brunkhorst B, Sun Y, Mueller SO, Lo K. A low-toxicity IL-2-based immunocytokine retains antitumor activity despite its high degree of IL-2 receptor selectivity. Clin. Cancer Res. 2011;17:3673–85.

64. Laurent J, Touvrey C, Gillessen S, Joffraud M, Vicari M, Bertrand C, Ongarello S, Liedert B, Gallerani E, Beck J, Omlin A, Sessa C, Quaratino S, Stupp R, Gnad-Vogt US, Speiser DE. T-cell activation by treatment of cancer patients with EMD 521873 (Selectikine), an IL-2/anti-DNA fusion protein. J. Transl. Med. 2013;7:11–5.

65. Junttila IS, Creusot RJ, Moraga I, Bates DL, Wong MT, Alonso MN, Suhoski MM, Lupardus P, Meier-Schellersheim M, Engleman EG, Utz PJ, Fathman CG, Paul WE, Garcia KC. Redirecting cell-type specific cytokine responses with engineered interleukin-4 superkines. Nature Chemical Biology 2012;8:990–8.

66. Levin AM, Bates DL, Ring AM, Krieg C, Lin JT, Su L, Moraga I, Raeber ME, Bowman GR, Novick P, Pande VS, Fathman CG, Boyman O, Garcia KC. Exploiting a natural conformational switch to engineer an interleukin-2 "superkine". Nature 2012;484:529–33.

67. Han KP, Zhu X, Liu B, Jeng E, Kong L, Yovandich JL, Vyas VV, Marcus WD, Chavaillaz PA, Romero CA, Rhode PR, Wong HC. IL-**15**:IL-15 receptor alpha superagonist complex: high-level co-expression in recombinant mammalian cells, purification and characterization. Cytokine 2011;56:804–10.

68. Vincent M, Bessard A, Cochonneau D, Teppaz G, Sole V, Maillasson M, Birkle S, Garrigue-Antar L, Quemener A, Jacques Y. Tumor targeting of the IL-15 superagonist RLI by an anti-GD2 antibody strongly enhances its antitumor potency. Int. J. Cancer 2013;133:757–65.

69. Elliott S, Lorenzini T, Asher S, Aoki K, Brankow D, Buck L, Busse L, Chang D, Fuller J, Grant J, Hernday N, Hokum M, Hu S, Knudten A, Levin N, Komorowski R, Martin F, Navarro R, Osslund T, Rogers G, Rogers N, Trail G, Egrie J. Enhancement of therapeutic protein *in vivo* activities through glycoengineering. Nat. Biotechnol. 2003;21:414–21.

70. Jarsch M, Brandt M, Lanzendorfer M, Haselbeck A. Comparative erythropoietin receptor binding kinetics of C.E.R.A. and epoetin-beta determined by surface plasmon resonance and competition binding assay. Pharmacology 2008;81:63–9.

71. Schellekens H. How similar do "biosimilars" need to be? Nat. Biotechnol. 2004;22:1357–9.

72. Lee JS, Ha TK, Lee SJ, Lee GM. Current state and perspectives on erythropoietin production. Appl. Microbiol. Biotechnol. 2012;95:1405–16.

73. Suzuki T, Ishii-Watabe A, Tada M, Kobayashi T, Kanayasu-Toyoda T, Kawanishi T, Yamaguchi T. Importance of neonatal FcR in regulating the serum half-life of therapeutic proteins containing the Fc domain of human IgG_1: a comparative study of the affinity of monoclonal antibodies and Fc-fusion proteins to human neonatal FcR. J. Immunol. 2010;184:1968–76.

74. Shimamoto G, Gegg C, Boone T, Queva C. Peptibodies: a flexible alternative format to antibodies. mAbs 2012;4:586–91.

75. Glaesner W, Vick AM, Millican R, Ellis B, Tschang SH, Tian Y, Bokvist K, Brenner M, Koester A, Porksen N, Etgen G, Bumol T. Engineering and characterization of the long-acting glucagon-like peptide-1 analogue LY2189265: an Fc fusion protein. Diabetes Metab. Res. 2010;26:287–96.

76. Mekhaiel D, Czajkowsky D, Andersen JT, Shi J, Sandlie I, McIntosh R, Pleass R. Polymeric human Fc-fusion proteins with modified effector functions. Sci. Rep. 2011;124:1–11.

77. Gaboriaud C, Juanhuix J, Gruez A, Lacroix M, Darnault C, Pignol D, Verger D, Fontecilla-Camps JC, Arlaud GJ. The crystal structure of the globular head of complement protein C1q provides a basis for its versatile recognition properties. J. Biol. Chem. 2003;278:46974–82.

78. Oganesyan V, Gao C, Shirinian L, Wu H, Dall'Acqua WF. Structural characterization of a human Fc fragment engineered for lack of effector functions. Acta Crystallogr. D Biol. Crystallogr. 2008;64:700–4.

79. Bonetto S, Spadola L, Buchanan A, Jermutus L, Lund J. Identification of cyclic peptides able to mimic the functional epitope of IgG_1-Fc for human Fc gammaRI. FASEB J. 2009;23:575–85.

80. Moore GL, Chen H, Karki S, Lazar GA. Engineered Fc variant antibodies with enhanced ability to recruit complement and mediate effector functions. MAbs. 2010;2:181–9.

81. Repp R, Kellner C, Muskulus A, Staudinger M, Nodehi SM, Glorius P, Akramiene D, Dechant M, Fey GH, van Berkel PH, van de Winkel JG, Parren PW, Valerius T, Gramatzki M, Peipp M. Combined Fc-protein- and Fc-glyco-engineering of scFv-Fc fusion proteins synergistically enhances CD16a binding but does not further enhance NK-cell mediated ADCC. J. Immunol. Methods 2011;373:67–78.

82. Wilkinson IC, Fowler SB, Machiesky L, Miller K, Hayes DB, Adib M, Her C, Borrok MJ, Tsui P, Burrell M, Corkill DJ, Witt S, Lowe DC, Webster CI. Monovalent IgG4 molecules: immunoglobulin Fc mutations that result in a monomeric structure. mAbs 2013;3:406–17.

83. Caravella J, Lugovskoy A. Design of next-generation protein therapeutics. Curr. Opin. Chem. Biol. 2010;14: 520–8.

84. Jevsevar S, Kunstelj M, Porekar VG. PEGylation of therapeutic proteins. Biotechnol. J. 2010;5:113–28.

85. Sleep D, Cameron J, Evans LR. Albumin as a versatile platform for drug half-life extension. Biochim. Biophys. Acta. 2013;1830:5526–34.

86. Madsbad S, Kielgast U, Asmar M, Deacon CF, Torekov SS, Holst JJ. An overview of once-weekly glucagon-like peptide-1 receptor agonists—available efficacy and safety data and perspectives for the future. Diabetes Obes. Metab. 2011;13:394–407.

87. Cordes AA, Platt CW, Carpenter JF, Randolph TW. Selective domain stabilization as a strategy to reduce fusion protein aggregation. J. Pharm. Sci. 2012;101:1400–9.

88. Andersen JT, Dalhus B, Cameron J, Daba MB, Plumridge A, Evans L, Brennan SO, Gunnarsen KS, Bjoras M, Sleep D, Sandlie I. Structure-based mutagenesis reveals the albumin-binding site of the neonatal Fc receptor. Nat. Commun. 2012;3:610.

89. Schellenberger V, Wang CW, Geething NC, Spink BJ, Campbell A, To W, Scholle MD, Yin Y, Yao Y, Bogin O, Cleland JL, Silverman J, Stemmer WP. A recombinant polypeptide extends the *in vivo* half-life of peptides and proteins in a tunable manner. Nat. Biotechnol. 2009;27:1186–90.

90. Schlapschy M, Binder U, Borger C, Theobald I, Wachinger K, Kisling S, Haller D, Skerra A. PASylation: a biological alternative to PEGylation for extending the plasma half-life of pharmaceutically active proteins. Protein Eng. Des. Sel. 2013;26:489–501.

91. Cleland JL, Geething NC, Moore JA, Rogers BC, Spink BJ, Wang CW, Alters SE, Stemmer WP, Schellenberger V. A novel long-acting human growth hormone fusion protein (VRS-317): enhanced *in vivo* potency and half-life. J. Pharm. Sci. 2012;101:2744–54.

92. Sarkar CA, Lowenhaupt K, Horan T, Boone TC, Tidor B, Lauffenburger DA. Rational cytokine design for increased lifetime and enhanced potency using pH-activated "histidine switching". Nat. Biotechnol. 2002;20: 908–13.

93. Sockolosky JT, Tiffany MR, Szoka FC. Engineering neonatal Fc receptor-mediated recycling and transcytosis in recombinant proteins by short terminal peptide extensions. Proc. Natl. Acad. Sci. U.S.A. 2012;109: 16095–100.

94. Bender NK, Heilig CE, Droll B, Wohlgemuth J, Armbruster FP, Heilig B. Immunogenicity, efficacy and adverse events of adalimumab in RA patients. Rheumatol. Int. 2007;27:269–74.

95. Casadevall N, Eckardt KU, Rossert J. Epoetin-induced autoimmune pure red cell aplasia. J. Am. Soc. Nephrol. 2005;16:S67–9.

96. Parfrey PS, Warden G, Barrett BJ. On peginesatide and anemia treatment in CKD. Am. J. Kidney Dis. 2013;368:1553–4.

97. Liu W, Onda M, Lee B, Kreitman RJ, Hassan R, Xiang L, Pastan I. Recombinant immunotoxin engineered for low immunogenicity and antigenicity by identifying and silencing human B-cell epitopes. Proc. Natl. Acad. Sci. U.S.A. 2012;109:11782–7.

98. Baker MP, Reynolds HM, Lumicisi B, Bryson CJ. Immunogenicity of protein therapeutics: the key causes, consequences and challenges. Self Nonself. 2010;1:314–22.

99. Parker AS, Choi Y, Griswold KE, Bailey-Kellogg C. Structure-guided deimmunization of therapeutic proteins. J. Comput. Biol. 2013;20:152–65.

100. Cantor JR, Yoo TH, Dixit A, Iverson BL, Forsthuber TG, Georgiou G. Therapeutic enzyme deimmunization by combinatorial T-cell epitope removal using neutral drift. Proc. Natl. Acad. Sci. U.S.A. 2011;108:1272–7.

101. Vlieghe P, Lisowski V, Martinez J, Khrestchatisky M. Synthetic therapeutic peptides: science and market. Drug Discov. Today 2010;15:40–56.

102. Mitchell JB, Smith J. D-amino acid residues in peptides and proteins. Proteins 2003;50:563–71.

103. Seebach D, Gardiner J. β-Peptidic peptidomimetics. Acc. Chem. Res. 2008;41:1366–75.

104. Revell JD, Lund PE, Linley JE, Metcalfe J, Burmeister N, Sridharan S, Jones C, Jermutus L, Bednarek MA. Potency optimization of Huwentoxin-IV on hNav1.7, a neurotoxin TTX-S sodium-channel antagonist from the venom of the Chinese bird-eating spider *Selenocosmia huwena*. Peptides 2013;44:40–6.

105. Klint J, Anangi R, Mobli M, Knapp O, Adams DJ, King GF. Spider-venom peptides that target the human NaV1.7 channel, potential analgesics for the treatment of chronic pain. Toxicon. 2012;60:110–1.

106. Brierley SM. Guanylate cyclase-C receptor activation, unexpected biology. Curr. Opin. Pharmacol. 2012;12: 632–40.

107. Gründemann C, Thell K, Lengen K, Garcia-Käufer M, Huang YH, Huber R, Craik DJ, Schabbauer G, Gruber CW. Cyclotides suppress human T-lymphocyte proliferation by an interleukin 2-dependent mechanism. PLoS ONE 2013;8:e68016.

108. Changa YS, Graves B, Guerlavais V, Tovar C, Packman K, To KH, Olson KA, Kesavan K, Gangurde P, Mukherjee A, et al. Stapled α-helical peptide drug development, a potent dual inhibitor of MDM2 and MDMX for p53-dependent cancer therapy. Proc. Natl. Acad. Sci. U.S.A. 2013;110:E3445–54.

109. Murage EN, Gao G, Bisello A, Ahn JM. Development of potent glucagon-like peptide-1 agonists with high enzyme stability via introduction of multiple lactam bridges. J. Med. Chem. 2010;53:6412–20.

110. Zhang L, Bulag G. Converting peptides into drug leads by lipidation. Curr. Med. Chem. 2012;19:1602–18.

111. Malm-Erjefält M, Bjørnsdottir I, Vanggaard J, Helleberg H, Larson U, Oosterhuis B, Jaap van Lier J, Zdravkovic M, Olsen AK. Metabolism and excretion of the once-daily human glucagon-like peptide-1 analog liraglutide in healthy male subjects and its *in vitro* degradation by dipeptidyl peptidase IV and neutral endopeptidase. Drug Metab. Dispos. 2010;38:1944–53.

112. Veronese FM, Pasut G. PEGylation, successful approach to drug delivery. Drug Discov. Today 2005;10: 1451–8.

113. Youn YS, Chae SY, Lee S, Jeon JE, Shin HG, Lee KC. Evaluation of therapeutic potentials of site-specific PEGylated glucagon-like peptide-1 isomers as a type 2 anti-diabetic treatment: insulinotropic activity, glucose-stabilizing capability, and proteolytic stability. Biochem. Pharmacol. 2007;73:84–93.

114. Santi DV, Schneider EL, Reid R, Robinson L, Ashley GW. Predictable and tunable half-life extension of thera-peutic agents by controlled chemical release from macromolecular conjugates. Proc. Natl. Acad. Sci. U.S.A. 2012;109:6211–6.

115. Hess S, Rotshild V, Hoffman A. Investigation of the enhancing mechanism of sodium N-[8-(2-hydroxybenzoyl) amino]caprylate effect on the intestinal permeability of polar molecules utilizing a voltage clamp method. Eur. J. Pharm. Sci. 2005;25:307–12.

116. Krauland A, Guggi D, Bernkop-Schnürch A. Oral peptide delivery, the potential of thiolated chitosan-insulin tablets on non-diabetic rats. J. Control. Release 2004;95:547–55.

117. Huang J, Ishino T, Chen G, Rolzin P, Osothprarop TF, Retting K, Li L, Jin P, Matin MJ, Huyghe B, Talukdar S, Bradshaw CW, Palanki M, Violand BN, Woodnutt G, Lappe RW, Ogilvie K, Levin N. Development of a novel long-acting antidiabetic FGF21 mimetic by targeted conjugation to a scaffold antibody. J. Pharmacol. Exp. Ther. 2013;346:270–80.

118. Angelini A, Diderich P, Morales-Sanfrutos J, Thurnheer S, Hacker D, Menin L, Heinis C. Chemical macrocycli-zation of peptides fused to antibody Fc fragments. Bioconjug. Chem. 2012;23:1856–63.

119. Quinlan BD, Gardner MR, Joshi VR, Chiang JJ, Farzan M. Direct expression and validation of phage-selected peptide variants in mammalian cells. J. Biol. Chem. 2013;288:18803–10.

120. Getz JA, Cheneval O, Craik DJ, Daugherty PS. Design of a cyclotide antagonist of neuropilin-1 and -2 that potently inhibits endothelial cell migration. ACS Chem. Biol. 2013;8:1147–54.

121. Bechara C, Sagan S. Cell-penetrating peptides, 20 years later, where do we stand? FEBS Lett. 2013;587: 1693–702.

122. Verdine GL, Hilinski GJ. Stapled peptides for intracellular drug targets. Methods Enzymol. 2012;503:3–33.

123. Cronican JJ, Beier KT, Davis TN, et al. A class of human proteins that deliver functional proteins into mamma-lian cells *in vitro* and *in vivo*. Chem. Biol. 2011;18:833–8.

124. Friedman AD, Claypool SE, Liu R. The smart targeting of nanoparticles. Curr. Pharm. Des. 2013;19:6315–29.

Biobetter Biologics

Alexandra Beumer Sassi[1], Radhika Nagarkar[2], Paul Hamblin[1]

[1]Biopharm R&D, GlaxoSmithKline, King of Prussia, PA, USA
[2]Biopharmaceutical Development, KBI Biopharma, Inc., Durham, NC, USA

INTRODUCTION

Biotherapeutics development has progressively increased in the past two decades.[1-3] This growth is driven by two main factors: (1) a significant benefit for patients due to highly selective medicines, and (2) a significant benefit for developers due to a high probability of success, multiple indication potential, extended revenue cycle, and significant financial returns. Despite this continued progress, the development of biopharmaceuticals is still characterized by high operating costs and lengthy timelines.

Recently, with several approved biotherapeutics coming off patent and continuing to do so in the next several years, a new market for biopharmaceutical products is being established. Investment growth in the development of follow-on biologics from both innovators and generic companies is being observed,[4] and these opportunities are becoming more and more attractive for competitors. For example, by as early as 2008, one company claimed to have developed a potential follow-on for Amgen's filgrastim, Neupogen® (approved for the treatment of neutropenia), for which the patent expired in December 2013. Market interest in follow-on biologics is also being stimulated by other products with patents that are anticipated to expire from 2013 to 2017, such as the monoclonal antibodies infliximab (Remicade®)

Novel Approaches and Strategies for Biologics, Vaccines and Cancer Therapies. DOI: 10.1016/B978-0-12-416603-5.00009-2

and adalimumab (Humira®).[4] Early on, developers considered the potential for abbreviated preclinical /clinical programs and reduced regulatory burden as significant advantages for follow-on biologics; however, the latter may not be true in all cases, as explained below.

The term *follow-on biologics* is widely used to include different biopharmaceutical categories such as biosimilars, biobetters, and next-generation biotherapeutics. Follow-on biologics are versions of the innovator drug succeeding its approval, usually manufactured and launched by a sponsor different from the innovator. Biosimilars (also known as biogenerics, or me-too biologics) have the same amino-acid sequence and molecular profile as the reference product. They also have no additional clinical advantage compared with the original drug.

Contrary to biosimilars, biobetters are designed to be improved versions of the innovator molecule with respect to price, patient convenience, product quality, safety, or efficacy. These improvements are achieved through purposeful modifications of the originator molecular profile. This chapter will focus on the development of such biobetters.

The term *biobetter* was popularized in the context of the Biologics Price Competition and Innovation Act (the Biosimilars Act), where the concept of biosimilars was formalized.[5] Modifications incorporated into biobetters may include molecular and functional changes impacting Fc interactions and glycosylation profiles to obtain a higher binding affinity, a longer half-life, or clinical result improvements. The modifications to the protein structure and potential changes in clinical outcomes are illustrated for a monoclonal antibody in Figure 9.1.

Definitions

The latest biotherapeutics entering the market have several optimized characteristics that improve upon the safety, efficacy, immunogenicity, and delivery of the first-generation drugs.[1,3,7–9] Among these innovative newer drugs, there are several classes such as biobetters, second- and third-generation monoclonal antibodies (mAbs), and next-generation therapeutics. Biobetters (also known as "biosuperiors" or "me better") are developed by changes in the molecular profile through chemical (e.g., PEGylation), molecular (e.g., amino acid substitutions), or functional changes that include, but are not limited to, increased half-life, reduced toxicity, reduced immunogenicity, and enhanced pharmacodynamic effects.[1] In this chapter, biobetters broadly refer to mAbs that may or may not have the same complement-determining region (CDR) as the first-generation molecule but are optimized with respect to their glycosylation profile and/or improved in their Fc functionality. Biobetters also encompass all biopharmaceutical molecular formats. On the process side, this class also encompasses manufacturing changes such as the change from a first-generation murine cell line to a commercial mammalian cell lines such as Chinese hamster ovary (CHO) cells to support high protein expression levels and generate biobetters with the improved posttranslational modifications. Overall, biobetters build upon the success of validated targets or pathways of drugs currently on the market. Table 9.1 contains a list of some of the biobetters molecules that have been recently approved or are under development.

Development Strategies

In general, development strategies such as stability enhancement, pharmacokinetic profile optimization, and improved safety of biopharmaceuticals fall into two major categories: (1)

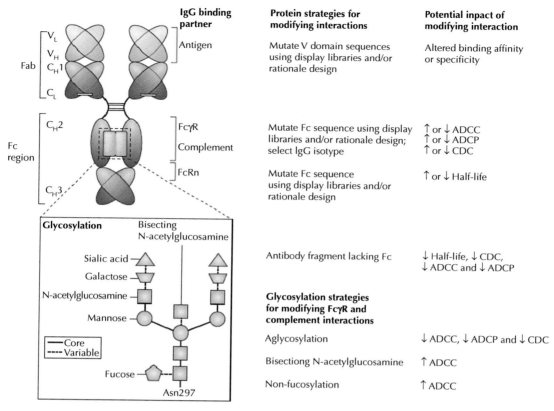

IgG binding partner	Protein strategies for modifying interactions	Potential inpact of modifying interaction
Antigen	Mutate V domain sequences using display libraries and/or rationale design	Altered binding affinity or specificity
FcγR / Complement	Mutate Fc sequence using display libraries and/or rationale design; select IgG isotype	↑ or ↓ ADCC ↑ or ↓ ADCP ↑ or ↓ CDC
FcRn	Mutate Fc sequence using display libraries and/or rationale design	↑ or ↓ Half-life
	Antibody fragment lacking Fc	↓ Half-life, ↓ CDC, ↓ ADCC and ↓ ADCP

Glycosylation strategies for modifying FcγR and complement interactions

Aglycosylation	↓ ADCC, ↓ ADCP and ↓ CDC
Bisectiong N-acetylglucosamine	↑ ADCC
Non-fucosylation	↑ ADCC

FIGURE 9.1 Engineering IgG structure and function. IgGs are approximately 150-kDa tetramers comprised of pairs of identical heavy and light chains linked by disulfide bonds (yellow bars). The heavy chains contain a variable domain (VH) and three constant domains (C_H1, C_H2 and C_H3), whereas the light chains contain a variable domain (VL) linked to a single constant domain (CL). A signature property of antibodies is highly selective antigen binding mediated by their variable domains. Human IgG, particularly IgG_1 and IgG_3, bound to an antigen on a target cell surface, can interact with Fc receptors for IgG (FcγRs) on effector cells and may support the destruction of target cells by antibody-dependent cell-mediated cytotoxicity (ADCC) or antibody-dependent cellular phagocytosis (ADCP), whereas interaction with the complement component C1q may support killing by complement-dependent cytotoxicity (CDC). Once in circulation, IgG antibodies can be taken up by vascular endothelial cells and other cells by pinocytosis. Subsequently, IgG can interact with the salvage receptor, neonatal FcR (FcRn), in a pH-dependent manner, with binding occurring in endosomes at pH 6.0 to 6.5, followed by recycling and release at the cell surface at pH 7.0 to 7.4. *Reprinted by permission from Macmillan Publishers Ltd: Nat. Rev. Immunol. Chan, A.C. and Carter, P.J. Therapeutic antibodies for autoimmunity and inflammation. 10(5): 301–16, copyright (2010).*

formulation approaches, and (2) protein engineering (molecule modifications). Formulation approaches have the advantage of modifying essential properties of the molecule without changing its mechanism of action. Thus, the application of purely formulation approaches can reduce the impact of development cycle time as well as the regulatory burden. One recent example is the new subcutaneous formulation of trastuzumab (Herceptin®, Genentech) that was approved by the European Commission in June 2013. Herceptin, first approved

TABLE 9.1   Preclinical, Clinical-Phase, and Approved Biobetter Molecules

Target/ Mechanism of Action	Originator (Trade Name/ Manufacturer)	Biobetter (Trade name/ Manufacturer)[a]	Current Phase	Indication	Notes
CD20	Rituximab (Rituzan®/ MabThera)	Afucosylated rituximab	Preclinical	Cancer therapy (not specific)	Two examples are rituximab GS4:0 aFuc hzIgG1, expressed in *Pichia pastoris*,[1] and BLX-300 expressed in a *Lemna* aquatic plant-based system.[10,11]
		Obinutuzumab	Granted breakthrough therapy designation by FDA, May 2013	Chronic lymphocytic leukemia and lymphoma (not approved)	Type II anti-CD20 IgG$_1$ antibody with reduced fucosylation[11,12]
CD80 and CD86	Abatacept (Orencia®/ Bristol-Myers Squibb)	Belatacept (Nulojix®/ Bristol-Myers Squibb)	Approved by FDA and EU in 2011	Kidney transplantation; graft rejection	Two amino acid substitutions (L104E and A29Y) to increase binding to both CD80 and CD86 and give rise to an overall 10-fold more potent inhibition of T-cell activation measured *in vitro* increased affinity to the target.[13,14]
Colony-stimulating factor	Filgrastim (Neupogen®/ Amgen)	Pegfilgrastim (Neulasta®/ Amgen)	Approved by FDA and EU in 2002	Chemotherapy-induced neutropenia	PEGylated filgrastim extends protein half-life.[13,14]
Depletion of plasma asparagine	L-Asparaginase	Pegaspargase (Oncaspar®/ Enzon Pharmaceuticals)	Approved by FDA in 1994	Acute lymphocytic leukemia for patients hypersensitive to L-asparaginase	PEGylated L-asparaginase, extends the protein half-life.[14]
Epidermal growth factor receptor (EGFR)	Cetuximab (Erbitux®/Eli Lilly)	Xtend™-EGFR, M428L/N434S	Preclinical	Not specified	Fc engineered, longer half-life[1]

Target	Protein	Product	Status	Indication	Description
Follicle-stimulating hormone (FSH) receptor	Human FSH	Corifollitropin alfa (Elonva®/Merck)	Approved by FDA in 2009 and by EU in 2010	Fertility treatment	Sustained follicle stimulant composed of the (subunit of human FSH and a hybrid (subunit formed by fusion of the human chorionic gonadotropin (subunit carboxy-terminal peptide with the (subunit of human FSH; increased half-life.[13-15]
HER2	Trastuzumab (Herceptin®/Genentech)	Modified trastuzumab	Phase III	Breast cancer	Subcutaneous formulation every 4 weeks[1,11]
		Afucosylated trastuzumab	Preclinical	Not specified	GFI5:0 aFuc hzIgG1 expressed in *Pichia pastoris*[1]
		Trastuzumab emtansine (Kadcyla®/Genentech)	Approved by FDA in 2013	HER2-positive metastatic breast cancer	Antibody–drug conjugate (ADC) comprised of trastuzumab linked to ImmunoGen's DM1 maytansinoid drug[11,12,14]
Human growth hormone receptor	Human growth hormone	Pegvisomant (Somavert®/Pfizer)	Approved by FDA in 2003 and by EU in 2001	Acromegaly	PEGylated growth hormone, extends the protein half-life[13,14]
Recombinant human growth hormone (rhGH)	Recombinant human growth hormone (rhGH)	rhGH fusion protein with XTEN (VRS-317)	Preclinical	Growth-hormone-deficient patients	Recombinant human growth hormone fusion protein with increased half-life[16]
Metabolizes uric acid to allantoin	Rasburicase	Pegloticase (Krystexxa®/Savient Pharmaceuticals)	Approved by FDA in 2010 and by EU in 2013	Refractory chronic gout	PEGylated recombinant porcine-like uricase extends protein half-life.[13,14]
Replaces adenosine deaminase	Adenosine deaminase	Pegademase bovine (Adagen®/Enzon Pharmaceuticals)	Approved by FDA in 1990	Severe combined immune deficiency (SCID)	PEGylated adenosine deamidase extends the protein half-life.[14]
Vascular endothelial growth factor A (VEGF-A)	Bevacizumab (Avastin®/Genentech)	Xtend™-VEGF, M428L/N434S	Preclinical	Not specified	Fc engineered, longer half-life[1]

[a] When available.

II. NOVEL APPROACHES FOR BIOLOGICS

in 1998 as targeted therapy for the treatment of human epidermal growth factor receptor 2 (HER2)-positive breast cancer was administered intravenously. The subcutaneous formulation employs technology developed by Halozyme Therapeutics involving the use of recombinant human hyaluronidase, which temporarily and reversibly degrades hyaluronan, enabling the 5-mL volume of the subcutaneous formulation of the drug to be rapidly dispersed and absorbed.[17] This represents a significant improvement in patient care. The approach of using recombinant human hyaluronidase in the formulation is also being investigated in clinical trials for other molecules such as rituximab and insulin.[11]

The use of hydrophilic polymers that would allow for a longer residence time *in situ*, potentially increasing the protein half-life, is another formulation approach being investigated at early stages of development.[18,19] Although such formulation approaches are still being explored to date, this is an emerging area and contributions to the field are still upcoming; therefore, trends in only molecule modification approaches for biobetter development are evaluated further in this chapter.

Within the biotherapeutics class, antibodies are the most abundant biologic commercially available. More than 25 antibodies have been approved for human therapy, and more than 240 are currently in clinical development.[6] Early monoclonal antibody therapies have delivered significant clinical values; however, the outcomes of these therapies still provide an opportunity for improvement. For example, in studies with rituximab, the first approved anti-CD20 chimeric monoclonal antibody for cancer treatment, only half of the patients showed clinical response.[20] In another Phase III clinical study with trastuzumab, median overall survival improved by only 5 months as compared with standard chemotherapy.[21]

There is a growing range of technologies available to support the identification and optimization of antibodies. The discovery of relevant human antibody targets has evolved from large phage display libraries to newer technologies, including yeast, ribosome, mRNA, mammalian, and *Escherichia coli* display libraries, as well as the direct cloning of human antibodies from human blood or bone marrow-derived cells.[6] The engineering and enhancement of antibody functions have been investigated as an alternative approach to overcome low efficacy or potential immunogenicity.[6] Such technologies may also enhance clinical potential via improvements in pharmacokinetics properties such as increased half-life. The availability of such well-established and broadly applicable technologies significantly enhances our ability to develop biobetter antibodies.[22] In summary, the opportunities for optimization of antibodies and potential development of biobetters rely on the growing range of technologies available to redesign antibodies to enhance their clinical potential via changes in pharmacokinetics and/or pharmacodynamics properties.

Regulatory Guidance

Currently, there are no specific regulatory guidances for biobetters. In the case of biosimilars, a sponsor may seek approval for a "biosimilar" product under the new section 351(k) of the Public Health Service (PHS) Act for the United States and under the guideline 437 from the Committee for Medicinal Products for Human use (CHMP) for the European Union. To demonstrate that a biological product is "biosimilar," the developer must provide data showing that the product is "highly similar" to the reference product. Despite any minor differences in clinically inactive components, there must be no clinically meaningful differences between the biological product and the reference product in terms of safety, purity, and potency.[23]

From a regulatory perspective, biobetters are assessed as new molecular entities and will be subject to the standards applied to all new drugs; however, biobetter programs may leverage innovator knowledge with respect to pharmacologic comparability, which may accelerate development timelines. The extent of differentiation from the innovator will impact the magnitude of data required for filing and the applicability of prior knowledge. Because there are no specific guidelines for biobetters, prospectively negotiating the required data package with regulators is critical.

Biobetter development is also considered attractive because the target biology has been "validated" through development of the innovator product, reducing the risk of development attrition from both business and clinical perspectives. The fact that biobetters are regulated as innovator products also enables the developer to derive benefit from patent protection and data exclusivity. New biologic entities are given data exclusivity of 12 years in the United States and 8 years in the European Union.[13] The main disadvantage is the time associated with following the regulatory pathway for submission of a new Biologic License Application (BLA) when compared to a biosimilar.[1] In addition, if the biologic has not come off patent, then the originator data available to sponsors are often sparse and difficult to obtain. From a commercial perspective, biobetters face a crowded marketplace where they must compete with the originator, biosimilars, and other biobetter products impacting product uptake and market share.

EMERGING TRENDS IN DEVELOPING BIOBETTER BIOLOGICS

New molecules emerging from optimization of an originator biopharmaceutical can sometimes be classified as second- and third-generation compounds. Second-generation therapeutics target the same antigen as the first-generation drug but possess an improved variable region. Improvements in the variable region can have several benefits, such as decreased immunogenicity. The earliest approved mAbs, such as Orthoclone OKT3, were murine antibodies that elicited an immune response and suffered from loss of efficacy due to formation of neutralizing antidrug antibodies. The shortcomings of murine antibodies were overcome by developing chimeric antibodies (e.g., infliximab) consisting of murine variable regions domains recombinantly fused to human constant domains.[24] Chimeric antibodies have further evolved into humanized and fully human second-generation drugs. These developments were made possible by the use of transgenic animals and *in vitro* protein engineering technologies such as phage display. Antibody engineering has also led to more efficacious second-generation therapeutics with affinity-matured CDRs that exhibit femtomolar dissociation constants to their target, more superior to those observed in a natural immune response.

Significant improvements in the pharmacokinetic (PK) profiles of protein drugs have been achieved via PEGylation and recombinant fusions with epitopes that increase the drug residence time in the body, thereby providing drugs that require infrequent dosing. Trends toward convenient subcutaneous delivery devices for patient self-administration have been made possible by high-concentration formulations of such efficacious second-generation mAbs. All of these improvements drastically change the structure and sequence of the mAb, yet target the same antigen as the first-generation drug; therefore, these alterations can be classified under second-generation therapeutics. Further enhancements in efficacy are attained by the use of non-native alternative drug formats such as antibody–drug conjugates and bispecific antibodies that simultaneously target multiple mechanisms associated with complex diseases.

Third-generation mAbs target a different epitope on the antigen or function through a different mechanism of action (MOA) with respect to the first-generation drug. Although, biobetters are the focus of this chapter, it is difficult to present the technological advances in biobetter development without discussing the other subclasses. The bulk of improvements in biobetter efficacy arise from alterations to the structure of the biologic. These structural modifications of biobetters as well as second-, third-, and next-generation biologic drugs are discussed in detail below.

Molecule Modification Approaches

Half-Life Improvement Using PEGylation and Recombinant Fusions

PEGYLATION

Covalent modification with a hydrophilic polymer such as polyethylene glycol (PEG) is a well-established protein engineering tool for enhancing the serum half-life of a drug. The circulatory half-life of a drug is governed by two major clearance pathways mediated by immune system recognition and by renal filtration. Of these, renal filtration forms an important mechanism of clearance wherein proteins smaller than 50 to 70 kDa easily pass through the kidneys simply by virtue of their small size.[25] The addition of a PEG chain dramatically increases the hydrodynamic size of the drug and thus excludes it from glomerular filtration. It is important to note that certain smaller proteins such as serum albumin (approximate MW 67 kDa) are retained by the kidneys due to electrostatic interactions with the negative charge on the glomerular membrane.[25] Some of the advantages of PEGylation include improved solubility, reduced aggregation propensity, decreased proteolytic degradation, and protection against exposure of immunogenic epitopes on the therapeutic protein.[26] One of the main disadvantages of pegylated therapeutics is a loss in bioactivity due to steric hindrance from the hydrated PEG chains in the target binding interface. This loss in biological activity can be minimized by applying site-specific PEGylation, controlling the degree of PEG branching, and monitoring the efficiency of the process.[25,27] PEG chains have been grafted on a wide array of molecules, including Fab' fragments (e.g., certolizumab pegol);[28,29] cytokines (e.g., IFN-γ2);[30,31] hormone analogs (e.g., pegvisomant);[32] enzymes (e.g., pegaspargase,[33] pegademase bovine[34]); peptides (e.g., GLP1,[35] pegloticase[36]); and aptamers (e.g., pegaptanib sodium.[37] The PEGylation of filgrastim and erythropoietin are discussed below.

PEGylation of filgrastim or granulocyte colony-stimulating factor (GCSF) has been successfully applied in both the biobetter and biosimilar arenas. GCSFs are growth factors used to treat neutropenia (loss of white blood cells) in patients undergoing chemotherapy. Because the presence of the PEG moiety reduces the renal clearance of pegfilgrastim, it is predominantly cleared through a self-regulating neutrophil-mediated mechanism dependent on the number of white blood cells. Thus, a single injection of the biobetter Neulasta® (pegfilgrastim) per chemotherapy cycle is as effective as the daily administration of Neupogen® (filgrastim).[38,39]

Erythropoietin (EPO), approved for clinical use since 1989, is a good example of applying PEGylation and glycoengineering (described below) to generate biobetters.[40–42] One of the best-studied and top-selling protein therapeutics, EPO is used in the treatment of anemia in oncology and chronic kidney disease. It contains approximately 40% of its weight in glycans (three N-linked and one O-linked). The naturally occurring glycans are mostly bianntenary, resulting in a short residence time in the body and frequent dosing. Of the current erythropoietins on the market, Epogen® and Arasnesp® are enriched during manufacturing for tetraantennary sialylated glycoforms to improve their *in vivo* metabolic stability.[43] Note that the second-generation drug Arasnesp has two additional glycosylation sites relative to Epogen. The pharmacokinetic improvement in a third-generation EPO called Mircera (methoxy polyethylene glycol-epoetin beta or continuous erythropoietin receptor activator) comes from conjugation of a PEG moiety on the N-terminal amino group or the α-amino group of largely Lys52 or Lys45. In these biobetters, the *in vitro* binding and potency are reduced relative to the unmodified molecule. The improvement in the *in vivo* efficacy arises from improved serum half-life.[41,44]

ALBUMIN FUSION

The long circulation time and unique properties of human serum albumin (HSA) are the reason for its successful application in PK improvement of small protein therapeutics. HSA, one of the most abundant proteins in blood, has a half-life of 19 days due to an FcRn mediated recycling, analogous to IgGs.[45] It also contains a single cysteine residue that is responsible for its antioxidant activity in blood. This antioxidant activity was also exploited by using HSA as an excipient in early formulations.[46,47] Due to these properties, recombinant albumin fusions of several therapeutics including insulin, human growth hormone, interferons, IL-2, Fab fragments, and single-chain variable fragments (scFv) have been explored. In addition to recombinant fusions, PK improvements can also be achieved by displaying epitopes capable of binding albumin *in vivo*. This covalent and noncovalent albumin binding for serum half-life enhancement can be demonstrated using glucagon-like peptide-1 (GLP-1) as an example. GLP1 peptide has been shown to help glycemic and body weight control in patients with type 2 diabetes;[48] however, it is not suitable for long-term use due to its poor *in vivo* stability associated with proteolytic degradation and renal clearance. To improve the half-life, an analog of GLP1 was made resistant to proteolysis by the enzyme DPP4. It was still subject to elimination by renal filtration. Different albumin binding strategies were further applied to GLP1 for PK improvement. Noncovalent binding of the GLP1 analog to plasma albumin was induced by attachment of a fatty acid chain in liraglutide. On the other hand, in albiglutide, two molecules of the GLP1 analog were covalently bound to HSA.[25] Albiglutide, a fusion of GLP1 analog to HSA, is a long-acting GLP1 receptor agonist compound currently in Phase III clinical development.[25] Albiglutide activates the receptor continuously at its recommended dose, enabling a pharmacokinetic profile that gives an important pharmacodynamic difference when compared to other GLP1 fusion proteins. Whereas short-acting GLP1 receptor agonists primarily lower postprandial blood glucose levels through inhibition of gastric emptying, the long-acting compounds such as albiglutide have a stronger effect on fasting glucose levels, which is mediated predominantly through their insulinotropic and glucagonostatic actions, making possible a better type 2 diabetes treatment.[48]

XTEN FUSION

To overcome the difficulties associated with the inherent polydispersity and conjugation of PEG to drugs, Schellenberger et al.[16,49-51] have designed hydrophilic polypeptides rich in glycine, glutamine, and serine that can be recombinantly expressed as a fusion to the therapeutic protein or peptide. The hydrophilic polypeptide constructs (XTEN) exhibit an extended unstructured conformation in solution that significantly increases the hydrodynamic radius of the fusion.[25,51] Similar to the PEG conjugates, improved prophylactic outcomes may arise from extended half-life of the drug in spite of reduced specific bioactivity determined *in vitro*.[50] This effect might be a useful characteristic for drugs where toxicity associated with peak dosing is a concern. Promising preclinical data for XTEN constructs with glucagon, GLP peptides, and growth hormone have been reported.[16,49-51]

CARBOXY-TERMINAL PEPTIDE FUSION

In contrast to the PEG and XTEN approaches to half-life extension, the carboxy-terminal peptide (CTP) fusion is a small naturally occurring peptide containing four *O*-glycosylation sites. CTP is contained within the protein human chorionic gonadotropin (hCG), a female hormone that helps maintain pregnancy. The CTP motif confers hCG with a significantly longer life-span compared to a second highly related hormone, luteinizing hormone (LH), which does not contain the CTP motif.[52] Due to the fact that the CTP sequence is naturally occurring, the motif has the potential to be non-immunogenic in humans when attached to other proteins.

The CTP technology has been successfully applied to follicle-stimulating hormone (FSH). Women who have fertility problems may get supplemental FSH to increase the likelihood of pregnancy. Previous formulations required daily FSH injections around the time of ovulation for seven days. The long-acting version of FSH is named corifollitropin alfa (FSH-CTP). A single injection of FSH-CTP achieved the same pregnancy rates as women receiving seven consecutive daily injections of FSH.[53] The broader application of the CTP technology is currently being investigated through a number of different therapeutic programs, including hGH, GLP1, Factor VIIa, and Factor IX.

Antibody–Drug Conjugates

Antibody–drug conjugates are non-native mAb formats classified as next-generation therapeutics in monoclonal antibody therapy. Their success can be attributed to their ability to combine two complementary approaches in cancer therapy.[54] In the first approach, the therapeutic such as a mAb functions in a targeted manner by binding to a specific antigen on the cancer cell, leading to a highly specific mechanism of action. For example, trastuzumab is specific for HER2-positive cells. However, this approach is not successful in certain heterogeneous tumors or in cases where, in response to the therapeutic, an alternate mechanism is upregulated that diminishes the result of the targeted therapy. In contrast, the second chemotherapy approach consists of a cytotoxic compound with low specificity to the target cell. The lack of specificity often reduces the therapeutic dose of the cytotoxic drug due to adverse events associated with its toxicity. By tagging the cytotoxic moiety onto a mAb, antibody–drug conjugates enable the targeted delivery of a highly toxic, nonspecific drug. One example is trastuzumab emtansine (Kadcyla®), an antibody–drug conjugate incorporating the HER2-targeted antitumor properties of trastuzumab with the cytotoxic activity of the microtubule-inhibitory agent DM1.[12,17] The details of the structure and components of antibody–drug conjugates are beyond the scope of this chapter and are reviewed elsewhere.[55]

Affinity Maturation

Affinity maturation is an important strategy in antibody optimization to generate safe and efficacious second-generation therapeutics.[56] Classically, therapeutic antibodies were obtained by immunizing mice or transgenic animals expressing human immunoglobulin genes with the desired antigen. Antigen-stimulated immune cells from these animals were transformed into hybridomas and subsequently screened to identify monoclonal antibodies with low nanomolar affinities for their target antigen. The development of efficacious antibodies with high specificity and affinity by *in vitro* affinity maturation is significant, as the possibility of smaller or infrequent dosing as well as the subsequent reduction in cost to the patient ensures a high success rate in the clinic. Note that, for certain solid tumor targets, high affinities are not desired because reduced therapeutic benefits are observed due to poor tumor penetration of the drug.[57] In addition to improvement in binding, specificity, and throughput associated with *in vitro* affinity maturation, limitations of immunogenicity linked to murine antibodies can also be overcome by selecting human single-domain or Fab fragments from non-immune combinatorial libraries using phase, yeast, or ribosome display technologies.[7,8,56,57]

Affinity maturation of palivizumab, the only approved monoclonal antibody for prophylaxis of respiratory syncytial virus (RSV), provides an interesting example. RSV is the leading cause of viral bronchiolitis and pneumonia in infants and children. Although palivizumab is effective in reducing hospitalizations resulting from RSV infection by 55% (compared to placebo), the development of a higher affinity antibody was expected to offer better prophylaxis. Initial attempts to generate a more potent version of palivizumab using a directed evolution approach yielded variants with 44-fold improved potency.[55] In subsequent *in vivo* studies, the same variants showed only a modest improvement in efficacy and a poor pharmacokinetic profile. These effects were attributed to a nonspecific binding profile. Further engineering was required to remove the nonspecific binding activity while retaining the improved potency.[58] The result was motavizumab (MEDI-524), an affinity-matured ultra-potent antibody that contains 13 amino-acid changes relative to palivizumab. Motavizumab has been compared head-to-head with palivizumab in Phase III clinical studies and was judged not to be inferior to palivizumab based on a 26% relative reduction in RSV hospitalizations compared with palivizumab.[59] However, skin reactions were higher in the motavizumab cohort compared to palivizumab, an observation that may have prompted MedImmune to discontinue development of motavizumab for the prophylaxis of RSV. Thus, improved antibody potency through affinity maturation may not guarantee improved clinical outcomes.

The success of affinity maturation can be demonstrated using the examples of abatacept and belatacept.[60–62] Both of these drugs were intended as immunosuppressants that target T-cell costimulation after organ transplantation. Abatacept is a fusion protein consisting of the extracellular domain of CTLA-4 recombinantly fused with the Fc of human IgG$_1$. CTLA-4 (CD152) is transiently expressed after T-cell activation and downregulates T-cell activation and proliferation by binding to CD80 and CD86 expressed by antigen-presenting cells.

Although abatacept is currently approved for treatment of rheumatoid arthritis, it was not very effective in inhibiting immune response in primate transplant models. This was shown to arise from the inability of abatacept to bind both CD80 and CD86 with high avidity. Abatacept inhibition of CD86 was 100-fold less as compared with CD80, and because CD80 and CD86 have overlapping function abatacept was ineffective in blocking T-cell activation. Using mutagenesis and surface plasmon resonance screening techniques, an affinity-matured molecule called belatacept was developed. Belatacept is derived from abatacept and contains two amino-acid substitutions (L104E and A29Y) to increase binding to both CD80 and CD86. Overall, belatacept displays tenfold more potent inhibition of T-cell activation relative to abatacept measured *in vitro*.

Thus, although affinity maturation can successfully yield optimized biobetter therapeutics with improved *in vitro* potency and the potential for enhanced efficacy, the case of palivizumab versus motavizumab provides a cautionary note.

Antibody Engineering

Fc receptors are a class of cell surface receptors that bind to the Fc portion of antibodies to form immune complexes and recruit the complement and/or effector system to defend the body against pathogens. Additionally, the neonatal receptor FcRn plays an important role in regulating the concentration of IgGs in the serum by a pH-dependent binding and recycling mechanism.[63] In this mechanism, IgGs in circulation are internalized by the cell wherein they bind FcRn in the slightly acidic (pH 6) environment of the endosome. The IgG–FcRn complex is protected from degradation and recycled back to the cell surface. Here, an increase in the pH to 7.4 results in the dissociation of the IgG–FcRn complex and releases the IgG back into circulation. Biobetter developers have utilized this FcRn-mediated control of IgG serum half-life to enhance the pharmacokinetic and clinical profile of mAbs.

Structurally, FcγR binds to the IgGs by making contacts within the C_H2 domains in the Fc region. Modifications of residues in this interface have been shown to diminish Fc binding. Moreover, glycosylation on Asn297 near this interface is also critical for FcR binding.[63] Glycosylation is one of the most important posttranslational modifications that can affect solubility, charge, folding, biological activity, and receptor function. Although the glycan can shield antigenic sequences to reduce immunogenicity, the presence of certain non-human carbohydrate moieties can induce an immune response.[64] Thus, glycoengineering is the modulation of biological activity by changing the structure and composition of the glycosylation profile of the mAb.

Better understanding of the biology of Fc receptors and the role of the glycan in Fc binding has resulted in the development of Fc- and glycoengineered biobetters with improved PK profile and precisely tuned effector functions. The application of these concepts in the modulation of antibody PK, target-mediated Ab clearance and antibody-dependent cell-mediated cytotoxicity (ADCC) is discussed below.

MODULATION OF ANTIBODY PHARMACOKINETICS

Improvements in the monoclonal antibody serum half-life through Fc engineering may lead to positive patient outcomes. A biobetter with these characteristics can allow for higher patient compliance by decreasing frequent dosing schedules. A number of groups have provided various molecular solutions to improve FcRn binding. Zalevsky and colleagues[65] demonstrated that increasing antibody (Fc-engineered cetuximab and bevacizumab) affinity to FcRn can be achieved using a double amino-acid change in the Fc region (M428L/N434S). Improved FcRn binding promotes half-life extension in cynomologus monkeys, translating into greater *in vivo* efficacy. Dall'Acqua and colleagues previously identified three residues in the Fc region that confer improved FcRn binding and prolonged serum half-life properties.[66,67] It is, however, critical to establish that Fc engineering will translate into improved convenience or superior exposure-dependent efficacy.

In a study conducted by Oganesavan et al.,[68] the effect of introducing the residues YTE (Fc/YTE) in a human Fc fragment on its interaction with the FcRn was investigated using x-ray crystallography. It is uncertain if the structural features observed in the fragment would occur in the full antibody; however, the results showed that Fc/YTE exhibited about an eight-fold increase in its binding to human FcRn at pH 6.0 when compared with its unmodified counterpart. One disadvantage of this approach is that the increase in binding affinity can decrease the stability of the mAb by destabilizing the C_H2 domain, as observed by a decrease in the melting temperature. Recent work has shown a novel Fc engineering approach that introduces different substitutions in each Fc domain asymmetrically, thus conferring optimal binding to FcγR with specificity, without compromising stability.[69] Although these studies have only been conducted *in vitro*, these novel Fc engineering approaches offer a great potential for biobetter development. The recent publication of the results of Phase I clinical studies incorporating the YTE technology into the anti-RSV antibody (MEDI-557) provides the first clinical data confirming that the preclinical models are predictive of pharmacokinetics in humans.[14]

MODULATION OF TARGET-MEDIATED DISPOSITION

For monoclonal antibodies where target-mediated clearance is a key factor in determining the serum half-life, Fc technologies that improve FcRn binding may have only a modest benefit. Igawa and coworkers[70] have taken a different approach to extending the half-life of tocilizumab (Actemra®). Tocilizumab inhibits the IL-6 receptor (IL-6R) and is subject to rapid target-mediated clearance, which drives a relatively frequent dosing interval. To reduce target-mediated clearance, they engineered tocilizumab to rapidly dissociate from IL-6R in the acidic environment of the endosome (pH 6), thus allowing the antibody to be recycled to the plasma. A Phase I study comparing tocilizumab with the engineered variant (SA237) has confirmed that SA237 has an improved pharmacokinetic/pharmacodynamic profile. Other groups have gone on to show the broader application of this technology to other antibodies predisposed to target-mediated clearance.[71]

Although anti-epidermal growth factor receptor (EGFR) antibodies have become clinically validated and commercially successful, they suffer from target-mediated clearance and skin reactions as a result of widespread expression of EGFR. One strategy to limit the widespread binding of EGFR antibodies is to mask the antibody with a short peptide sequence such that the antibody remains inert in healthy tissue.[72] Unmasking occurs in the tumor microenvironment, where increased protease activity clips off a short peptide sequence designed to block the antibody–target interaction. Although it is relatively early in the development of this approach, the results from preclinical models and *in vitro* studies with the masked EGFR antibodies look encouraging.

MODULATION OF ADCC AND GLYCOENGINEERING

Adaptive immunity involves the engagement of effector functions mediated through the binding of the Fc portion of the antibody–antigen complex to activating and inhibitory Fcγ receptors on immune cells, such as natural killer (NK) cells.[73,74] ADCC, one of these effector functions, is modulated in part through the activating Fc receptor FcγIIIa, which is expressed on NK cells.[74] Crystal structures of the Fc portion of human IgG and FcγIIIa reveal that, in addition to protein–protein contacts, there are also significant interactions between the carbohydrate on the IgG and the Fcγ receptor.[75] Therefore, the composition of the N-linked glycosylation on Asn297 in the Fc region of IgGs is thought to govern binding affinity to Fcγ receptors and in turn the degree of ADCC induced by the IgG.[76] The glycan structure of human IgGs consists of a complex heptapolysaccharide composed of N-acetyl glucosamine (GlcNAc) and mannose, with variable numbers of fucose, galactose, bisecting GlcNAc residues, and sialic acids.[75,77] The major human glycans containing a core fucose moiety with zero, one, or two terminal galactose residues are referred to as G_0, G_1, and G_2, respectively. Complex oligosaccharides without core fucosylation and high mannose structure also occur naturally to a smaller extent. Because the posttranslation modification machinery varies among bacteria, plant, yeast, and mammalian cells, early antibody development focused on matching the glycan composition of the recombinant antibodies produced in host cell lines with those found in naturally occurring human IgGs. The GlycoFi technology (Merck) utilized to generate a human IgG glycan in a *Pichia* cell line is an excellent example.[74] Thus, the ability to precisely tune the glycan composition has enabled biobetter developers to modulate biological function via the enhancement or abrogation of ADCC, thereby improving the therapeutic efficacy of mAbs. This field of work is broadly referred to as glycoengineering.

Different IgG glycoforms vary in their ability to induce ADCC. For example, reduced core fucosylation dramatically increases IgG binding to the receptor FcγIIIa and increases ADCC. Afucosylation has been achieved through the use of fucosyltransferase knockout cell lines as well as the coexpression of fucosyltransferase-interfering RNA in host plant and CHO cells.[78] The structural basis for the high ADCC observed for afucosylated mAbs is that the fucose at Asn297 blocks the interaction of the carbohydrate at Asn162 on FcγIIIa with IgG_1.[75] Afucosylated mAbs thus exhibit higher affinity, selectively for FcγIIIa and FcγIIIb, as the other Fcγ receptors are not glycosylated at that location. Although afucosylation does not alter the affinity for FcRn, changes in the glycan composition may affect clearance through non-target-mediated mechanisms.[79] These glycoengineering concepts were applied in obinutuzumab (GA101, Roche), an anti-CD20 glycoengineered mAb with promising Phase III clinical results compared to rituximab (Rituxan®, MabThera). Obinutuzumab is a type II anti-CD20 third-generation antibody for two reasons.[80] First, it has been glycoengineered to contain a non-fucosylated glycan.[77] Additional ADCC improvement in GA101 is also achieved through the presence of a bisecting GlcNAc. As a result, unlike type I CD20 antibodies such as rituximab, obinutuzumab strongly induces ADCC but does not induce CDC. Second, it recognizes an overlapping epitope and binds to CD20 in a different orientation relative to type I CD20 antibodies.[81] Thus, the GlycoMab technology (Roche/GlycArt) uses bisecting, non-fucosylated glycans to achieve a 10- to 10,000-fold enhancement in ADCC relative to the unmodified mAb. Another biobetter being developed using the GlycoMab technology is GA201,[82,83] which is also glycoengineered to contain bisected, afucosylated carbohydrate variants. GA201 is an anti-EGFR recombinant humanized IgG$_1$ that exhibits enhanced ADCC relative to anti-EGFR monoclonal antibodies, such as cetuximab (Erbitux®) and panitumumab (Vectibix®), for the treatment of certain cancers.[82] however, Roche recently discontinued the development of GA201.

Enhancing ADCC activity by modifying the amino-acid sequence of the Fc domain has been extensively studied. Mutations in the Fc domain (such as S298A, E333A, K334A, F243L, R292P, Y300L, V305I, and P396L) have been shown to improve binding to FcγRIIIa and enhance capacity for ADCC *in vitro* and in some limited studies *in vivo*.[22] However, it is still not known whether the improvement of effector functions observed in preclinical studies will be accurately reflected in patients due to the lack of appropriate animal models.

Although enhancement of Fc function is commonly used for improvement of antitumor activity in monoclonal antibodies through ADCC, binding to the Fcγ receptor can be blocked when it is therapeutically beneficial such as in autoimmune or inflammatory diseases (e.g., rheumatoid arthritis and lupus).[63] Removal of the glycan (i.e., aglycosylation of the monoclonal antibodies) may be used to modulate ADCC.[77] Aglycosylation is thought to result in loss of ADCC but enhanced complement-dependent cytotoxicity (CDC) due to a compaction of structure in the Fc region.[84]

Glycoengineering is also being used to improve the ADCC activity of other clinically validated cancer immunotherapeutics. TrasGEX™ and CetuGEX™ (Glycotope) are ADCC-enhanced version of trastuzumab and cetuximab, respectively, and are currently in the early stages of clinical development. In summary, glycoengineering has been shown to be a powerful tool to tune the cytotoxic activity of mAbs.

MANUFACTURING PROCESS IMPROVEMENTS

In the case of biosimilars, manufacturing presents one of the biggest obstacles for developers, because small differences in cell line, production methods, and purification steps can alter the final protein structure as well as its activity and safety. For biobetters, changes in the manufacturing process do not automatically impose an unplanned alteration of the final protein structure. As an example, Xyntha®, a recombinant B-domain-deleted coagulation factor VIII, is being manufactured with a few changes in the process when compared to the originator molecule. The same CHO cell line is used for the originator and biobetter manufacture; however, details of both upstream and downstream processing have been revised. The primary manufacturing alterations include the use of a chemically defined culture medium containing recombinant insulin, the replacement of an immunoaffinity purification step with an affinity step dependent upon a synthetic ligand, and the introduction of a nanofiltration step. These changes have been made to reduce the risk of viral contamination and represent an improvement in safety in the biobetter process when compared to the originator.[85]

Posttranslational processing (such as glycosylation) also impacts the outcome of the biopharmaceutical during manufacturing process. Glycosylation variation, as previously discussed, can alter *in vivo* functions and stability. Biobetter molecules obtained by the manipulation of oligosaccharide structure via the overexpression of appropriate glycosyltransferases possess enhanced glycan quality, leading to improved ADCC and CDC functions.[86]

CONCLUSIONS

Significant improvements have been made in the development of biologics, leading to safer molecules with greater efficacy and allowing for better patient compliance. Although some of the technological advances have been implemented more than 20 years ago (e.g., pegademase bovine), the term biobetter is new and has been around for only a few years; it defines biopharmaceutical molecules that are developed by changes in the molecular profile through chemical, molecular, or functional changes. These changes add considerable enhancements to the modified biologic that include, but are not limited to, increased half-life, reduced toxicity, reduced immunogenicity, and enhanced pharmacodynamic effects. It is worth noting that, although some biobetter technologies are very mature (e.g., PEGylation, CTP fusion) and have yielded commercially successfully next-generation molecules, others are only in the early stages of preclinical or clinical development (e.g., YTE, XTEN).

There is some controversy within the biopharmaceutical field regarding the exact definition of biobetters. In some instances, the term is more broadly defined and covers second- and third-generation molecules. This chapter focused on the most common development strategies that have been made to an originator molecule and have truly showed an improvement in that molecule. Such modification approaches include PEGylation, recombinant fusions, antibody–drug conjugate, affinity maturation, and antibody engineering. Despite the differences in defining biobetters, it is clear that several advances are being made in biological discovery, optimization, and formulation.

Acknowledgments

The authors would like to thank Dr. Roxana Ivanescu, Dr. Rick Caimi, and Dr. Andrew Hagarman for critical review of this manuscript and for their insightful suggestions.

References

1. Beck A. Biosimilar, biobetter and next generation therapeutic antibodies. MAbs. 2011;3(2):107–10.
2. Beck A, Wurch T, Bailly C, Corvaia N. Strategies and challenges for the next generation of therapeutic antibodies. Nat. Rev. Immunol. 2010;10(5):345–52.
3. Carter PJ. Introduction to current and future protein therapeutics: a protein engineering perspective. Exp. Cell Res. 2011;317(9):1261–9.
4. Hughes B. Gearing up for follow-on biologics. Nat. Rev. Drug Discov. 2009;8(3):181.
5. USFDA. Title VII—Improving Access to Innovative Medical Therapies, Subtitle A—Biologics Price Competition and Innovation. Washington, DC: U.S. Food and Drug Administration, 2009.
6. Chan AC, Carter PJ. Therapeutic antibodies for autoimmunity and inflammation. Nat. Rev. Immunol. 2010;10(5):301–16.
7. Campbell J, Lowe D, Sleeman MA. Developing the next generation of monoclonal antibodies for the treatment of rheumatoid arthritis. Br. J. Pharmacol. 2011;162(7):1470–84.
8. Carter PJ. Potent antibody therapeutics by design. Nat. Rev. Immunol. 2006;6(5):343–57.
9. Beck A, Sanglier-Cianferani S, Van Dorsselaer A. Biosimilar, biobetter, and next generation antibody characterization by mass spectrometry. Anal. Chem. 2012;84(11):4637–46.
10. Gasdaska JR, Sherwood S, Regan JT, Dickey LF. An afucosylated anti-CD20 monoclonal antibody with greater antibody-dependent cellular cytotoxicity and B-cell depletion and lower complement-dependent cytotoxicity than rituximab. Mol. Immunol. 2012;50(3):134–41.
11. U.S. National Institutes of Health, www.clinicaltrials.gov.
12. Reichert JM. Antibodies to watch in 2013: mid-year update. MAbs. 2013;5(4):513–7.

13. European Medicines Agency, http://www.ema.europa.eu/ema/.
14. Robbie GJ, Criste R, Dall'Acqua WF, Jensen K, Patel NK, Losonsky GA, et al. A novel investigational Fc-modified humanized monoclonal antibody, motavizumab-YTE, has an extended half-life in healthy adults. Antimicrob. Agents Chemother. 2013;57(12):6147–53.
15. Verbost P, Sloot WN, Rose UM, de Leeuw R, Hanssen RG, Verheijden GF. Pharmacologic profiling of corifollitropin alfa, the first developed sustained follicle stimulant. Eur. J. Pharmacol. 2010;651(1-3):227–33.
16. Cleland JL, Geething NC, Moore JA, Rogers BC, Spink BJ, Wang CW, et al. A novel long-acting human growth hormone fusion protein (vrs-317): enhanced *in vivo* potency and half-life. J. Pharm. Sci. 2012;101(8):2744–54.
17. Launay-Vacher V. An appraisal of subcutaneous trastuzumab: a new formulation meeting clinical needs. Cancer Chemother. Pharmacol. 2013;72(6):1361–7.
18. Walsh S, Kokai-Kun J, Shah A, Mond J. Extended nasal residence time of lysostaphin and an anti-staphylococcal monoclonal antibody by delivery in semisolid or polymeric carriers. Pharm. Res. 2004;21(10):1770–5.
19. Chan YP, Meyrueix R, Kravtzoff R, Nicolas F, Lundstrom K. Review on Medusa: a polymer-based sustained release technology for protein and peptide drugs. Expert Opin. Drug Deliv. 2007;4(4):441–51.
20. McLaughlin P, Grillo-Lopez AJ, Link BK, Levy R, Czuczman MS, Williams ME, et al. Rituximab chimeric anti-CD20 monoclonal antibody therapy for relapsed indolent lymphoma: half of patients respond to a four-dose treatment program. J. Clin. Oncol. 1998;16(8):2825–33.
21. Slamon DJ, Leyland-Jones B, Shak S, Fuchs H, Paton V, Bajamonde A, et al. Use of chemotherapy plus a monoclonal antibody against HER2 for metastatic breast cancer that overexpresses HER2. N. Engl. J. Med. 2001;344(11):783–92.
22. Kubota T, Niwa R, Satoh M, Akinaga S, Shitara K, Hanai N. Engineered therapeutic antibodies with improved effector functions. Cancer Sci. 2009;100(9):1566–72.
23. USFDA. Implementation of the Biologics Price Competition and Innovation Act of 2009. Washington, DC: U.S. Food and Drug Administration; 2011. (http://www.fda.gov/Drugs/GuidanceComplianceRegulatoryInformation/ucm215089.htm).
24. Knight DM, Trinh H, Le J, Siegel S, Shealy D, McDonough M, et al. Construction and initial characterization of a mouse–human chimeric anti-TNF antibody. Mol. Immunol. 1993;30(16):1443–53.
25. Kontos S, Hubbell JA. Drug development: longer-lived proteins. Chem. Soc. Rev. 2012;41(7):2686–95.
26. Piedmonte DM, Treuheit MJ. Formulation of Neulasta® (pegfilgrastim). Adv. Drug Deliv. Rev. 2008;60(1):50–8.
27. Jevsevar S, Kunstelj M, Porekar VG. PEGylation of therapeutic proteins. Biotechnol. J. 2010;5(1):113–28.
28. van Schouwenburg PA, Rispens T, Wolbink GJ. Immunogenicity of anti-TNF biologic therapies for rheumatoid arthritis. Nat. Rev. Rheumatol. 2013;9(3):164–72.
29. Nesbitt A, Fossati G, Bergin M, Stephens P, Stephens S, Foulkes R, et al. Mechanism of action of certolizumab pegol (CDP870): *in vitro* comparison with other anti-tumor necrosis factor alpha agents. Inflamm. Bowel Dis. 2007;13(11):1323–32.
30. Fried MW, Shiffman ML, Reddy KR, Smith C, Marinos G, Goncales FL, et al. Peginterferon alfa-2a plus ribavirin for chronic hepatitis C virus infection. N. Engl. J. Med. 2002;347(13):975–82.
31. Manns MP, McHutchison JG, Gordon SC, Rustgi VK, Shiffman M, Reindollar R, et al. Peginterferon alfa-2b plus ribavirin compared with interferon alfa-2b plus ribavirin for initial treatment of chronic hepatitis C: a randomised trial. Lancet 2001;358(9286):958–65.
32. van der Lely AJ, Hutson RK, Trainer PJ, Besser GM, Barkan AL, Katznelson L, et al. Long-term treatment of acromegaly with pegvisomant, a growth hormone receptor antagonist. Lancet 2001;358(9295):1754–9.
33. Willer A, Gerss J, Konig T, Franke D, Kuhnel HJ, Henze G, et al. Anti-*Escherichia coli* asparaginase antibody levels determine the activity of second-line treatment with pegylated *E. coli* asparaginase: a retrospective analysis within the ALL-BFM trials. Blood 2011;118(22):5774–82.
34. Bax BE, Bain MD, Fairbanks LD, Webster ADB, Chalmers RA. *In vitro* and *in vivo* studies with human carrier erythrocytes loaded with polyethylene glycol-conjugated and native adenosine deaminase. Br. J. Haematol. 2000;109(3):549–54.
35. Lee SH, Lee S, Youn YS, Na DH, Chae SY, Byun Y, et al. Synthesis, characterization, and pharmacokinetic studies of PEGylated glucagon-like peptide-1. Bioconjug. Chem. 2005;16(2):377–82.
36. Terkeltaub R. Update on gout: new therapeutic strategies and options. Nat. Rev. Rheumatol. 2010;6(1):30–8.
37. Ng EWM, Shima DT, Calias P, Cunningham ET, Guyer DR, Adamis AP. Pegaptanib, a targeted anti-VEGF aptamer for ocular vascular disease. Nat. Rev. Drug Discov. 2006;5(2):123–32.

38. Renwick W, Pettengell R, Green M. Use of filgrastim and pegfilgrastim to support delivery of chemotherapy twenty years of clinical experience. Biodrugs 2009;23(3):175–86.

39. Zhai YQ, Zhao YJ, Lei JD, Su ZG, Ma GH. Enhanced circulation half-life of site-specific PEGylated rhG-CSF: optimization of PEG molecular weight. J. Biotechnol. 2009;142(3-4):259–66.

40. Nett JH, Gomathinayagam S, Hamilton SR, Gong B, Davidson RC, Du M, et al. Optimization of erythropoietin production with controlled glycosylation-PEGylated erythropoietin produced in glycoengineered *Pichia pastoris*. J. Biotechnol. 2012;157(1):198–206.

41. Liu LM, Li HJ, Hamilton SR, Gomathinayagam S, Rayfield WJ, Van Maanen M, et al. The impact of sialic acids on the pharmacokinetics of a PEGylated erythropoietin. J. Pharm. Sci. 2012;101(12):4414–8.

42. Reichel C. Recent developments in doping testing for erythropoietin. Anal. Bioanal. Chem. 2011;401(2):463–81.

43. Macdougall IC, Padhi D, Jang G. Pharmacology of darbepoetin alfa. Nephrol. Dial. Transplant. 2007;22:2–9.

44. Kiss Z, Elliott S, Jedynasty K, Tesar V, Szegedi J. Discovery and basic pharmacology of erythropoiesis-stimulating agents (ESAs), including the hyperglycosylated ESA, darbepoetin alfa: an update of the rationale and clinical impact. Eur. J. Clin. Pharmacol. 2010;66(4):331–40.

45. Muller D, Karle A, Meibburger B, Hofig I, Stork R, Kontermann RE. Improved pharmacokinetics of recombinant bispecific antibody molecules by fusion to human serum albumin. J. Biol. Chem. 2007;282(17):12650–60.

46. Park SS, Park J, Ko J, Chen L, Meriage D, Crouse-Zeineddini J, et al. Biochemical assessment of erythropoietin products from Asia versus US epoetin alfa manufactured by Amgen. J. Pharm. Sci. 2009;98(5):1688–99.

47. Taguchi K, Victor TGC, Maruyama T, Otagiri M. Pharmaceutical aspects of the recombinant human serum albumin dimer: structural characteristics, biological properties, and medical applications. J. Pharm. Sci. 2012;101(9):3033–46.

48. Meier JJ. GLP-1 receptor agonists for individualized treatment of type 2 diabetes mellitus. Nat. Rev. Endocrinol. 2012;8(12):728–42.

49. Alters SE, McLaughlin B, Spink B, Lachinyan T, Wang CW, Podust V, et al. GLP2-2G-XTEN: a pharmaceutical protein with improved serum half-life and efficacy in a rat Crohn's disease model. PLoS ONE. 2012;7(11):e50630.

50. Geething NC, To W, Spink BJ, Scholle MD, Wang CW, Yin Y, et al. Gcg-XTEN: an improved glucagon capable of preventing hypoglycemia without increasing baseline blood glucose. PLoS ONE. 2010;5(4):e10175.

51. Schellenberger V, Wang CW, Geething NC, Spink BJ, Campbell A, To W, et al. A recombinant polypeptide extends the *in vivo* half-life of peptides and proteins in a tunable manner. Nat. Biotechnol. 2009;27(12):1186–90.

52. Fares FA, Levi F, Reznick AZ, Kraiem Z. Engineering a potential antagonist of human thyrotropin and thyroid-stimulating antibody. J. Biol. Chem. 2001;276(7):4543–8.

53. Devroey P, Boostanfar R, Koper NP, Mannaerts BM, Ijzerman-Boon PC, Fauser BC. A double-blind, non-inferiority RCT comparing corifollitropin alfa and recombinant FSH during the first seven days of ovarian stimulation using a GnRH antagonist protocol. Hum. Reprod. 2009;24(12):3063–72.

54. Flygare JA, Pillow TH, Aristoff P. Antibody–drug conjugates for the treatment of cancer. Chem. Biol. Drug Des. 2013;81(1):113–21.

55. Wu AM, Senter PD. Arming antibodies: prospects and challenges for immunoconjugates. Nat. Biotechnol. 2005;23(9):1137–46.

56. Schier R, Bye J, Apell G, McCall A, Adams GP, Malmqvist M, et al. Isolation of high-affinity monomeric human anti-c-erbB-2 single chain Fv using affinity-driven selection. J. Mol. Biol. 1996;255(1):28–43.

57. Dufner P, Jermutus L, Minter RR. Harnessing phage and ribosome display for antibody optimisation. Trends Biotechnol. 2006;24(11):523–9.

58. Wu H, Pfarr DS, Johnson S, Brewah YA, Woods RM, Patel NK, et al. Development of motavizumab, an ultra-potent antibody for the prevention of respiratory syncytial virus infection in the upper and lower respiratory tract. J. Mol. Biol. 2007;368(3):652–65.

59. Carbonell-Estrany X, Simoes EA, Dagan R, Hall CB, Harris B, Hultquist M, et al. Motavizumab for prophylaxis of respiratory syncytial virus in high-risk children: a noninferiority trial. Pediatrics 2009;125(1):e35–51.

60. Larsen CP, Pearson TC, Adams AB, Tso P, Shirasugi N, Strobert E, et al. Rational development of LEA29Y (belatacept), a high-affinity variant of CTLA4-lg with potent immunosuppressive properties. Am. J. Transplant. 2005;5(3):443–53.

61. Vincenti F, Charpentier B, Vanrenterghem Y, Rostaing L, Bresnahan B, Darji P, et al. A Phase III study of belatacept-based immunosuppression regimens versus cyclosporine in renal transplant recipients (BENEFIT study). Am. J. Transplant. 2010;10(3):535–46.

62. Vincenti F, Larsen C, Durrbach A, Wekerle T, Nashan B, Blancho G, et al. Costimulation blockade with belatacept in renal transplantation. New Engl. J. Med. 2005;353(8):770–81.

63. Hogarth PM, Pietersz GA. Fc receptor-targeted therapies for the treatment of inflammation, cancer and beyond. Nat. Rev. Drug Discov. 2012;11(4):311–31.

64. van Beers MMC, Bardor M. Minimizing immunogenicity of biopharmaceuticals by controlling critical quality attributes of proteins. Biotechnol. J. 2012;7(12):1473–84.

65. Zalevsky J, Chamberlain AK, Horton HM, Karki S, Leung IW, Sproule TJ, et al. Enhanced antibody half-life improves *in vivo* activity. Nat Biotechnol. 2010;28(2):157–9.

66. Dall'Acqua WF, Kiener PA, Wu H. Properties of human IgG$_1$s engineered for enhanced binding to the neonatal Fc receptor (FcRn). J. Biol. Chem. 2006;281(33):23514–24.

67. Dall'Acqua WF, Woods RM, Ward ES, Palaszynski SR, Patel NK, Brewah YA, et al. Increasing the affinity of a human IgG$_1$ for the neonatal Fc receptor: biological consequences. J. Immunol. 2002;169(9):5171–80.

68. Oganesyan V, Damschroder MM, Woods RM, Cook KE, Wu H, Dall'Acqua WF. Structural characterization of a human Fc fragment engineered for extended serum half-life. Mol. Immunol. 2009;46(8-9):1750–5.

69. Mimoto F, Igawa T, Kuramochi T, Katada H, Kadono S, Kamikawa T, et al. Novel asymmetrically engineered antibody Fc variant with superior FcgammaR binding affinity and specificity compared with afucosylated Fc variant. MAbs. 2013;5(2):229–36.

70. Igawa T, Tsunoda H, Tachibana T, Maeda A, Mimoto F, Moriyama C, et al. Reduced elimination of IgG antibodies by engineering the variable region. Protein Eng. Des. Sel. 2010;23(5):385–92.

71. Chaparro-Riggers J, Liang H, DeVay RM, Bai L, Sutton JE, Chen W, et al. Increasing serum half-life and extending cholesterol lowering *in vivo* by engineering antibody with pH-sensitive binding to PCSK9. J. Biol. Chem. 2012;287(14):11090–7.

72. Erster O, Thomas JM, Hamzah J, Jabaiah AM, Getz JA, Schoep TD, et al. Site-specific targeting of antibody activity *in vivo* mediated by disease-associated proteases. J. Control Rel. 2012;161(3):804–12.

73. Sazinsky SL, Ott RG, Silver NW, Tidor B, Ravetch JV, Wittrup KD. Aglycosylated immunoglobulin G(1) variants productively engage activating Fc receptors. Proc. Natl. Acad. Sci. U.S.A. 2008;105(51):20167–72.

74. Li HJ, Sethuraman N, Stadheim TA, Zha DX, Prinz B, Ballew N, et al. Optimization of humanized IgGs in glycoengineered *Pichia pastoris*. Nat. Biotechnol. 2006;24(2):210–5.

75. Ferrara C, Grau S, Jager C, Sondermann P, Brunker P, Waldhauer I, et al. Unique carbohydrate-carbohydrate interactions are required for high affinity binding between Fc gamma RIII and antibodies lacking core fucose. Proc. Natl. Acad. Sci. U.S.A. 2011;108(31):12669–74.

76. Yu XJ, Baruah K, Harvey DJ, Vasiljevic S, Alonzi DS, Song BD, et al. Engineering hydrophobic protein–carbohydrate interactions to fine-tune monoclonal antibodies. J. Am. Chem. Soc. 2013;135(26):9723–32.

77. Hristodorov D, Fischer R, Linden L. With or without sugar? (A)glycosylation of therapeutic antibodies. Mol. Biotechnol. 2013;54(3):1056–68.

78. Shen Y, Liu HC. Methods to determine the level of afucosylation in recombinant monoclonal antibodies. Anal. Chem. 2010;82(23):9871–7.

79. Junttila TT, Parsons K, Olsson C, Lu YM, Xin Y, Theriault J, et al. Superior *in vivo* efficacy of afucosylated trastuzumab in the treatment of HER2-amplified breast cancer. Cancer Res. 2010;70(11):4481–9.

80. Robak T, Robak E. New anti-CD20 monoclonal antibodies for the treatment of B-cell lymphoid malignancies. Biodrugs. 2011;25(1):13–25.

81. van Oers MHJ. CD20 antibodies: type II to tango? Blood 2012;119(22):5061–3.

82. Gerdes CA, Nicolini VG, Herter S, van Puijenbroek E, Lang S, Roemmele M, et al. GA201 (RG7160): a novel, humanized, glycoengineered anti-EGFR antibody with enhanced ADCC and superior *in vivo* efficacy compared with cetuximab. Clin. Cancer Res. 2013;19(5):1126–38.

83. Paz-Ares LG, Gomez-Roca C, Delord JP, Cervantes A, Markman B, Corral J, et al. Phase I pharmacokinetic and pharmacodynamic dose-escalation study of RG7160 (GA201), the first glycoengineered monoclonal antibody against the epidermal growth factor receptor, in patients with advanced solid tumors. J. Clin. Oncol. 2011;29(28):3783–90.

84. Hale G, Rebello P, Al Bakir I, Bolam E, Wiczling P, Jusko WJ, et al. Pharmacokinetics and antibody responses to the CD3 antibody otelixizumab used in the treatment of type 1 diabetes. J. Clin. Pharmacol. 2010;50(11):1238–48.

85. Walsh G. Biopharmaceutical benchmarks 2010. Nat. Biotechnol. 2010;28(9):917–24.

86. Rita Costa A, Elisa Rodrigues M, Henriques M, Azeredo J, Oliveira R. Guidelines to cell engineering for monoclonal antibody production. Eur. J. Pharm. Biopharm. 2009;74(2):127–38.

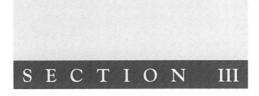

Vaccines Against Non-Infectious, Non-Cancer Novel Targets

Deborah A. Garside[1], Reinaldo Acevedo[2], Manal Alsaadi[3],
Natalie Nimmo[4], Ayman Gebril[4], Dimitrios Lamprou[4],
Alexander B. Mullen[4], Valerie A. Ferro[4]

[1]Imperial College London, Faculty of Medicine, London, UK
[2]Research and Development vice-presidency of Finlay Institute, Havana, Cuba
[3]University of Tripoli, Faculty of Pharmacy, Tripoli, Libya
[4]University of Strathclyde, Strathclyde Institute of Pharmacy and Biomedical Science, Glasgow, UK

OUTLINE

Novel Approaches and Strategies for Biologics, Vaccines and Cancer Therapies. DOI: 10.1016/B978-0-12-416603-5.00010-9

OVERVIEW OF NON-INFECTIOUS, NON-CANCER VACCINE TARGETS

Vaccines have had a major role in preventative medicine and in controlling and even eradicating many infectious diseases caused mainly by bacterial and viral pathogens.[1] Protection provided by vaccination against these diseases has generally been due to production of antigen-specific antibodies. This has had a major impact on mortality rates and improvement in the quality of life of millions of people. Other diseases have also benefited from vaccine technology, notably cancers caused by viruses for which there are several prophylactic vaccines on the market.[2] The purpose of this review is to consider non-infectious and non-cancer vaccine targets, new tools used to enable this type of vaccine to be developed, and relevant ethical issues that have arisen. For convenience these have been broadly considered under the various physiological systems, although there is some cross-over.

REPRODUCTIVE SYSTEM

Historically, the first vaccines targeted against non-infectious diseases were the contraceptive or antifertility vaccines developed in the 1970s and 1980s.[3-5] Although research in this field reached a pinnacle in the 1990s, a lack of funding and interest by pharmaceutical companies hindered further progress; however, some candidate antigens have been shown to be suitable for anticancer applications, which has allowed the research to continue.[6] This has enabled antifertility vaccine research and development (R&D) to continue at a preclinical level until the unmet need for contraceptives outweighs the lack of interest by funding bodies.

The Need for Contraceptive Vaccines

Contraceptives have differing requirements, depending on global location. In developing countries, there is a need for population control and reduction of maternal deaths, which are high compared to developed countries.[7] Any methods of contraception designed to meet this need must be effective and inexpensive and should minimize the need for medical attention in the absence of skilled health personnel.[8] On the other hand, in developed countries, the focus has been on reducing teenage pregnancy and abortion rates; in this case, contraceptives have to minimize human error, particularly in young adults, as some of the most common reasons for contraceptive failure include forgetting to use an oral contraceptive or a barrier method.[9] In both cases, a long-term contraceptive would be ideal.

Most currently available long-term methods are hormone based and mainly devised for female use. These include hormone-based injections, transdermal patches, and combined hormonal release rings; however, long-term steroid contraceptives have well-recorded side-effects. Despite the need for alternative methods, there have been few novel human contraceptives developed in the last 50 years.[10] Immunocontraceptive vaccines, developed against reproductive hormones or gametes, have been tantalizingly close to market, but as yet are currently licensed for use in animals only.[10,11] An example of this is the vaccines based on gonadotropin-releasing hormone (GnRH) or luteinizing hormone-releasing hormone (LHRH), which controls secretion of the gonadotropins, luteinizing hormone (LH), and follicle-stimulating hormone (FSH); gamete release from the ovaries; and secretion of hormones that maintain the thickness of the endometrial lining (Figure 10.1). Vaccination with GnRH thus results in total endocrine disruption, which can impact on libido and menstrual cycle; hence, developments have been mainly used to control female reproduction in animals.[12]

Another hormone that has had a long history in immunocontraceptive development is human chorionic gonadotropin (hCG), which is secreted in the female reproductive tract upon conception to aid implantation of the fertilized egg to the endometrial lining. Vaccination against hCG is intended to target the egg at implantation, resulting in a localized vaccine that would only take effect in the event of conception, minimizing systemic side-effects. This particular target has had a checkered history, initially caused by problems with achieving suitable levels of neutralizing antibodies and later with maintaining the vaccine response for a sufficient length of time.[13] This leaves the possibility of this molecule being developed for contraceptive use unlikely. Nevertheless, there is promise of a role in the treatment of advanced-stage terminal cancers expressing hCG.[6]

Disappointing results from hormone immunocontraceptive research led to the search for non-hormone targets. Sperm proteins are attractive vaccine targets as they are highly immunogenic and are often sperm specific and hence do not affect other biological processes.[14] Proteins have been chosen based on their sperm specificity, surface expression, involvement in fertility, and ability to raise long-lasting antibodies capable of inhibiting fertility. The anti-sperm proteins are considered in more detail in the next section.

Male-Associated Reproductive Targets

The development of antifertility vaccines for reproductive-related purposes in the male is primarily for contraception, although some vaccines have been developed for antiprostate cancer therapies in humans[15] and in animals to control testosterone levels.[16] Immunocontraception involves harnessing the immune system to disrupt the male reproductive process by targeting the key components: male reproductive hormones and sperm (see Figure 10.1). The former has been a significantly researched area and consists of hormonal targets that are common to both the male and female reproductive process, such as GnRH, FSH, and LH.[13] Interestingly, there has been little vaccine research targeting the key male reproductive hormone, testosterone. Most early research was carried out in the 1970s and demonstrated that testosterone immunization resulted in an increased production of the hormone via negative feedback.[17] Inhibiting testosterone function has therefore generally been achieved by developing vaccines that inhibit the action of GnRH and LH, both of which are responsible for the control of testosterone production.

Commercial vaccines against GnRH include Pfizer's Improvac™, which is used to prevent boar taint in male farmed pigs.[16] Similarly, GonaCon™ was developed as a reproductive inhibitor in wild animals by the U.S. Department of Agriculture, National Wildlife Research Center.[18] Although registered with the U.S. Environmental Protection Agency for use in white-tailed deer and wild horses,[19] GonaCon has also been used in the management of free-ranging species, including squirrels, black-tailed prairie dogs, bison, domestic cats, and domestic and feral swine.[18] Efforts to develop anti-LH and FSH vaccines have generally been unsuccessful and have largely been dropped as potential male reproductive vaccine targets in humans.[13]

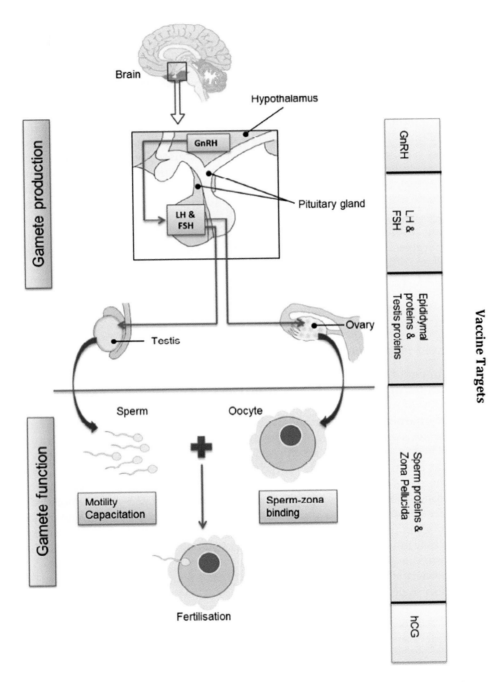

FIGURE 10.1 Reproductive axis in both male and female reproduction, showing antifertility vaccine targets.

TABLE 10.1 Sperm Targets and Function Affected by Antibody Binding

Sperm Target	Sperm Function Affected	Refs.
Acrosin	Sperm–egg binding	Howes and Jones[26]
CatSper1	Intracellular Ca^{2+} concentration, motility	Chen et al.,[44] Li et al.[170]
Eppin	Sperm motility	Chen et al.[44]
ESP	Sperm–egg binding	Lv et al.[171]
LDHC4	Sperm motility	Goldberg and Herr[172]
hCRISP1	Sperm–egg binding	Ellerman et al.[173]
Izumo	Sperm–egg fusion, fertilization	Wang et al.[174]
PH20	Sperm–egg interaction	Primakoff et al.[175]
Proacrosin	Sperm–egg binding	Garcia et al.[27]
SAGA-1	Sperm–egg binding	Parry et al.[176]
SAMP14	Sperm–egg interaction	Shetty et al.[177]
SPAG9	Sperm–egg fusion, fertilisation	Shankar et al.[178]
SFP2	Sperm motility	Khan et al.[38]
SP17	Sperm motility	Lea et al.[179]
SP10	Sperm–egg binding	Herr et al.[180]
TSA-1	Sperm motility, capacitation	Santhanam and Naz[181]

Currently, the focus has moved away from hormone targets onto those involved in sperm development and function. These include sperm and epididymal proteins and other potential male reproductive targets as detailed below.

Sperm Proteins

To date, numerous sperm proteins have been investigated for their immunocontraceptive potential, many of which are listed in Table 10.1. Some recent targets are also detailed below, and their general location on spermatozoa is shown in Figure 10.2.

SP10

One of the early sperm specific proteins investigated as a possible contraceptive target was SP10, a human intra-acrosomal protein.[20] Functional studies have shown that SP10 is involved in sperm–oolemma binding, but not sperm–zona pellucida (ZP) binding during fertilization in the human.[21] However, a monoclonal antibody to human SP10 only inhibited the binding of human sperm to hamster oolemma, not to human ZP *in vitro*. More recently, the use of a recombinant SP10 protein has been used to immunize male mice,[22] resulting in sterility for up to three months, while testosterone levels and sperm characteristics remained normal.

CATSPER

CatSper is a voltage-sensitive calcium channel that is expressed in the testis and has a significant role in sperm function. CatSper (1–4) ion channel subunit genes cause sperm cell hyperactivation and hence facilitate male fertility. In initial experiments, researchers

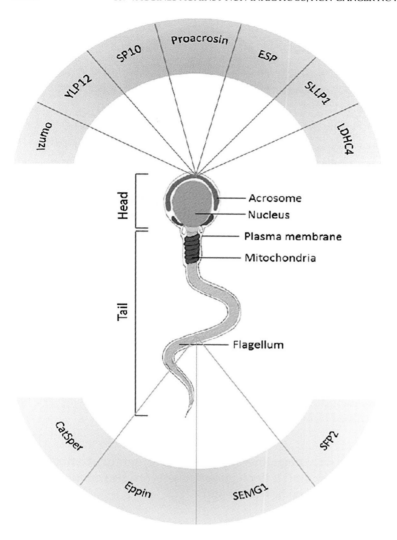

FIGURE 10.2   Sperm protein location.

investigated a small extracellular loop as a key target for the generation of antibodies, with the aim of blocking the ion channel, thus inhibiting sperm function.[23] Vaccination studies in mice using the extracellular fragment cloned into pET-32a and pEGFP-N1 plasmids has enabled antigen-specific antibodies to be produced, enabling a significant reduction of fertility with no evident adverse effects or abnormal mating behavior.[24,25]

PROACROSIN (DNA IMMUNIZATION)

Fertilization is determined to a large extent by compatibility between ligand and receptor molecules on the surface of sperm and oocytes. On the ZP, sperm receptor activity is associated with glycoproteins ZP3 (primary receptor for acrosome-intact sperm) and ZP2 (secondary receptor for acrosome-reacted sperm). Proacrosin is a molecule that is located under the acrosomal cap of the sperm that acts as a secondary ligand after the acrosome reaction.[26] It binds to the oocyte receptor ZP2, and as a serine protease it is capable of lysing the ZP locally. As such, it has been investigated as a possible vaccine target for inhibiting sperm–oocyte binding. In recent vaccine-related studies, mice administered human proacrosin cDNA (pSF2-Acro) developed high levels of specific antibodies that recognized the sperm acrosomal cap. The number of fertile mice was lower, and a negative correlation between antibody levels and smaller litter size was found, while antiproacrosin/acrosin neutralizing antibodies have been shown to inhibit sperm–ZP binding.[27]

YLP(12)

Another target arising from research into human sperm–ZP interaction is a synthetic dodecamer sequence, YLP(12).[28] The peptide sequence is localized on the acrosomal region of human sperm, and sperm–ZP interactions of this sort may find applications in contraceptive vaccine development.

EQUATORIAL SEGMENT PROTEIN

Wolkowicz et al.[29] first described the sperm-specific human equatorial segment protein (hESP) protein and showed that it was localized on the equatorial segment of the acrosome. It was also shown to be involved in acrosome biogenesis and is able to crossreact with sera from patients (both male and female). Antisera raised against recombinant hESP prevented the binding and fusion of human sperm in a hamster egg penetration assay.[30] These characteristics have made it a new contender for investigation as a possible immunocontraceptive target.

IZUMO

Inoue et al.[31] were the first to identify Izumo on the surface of mouse sperm. Izumo is required for egg–sperm fusion. It is a sperm membrane protein also found in human sperm—the addition of an antibody against human Izumo left the sperm unable to fuse with ZP-free hamster eggs.[31] Furthermore, immune-infertile female sera have circulating isoantibodies against Izumo, which may help improve clinical applications in diagnosis and treatment of infertility, as well as contraceptive vaccine development.[32] Recent investigations have identified three novel proteins showing significant homology to the N-terminal domain of Izumo: Izumo 2, Izumo 3, and Izumo 4 (Izumo 1 is the original Izumo).[33] These proteins have been shown to form complexes on sperm that may be essential for sperm–egg fusion.[34]

SLLP1

Mandal et al.[35] first reported the presence of this non-bacteriolytic, lysozyme-like protein in the acrosome of human sperm. SLLP1 was also found in mouse spermatozoa following the acrosome reaction and has a role in sperm–egg binding and fertilization.[36] Further research in the female confirmed the presence of an oocyte-specific membrane metalloproteinase, SAS1B (sperm acrosomal SLLP1 binding), that was found to bind SLLP1.[37] SAS1B knockout female mice showed a 34% reduction in fertility, indicating that SAS1B–SLLP1 had been identified as a pair of novel sperm–egg binding partners involving the oolemma and intraacrosomal compartment during fertilization.

SPERM FLAGELLAR PROTEIN 2

Sperm flagellar protein 2 (SFP2) has been identified as a novel sperm target.[38] When mice were immunized against two synthetic peptides of SFP2, the incubation of rodent and human sperm with the immune sera of peptide 1 caused significant reduction in the function of sperm *in vitro*. Additionally, only peptide 1 induced high titers of antibodies in all the immunized mice, which resulted in a reduced fertility rate down to 20%. These are early data, and the target needs to be studied in more depth, but the investigations indicate that this may be a new vaccine target worth investigating further.

Testis-Associated Targets

LACTATE DEHYDROGENASE C4

Lactate dehydrogenase C4 (LDHC4) is a key enzyme for sperm metabolism. It is highly immunogenic and is distributed specifically in the testis. LDHC4 catalyzes the conversion of lactate to pyruvate and is not expressed until puberty. It has been studied for many years, but advances in vaccine development have renewed interest in LDHC4, including development of DNA vaccines and use of mucosal vaccination.[39]

Epididymal Proteins

Spermatozoa gain motile function and are able to recognize and fertilize an egg when they have progressed through the epididymis. As such, identifying targets that prevent this process are expected to inhibit sperm function. However, to date attempts to interfere with this process have not been successful.[40] The epididymal vaccine targets are not as numerous as those located on the sperm, but some of the recent novel targets are detailed below.

EPIDIDYMAL PROTEASE INHIBITOR

Epididymal protease inhibitor (Eppin) is one of the most promising epididymal targets. It is an antimicrobial cysteine-rich protein that is important for sperm motility. Eppin is abundantly expressed in rat testis and epididymis. Reverse-transcriptase polymerase chain reaction (PCR) studies have also demonstrated that Eppin mRNA is found in Sertoli cells and spermatogenic cells. Spermatozoa-associated Eppin is thought to be secreted primarily by epithelial cells of the epididymis. Surgical castration downregulates Eppin mRNA and protein expression in the caput and cauda epididymis. This effect can be reversed using testosterone replacement.[41] Antibodies to Eppin raised in male monkeys have provided an effective and reversible contraceptive by disrupting Eppin's interaction with semenogelin during ejaculation.[42,43] Protein prime-peptide studies have shown that all of the animals injected with rhEppin followed by an epitope-based peptide boost induced antigen-specific IgG$_{2b}$ and IgG$_1$ antibodies.[44] More importantly, the IgA levels in epididymal lavages were higher and correlated well with cytokine profiles in splenocyte cultures. Furthermore, peptide competition assays demonstrated that a rhEppin-alone prime-boost vaccination led to a broader B-cell response, while a protein prime-epitope-peptide boost strategy induced an immune response mainly against the epitope. The results from the antibody studies indicate that such immunization strategies may drive a highly specific humoral response.

SEMENOGELIN 1

During ejaculation, semenogelin 1 (SEMG1) from seminal vesicles binds to Eppin, activating a series of events that include modulating prostate-specific antigen (PSA) enzyme activity, providing antimicrobial protection, and binding SEMG, thereby inhibiting sperm motility.[45] As PSA hydrolyzes SEMG in the ejaculate, spermatozoa gain progressive motility. The immunization of male monkeys with recombinant Eppin results in complete, but reversible, contraception, demonstrating that it has a key role in male fertility.[43]

The Future View of Reproductive Targets

It is less likely that novel targets will be identified in the female reproductive tract for future immunocontraceptive design, but the list of novel male reproductive targets being investigated for immunocontraception continues to grow and gene knockout technology has provided a important tool for identifying candidate sperm targets. Since 2004, over 100 genes have been identified whose deletion has demonstrated an effect on male fertility in mice. However, the majority of these knockouts also demonstrated an effect on non-reproductive organs concomitant with an antifertility effect.[46] Only a few knockout genes or proteins induced a specific effect on fertility without additional serious side-effects. It is these few genes or proteins that may provide novel targets for contraceptive vaccines.

Although there are several novel male vaccine targets for reproductive activity, it should be noted that many of these have only been investigated for their role in the female reproductive tract to prevent sperm function. Few male targets have been investigated for their ability to inhibit sperm function when administered to the male. This is probably due to the patchy understanding of the immunology of the male reproductive tract and also to the quantity of sperm that must be neutralized in the male. As a better understanding of immunology grows, more novel vaccine targets will arise. Current research is beginning to provide a better understanding of the blood–testis barrier and the immunological roles of both the testis and epididymis.[47,48] This will help facilitate the development of new contraceptive targets in the male. One approach may be to combine different targets in order to improve the chances of better disrupting spermatozoa function.

Another approach that may be the focus of future research is the development of multipurpose vaccines to increase the versatility of the immunocontraceptive, while also reducing any side-effects seen with multiple single-platform vaccinations. In particular, there may be a growing need to provide effective protection against cancers and/or sexually transmitted infections while providing effective birth control. Multipurpose immunocontraceptives may also prove attractive to the pharmaceutical industry.

More recently, the mucosal system has also been suggested as a targeted route of vaccine delivery,[49] including for delivery of contraceptive vaccines.[50] However, a greater understanding of the mucosal immune system is required before the challenges of mucosal vaccination can be overcome (reviewed by Gebril et al.[51]).

NEUROENDOCRINE SYSTEM

While the early antireproductive vaccines (such as GnRH, LH, FSH) targeted the brain, it was soon clear that shutting down the hypothalamic–pituitary axis could have profound effects on the endocrine, reproductive, and immune systems. Today, there is a realization that vaccination against a seemingly simple target can have adverse consequences, and the next targets examined highlight this.

Alzheimer Vaccines Targeting Proteinopathy

Alzheimer disease (AD) has provided non-infectious vaccine targets, and research in this area has been progressing for the last few decades. This was conceptualized following the discovery of the role of amyloid β-protein (Aβ) in the plaques found in AD, and pharmaceutical interest focused on producing antibodies against Aβ in both active and passive immunization strategies; only active are discussed in this section. Plaques are one of the two pathophysiological hallmarks of AD, and these develop in the early stages of the disease, while neurofibrillary tangles are evident later on and correlate with cognitive decline,[52] although the mechanism of action has yet to be established. The first experiments carried out by Schenk et al.[53] immunized mice with an Aβ peptide on a monthly basis for nearly a year, which resulted in antibody production that significantly reduced plaque burden. These early studies were abandoned due to observations of adverse events in clinical trials (e.g., meningoencephalitis in approximately 6% of treated patients[54]). Subsequent studies demonstrated that this was caused by T-cell responses to epitopes at the C-terminus.[55] Other studies showed that immunization against the amino-terminal and central domains of Aβ resulted in improved cognition tests in preclinical models of AD, independent of plaque removal.[54] Several clinical trials have since been carried out in patients or are in development (Table 10.2). The most recent candidate peptide antigens contain only B-cell epitopes to minimize adverse T-cell

TABLE 10.2   Aβ Active Immunization Clinical Trials Completed or in Progress

Antigen	Trial	Comments	Refs.
AN1792/AIP-001 (Elan/Wyeth)	Phase IIA (NCT00021723)	Stopped early due to adverse effects caused by T-cell responses. Follow-on studies show correlation between antibody response and plaque burden	Bayer et al.,[182] Gilman et al.,[183] Vellas et al.[184]
ACC-001; N-terminal Aβ1–6 peptide linked to a carrier protein in QS21 adjuvant (Pfizer/Janssen AIP)	Phase II (NCT00479557)	Completed January 2013	Ryan and Grundman[185]
	Phase II (NCT01284387)	Completed February 2014	
Affitope AD02; Six amino acid peptide, Aβ1–6, that mimic N-terminus of native Aβ (AFFiRiS AG)	Phase II (NCT01117818)	Completed December 2013	Schneeberger et al.[186]
CAD-106; Aβ1–6 conjugated to a virus-like particle (Novartis/Cytos)	Phase II (NCT01097096)	Completed December 2012	Winblad et al.[187]
UB311 Aβ1–14 in UBITh (United Biomedical)	Phase I (NCT00965588)	Completed April 2011	Wang et al.[188]
V950 (Merck); Aβ N-terminus peptides and ISCO-MATRIX	Phase I (NCT00464334)	Completed January 2012	Savage et al.[189]

TABLE 10.3   Clinical and Preclinical Anti-Tau Immunization Studies

Antigen	Experimental Details	Outcomes	Refs.
AADvac1, a tau peptide-KLH conjugate vaccine (Axon Neuroscience SE)	Phase I (NCT01850238)	Estimated completion March 2015	—
Whole recombinant human tau	C57BL/6 wild-type mice immunized with antigen in complete Freund's adjuvant supplemented with *Mycobacterium* tuberculosis; administration of pertussis toxin and a booster 1 week later	Anti-tau antibodies and adverse encephalitis events were reported	Rosenmann et al.[190]
Three short tau phosphopeptides comprising phosphorylation sites Ser202/Thr205 (PHF1), Thr212/Ser214 (AT100), and Thr231 (AT180)	Three-month-old K257T/P301S double-mutant, tau-expressing mice immunized	Pathology was prevented and tau phosphorylation was significantly reduced	Boimel et al.[191]
Thirty amino-acid peptides comprising a PHF1 phospho-epitope of tau (Ser396/Ser404) in aluminum adjuvant	Two-month-old P301L tau transgenic JNPL3 mice immunized monthly for up to 8 months	Tau phosphorylation was reduced, although total tau levels were not reduced	Asuni et al.[192]
PHF1 phospho-epitope of tau (Ser396/Ser404) i.p. in aluminum adjuvant	Three-month-old htau mouse model immunized with first three injections every 2 weeks until 7 to 8 months of age; subsequent administrations at monthly intervals	Tau pathology was reduced	Boutajangout et al.[193]

responses. Preclinical studies are also ongoing with DNA encoding the Aβ1-42 peptide.[56] Active immunization may also be effective in intracellular neurofibrillary tangles containing hyperphosphorylated tau protein in animal models of AD,[57,58] as there seems to be crosstalk between Aβ and tau[59] (Table 10.3). Although the literature on preclinical studies describes examples of effective Aβ clearance, the clinical reality is fraught with adverse effects, and the development of safe, efficacious treatments is still a long way to fruition. Nevertheless, the potential for a new vaccine in this field is promising as evidenced by Pharma activity.

The Search for Other Neurodegenerative Vaccines

The relative success with Alzheimer vaccines has encouraged researchers to seek treatments for other brain conditions associated with neurodegeneration, specifically where proteinopathy can be identified, such as in Parkinson's disease (PD). In this case, the target is to prevent the accumulation and aggregation of the misfolded protein, α-synuclein (aSyn).[60] AFFiRiS AG is using the same principles as applied to their AD vaccines, and their anti-PD vaccine is based on the use of short antigens to avoid activating aSyn-specific T cells and, thus, cellular autoimmunity. Their first vaccine, AFFITOPEPD01A, has entered clinical trials (NCT01568099, NCT01885494).

Neuro-Targeted Vaccines to Treat Addictions and Substance Abuse

Vaccines are being developed against targets such as nicotine,[61] cocaine,[62] heroin,[63] opiates,[64] and methamphetamine.[65] Substance abuse is a major health problem worldwide; studies carried out on drug dependence and implications for treatment estimate that 5 million deaths can be associated with smoking,[66] which costs US$67 billion each year in terms of crime, lost job productivity, and other social problems.[67] The main problem associated with these vaccines is induction of sufficiently high antibody titers that are capable of blocking the drugs from entering the bloodstream. The concept is for antibodies to bind to the drugs to prevent them from reaching the brain, thus interrupting the pleasure and reward-inducing effects, with the idea being that this will result in higher efficiency and fewer side-effects.[68] As nicotine is a small molecule, the main strategy consists of conjugation of the molecule to carrier proteins and use of delivery systems (Table 10.4). To date, the results have been disappointing, and this is another example of why we need better preclinical disease models to improve translational studies (reviewed by Caponnetto et al.,[68] Hartmann-Boyce,[69] and Fahim et al.[70]). Other strategies are being applied to heroin, as this molecule is rapidly metabolized to 6-acetylmorphine and morphine. In this case, a multi-haptenic structure has been designed to represent the metabolites of heroin.[71] The advantage of this approach is that, because the vaccine does not target opioid receptors, it can be used together with other therapeutic options; also, it allows for minimal medical supervision and increased patient compliance.

Vaccines to Treat Stress and Depression

As can be seen from the neurodegenerative disorders, novel targets for vaccination arise where a protein can be found to cause a particular affliction. On the other hand, indirect targets are emerging that show that modulation of the immune system may provide signals that can produce novel vaccines to treat stress and depression. Although the mechanisms of such vaccines are not fully understood, the beneficial effects of these types of vaccines are considered worth pursuing. For example, research is ongoing to modulate immune surveillance at the choroid plexus at the periphery of the brain. Actively immunizing against central nervous

TABLE 10.4   Progress in Development of Antinicotine Vaccines

Vaccine Candidate	Producer	Carrier Protein	Stage	Refs.
NicVAX™	Nabi/GlaxoSmithKline (United Kingdom)	*Pseudomonas aeruginosa* exoprotein A (rEPA)	Phase III completed	Hartmann-Boyce et al.[69]
Nic002	Cytos/Novartis (Switzerland)	Virus-like particle (VLP)	Phase II completed	Cornuz et al.[194]
Niccine™	Independent Pharmaceutica (Sweden)	Tetanus toxoid	Phase II completed	Tonstad et al.[195]
TA-NIC	Xenova/Celtic Pharma, (United Kingdom)	CTB (recombinant B subunit of cholera toxin)	Phase II completed	Caponnetto et al.[68]

system (CNS)-derived peptides has been shown to result in modulation of hippocampal plasticity and cause a reduction in anxiety levels.[72]

Other research relates to the observation that immune activation can have an impact on depression; this was seen in patients treated with interferon γ (IFN-γ) or interleukin 2 (IL-2) who also developed depressive symptoms.[73,74] Lowry et al.[75] have demonstrated that vaccination with antigens derived from the non-pathogenic *Mycobacterium vaccae* activates a specific subset of serotonergic neurons that alters stress-related emotional behavior in a rodent model. This may be backed up by the growing evidence of depression related to vaccination and the known impact of stress on efficacy of vaccination.[76,77] Similarly, immune-modulation of gut microbiota and controlling inflammatory mediators through vaccination are also being suggested as a means of treating depression (reviewed by Rook et al.[78]). A recent paper suggested that vaccination against heat-shock proteins that induces T-regulatory (Treg) activity can have an impact not only on ameliorating depression, but also in treating autoimmune disease, neurodegenerative diseases, and inflammatory conditions.[79] This shows that we have a lot to learn about the role of the immune system on the impact of health status.

Ethics and Legal Considerations of Brain-Targeted Diseases

Neurodegenerative-Targeted Vaccines

Although the ethical principles of vaccine research have been established for a considerable time and govern provision of access to care and treatment to participants in biomedical research, the application of these ethical principles can present unique issues in relation to vaccines for the treatment of neurodegenerative disease. The main code for participation in research is an ability of the potential participant to be capable of providing informed consent—that is, demonstrating an ability to understand what the nature and purpose of the research may be and to comprehend the potential risks or benefits of participation. However, it is known that the prevalence of incapacity can be considerable in certain disease states, particularly those where there is a neurodegenerative component,[80] resulting in the potential exclusion of patient populations who would be the target population for recruitment to such vaccine trials over fears of inability to provide informed consent. This has been recognized as a potential problem limiting the ability to conduct research in an elderly population where neurodegenerative disease is more common.[81] This has led to researchers looking at the validity of surrogate consent, usually by a close family member acting as a proxy for the wishes of the cognitively impaired individual. The concept of surrogate consent is already widely accepted and applied to the administration of vaccines in children where parents provide consent to treat in the best interests of the child. Research within the context of neurodegenerative disease has indicated that a majority of the older general public broadly supports a policy of surrogate consent for diseases such as AD and are comfortable with the possibility that their surrogates may not always exactly execute their wishes in relation to future research participation.[82,83] Nonetheless, there is an ongoing need for consensus by medical, regulatory authorities and the wider public on how best to overcome the existing ethical reservations relating to enrolment of incapacitated individuals into vaccine research which may directly benefit them if successful.

Substance Abuse Vaccines

Vaccines against substance abuse raise ethical and legal concerns, which can vary depending upon the potential vaccination group in question. For example, vaccination of adults with a preexisting substance misuse problem can raise a number of issues. One potential problem is that vaccinated individuals may modify their behaviors in a way that ultimately places them at greater risk; for example, they may think that their tolerance to the vaccinated drug or to other drugs of misuse has been enhanced and therefore take larger doses than normal, with a resultant rise in potentially toxic side-effects. In contrast, there may be a desire for parents to vaccinate their children against potential substances of misuse, and their desire to protect their child raises the ethical dilemmas of the ability of an individual, the child, to make an autonomous choice at a later stage to consume what may be a legally permitted drug (e.g., cigarettes) or the ethics of vaccinating someone against a substance which they may not have misused in the first instance. There is also the need to balance the practicalities of vaccination against drugs of misuse which require frequent booster vaccinations to maintain effective antibodies against the drugs versus the potential to cause anxiety or harm as a direct consequence of ongoing vaccination.[84]

IMMUNE SYSTEM

Current Strategies in Allergen Vaccine Development

The immune response is regulated by several mechanisms to protect the body from exogenous and endogenous attacks. In particular, danger signals are recognized by the immune system, which enables a proper response to pathogenic stimuli.[85] Allergies are caused by different factors such as the nature of the allergen, administration route, genetics, and coexistence with other infectious diseases or even commensal bacteria flora.[86] About 25% of the population is affected by allergies, although some estimates are even higher (30 to 40%, as reported by the World Allergy Organization[87]), the majority from industrialized countries.[88] Allergies induce rhinitis, asthma, food intolerance, skin inflammation, ocular discomfort, and toxin- or venom-induced anaphylaxis.[89] Respiratory allergies such as rhinitis, conjunctivitis, and asthma often coexist in the same patient, especially rhinitis and asthma, which are considered part of a common syndrome.[90]

Immune Response to Allergens

Major allergens identified from pollen, house dust mites, pets, molds, food, and insects are mainly protein, glycoprotein, or lipoprotein in nature.[91] A detailed description of how allergens cause allergic reactions and the different allergy phases are described by Galli et al.,[92] but it is generally accepted that the mechanisms triggering allergic reactions are related to recurrent exposure to allergens, which boost production of allergen-specific IgE antibodies. These antibodies bind to high-affinity receptors for IgE FcγRI receptors located on the surface of mast cells and basophils, which secrete inflammatory mediators. The serial activation of FcγRI receptors leads to sensitization of patients to a specific allergen.[93,94] A Th2 immune response is responsible for the induction of IgE-mediated allergy, particularly because this committed T-cell pattern produces cytokines such as IL-4, IL-5, IL-9, and IL-13. These cytokines play a crucial role in the maintenance of high allergen-specific IgE levels, stimulate eosinophil progenitors in bone marrow, induce inflammatory cell influx into inflamed tissue, and result in production of mucus and smooth muscle contraction.[95] Allergen-specific immunotherapy (A-SIT) is considered the only form of treatment that can alter the immunological basis of allergic diseases with long-term effects.[90] It is carried out with the administration of increasing doses of allergens in order to obtain hyposensitization and long-term relief of symptoms occurring after natural allergen exposure.[96] Increasing doses of allergens are required for the best therapeutic results, and treatments may take as long as one to three years. The aim of A-SIT is to modify peripheral and mucosal Th2 responses to a particular allergen in favor of Th1 and Treg responses. The latter may be a key early event, and IL-10-producing Treg cells may be detectable within a few weeks of the first injection. IL-10 inhibits mast cell, eosinophil, and T-cell responses, in addition to acting on B cells to favor the induction of IgG_4, which blocks the binding of IgE to the allergen and subsequent degranulation of mast cells and basophils.[97,98] In any case, Th1 and/or Treg commitment downmodulates allergenic cytokines such as IL-4, IL-5, and IL-19 and reduce specific IgE secretion, which is translated into an improved environment to eliminate or reduce allergic reactions.[99] Several other T cells (Th17, Th22, and Th23) have been associated with the physiopathology of allergy, and an extensive analysis of this topic has been reviewed elsewhere.[86,100]

Traditionally, aqueous extracts from different allergenic sources have been used in A-SIT; therefore, most licensed vaccines contain purified or semi-purified antigens. However, IgE-mediated reactions and T-cell reactions, among others, have been reported to be due to the use of extracts containing complex mixtures of allergens.[101] A new phase in the development of allergen vaccines has begun with the design of more defined allergenic molecules, including synthetic peptides and recombinant proteins,[98,102] as described below.

Recent Antigen Modifications to Improve Vaccine Efficacy

SYNTHETIC PEPTIDE VACCINES

Sequencing and molecular cloning of allergen antigens began more than 30 years ago, and since then several approaches have been used to target allergen specific T cells. Synthetic peptides, comprised of linear sequences from small allergens, may bind to receptors from specific T cells and induce very low reactivity to specific IgE.[103] Synthetic peptides derived from Fel d1 (a major allergen identified in cats)[104] and bee venom have been evaluated.[105] However, new clinical studies are needed to define the mechanisms involved. A possible drawback of the peptide vaccine strategy lies in the use of single or multiple peptides in contrast to the diverse repertoire of T cells, which may be engaged or activated by "natural" allergens. An alternative to synthetic peptide vaccines is the use of recombinant vaccines

RECOMBINANT PROTEIN VACCINES

Production of extracts is limited by the low consistency of the batches produced and problems related to the evaluation of their quality.[106] Vaccines constructed using recombinant proteins may overcome these problems. Two main protein approaches have been described in this field: recombinant hypoallergens and recombinant wild-type allergens.[98] The first type uses molecular biology techniques to introduce mutations, deletions, or oligomerizations in the allergen sequence.[106] This type of recombinant protein is characterized by strongly reduced IgE reactivity, whereas wild-type recombinant proteins are produced as a copy of the original allergen. Several manipulations of this protein, such as the introduction of mutations into the sequence, production of larger non-allergenic fragments, and reassembly of sequences, can also be made to enhance their immunogenicity or to conjugate them to other relevant immunogenic peptides.[98,103] Both types of protein have been produced mainly in *Escherichia coli* and share the immunotherapeutic mechanism of induction of allergen-specific IgG (IgG₄) that inhibits the binding of IgE to the allergen.[107] Clinical studies have been carried out comparing wild-type recombinant Bet v 1 (birch pollen allergen) with the purified natural extract (nBet v 1). These have demonstrated higher induction of IgG-blocking antibodies by the recombinant formulation.[108]

NUCLEIC ACID VACCINES

Vaccination with DNA uses a different approach to develop vaccine candidates for A-SIT. Huang et al.[109] demonstrated that immunization with a DNA plasmid encoding Bermuda grass pollen allergen, Cynd 1, induced Th1 responses and suppressed specific IgE antibody. However, some concerns exist regarding the possibility of an uncontrolled production of allergens in patients treated with DNA vaccines. A possible solution is to encode hypoallergenic fragments of DNA[110] or to improve the immunization with RNA, which induces a transient production of allergens.[111] In any case, further studies will be needed to choose the best strategy. An alternative is the resurgence of allergen-encoding mRNA vaccines that can elicit long-lasting protection from sensitization and induce immunity that is similar to the natural protective response that is acquired in the presence of microbial burden in infants. This means they can be used to protect at-risk children who have not yet been sensitized to allergens.[112]

Enhancements Used to Improve Vaccine Targeting in Allergen Research

Adjuvants are essential in vaccine formulations and are described as components that increase the specific immune response to a given antigen.[113] These can be divided into immune stimulators and delivery systems, although some substances can act by both mechanisms.[114] Therapeutic vaccines have benefited from new approaches in the field of adjuvant research, as have allergen vaccines.

IMMUNE STIMULATORS

Several immune stimulator components from bacteria and viruses have been identified, including lipopolysaccharide (LPS) in cell walls of bacteria as well as unmethylated motifs of bacterial DNA (CpG), which can activate Toll-like receptors (TLRs) on the surface or in the cytosolic compartments of antigen-presenting cells (APCs).[115] APC activation increases cytokine expression, antigen presentation, and other events that cause the maturation of APCs. Activated APCs control the activation of T and B cells, as well as the commitment of CD4+ T cells in Th1, Th2, Treg, and Th17 cells.[116] Activation of TLR 9 by CpG oligodeoxynucleotides (ODNs) inhibits a Th2 response and favors a Th1 pattern. A formulation of ODN-1018 conjugated to Amb a 1 (a pollen allergen) has been evaluated in clinical trials. The induction of allergen-specific neutralizing IgG antibodies and reduced seasonal boost in IgE production have encouraged evaluation of new formulations.[117] An example of this is the use of detoxified LPS from *Salmonella minnesota*, known as monophosphoril lipid A (MPL), which has been evaluated with pollen allergens. MPL is thought to be a Th1-inducing adjuvant. Engagement of MPL with TLR4 in APCs stimulates the secretion of cytokines such as IL-12, which is closely related to the reduced induction of IgE and switching to IgG_1 and IgG_4 in humans.[118] Pollinex Quatro™ (Allergy Therapeutics), licensed in Europe and Canada, contains MPL and is used for the treatment of allergy to grass, tree, or ragweed pollen.[119] This vaccine is administered with a very short therapeutic schedule (four doses weekly), sufficient to produce an effective immunotherapeutic action.[120] This is one of the greatest advantages of this formulation, which increases the compliance and adherence of patients to the treatment regimen. Another bacterial-derived immune stimulant is Adjuvant Finlay Proteoliposome 1 (AFPL1), an outer membrane vesicle or proteoliposome derived from *Neisseria meningitidis* serogroup B that contains LPS and porins that are thought to activate TLR4 and TLR2, respectively. This activation promotes the induction of a Th1 pattern of response.[121] Subcutaneous immunization of mice with *Dermatophagoides siboney* (a dust mite species) and AFPL1 adsorbed onto aluminum hydroxide induces high IgG_{2a} titers and IFN-γ, with a reduction in specific IgE levels.[122] Currently, a Phase I clinical trial with this vaccine candidate is under evaluation.[123]

DELIVERY SYSTEMS

Delivery systems are vehicles that carry antigens or "allergens" and also immune stimulators to APCs. Aluminum salts are an example of a depot adjuvant, and many allergens have been adsorbed onto aluminum hydroxide. A depot effect promotes the presentation of allergens to APCs, although Th2 responses have been reported associated with stimulation of inflammasome signaling.[124] For this reason, alum adjuvants have been used less in novel vaccine strategies, although the combination of aluminum salts with potent immune stimulators, such as LPS, MPL, or AFPL1, may switch the Th2 response to a Th1 pattern.[121,125] The amino acid L-tyrosine has also been used as a depot adjuvant. Pollinex Quatro contains pollen allergens and MPL adsorbed onto a L-tyrosine depot. This amino acid is normally found in blood at physiological levels of 0.5 mg/kg of an adult person and is administered at 0.3 mg/kg with the vaccine, so no important adverse reactions have been reported. The depot is weakly soluble at neutral pH and allows the adsorption and slow release of the allergen and the immune stimulator when administered via the subcutaneous route.[126] Non-depot-forming adjuvants include nanoparticles composed of poly-lactide-*co*-glycolic acids (PLGA). Immunization with PLGA nanoparticles loaded with the birch pollen antigen Bet v1 have been shown to reduce the Th2 response, showing an increase in antigen-specific IgG_{2a} and IFN-γ, which demonstrates the potential of PLGA in A-SIT.[127,128] Similar approaches with polymeric nanoparticles have been developed with polyanhydrides. Gantrez™ AN copolymers are a commercial product (Ashland, Covington, KY) that has been shown to have strong bioadhesive interaction with gut mucosa. The copolymers have been applied via the oral route for immunotherapy treatment with allergenic proteins from rye grass (*Lollium perenne*) pollen.[129] Other nano- and microparticles used with allergens have been developed with the polysaccharide chitosan.[130] Due to the low cost of production, biocompatibility, biodegradability, nontoxicity, and bioadhesive characteristics of chitosan, most products containing the polymer have been licensed mainly for mucosal applications. Oral immunization with chitosan nanoparticles entrapping the gene Ara h2 (the major allergen found in peanuts) has been shown to induce protective immunity in a peanut allergy mouse model, with significant reduction in the levels of antigen-specific IgE, plasma histamine, and the induction of specific

IgA antibodies.[131] Bacterial- and viral-derived particles have also been used to deliver allergens, including AFPL1[122,132] and virus-like particles (VLPs).[133,134] VLPs have been used with peptides from the major dust mite allergen *Dermatophagoides pteronyssinus* (Der p 1)[135] and the cat allergen Fel d 1.[136] These studies have been shown to induce a decrease in allergic reaction. More recently, the combination of VLPs with the immune stimulator CpG has demonstrated enormous potential in the design of therapeutic vaccines against allergies.[137]

DIFFERENT ROUTES OF ADMINISTRATION

Administration routes other than subcutaneous immunotherapy (SCIT) have also been investigated. Sublingual immunotherapy (SLIT) has the advantage of convenient administration, permitting self-administration of drops or tablets containing the allergen extract.[98] SLIT has also been reported to be safer than SCIT in terms of side effects and has gained popularity in Europe.[138] Examples of SLIT products approved in Europe include the timothy grass immunotherapy tablets (S-AIT) Grazax®[139] and Staloral® drops.[140] However, recent studies have indicated that SLIT may not be advantageous over SCIT. Although S-AIT has shown efficacy in studies conducted in Europe,[139,141,142] a Phase III trial in the United States showed no immunological benefit in comparison to the placebo group.[143] A direct comparison between SLIT and SCIT in a metaanalysis study also showed clear evidence that SCIT was better than SLIT.[144] The mechanisms of action are not very well understood. The original rationale of SLIT was to achieve an immediate and rapid absorption of the vaccine through the oral mucosa; however, it has been demonstrated that direct absorption of relevance does not occur through the sublingual mucosa.[145] Several studies propose that the allergen is captured within the oral mucosa by oral Langerhans cells and subsequently these cells mature and migrate to proximal draining lymph nodes, where production of blocking IgG antibodies and the induction of T-lymphocyte producers of suppressive cytokines IL-10 and transforming growth factor (TGF) are stimulated.[146,147] Currently, application of oral immunotherapy for the treatment of food allergies (such as bovine milk and peanut allergy) is also being investigated.[148,149] The use of transgenic rice to express mite allergen has also been demonstrated by Suzuki et al.,[150] who reported that Th2-type cytokines produced by peripheral CD4+ T cells *in vitro* were significantly reduced following oral vaccination in a murine asthma model.[151] Other routes of administration include epicutaneous immunotherapy (EPIT). Mondoulet et al.[152] demonstrated that EPIT was comparable to SLIT in mice sensitized to timothy grass allergen. In a clinical trial involving patients with grass-pollen-induced rhinoconjunctivitis, EPIT was found to be safe and efficacious in a dose-dependent manner.[153] However, it was also found that drug-related adverse events occurred by increasing allergen doses. EPIT has also demonstrated promising results for food and inhalant allergies.[154]

LATEST DEVELOPMENTS IN ALLERGEN VACCINES

The immediate focus is to increase compliance by reducing the length of treatment time. Intralymphatic (ILIT) has been shown to produce improved clinical benefits with shorter treatment times (three injections compared with a 3-year schedule for SCIT). Furthermore, there is a trend toward development of mucosal treatment regimens to reduce treatment time and increase the convenience of administration. In addition to targeting allergens, there are also attempts being made to target the underlying functional and immunological abnormalities associated with respiratory diseases. Takeda et al.[155] demonstrated the possibility of employing vaccination in suppressing airway hyperresponsiveness (AHR) and inflammation associated with asthma after establishment of the disease. In this study, vaccination using ovalbumin (OVA) coupled to liposome–DNA complexes (CDLC) was shown to significantly suppress AHR in mice previously sensitized and challenged with OVA. This effect was attributed to the vaccine being able to elicit strong CD4+ and CD8+ T-cell responses and activation of Th1 immunity.

FUTURE TRENDS

Snapshot of Other Emerging Vaccine Targets

The targets shown in Table 10.5 provide a snapshot of vaccine developments that may take off in the near future, but are still at a very early stage of research.

Application of New Technologies to Improve Vaccine Development

New technologies that are driving the next generation of vaccines have broadly been divided into three categories: antigen discovery, development of effective adjuvants and delivery systems, and understanding immune responses. In parallel, new cutting-edge tools are being developed to elucidate new information that encompasses all three categories; the examples highlighted here involve genomics and proteomics, individual cell monitoring, and nanoscale sampling.

TABLE 10.5   Future Novel Targets

Condition Targeted	Details	Refs.
Hypertension	Mice immunized with angiotensin II peptide conjugated to keyhole limpet hemocyanin showed reduced systolic blood pressure	Nakagami et al.[196]
Artherosclerosis	Lipoprotein(a) in low-density lipoprotein is targeted	Nakagami et al.[196]
Coeliac disease	NexVax2 vaccine consisting of three gluten peptides induces T-cell immune tolerance in HLA-DQ2-positive patients	Crespo Perez et al.[197]
Type 1 diabetes	Auto-antigen vaccination	Clemente-Casares et al.[198]
Obesity	Anti-ghrelin immunization	Andrade et al.[199]
Chronic kidney disease	DNA vaccination against various self-antigens (chemokines, costimulatory molecules, T-cell receptors)	Wang et al.[200]
Multiple sclerosis	A new class of vaccines known as tolerogenic vaccines is being developed that induce immunological tolerance in order to suppress the immune system (e.g., inflammatory responses, autoimmunity)	Mannie and Curtis[201]
Rheumatoid arthritis	Immunization against tumour necrosis factor alpha (TNFα)	Jia et al.[202]

Antigen Discovery

One major approach to mining for new antigens from bacterial species is known as reverse vaccinology. In this approach, the sequences of the whole genome of microorganisms are examined. Proteins that are predicted to be surface exposed or secreted are cloned and expressed. Each protein is then screened for its ability to produce antibodies in mice that can kill or neutralize the target pathogen.[156] It is conceivable that such a technique may be applicable to non-infectious target proteins.

Adjuvants and Delivery Systems

In this chapter, we have already examined development of immune stimulators and delivery systems in allergy vaccines. Because it is likely that mucosal vaccines will dominate the future, delivery systems are likely to be developed for mucosal administration, and these are reviewed in detail elsewhere.[51]

Understanding Immune Responses

As with vaccines that target infections and cancer, safety is paramount for non-infectious targets as well. This is particularly important when the vaccines cause profound effects in physiological systems that can impact badly when things go wrong. Therefore, it is critical that we hasten our understanding of the immune response. To this end, rationale design is relying on computer-aided modeling, focusing on antibody modeling of the antigen-binding site or complementary-determining regions and prediction of the relative orientations of the variable heavy and light chains in the antibody molecules.[157]

Tools for Understanding Vaccines

The complication and importance of vaccines create a unique challenge for formulation and physicochemical characterization. Vaccines may consist of one or more types of antigenic component, polysaccharides, proteins, polynucleotides, and particle conjugates.[158] Therefore, it is important to use state-of-the-art techniques in order to understand the physicochemical stability of vaccine preparations and their morphology, as small changes such as size, shape, and surface properties influence their biodistribution and release.[159] There are several such analytical tools that are available for the study of physicochemical parameter characterization of vaccines. Atomic force microscopy (AFM) has been used to study protein–protein, drug–protein, and particle–surface interactions[160] and particle stability.[161] Most importantly, AFM has been used to investigate the mechanical properties and their response to nanoparticles by measuring the nanomechanical properties such as surface roughness, stiffness, rigidity, Young's modulus, deformation, and dissipation.[162]

Circular dichroism (CD) spectroscopy uses the different ways that individual types of molecules absorb light in order to investigate their structure and has a wide range of applications, including investigating the secondary structure of proteins and for structural studies of small organic molecules, proteins, and DNA.[163,164] Contact-angle goniometry (CAG) could be used to investigate any changes in the hydrophilicity or hydrophobicity of different formulations and changes in the surface energy of the final product.[163]

Differential scanning calorimetric (DSC) provides the ability to determine stabilizing conditions of a protein-based vaccine during formulation development and can also be used to assess a change in the protein or polynucleotide present.[165] Isothermal titration calorimetry

(ITC) is an advanced technique for measuring and probing the thermodynamics of vaccine formulation interactions and is used to determine many binding parameters (such as n, KD, ΔH, ΔS) in a single experiment without the need for labels.[166] Particle size analyzers and zeta potential equipment are also important, as surface charge and particle sizing can be determined in a few seconds. Moreover, transmission electron microscopy (TEM) and scanning electron microscopy (SEM) could also be used to investigate size and morphology; they are more accurate and have higher resolution.

Nuclear magnetic resonance (NMR) is a technique that reveals high-resolution structural information in liquid form and could help to investigate the structure, dynamics, and topology of drug–protein interactions.[167] Raman confocal microscopy has the capability of collecting information such as fingerprint spectra, three-dimensional structural changes on orientation and conformation, intermolecular interactions, and dynamics. Rheometry could be used to study the stiffness and spectroscopic changes as we "push" micro or nano formulations. Surface plasmon resonance (SPR) provides information on affinity, kinetics, and specificity of molecular interactions.[168] Moreover, the chemical composition of the surface of micro- and nanoparticles before and after adsorption of vaccine antigens can be measured using x-ray photoelectron spectroscopy (XPS) and time-of-flight secondary ion mass spectrometry (TOF-SIMS).[169]

CONCLUSIONS

New targets are continuously being identified as knowledge of disease states and the immune system increases. Advances in tools to progress understanding of molecular interactions and antigen discovery are critical. More importantly, however, we require better preclinical models to test the vaccines in order to avoid adverse effects and to accelerate product development. As new targets are identified, ethical and legal considerations will also become important features in vaccine design. Overall, though, the future for non-infectious/non-cancer vaccine developments is promising.

References

1. Koff WC, Burton DR, Johnson PR, Walker BD, King CR, Nabel GJ, Ahmed R, Bhan MK, Plotkin SA. Accelerating next-generation vaccine development for global disease prevention. Science 2013;340(6136):1232910.
2. Mbulaiteye SM, Buonaguro FM. Infections and cancer: debate about using vaccines as a cancer control tool. Infect. Agents Cancer 2013;8(1):16.
3. Das C, Talwar GP, Ramakrishnan S, Salahuddin M, Kumar S, Hingorani V, Coutinho E, Croxatto H, Hemmingson E, Johansson E, Luukkainen T, Shahani S, Sundaram K, Nash H, Segal SJ. Discriminatory effect of anti-Pr-beta-hCG-TT antibodies on the neutralization of the biological activity of placental and pituitary gonadotropins. Contraception 1978;18(1):35–50.
4. Goldberg E, Wheat TE, Powell JE, Stevens VC. Reduction of fertility in female baboons immunized with lactate dehydrogenase C4. Fertil. Steril. 1981;35(2):214–7.
5. Isojima S, Koyama K, Takada Y, Shigeta M, Tsuji Y, Hasegawa A. The development of a contraceptive vaccine by purification of antigens from gametes. Am. J. Reprod. Immunol. Microbiol. 1986;10(3):90–2.
6. Talwar GP. A unique vaccine for control of fertility and therapy of advanced-stage terminal cancers ectopically expressing human chorionic gonadotropin. Ann. N.Y. Acad. Sci. 2013;1283:50–6.
7. Hogan MC, Foreman KJ, Naghavi M, Ahn SY, Wang M, Makela SM, Lopez AD, Lozano R, Murray CJ. Maternal mortality for 181 countries, 1980-2008: a systematic analysis of progress towards Millennium Development Goal 5. Lancet 2010;375(9726):1609–23.

8. Alvarez JL, Gil R, Hernandez V, Gil A. Factors associated with maternal mortality in Sub-Saharan Africa: an ecological study. BMC Public Health 2009;9:462.
9. Brown S, Guthrie K. Why don't teenagers use contraception? A qualitative interview study. Eur. J. Contracept. Reprod. Health Care 2010;15(3):197–204.
10. McLaughlin EA, Aitken RJ. Is there a role for immunocontraception? Mol. Cell. Endocrinol. 2011;335(1): 78–88.
11. Ferro VA, Mordini E. Peptide vaccines in immunocontraception. Curr. Opin. Mol. Ther. 2004;6(1):83–9.
12. Schulman ML, Botha AE, Muenscher SB, Annandale CH, Guthrie AJ, Bertschinger HJ. Reversibility of the effects of GnRH-vaccination used to suppress reproductive function in mares. Equine Vet. J. 2013;45(1):111–3.
13. Ferro VA, Garside DA. Reproductive component vaccine developments for contraceptive and non-contraceptive uses. Expert Opin. Ther. Pat. 2011;21(9):1473–82.
14. Garside DA, Gebril A, Alsaadi M, Nimmo N, Mullen AB, Ferro VA. An update on the potential for male contraception: emerging options. Open Access J. Contraception 2013;4:1–11.
15. Aguilar FF, Barranco JJ, Fuentes EB, Aguilera LC, Saez YL, Santana MDC, Vazquez EP, Baker RB, Acosta OR, Perez HG, Nieto GG. Very small size proteoliposomes (VSSP) and montanide combination enhance the humoral immuno response in a GnRH based vaccine directed to prostate cancer. Vaccine 2012;30(46):6595–9.
16. Dunshea FR, Colantoni C, Howard K, McCauley I, Jackson P, Long KA, Lopaticki S, Nugent EA, Simons JA, Walker J, Hennessy DP. Vaccination of boars with a GnRH vaccine (Improvac) eliminates boar taint and increases growth performance. J. Anim. Sci. 2001;79(10):2524–35.
17. Wickings EJ, Becher A, Nieschlag E. Testosterone metabolism in rabbits actively immunized with testosterone. Endocrinology 1976;98(5):1142–6.
18. Miller LA, Fagerstone KA, Wagner RA, Finkler M. Use of a GnRH vaccine, GonaCon, for prevention and treatment of adrenocortical disease (ACD) in domestic ferrets. Vaccine 2013;31(41):4619–23.
19. Fagerstone KA, Miller LA, Killian G, Yoder CA. Review of issues concerning the use of reproductive inhibitors, with particular emphasis on resolving human-wildlife conflicts in North America. Integr. Zool. 2010;5(1):15–30.
20. Srinivasan J, Tinge S, Wright R, Herr JC, Curtiss R. Oral immunization with attenuated Salmonella expressing human sperm antigen induces antibodies in serum and the reproductive tract. Biol. Reprod. 1995;53(2):462–71.
21. Hamatani T, Tanabe K, Kamei K, Sakai N, Yamamoto Y, Yoshimura Y. A monoclonal antibody to human SP-10 inhibits in vitro the binding of human sperm to hamster oolemma but not to human Zona pellucida. Biol Reprod. 2000;62(5):1201–8.
22. Goyal S, Manivannan B, Kumraj GR, Ansari AS, Lohiya NK. Evaluation of efficacy and safety of recombinant sperm-specific contraceptive vaccine in albino mice. Am. J. Reprod. Immunol. 2013;69(5):495–508.
23. Zheng L, Wang H, Li B, Zeng X. Sperm-specific ion channels: targets holding the most potential for male contraceptives in development. Contraception 2013;88(4):485–92.
24. Nazari M, Mirshahi M, Mowla SJ, Bamdad T, Sarikhani S. Investigation in vitro expression of CatSper sub fragment followed by production of polyclonal antibody: potential candidate for the next generation of non hormonal contraceptive. Cell J. 2012;14(3):215–24.
25. Li HG, Ding XF, Guo CC, Guan HT, Xiong CL. Immunization of male mice with B-cell epitopes in transmembrane domains of CatSper1 inhibits fertility. Fertil. Steril. 2012;97(2):445–52.
26. Howes L, Jones R. Interactions between zona pellucida glycoproteins and sperm proacrosin/acrosin during fertilization. J. Reprod. Immunol. 2002;53(1-2):181–92.
27. Garcia L, Veiga MF, Lustig L, Vazquez-Levin MH, Veaute C. DNA immunization against proacrosin impairs fertility in male mice. Am. J. Reprod. Immunol. 2012;68(1):56–67.
28. Naz RK. Molecular and immunological characteristics of sperm antigens involved in egg binding. J. Reprod. Immunol. 2002;53(1-2):13–23.
29. Wolkowicz MJ, Shetty J, Westbrook A, Klotz K, Jayes F, Mandal A, Flickinger CJ, Herr JC. Equatorial segment protein defines a discrete acrosomal subcompartment persisting throughout acrosomal biogenesis. Biol. Reprod. 2003;69(3):735–45.
30. Wolkowicz MJ, Digilio L, Klotz K, Shetty J, Flickinger CJ, Herr JC. Equatorial segment protein (ESP) is a human alloantigen involved in sperm–egg binding and fusion. J. Androl. 2008;29(3):272–82.
31. Inoue N, Ikawa M, Isotani A, Okabe M. The immunoglobulin superfamily protein Izumo is required for sperm to fuse with eggs. Nature 2005;434(7030):234–8.
32. Clark S, Naz RK. Presence and incidence of izumo antibodies in sera of immunoinfertile women and men. Am. J. Reprod. Immunol. 2013;69(3):256–63.

33. Ellerman DA, Pei JM, Gupta S, Snell WJ, Myles D, Primakoff P. Izumo is part of a multiprotein family whose members form large complexes on mammalian sperm. Mol. Reprod. Dev. 2009;76(12):1188–99.

34. Kim E, Kim JS, Lee Y, Song BS, Sim BW, Kim SU, Saitoh T, Yazawa H, Nunoya T, Chang KT. Molecular cloning, characterization of porcine IZUMO1, an IgSF family member. Reprod. Domest. Anim. 2013;48(1):90–7.

35. Mandal A, Klotz KL, Shetty J, Jayes FL, Wolkowicz MJ, Bolling LC, Coonrod SA, Black MB, Diekman AB, Haystead TA, Flickinger CJ, Herr JC. SLLP1, a unique, intra-acrosomal, non-bacteriolytic, c lysozyme-like protein of human spermatozoa. Biol. Reprod. 2003;68(5):1525–37.

36. Herrero MB, Mandal A, Digilio LC, Coonrod SA, Maier B, Herr JC. Mouse SLLP1, a sperm lysozyme-like protein involved in sperm–egg binding and fertilization. Dev. Biol. 2005;284(1):126–42.

37. Sachdev M, Mandal A, Mulders S, Digilio LC, Panneerdoss S, Suryavathi V, Pires E, Klotz KL, Hermens L, Herrero MB, Flickinger CJ, van Duin M, Herr JC. Oocyte specific oolemmal SAS1B involved in sperm binding through intra-acrosomal SLLP1 during fertilization. Dev. Biol. 2012;363(1):40–51.

38. Khan SA, Jadhav SV, Suryawanshi AR, Bhonde GS, Gajbhiye RK, Khole VV. Evaluation of contraceptive potential of a novel epididymal sperm protein SFP2 in a mouse model. Am. J. Reprod. Immunol. 2011;66(3):185–98.

39. Chen Y, Zhang D, Xin N, Xiong YZ, Chen P, Li B, Tu XD, Lan FH. Construction of sperm-specific lactate dehydrogenase DNA vaccine and experimental study of its immunocontraceptive effect on mice. Sci. China C Life Sci. 2008;51(4):308–16.

40. Hinton BT, Cooper TG. The epididymis as a target for male contraceptive development. In: Habenicht U-F, Aitken RJ, editors. The Epididymis as a Target for Male Contraceptive Development. Berling: Springer; 2010. p. 117–37.

41. Silva EJ, Patrao MT, Tsuruta JK, O'Rand MG, Avellar MC. Epididymal protease inhibitor (EPPIN) is differentially expressed in the male rat reproductive tract and immunolocalized in maturing spermatozoa. Mol. Reprod. Dev. 2012;79(12):832–42.

42. O'Rand MG, Widgren EE, Wang Z, Richardson RT. Eppin: an epididymal protease inhibitor and a target for male contraception. Soc. Reprod. Fertil. Suppl. 2007;63:445–53.

43. O'Rand MG, Widgren EE, Hamil KG, Silva EJ, Richardson RT. Epididymal protein targets: a brief history of the development of epididymal protease inhibitor as a contraceptive. J. Androl. 2011;32(6):698–704.

44. Chen Z, He W, Wu Y, Yan P, He H, Zhang J, Yang X, Shen Z, Liang Z, Li J. A highly specific antibody response after protein prime-peptide boost immunization with Eppin/B-cell epitope in mice. Hum. Vaccin. 2011;7(8):849–55.

45. Robert M, Gagnon C. Sperm motility inhibitor from human seminal plasma: association with semen coagulum. Mol. Hum. Reprod. 1995;1(6):292–7.

46. Naz RK, Engle A, None R. Gene knockouts that affect male fertility: novel targets for contraception. Front. Biosci. 2009;14:3994–4007.

47. Hedger MP. Immunophysiology and pathology of inflammation in the testis and epididymis. J. Androl. 2011;32(6):625–40.

48. Mital P, Hinton BT, Dufour JM. The blood-testis and blood-epididymis barriers are more than just their tight junctions. Biol. Reprod. 2011;84(5):851–8.

49. Rajapaksa TE, Lo DD. Microencapsulation of vaccine antigens and adjuvants for mucosal targeting. Curr. Immunol. Rev. 2010;6(1):29–37.

50. Krishna SV, Ashok V, Chatterjee A. A review on vaginal drug delivery systems. Int. J. Biol. Pharm. Allied Sci. 2012;1(2):152–67.

51. Gebril A, Alsaadi M, Acevedo R, Mullen AB, Ferro VA. Optimizing efficacy of mucosal vaccines. Expert Rev. Vaccines 2012;11(9):1139–55.

52. Serrano-Pozo A, Frosch MP, Masliah E, Hyman BT. Neuropathological alterations in Alzheimer disease. Cold Spring Harb. Perspect. Med. 2011;1(1):a006189.

53. Schenk D, Barbour R, Dunn W, Gordon G, Grajeda H, Guido T, Hu K, Huang J, Johnson-Wood K, Khan K, et al. Immunization with amyloid-beta attenuates Alzheimer-disease-like pathology in the PDAPP mouse. Nature 1999;400(6740):173–7.

54. Schenk D, Basi GS, Pangalos MN. Treatment strategies targeting amyloid beta-protein. Cold Spring Harb. Perspect. Med. 2012;2(9):a006387.

55. Monsonego A, Zota V, Karni A, Krieger JI, Bar-Or A, Bitan G, Budson AE, Sperling R, Selkoe DJ, Weiner HL. Increased T cell reactivity to amyloid beta protein in older humans and patients with Alzheimer disease. J. Clin Invest. 2003;112(3):415–22.

56. Qu B, Rosenberg RN, Li L, Boyer PJ, Johnston SA. Gene vaccination to bias the immune response to amyloid-beta peptide as therapy for Alzheimer disease. Arch. Neurol. 2004;61(12):1859–64.

57. Panza F, Frisardi V, Solfrizzi V, Imbimbo BP, Logroscino G, Santamato A, Greco A, Seripa D, Pilotto A. Immunotherapy for Alzheimer's disease: from anti-beta-amyloid to tau-based immunization strategies. Immunotherapy 2012;4(2):213–38.

58. Troquier L, Caillierez R, Burnouf S, Fernandez-Gomez FJ, Grosjean ME, Zommer N, Sergeant N, Schraen-Maschke S, Blum D, Buee L. Targeting phospho-Ser422 by active Tau Immunotherapy in the THYTau22 mouse model: a suitable therapeutic approach. Curr. Alzheimer Res. 2012;9(4):397–405.

59. Oddo S, Vasilevko V, Caccamo A, Kitazawa M, Cribbs DH, LaFerla FM. Reduction of soluble Abeta and tau, but not soluble Abeta alone, ameliorates cognitive decline in transgenic mice with plaques and tangles. J. Biol. Chem. 2006;281(51):39413–23.

60. Schneeberger A, Mandler M, Mattner F, Schmidt W. Vaccination for Parkinson's disease. Parkinsonism Relat. Disord. 2012;18(Suppl. 1):S11–3.

61. Raupach T, Hoogsteder PH, Onno van Schayck CP. Nicotine vaccines to assist with smoking cessation: current status of research. Drugs 2012;72(4):e1–16.

62. Kosten T, Domingo C, Orson F, Kinsey B. Vaccines against stimulants: cocaine and methamphetamine. Br. J. Clin. Pharmacol. 2013;77(2):368–74.

63. Stowe GN, Schlosburg JE, Vendruscolo LF, Edwards S, Misra KK, Schulteis G, Zakhari JS, Koob GF, Janda KD. Developing a vaccine against multiple psychoactive targets: a case study of heroin. CNS Neurol. Disord. Drug Targets 2011;10(8):865–75.

64. McLemore GL, Lewis T, Jones CH, Gauda EB. Novel pharmacotherapeutic strategies for treatment of opioid-induced neonatal abstinence syndrome. Semin. Fetal Neonatal. Med. 2013;18(1):35–41.

65. Kosten TR, Domingo CB. Can you vaccinate against substance abuse? Expert Opin. Biol. Ther. 2013;13(8):1093–7.

66. Doll R, Peto R, Boreham J, Sutherland I. Mortality in relation to smoking: 50 years' observations on male British doctors. BMJ 2004;328(7455):1519.

67. McLellan AT, Lewis DC, O'Brien CP, Kleber HD. Drug dependence, a chronic medical illness: implications for treatment, insurance, and outcomes evaluation. JAMA 2000;284(13):1689–95.

68. Caponnetto P, Russo C, Polosa R. Smoking cessation: present status and future perspectives. Curr. Opin. Pharmacol. 2012;12(3):229–37.

69. Hartmann-Boyce, J., Cahill, K., Hatsukami, D., and Cornuz, J. Nicotine vaccines for smoking cessation. *Cochrane Database Syst. Rev.* 2012; **8:** CD007072.

70. Fahim RE, Kessler PD, Kalnik MW. Therapeutic vaccines against tobacco addiction. Expert Rev. Vaccines 2013;12(3):333–42.

71. Schlosburg JE, Vendruscolo LF, Bremer PT, Lockner JW, Wade CL, Nunes AAK, Stowe GN, Edwards S, Janda KD, Koob GF. Dynamic vaccine blocks relapse to compulsive intake of heroin. Proc. Natl. Acad. Sci. U.S.A. 2013;110(22):9036–41.

72. Schwartz M, Baruch K. Vaccine for the mind: Immunity against self at the choroid plexus for erasing biochemical consequences of stressful episodes. Hum. Vaccin. Immunother. 2012;8(10):1465–8.

73. Capuron L, Miller AH. Cytokines and psychopathology: lessons from interferon-alpha. Biol. Psychiatry 2004;56(11):819–24.

74. Capuron L, Ravaud A, Miller AH, Dantzer R. Baseline mood and psychosocial characteristics of patients developing depressive symptoms during interleukin-2 and/or interferon-alpha cancer therapy. Brain Behav. Immun. 2004;18(3):205–13.

75. Lowry CA, Hollis JH, de Vries A, Pan B, Brunet LR, Hunt JR, Paton JF, van Kampen E, Knight DM, Evans AK, Rook GA, Lightman SL. Identification of an immune-responsive mesolimbocortical serotonergic system: potential role in regulation of emotional behavior. Neuroscience 2007;146(2):756–72.

76. Glaser R, Robles TF, Sheridan J, Malarkey WB, Kiecolt-Glaser JK. Mild depressive symptoms are associated with amplified and prolonged inflammatory responses after influenza virus vaccination in older adults. Arch. Gen. Psychiatry 2003;60(10):1009–14.

77. Kiecolt-Glaser JK, Glaser R, Gravenstein S, Malarkey WB, Sheridan J. Chronic stress alters the immune response to influenza virus vaccine in older adults. Proc. Natl. Acad. Sci. U.S.A. 1996;93(7):3043–7.

78. Rook GA, Raison CL, Lowry CA. Can we vaccinate against depression? Drug Discov. Today 2012;17(9-10):451–8.

79. McCarty MF, Al-Harbi SA. Vaccination with heat-shocked mononuclear cells as a strategy for treating neurodegenerative disorders driven by microglial inflammation. Med. Hypotheses 2013;81(5):773–6.

80. Sessums LL, Zembrzuska H, Jackson JL. Does this patient have medical decision-making capacity? JAMA 2011;306(4):420–7.

81. Taylor JS, DeMers SM, Vig EK, Borson S. The disappearing subject: exclusion of people with cognitive impairment and dementia from geriatrics research. J. Am. Geriatr. Soc. 2012;60(3):413–9.

82. Kim SYH, Kim HM, Knopman DS, De Vries R, Damschroder L, Appelbaum PS. Effect of public deliberation on attitudes toward surrogate consent for dementia research. Neurology 2011;77(24):2097–104.

83. Kim SYH, Kim HM, Ryan KA, Appelbaum PS, Knopman DS, Damschroder L, De Vries R. How important is 'accuracy' of surrogate decision-making for research participation? PLoS ONE 2013;8(1):e54790.

84. Lev O, Wilfond BS, McBride CM. Enhancing children against unhealthy behaviors—an ethical and policy assessment of using a nicotine vaccine. Public Health Ethics 2013;6(2):197–206.

85. Matzinger P. The danger model: a renewed sense of self. Science 2002;296(5566):301–5.

86. Akkoc T, Akdis M, Akdis CA. Update in the mechanisms of allergen-specific immunotheraphy. Allergy Asthma Immunol. Res. 2011;3(1):11–20.

87. Walter G, Holgate S, Pawankar R, Lockey R. WAO White Book on Allergy 2011-2012: Executive Summary. Milwaukee, WI: World Allergy Organization; 2011.

88. Martino DJ, Prescott SL. Silent mysteries: epigenetic paradigms could hold the key to conquering the epidemic of allergy and immune disease. Allergy 2010;65(1):7–15.

89. Warner JO, Kaliner MA, Crisci CD, Del Giacco S, Frew AJ, Liu GH, Maspero J, Moon HB, Nakagawa T, Potter PC, Rosenwasser LJ, Singh AB, Valovirta E, Van Cauwenberge P. Allergy practice worldwide: a report by the World Allergy Organization Specialty and Training Council. Int. Arch. Allergy Immunol. 2006;139(2):166–74.

90. Papadopoulos NG, Agache I, Bavbek S, Bilo BM, Braido F, Cardona V, Custovic A, Demonchy J, Demoly P, Eigenmann P, et al. Research needs in allergy: an EAACI position paper, in collaboration with EFA. Clin. Transl. Allergy 2012;2(1):21.

91. Valenta R. Biochemistry of allergens and recombinant allergens. 2nd ed. In: Kay AB, Kaplan AP, Bousquet J, Holt PG, editors. Allergy and Allergic Diseases, Vol. 1. Oxford: Wiley-Blackwell; 2009. p. 895–912.

92. Galli SJ, Tsai M, Piliponsky AM. The development of allergic inflammation. Nature 2008;454(7203):445–54.

93. Niederberger V, Ring J, Rakoski J, Jager S, Spitzauer S, Valent P, Horak F, Kundi M, Valenta R. Antigens drive memory IgE responses in human allergy via the nasal mucosa. Int. Arch. Allergy Immunol. 2007;142(2):133–44.

94. Rebouças JDS, Irache JM, Camacho AI, Esparza I, Del Pozo V, Sanz ML, Ferrer M, Gamazo C. Development of poly(anhydride) nanoparticles loaded with peanut proteins: the influence of preparation method on the immunogenic properties. Eur. J. Pharm. Biopharm. 2012;82(2):241–9.

95. Larche M, Akdis CA, Valenta R. Immunological mechanisms of allergen-specific immunotherapy. Nat. Rev. Immunol. 2006;6(10):761–71.

96. Frew AJ. Allergen immunotherapy. J. Allergy Clin. Immunol. 2010;125(2, Suppl. 2):S306–13.

97. van Neerven RJ, Knol EF, Ejrnaes A, Wurtzen PA. IgE-mediated allergen presentation and blocking antibodies: regulation of T-cell activation in allergy. Int. Arch. Allergy Immunol. 2006;141(2):119–29.

98. Valenta R, Campana R, Marth K, van Hage M. Allergen-specific immunotherapy: from therapeutic vaccines to prophylactic approaches. J. Intern. Med. 2012;272(2):144–57.

99. Akdis CA. Therapies for allergic inflammation: refining strategies to induce tolerance. Nat. Med. 2012;18(5):736–49.

100. Soyer OU, Akdis M, Ring J, Behrendt H, Crameri R, Lauener R, Akdis CA. Mechanisms of peripheral tolerance to allergens. Allergy 2013;68(2):161–70.

101. Bernstein DI, Wanner M, Borish L, Liss GM. Twelve-year survey of fatal reactions to allergen injections and skin testing: 1990-2001. J. Allergy Clin. Immunol. 2004;113(6):1129–36.

102. Linhart B, Valenta R. Mechanisms underlying allergy vaccination with recombinant hypoallergenic allergen derivatives. Vaccine 2012;30(29):4328–35.

103. Valenta R, Ferreira F, Focke-Tejkl M, Linhart B, Niederberger V, Swoboda I, Vrtala S. From allergen genes to allergy vaccines. Annu. Rev. Immunol. 2010;28:211–41.

104. Oldfield WL, Larche M, Kay AB. Effect of T-cell peptides derived from Fel d 1 on allergic reactions and cytokine production in patients sensitive to cats: a randomised controlled trial. Lancet 2002;360(9326):47–53.

III. NOVEL APPROACHES FOR VACCINES

105. Muller U, Akdis CA, Fricker M, Akdis M, Blesken T, Bettens F, Blaser K. Successful immunotherapy with T-cell epitope peptides of bee venom phospholipase A2 induces specific T-cell anergy in patients allergic to bee venom. J. Allergy Clin. Immunol. 1998;101(6, Pt. 1):747–54.

106. Focke M, Swoboda I, Marth K, Valenta R. Developments in allergen-specific immunotherapy: from allergen extracts to allergy vaccines bypassing allergen-specific immunoglobulin E and T cell reactivity. Clin. Exp. Allergy 2010;40(3):385–97.

107. Reisinger J, Horak F, Pauli G, van Hage M, Cromwell O, Konig F, Valenta R, Niederberger V. Allergen-specific nasal IgG antibodies induced by vaccination with genetically modified allergens are associated with reduced nasal allergen sensitivity. J. Allergy Clin. Immunol. 2005;116(2):347–54.

108. Pauli G, Larsen TH, Rak S, Horak F, Pastorello E, Valenta R, Purohit A, Arvidsson M, Kavina A, Schroeder JW, Mothes N, Spitzauer S, Montagut A, Galvain S, Melac M, Andre C, Poulsen LK, Malling HJ. Efficacy of recombinant birch pollen vaccine for the treatment of birch-allergic rhinoconjunctivitis. J. Allergy Clin. Immunol. 2008;122(5):951–60.

109. Huang CF, Chu CH, Wu CC, Chang ZN, Chue FL, Peng HJ. Induction of specific Th1 responses and suppression of IgE antibody formation by vaccination with plasmid DNA encoding Cyn d 1. Int Arch Allergy Immunol. 2012;158(2):142–50.

110. Hochreiter R, Stepanoska T, Ferreira F, Valenta R, Vrtala S, Thalhamer J, Hartl A. Prevention of allergen-specific IgE production and suppression of an established Th2–type response by immunization with DNA encoding hypoallergenic allergen derivatives of Bet v 1, the major birch-pollen allergen. Eur. J. Immunol. 2003;33(6): 1667–76.

111. Roesler E, Weiss R, Weinberger EE, Fruehwirth A, Stoecklinger A, Mostbock S, Ferreira F, Thalhamer J, Scheiblhofer S. Immunize and disappear-safety-optimized mRNA vaccination with a panel of 29 allergens. J. Allergy Clin. Immunol. 2009;124(5):1070–7.

112. Weiss R, Scheiblhofer S, Roesler E, Weinberger E, Thalhamer J. mRNA vaccination as a safe approach for specific protection from type I allergy. Expert Rev. Vaccines 2012;11(1):55–67.

113. Reed SG, Bertholet S, Coler RN, Friede M. New horizons in adjuvants for vaccine development. Trends Immunol. 2009;30(1):23–32.

114. EMA. *EMA 2004: Guideline on Adjuvants in Vaccines*, EMEA/CPMP/VEG/17/03/2004v5/Consultation. London: European Medicines Agency.

115. Song DH, Lee JO. Sensing of microbial molecular patterns by Toll-like receptors. Immunol. Rev. 2012;250(1): 216–29.

116. Zhu J, Yamane H, Paul WE. Differentiation of effector CD4 T cell populations (*). Annu. Rev. Immunol. 2010;28:445–89.

117. Creticos PS, Schroeder JT, Hamilton RG, Balcer-Whaley SL, Khattignavong AP, Lindblad R, Li H, Coffman R, Seyfert V, Eiden JJ, Broide D. Immunotherapy with a ragweed-toll-like receptor 9 agonist vaccine for allergic rhinitis. N. Engl. J. Med. 2006;355(14):1445–55.

118. Mothes N, Heinzkill M, Drachenberg KJ, Sperr WR, Krauth MT, Majlesi Y, Semper H, Valent P, Niederberger V, Kraft D, Valenta R. Allergen-specific immunotherapy with a monophosphoryl lipid A-adjuvanted vaccine: reduced seasonally boosted immunoglobulin E production and inhibition of basophil histamine release by therapy-induced blocking antibodies. Clin. Exp. Allergy 2003;33(9):1198–208.

119. Patel P, Salapatek AM. Pollinex Quattro: a novel and well-tolerated, ultra short-course allergy vaccine. Expert Rev. Vaccines 2006;5(5):617–29.

120. Drachenberg KJ, Wheeler AW, Stuebner P, Horak F. A well-tolerated grass pollen-specific allergy vaccine containing a novel adjuvant, monophosphoryl lipid A, reduces allergic symptoms after only four preseasonal injections. Allergy 2001;56(6):498–505.

121. Perez O, Lastre M, Cabrera O, del Campo J, Bracho G, Cuello M, Balboa J, Acevedo R, Zayas C, Gil D, Mora N, Gonzalez D, Perez R, Gonzalez E, Barbera R, Fajardo EM, Sierra G, Solis RL, Campa C. New vaccines require potent adjuvants like AFPL1 and AFCo1. Scand. J. Immunol. 2007;66(2-3):271–7.

122. Lastre M, Perez O, Labrada A, Bidot I, Perez J, Bracho G, del Campo J, Perez D, Facenda E, Zayas C, Rodriguez C, Sierra G. Bacterial derived proteoliposome for allergy vaccines. Vaccine 2006;24(Suppl. 2). S2-34–5.

123. RPCEC. Inmunoterapia Subcutánea con PROLINEM-Asma-Adultos-Fase I. Subcutaneous immunotherapy with PROLINEM clinical trial Phase I, Adults Cuban Public Registry of Clinical Trials; 2013.

124. Eisenbarth SC, Colegio OR, O'Connor W, Sutterwala FS, Flavell RA. Crucial role for the Nalp3 inflammasome in the immunostimulatory properties of aluminium adjuvants. Nature 2008;453(7198):1122–6.

125. Moschos SA, Bramwell VW, Somavarapu S, Alpar HO. Modulating the adjuvanticity of alum by co-administration of muramyl di-peptide (MDP) or Quil-A. Vaccine 2006;24(8):1081–6.
126. Baldrick P, Richardson D, Wheeler AW. Review of L-tyrosine confirming its safe human use as an adjuvant. J. Appl. Toxicol. 2002;22(5):333–44.
127. Scholl I, Weissenbock A, Forster-Waldl E, Untersmayr E, Walter F, Willheim M, Boltz-Nitulescu G, Scheiner O, Gabor F, Jensen-Jarolim E. Allergen-loaded biodegradable poly(D,L-lactic-co-glycolic) acid nanoparticles down-regulate an ongoing Th2 response in the BALB/c mouse model. Clin. Exp. Allergy 2004;34(2):315–21.
128. Scholl I, Kopp T, Bohle B, Jensen-Jarolim E. Biodegradable PLGA particles for improved systemic and mucosal treatment of type I allergy. Immunol. Allergy Clin. North Am. 2006;26(2):349–64. ix.
129. Gomez S, Gamazo C, Roman BS, Ferrer M, Sanz ML, Irache JM. Gantrez AN nanoparticles as an adjuvant for oral immunotherapy with allergens. Vaccine 2007;25(29):5263–71.
130. Morris G, Kok S, Harding S, Adams G. Polysaccharide drug delivery systems based on pectin and chitosan. Biotechnol. Genet. Eng. Rev. 2010;27:257–84.
131. Roy K, Mao HQ, Huang SK, Leong KW. Oral gene delivery with chitosan—DNA nanoparticles generates immunologic protection in a murine model of peanut allergy. Nat. Med. 1999;5(4):387–91.
132. Rodriguez T, Perez O, Menager N, Ugrinovic S, Bracho G, Mastroeni P. Interactions of proteoliposomes from serogroup B Neisseria meningitidis with bone marrow-derived dendritic cells and macrophages: adjuvant effects and antigen delivery. Vaccine 2005;23(10):1312–21.
133. Storni T, Ruedl C, Schwarz K, Schwendener RA, Renner WA, Bachmann MF. Nonmethylated CG motifs packaged into virus-like particles induce protective cytotoxic T cell responses in the absence of systemic side effects. J. Immunol. 2004;172(3):1777–85.
134. Vekemans J, Ballou WR. *Plasmodium falciparum* malaria vaccines in development. Expert Rev. Vaccines 2008;7(2):223–40.
135. Kundig TM, Senti G, Schnetzler G, Wolf C, Prinz Vavricka BM, Fulurija A, Hennecke F, Sladko K, Jennings GT, Bachmann MF. Der 1 peptide on virus-like particles is safe and highly immunogenic in healthy adults. J. Allergy Clin. Immunol. 2006;117(6):1470–6.
136. Schmitz N, Dietmeier K, Bauer M, Maudrich M, Utzinger S, Muntwiler S, Saudan P, Bachmann MF. Displaying Fel d1 on virus-like particles prevents reactogenicity despite greatly enhanced immunogenicity: a novel therapy for cat allergy. J. Exp. Med. 2009;206(9):1941–55.
137. Klimek L, Schendzielorz P, Mueller P, Saudan P, Willers J. Immunotherapy of allergic rhinitis: new therapeutic opportunities with virus-like particles filled with CpG motifs. Am. J. Rhinol. Allergy 2013;27(3):206–12.
138. Grönlund H, Gafvelin G. Recombinant Bet v 1 vaccine for treatment of allergy to birch pollen. Hum. Vaccin. 2010;6(12):970–7.
139. Senna GE, Calderon M, Milani M. Allergy immunotherapy tablet: Grazax® for the treatment of grass pollen allergy. Exp. Rev. Clin. Immunol. 2011;7(1):21–7.
140. Frati F, Scurati S, Puccinelli P, David M, Hilaire C, Capecce M, Marcucci F, Incorvaia C. Development of a sublingual allergy vaccine for grass pollinosis. Drug Des. Devel. Ther. 2010;4:99–105.
141. Nelson H, Lehmann L, Blaiss MS. Treatment of seasonal allergic rhinoconjunctivitis with a once-daily SQ-standardized grass allergy immunotherapy tablet. Curr. Med. Res. Opin. 2012;28(6):1043–51.
142. Reich K, Gessner C, Kroker A, Schwab JA, Pohl W, Villesen H, Wüstenberg E, Emminger W. Immunologic effects and tolerability profile of in-season initiation of a standardized-quality grass allergy immunotherapy tablet: a Phase III, multicenter, randomized, double-blind, placebo-controlled trial in adults with grass pollen-induced rhinoconjunctivitis. Clin. Ther. 2011;33(7):828–40.
143. Murphy K, Gawchik S, Bernstein D, Andersen J, Rud Pedersen M. A phase 3 trial assessing the efficacy and safety of grass allergy immunotherapy tablet in subjects with grass pollen-induced allergic rhinitis with or without conjunctivitis, with or without asthma. J. Negat. Results Biomed. 2013;12(1):10.
144. Di Bona D, Plaia A, Leto-Barone MS, La Piana S, Di Lorenzo G. Efficacy of subcutaneous and sublingual immunotherapy with grass allergens for seasonal allergic rhinitis: a meta-analysis-based comparison. J. Allergy Clin. Immunol. 2012;130(5):1097–107.
145. Passalacqua G, Durham SR. Allergic rhinitis and its impact on asthma update: allergen immunotherapy. J. Allergy Clin. Immunol. 2007;119(4):881–91.
146. Samsom JN, van Berkel LA, van Helvoort JM, Unger WW, Jansen W, Thepen T, Mebius RE, Verbeek SS, Kraal G. Fc gamma RIIB regulates nasal and oral tolerance: a role for dendritic cells. J. Immunol. 2005;174(9): 5279–87.

147. van Helvoort JM, Samsom JN, Chantry D, Jansen W, Schadee-Eestermans I, Thepen T, Mebius RE, Kraal G. Preferential expression of IgG2b in nose draining cervical lymph nodes and its putative role in mucosal tolerance induction. Allergy 2004;59(11):1211–8.

148. Varshney P, Jones SM, Scurlock AM, Perry TT, Kemper A, Steele P, Hiegel A, Kamilaris J, Carlisle S, Yue X, Kulis M, Pons L, Vickery B, Burks AW. A randomized controlled study of peanut oral immunotherapy: clinical desensitization and modulation of the allergic response. J. Allergy Clin. Immunol. 2011;127(3):654–60.

149. Brozek JL, Terracciano L, Hsu J, Kreis J, Compalati E, Santesso N, Fiocchi A, Schunemann HJ. Oral immunotherapy for IgE-mediated cow's milk allergy: a systematic review and meta-analysis. Clin. Exp. Allergy 2012;42(3):363–74.

150. Suzuki K, Kaminuma O, Yang L, Takai T, Mori A, Umezu-Goto M, Ohtomo T, Ohmachi Y, Noda Y, Hirose S, Okumura K, Ogawa H, Takada K, Hirasawa M, Hiroi T, Takaiwa F. Prevention of allergic asthma by vaccination with transgenic rice seed expressing mite allergen: induction of allergen-specific oral tolerance without bystander suppression. Plant Biotechnol. J. 2011;9(9):982–90.

151. Suzuki K, Kaminuma O, Yang L, Motoi Y, Takai T, Ichikawa S, Okumura K, Ogawa H, Mori A, Takaiwa F, Hiroi T. Development of transgenic rice expressing mite antigen for a new concept of immunotherapy. Int. Arch. Allergy Immunol. 2009;149(Suppl. 1):21–4.

152. Mondoulet L, Dioszeghy V, Ligouis M, Dhelft V, Puteaux E, Dupont C, Benhamou P-H. Epicutaneous immunotherapy compared with sublingual immunotherapy in mice sensitized to pollen (*Phleum pratense*). ISRN Allergy 2012;2012:375735.

153. Senti G, von Moos S, Tay F, Graf N, Sonderegger T, Johansen P, Kündig TM. Epicutaneous allergen-specific immunotherapy ameliorates grass pollen-induced rhinoconjunctivitis: a double-blind, placebo-controlled dose escalation study. J. Allergy Clin Immunol. 2012;129(1):128–35.

154. Cox L, Compalati E, Kundig T, Larche M. New directions in immunotherapy. Curr. Allergy Asthma Rep. 2013;13(2):178–95.

155. Takeda K, Miyahara N, Kodama T, Taube C, Balhorn A, Dakhama A, Kitamura K, Hirano A, Tanimoto M, Gelfand EW. S-carboxymethylcysteine normalises airway responsiveness in sensitised and challenged mice. Eur. Respir. J. 2005;26(4):577–85.

156. Delany I, Rappuoli R, Seib KL. Vaccines, reverse vaccinology, and bacterial pathogenesis. Cold Spring Harb. Perspect. Med. 2013;3(5):a012476.

157. Kuroda D, Shirai H, Jacobson MP, Nakamura H. Computer-aided antibody design. Protein Eng. Des. Sel. 2012;25(10):507–21.

158. Volkin DB, Burke CJ, Sanyal G, Middaugh CR. Analysis of vaccine stability. Dev. Biol. Stand. 1996;87:135–42.

159. Petros RA, DeSimone JM. Strategies in the design of nanoparticles for therapeutic applications. Nat. Rev. Drug Discov. 2010;9(8):615–27.

160. Quinn AS, Rand JH, Wu XX, Taatjes DJ. Viewing dynamic interactions of proteins and a model lipid membrane with atomic force microscopy. Methods Mol Biol. 2013;931:259–93.

161. Grama C, Venkatpurwar V, Lamprou D, Ravi Kumar MNV. Towards scale-up and regulatory shelf-stability testing of curcumin encapsulated polyester nanoparticles. Drug Deliv. Transl. Res. 2013;3(3):286–93.

162. Lamprou DA, Venkatpurwar V, Kumar MNVR. Atomic force microscopy images label-free, drug encapsulated nanoparticles *in vivo* and detects difference in tissue mechanical properties of treated and untreated: a tip for nanotoxicology. PLoS ONE 2013;8(5):e64490.

163. Couston RG, Lamprou DA, Uddin S, van der Walle CF. Interaction and destabilization of a monoclonal antibody and albumin to surfaces of varying functionality and hydrophobicity. Int. J. Pharm. 2012;438(1-2):71–80.

164. Maddux NR, Joshi SB, Volkin DB, Ralston JP, Middaugh CR. Multidimensional methods for the formulation of biopharmaceuticals and vaccines. J. Pharm Sci. June 6, 2011. Epub ahead of print.

165. Le Tallec D, Doucet D, Elouahabi A, Harvengt P, Deschuyteneer M, Deschamps M. Cervarix, the GSK HPV-16/HPV-18 AS04-adjuvanted cervical cancer vaccine, demonstrates stability upon long-term storage and under simulated cold chain break conditions. Hum. Vaccin. 2009;5(7):467–74.

166. Jelesarov I, Bosshard HR. Isothermal titration calorimetry and differential scanning calorimetry as complementary tools to investigate the energetics of biomolecular recognition. J. Mol Recognit. 1999;12(1):3–18.

167. Xu Q, Klees J, Teyral J, Capen R, Huang M, Sturgess AW, Hennessey JP Jr, Washabaugh M, Sitrin R, Abeygunawardana C. Quantitative nuclear magnetic resonance analysis and characterization of the derivatized Haemophilus influenzae type b polysaccharide intermediate for PedvaxHIB. Anal. Biochem. 2005;337(2):235–45.

168. Hearty S, Conroy PJ, Ayyar BV, Byrne B, O'Kennedy R. Surface plasmon resonance for vaccine design and efficacy studies: recent applications and future trends. Expert Rev. Vaccines 2010;9(6):645–64.

169. Chesko J, Kazzaz J, Ugozzoli M, Singh M, O'Hagan DT, Madden C, Perkins M, Patel N. Characterization of antigens adsorbed to anionic PLG microparticles by XPS and TOF-SIMS. J. Pharm. Sci. 2008;97(4): 1443–53.

170. Li B, Jia Z, Wang T, Wang W, Zhang C, Chen P, Ma K, Zhou C. Interaction of Wnt/beta-catenin and notch signaling in the early stage of cardiac differentiation of P19CL6 cells. J. Cell Biochem. 2012;113(2):629–39.

171. Lv ZM, Wang M, Xu C. Antifertility characteristics of the N-terminal region of mouse equatorial segment protein. Anat. Rec. (Hoboken) 2010;293(1):171–81.

172. Goldberg E, Herr J. LDH-C4 as a contraceptive vaccine. In: Gupta S, editor. LDH-C4 as a Contraceptive Vaccine. Amsterdam: Springer; 1999. p. 309–15.

173. Ellerman DA, Cohen DJ, Munoz MW, Da Ros VG, Ernesto JI, Tollner TL, Cuasnicu PS. Immunologic behavior of human cysteine-rich secretory protein 1 (hCRISP1) in primates: prospects for immunocontraception. Fertil. Steril. 2010;93(8):2551–6.

174. Wang M, Lv ZM, Shi JL, Hu YQ, Xu C. Immunocontraceptive potential of the Ig-like domain of Izumo. Mol. Reprod. Dev. 2009;76(8):794–801.

175. Primakoff P, Lathrop W, Woolman L, Cowan A, Myles D. Fully effective contraception in male and female guinea pigs immunized with the sperm protein PH-20. Nature 1988;335(6190):543–6.

176. Parry S, Wong NK, Easton RL, Panico M, Haslam SM, Morris HR, Anderson P, Klotz KL, Herr JC, Diekman AB, Dell A. The sperm agglutination antigen-1 (SAGA-1) glycoforms of CD52 are O-glycosylated. Glycobiology 2007;17(10):1120–6.

177. Shetty J, Wolkowicz MJ, Digilio LC, Klotz KL, Jayes FL, Diekman AB, Westbrook VA, Farris EM, Hao Z, Coonrod SA, Flickinger CJ, Herr JC. SAMP14, a novel, acrosomal membrane-associated, glycosylphosphatidylinositol-anchored member of the Ly-6/urokinase-type plasminogen activator receptor superfamily with a role in sperm–egg interaction. J. Biol. Chem. 2003;278(33):30506–15.

178. Shankar S, Mohapatra B, Suri A. Cloning of a novel human testis mRNA specifically expressed in testicular haploid germ cells, having unique palindromic sequences and encoding a leucine zipper dimerization motif. Biochem. Biophys. Res. Commun. 1998;243(2):561–5.

179. Lea IA, van Lierop MJC, Widgren EE, Grootenhuis A, Wen Y, van Duin M, O'Rand MG. A chimeric sperm peptide induces antibodies and strain-specific reversible infertility in mice. Biol. Reprod. 1998;59(3):527–36.

180. Herr JC, Flickinger CJ, Homyk M, Klotz K, John E. Biochemical and morphological characterization of the intraacrosomal antigen Sp-10 from human sperm. Biol. Reprod. 1990;42(1):181–93.

181. Santhanam R, Naz RK. Novel human testis-specific cDNA: molecular cloning, expression and immunobiological effects of the recombinant protein. Mol. Reprod. Dev. 2001;60(1):1–12.

182. Bayer AJ, Bullock R, Jones RW, Wilkinson D, Paterson KR, Jenkins L, Millais SB, Donoghue S. Evaluation of the safety and immunogenicity of synthetic Abeta42 (AN1792) in patients with AD. Neurology 2005;64(1): 94–101.

183. Gilman S, Koller M, Black RS, Jenkins L, Griffith SG, Fox NC, Eisner L, Kirby L, Rovira MB, Forette F, Orgogozo JM. Clinical effects of Abeta immunization (AN1792) in patients with AD in an interrupted trial. Neurology 2005;64(9):1553–62.

184. Vellas B, Black R, Thal LJ, Fox NC, Daniels M, McLennan G, Tompkins C, Leibman C, Pomfret M, Grundman M. Long-term follow-up of patients immunized with AN1792: reduced functional decline in antibody responders. Curr. Alzheimer Res. 2009;6(2):144–51.

185. Ryan JM, Grundman M. Anti-amyloid-beta immunotherapy in Alzheimer's disease: ACC-001 clinical trials are ongoing. J. Alzheimers Dis. 2009;17(2):243.

186. Schneeberger A, Mandler M, Otawa O, Zauner W, Mattner F, Schmidt W. Development of AFFITOPE vaccines for Alzheimer's disease (AD)—from concept to clinical testing. J. Nutr. Health Aging. 2009;13(3):264–7.

187. Winblad B, Andreasen N, Minthon L, Floesser A, Imbert G, Dumortier T, Maguire RP, Blennow K, Lundmark J, Staufenbiel M, Orgogozo JM, Graf A. Safety, tolerability, and antibody response of active Abeta immunotherapy with CAD106 in patients with Alzheimer's disease: randomised, double-blind, placebo-controlled, first-in-human study. Lancet Neurol. 2012;11(7):597–604.

188. Wang CY, Finstad CL, Walfield AM, Sia C, Sokoll KK, Chang TY, Fang XD, Hung CH, Hutter-Paier B, Windisch M. Site-specific UBITh amyloid-beta vaccine for immunotherapy of Alzheimer's disease. Vaccine 2007;25(16):3041–52.

189. Savage MJ, Wu G, McCampbell A, Wessner KR, Citron M, Liang X, Hsieh S, Wolfe AL, Kinney GG, Rosen LB, Renger JJ. A novel multivalent Abeta peptide vaccine with preclinical evidence of a central immune response that generates antisera recognizing a wide range of Abeta peptide species. Alzheimers Dement. 2010;6(4):S142.

190. Rosenmann H, Grigoriadis N, Karussis D, Boimel M, Touloumi O, Ovadia H, Abramsky O. Tauopathy-like abnormalities and neurologic deficits in mice immunized with neuronal tau protein. Arch. Neurol. 2006;63(10):1459–67.

191. Boimel M, Grigoriadis N, Lourbopoulos A, Haber E, Abramsky O, Rosenmann H. Efficacy and safety of immunization with phosphorylated tau against neurofibrillary tangles in mice. Exp. Neurol. 2010;224(2):472–85.

192. Asuni AA, Boutajangout A, Quartermain D, Sigurdsson EM. Immunotherapy targeting pathological tau conformers in a tangle mouse model reduces brain pathology with associated functional improvements. J. Neurosci. 2007;27(34):9115–29.

193. Boutajangout A, Quartermain D, Sigurdsson EM. Immunotherapy targeting pathological tau prevents cognitive decline in a new tangle mouse model. J. Neurosci. 2010;30(49):16559–66.

194. Cornuz J, Zwahlen S, Jungi WF, Osterwalder J, Klingler K, van Melle G, Bangala Y, Guessous I, Muller P, Willers J, Maurer P, Bachmann MF, Cerny T. A vaccine against nicotine for smoking cessation: a randomized controlled trial. PLoS ONE 2008;3(6):e2547.

195. Tonstad S, Heggen E, Giljam H, Lagerbäck P-Å, Tønnesen P, Wikingsson LD, Lindblom N, de Villiers S, Svensson TH, Fagerström K-O. Niccine®, a nicotine vaccine, for relapse prevention: a Phase II, randomized, placebo-controlled, multicenter clinical trial. Nicotine Tob. Res. 2013;15(9):1492–501.

196. Nakagami F, Koriyama H, Nakagami H, Osako MK, Shimamura M, Kyutoku M, Miyake T, Katsuya T, Rakugi H, Morishita R. Decrease in blood pressure and regression of cardiovascular complications by angiotensin II vaccine in mice. PLoS ONE 2013;8(3):e60493.

197. Crespo Perez L, Castillejo de Villasante G, Cano Ruiz A, Leon F. Non-dietary therapeutic clinical trials in coeliac disease. Eur. J. Intern. Med. 2012;23(1):9–14.

198. Clemente-Casares X, Tsai S, Huang C, Santamaria P. Antigen-specific therapeutic approaches in type 1 diabetes. Cold Spring Harb. Perspect. Med. 2012;2(2):a007773.

199. Andrade S, Pinho F, Ribeiro AM, Carreira M, Casanueva FF, Roy P, Monteiro MP. Immunization against active ghrelin using virus-like particles for obesity treatment. Curr. Pharm. Des. 2013;19(36):6551–8.

200. Wang YM, Zhou JJ, Wang Y, Watson D, Zhang GY, Hu M, Wu H, Zheng G, Durkan AM, Harris DC, Alexander SI. Daedalic DNA vaccination against self antigens as a treatment for chronic kidney disease. Int. J. Clin. Exp. Pathol. 2013;6(3):326–33.

201. Mannie MD, Curtis AD 2nd. Tolerogenic vaccines for multiple sclerosis. Hum. Vaccin. Immunother. 2013;9(5):1032–8.

202. Jia T, Pan Y, Li J, Wang L. Strategies for active TNF-alpha vaccination in rheumatoid arthritis treatment. Vaccine 2013;31(38):4063–8.

Winning a Race Against Evolving Pathogens with Novel Platforms and Universal Vaccines

Jan ter Meulen[1], Danilo Casimiro[2], Beth-Ann Coller[3], Jon Heinrichs[2], Akhilesh Bhambhani[4]

[1]Immune Design, Seattle, WA, USA
[2]Merck Research Laboratories, Vaccine Research, West Point, PA, USA
[3]Merck Research Laboratories, Vaccine Research, Global Clinical Development, North Wales, PA, USA
[4]Merck Research Laboratories, Bioprocess R&D, Formulation Development, West Point, PA, USA

OUTLINE

Novel Approaches and Strategies for Biologics, Vaccines and Cancer Therapies. DOI: 10.1016/B978-0-12-416603-5.00011-0

SEASONAL AND PANDEMIC INFLUENZA VACCINES

Introduction

Seasonal influenza can cause as many as 49,000 deaths and more than 200,000 hospitalizations annually in the United States, resulting in $27 billion in health costs and enormous economic costs in lost work time. It has been estimated that the annual toll of seasonal epidemics worldwide is 250,000 to 500,000 deaths (www.who.int/mediacentre/factsheets/2003/fs211/en). Pandemic influenza occurred in 1918, 1957, 1968, and 2009 due to the introduction of novel influenza A viruses from both avian and swine reservoirs. Although the highly lethal avian H5N1 subtype has thus far not achieved effective human-to-human transmissibility, this or other zoonotic influenza viruses continue to pose major pandemic threats.[1] Vaccination remains the most effective means to control seasonal influenza.

Influenza viruses are members of the RNA virus family Orthomyxoviridae. Based on their nucleocapsid and matrix protein antigens, they are divided into three distinct immunological types: A, B, and C. Antigenic variation of the envelope glycoproteins hemagglutinin (HA) and neuraminidase (NA) provides the basis for further classification of influenza A viruses into 16 HA and 9 NA subtypes. The usefulness of current seasonal influenza virus vaccines, which are based on HA and NA preparations from virus grown in eggs or tissue culture, is limited by the narrow breadth of protection they provide.[2] Because influenza viruses are able to evade the human herd immunity by constantly changing antigenic regions in the HA and NA, annual reformulation of influenza vaccines based on surveillance data of circulating influenza strains and antigenic relatedness is necessary. Mismatches between vaccine strains and circulating viruses occur and reduce the effectiveness of the vaccines. A recent metaanalysis of 30 studies representing 88,468 study participants (children and non-elderly adults) revealed that summary vaccine efficacy was 65% against any strain, 78% against matched strains, and 55% against not-matched strains. Both live-attenuated and inactivated vaccines showed similar levels of protection against not-matched strains (60 and 55%, respectively). Live-attenuated vaccines performed better than inactivated vaccines in children (80 versus 48%), whereas inactivated vaccines performed better than live-attenuated vaccines in adults (59 versus 39%). There was a large difference in efficacy against influenza A (69%) and influenza B (49%) types for not-matched strains.[3] It is estimated, however, to be significantly lower in the elderly (>65 years) and very young (<2 years).[4] The development of vaccines with broader coverage and improved efficacy is furthermore warranted by the pandemic threat from avian viruses such as H7N9 and other zoonotic influenza viruses.

The presence of anti-influenza neutralizing antibodies is the principal correlate of natural protection in humans, and HA, the most abundant surface glycoprotein of influenza virus, is the primary target in a natural infection. By binding to the HA protein, neutralizing antibodies can either prevent the attachment of the virus to the sialic acid receptor on the surfaces of epithelial cells or inhibit the subsequent membrane fusion step of entry in the host cell. The serological criteria used for approval of seasonal influenza vaccines are a seroconversion rate (i.e., percent of subjects with a minimum fourfold rise in hemagglutination inhibition [HI] titer) for persons younger than 65 of >40% and seroprotection rate (i.e., percent of subjects with HI titer >1:40) for this same age group of ≥70%.

Neutralizing antibodies to the second most abundant surface glycoprotein, neuraminidase (NA), also contribute to protection. In addition to neutralizing antibodies, non-neutralizing antibodies as well as CD4+ cells and cytotoxic T cells are also believed to play a role in protection. Although these have been extensively studied in animal models, their role in protecting humans from infection is less clear. Important antigens are the highly conserved external portion of the matrix protein M2 (M2e) as a target for antibody-dependent cellular cytotoxicity (ADCC) and the also highly conserved nucleoprotein and matrix protein 1 (M1), which contains known human T-cell epitopes. Higher frequencies of preexisting T cells to conserved CD8 epitopes were found in individuals who developed less severe pandemic H1N1 influenza infection, with total symptom score having the strongest inverse correlation with the frequency of interferon-γ (IFN-γ)+ interleukin-2 (IL-2)– CD8+ T cells. In the absence of cross-reactive neutralizing antibodies, CD8+ T cells specific to conserved viral epitopes correlated with cross-protection against symptomatic influenza.[5]

Combination vaccines that target HA and one or more viral proteins including NA are in clinical development using a variety of delivery strategies (DNA, protein, virus-like particles, or viral vector-based) and a number of different adjuvant strategies. The challenges for the successful licensure of such novel vaccines include a lack of knowledge of correlates or surrogates of protection in humans, the lack of standardized assays that measure non anti-HA based immune responses, and the lack of reagents and procedures that can be used to measure vaccine potency for standardization of novel target vaccines.[6]

Influenza vaccines based on a mechanism other than virus neutralization have been shown to prevent or reduce mortality in animal challenge experiments, but not to prevent disease symptoms, such as weight loss. Although such disease-modifying vaccination approaches may be acceptable in a pandemic situation to prevent excess mortality, they are not considered a viable alternative to the currently used seasonal influenza vaccines, which achieve sterilizing immunity and prevent mortality and morbidity. The development of improved influenza vaccine, whether adjuvanted and/or rationally designed, will crucially depend on a better understanding of the immune correlates of protection in humans.[7]

Enhancing Immune Responses to Influenza Virus Vaccines Using Novel Adjuvants

Current efforts to improve immunogenicity and efficacy of influenza vaccine focus mainly on quadrivalent seasonal formulations, higher antigen doses, novel adjuvants, and novel routes of administration. In 1978, the first trivalent vaccine included two influenza A strains and one influenza B strain. Currently, there are two influenza B lineages circulating, and several inactivated quadrivalent influenza vaccines containing two B strains are available.[8]

Of the many "novel" (i.e., non-aluminum based adjuvants) in development, squalene-based oil-in-water (o/w) emulsions are the most successful ones in clinical use with influenza vaccines. These adjuvants enhance seroprotective antibody titers to homologous and heterologous strains of virus and result in significant dose sparing. All major influenza vaccine manufacturers are using oil-in-water emulsions in licensed seasonal or pre-pandemic vaccines, including MF59® (Novartis), ASO3 (GlaxoSmithKline), and AF03 (Sanofi). These adjuvants contain shark-derived squalene that is microfluidized in buffer and surfactants to generate oil particles averaging 100 to 160 nm in diameter suspended in water. All induce seroprotective antibody responses to inactivated H5N1 vaccines that exceed approvable end-point criteria in humans and mediate a significant dose sparing effect, including in the pediatric population.[9-11]

Oil-in-water emulsions are also being explored to increase immune responses to seasonal influenza vaccines in young children and the elderly. In a study performed with an MF59 adjuvanted trivalent inactivated vaccine (ATIV) in children, the efficacy rates for ATIV were 79% (95% CI, 55 to 90) in children 6 to less than 36 months of age and 92% (95% CI, 77 to 97) in those 36 to less than 72 months of age, as compared with 40% (95% CI, −6 to 66) and 45% (95% CI, 6 to 68), respectively, for TIV.[11] Although adjuvantation clearly enhances both immunogenicity and efficacy of seasonal influenza vaccines in children,[12] a recent large-scale study in the elderly involving 43,802 participants showed that, despite improved immunogenicity, an AS03-adjuvanted TIV is not superior to a non-adjuvanted TIV for the prevention of influenza in people ages 65 years or older.[13] The study suggested furthermore that the benefit of influenza vaccination in elderly people might vary depending on influenza subtypes; the greatest efficacy was recorded against the H3N2 subtype.

Emulsions induce a chemokine gradient at the site of injection that recruits leukocyte infiltration and antigen transport to local lymph nodes, and their induction of broadly reactive CD4 T cells predicts the rise of neutralizing antibody titers after booster immunizations.[14,15] In adults and children, MF59 selectively enhanced antibody responses to the hemagglutinin 1 (HA1) globular head relative to the more conserved HA2 domain in terms of increased antibody titers as well as a more diverse antibody epitope repertoire. Antibody affinity was significantly increased and antibody affinity maturation after each sequential vaccination was improved. Thus, MF59 quantitatively and qualitatively enhances functional antibody responses to HA-based vaccines by improving both epitope breadth and binding affinity.[16]

Despite their utility and the fact these o/w emulsions are approved in the European Union and have been administered to tens of millions of subjects without obvious problems, vaccines containing emulsion-based adjuvants have not been approved in the United States. Unexpectedly, Sweden, Finland, and recently also the United Kingdom reported an increase of narcolepsy up to 14-fold in children and 3- to 5-fold in adults in temporal association with having been vaccinated with the AS03-adjuvanted H1N1 vaccine Pandemrix in 2009.[17,18] In Finland, a total of 98 cases of narcolepsy were registered subsequent to vaccination with Pandemrix, and the increased risk of narcolepsy attributed to vaccination with Pandemrix in adults was 1/100 000, whereas in children it was 6/100 000 (http://www.thl.fi/doc/en/33516). For perspective, approximately half of the Finnish population was vaccinated with Pandemrix, and the vaccine prevented 80 000 swine flu infections as well as approximately 50 deaths caused by swine flu virus during the first year following the vaccination. The risk in adults has also been studied in a collaborative European-wide case-control study in the Netherlands, Italy, Norway, the United Kingdom, and Denmark, but so far no increase has been observed in these countries. In October 2012, the European Medicines Agency (EMA) Committee on Human Medicinal Products (CHMP) concluded that, on the basis of the current evidence, the role of the Pandemrix antigen and its adjuvant on the association between Pandemrix and narcolepsy remains unknown. Studies to elucidate a possible causality, including the presence of HLA-DQB1-0602 as a genetic risk factor, are still ongoing. Chronic neurological disorders were not observed with other H1N1 pandemic vaccines adjuvanted with o/w emulsions.

A number of other novel adjuvants have been tested successfully in animal immunogenicity and challenge studies, such as saponins and toll-like receptor 4 agonists; for some of these, substantial safety databases are available that will accelerate their evaluation with influenza vaccines in clinical trials.[19]

Design of Recombinant Antigens for Improved and "Universal" Influenza Vaccines

To overcome the requirement of having to generate annually new reassortant influenza viruses that represent antigenically the circulating virus strains and are adapted to growth in embryonated eggs or cell culture, a variety of approaches are currently being explored to develop recombinant vaccines based on HA and/or conserved proteins (NP, M2), including DNA and RNA immunization, vectored approaches (e.g., adenovirus) and recombinant proteins. All recombinant approaches allow in theory the design of antigens with enhanced breath of protection, which is especially relevant for the development of pre-pandemic vaccines. To date, the only licensed influenza vaccine based on recombinantly expressed HA protein is Flublok®, which is manufactured in insect cells and currently licensed in the United States for adults 18 to 49 years of age.[20] Unexpectedly, the receptor-binding domain of influenza virus HA produced in *Escherichia coli* also folds into its native, immunogenic structure, and fusion of this domain to the TLR5-agonist flagellin resulted in a self-adjuvanting protein that induced potent neutralizing antibody responses in both young adults and the elderly in humans.[21,22]

Influenza HA consists of a membrane-distal globular head domain that contains the receptor-binding site and is comprised exclusively of the HA1 subunit. The viral membrane proximal, elongated, stem domain (or stalk) is composed of both HA1 and HA2 subunits, but primarily of the latter. There are two major phylogenetic HA groups: group 1 (subtypes H1, H2, H5, H6, H8, H9, H11, H12, H13, and H16) and group 2 (subtypes H3, H4, H7, H10, H14 and H15). The majority of influenza virus neutralizing antibodies are directed against the highly variable globular head domain of the protein. They inhibit receptor binding and have hemagglutination inhibition activity that is generally strain specific. The stalk domain of the HA is relatively well conserved but far less immunogenic; recently, broadly neutralizing antibodies against this domain of the HA have been isolated, suggesting that a vaccine based on the induction of such antibodies could provide heterosubtypic protection.[23] These antibodies can be found in humans who have been exposed to influenza viruses via either vaccination or infection but they seem to be rare in nature, and *in vivo* levels of these antibodies are likely to be too low to afford protection. These antibodies are HI negative and mediate their neutralizing activity through other mechanisms, such as blocking of fusion of the viral and cellular membranes. Because the sequence identity of the stalk domains of members from the two groups of HAs is low, it is likely that a universal vaccine based on the influenza stalk will have to include a group 1, a group 2, and an influenza B stalk antigen. A number of rational design approaches are currently being pursued to direct the antibody response against the stalk, including expression of recombinant HA constructs in *Escherichia coli*, expression of head/stalk chimeric HAs in mammalian cells, and display of HA on self-assembling ferritin nanoparticles expressed in mammalian cells.[24-26] Some of these approaches generate fairly broadly neutralizing antibodies and protect mice in experimental challenge, but none has been tested in humans yet. As a caveat to stalk-based influenza vaccines, recent studies have raised the possibility of an antibody-dependent enhancement of influenza virus pathogenicity induced by non-neutralizing cross-reactive antibodies.[27]

In summary, heterosubtypic, neutralizing antibodies directed against the stem of the influenza virus hemagglutinin can be induced in animals through a number of antigen design approaches. Provided that these antigens induce measurable neutralizing responses in humans, can be manufactured, and are safe, they may be useful either as add-ons to seasonal vaccines or as prepandemic vaccines in their own right.

HUMAN IMMUNODEFICIENCY VIRUS VACCINES

Human immunodeficiency virus (HIV) infection remains one of the largest global infectious disease killer. In 2012, about 35.3 million people, including 3.3 million children under the age of 15 years, were living with the human immunodeficiency virus.[28] Despite the advances in HIV treatment and control, about 2.3 million new cases and 1.6 million deaths were reported in 2012. Hence, a vaccine against HIV/AIDS remains an important public health priority in order to curtail this epidemic.

The development of an effective vaccine against HIV/AIDS has several challenges. Fundamentally, chronic infection with HIV-1 results in significant damage to the immune system, resulting in comorbidities and, without sufficient antiviral (AV) intervention, mortality. Additionally, the RNA virus is able to evade the host immune control through various mechanisms including downregulation of MHCI presentation[29] and rapid viral evolution to escape both neutralizing antibodies and T cell-mediated lysis.[30,31] These immune evasion mechanisms have, in part, had a significant role in the lack of efficacy seen with several vaccine approaches tested in clinical trials. However, the relatively high level of attention and research and development (R&D) investment in recent years to understand the outcomes of those clinical efficacy trials have yielded an understanding of how the immune system could control HIV infection, which in turn could contribute to the development of effective vaccine approaches.

Vaccine Principle

The host control of chronic infections can be mediated by many arms of the immune system. In principle, the prevention of acquisition is largely mediated by antibodies able to block one or more aspects of viral entry and infection of target cells (e.g., binding of virus to cellular receptors, membrane fusion). The ability of a vaccine to elicit a potent neutralizing antibody response is challenged by (1) large Env sequence variability within clade and between virus clades, and (2) if the vaccine protection is partial, potential ability of the founder viruses to mutate and evade the incident antibody specificities. There are other means by which antibodies can mediate control of HIV infection. Binding antibodies may aggregate virions, retard mobility of the virus through the cervical mucus, inhibit transcytosis, and/or mediate Fc receptor-mediated antibody inhibition. Weinhold and coworkers[32] showed that CD4+ T-cell lines with gp120 bound to their CD4 receptors were susceptible to lysis by peripheral blood mononuclear cells (PBMCs) from HIV-infected individuals, but not from uninfected people, and this killing was mediated by natural killer (NK) cells that recognized infected CD4 T cells through anti-gp120 antibodies bound to their Fc receptor. The containment of a persistent infection by the immune system can in turn be mediated by cellular immune responses. This is relevant to many herpesvirus infections in which viral reactivations are associated with severe diseases in an immunocompromised patient population.[33] In the case of HIV-1, it has been well documented that elite HIV controllers (HIV-positive people having undetectable HIV viral load without the use of HIV medications[34]) are associated with specific MHC-I alleles and efficacies of the T-cell clones to kill HIV infected cells. Additional population analyses of the CD8 T-cell responses and viral loads in untreated HIV-infected subjects also reveal those antigens (e.g., Gag) that are more associated with lower viremia.[35]

Vaccine Efficacy Trials

A trial to test the field efficacy of an HIV-1 vaccine is a very large and serious undertaking and is typically enabled by multilateral collaborations, involving the federal government agencies, foreign governments, non-industry laboratories, and private industry partners, among others. The area of HIV-1 vaccine R&D has benefited from clinical trials that evaluated the efficacies of four different vaccine approaches against HIV-1 infection and disease markers. The clinical efficacy is assessed using the primary endpoint of prevention of HIV-1 acquisition and secondary endpoints such as CD4 counts, viral loads, onset of AIDS, and antiretroviral treatment. Although an HIV-1 vaccine remains a distant possibility, these studies have provided important information regarding the science of protective immunity against HIV-1 as well as operational conduct of future clinical efficacy trials. Below, we outline the studies and study results of the four vaccine approaches.

HIV Env Vaccine

The first vaccine to enter into a clinical efficacy trial was a bivalent gp120 vaccine based on sequences from clade B and CDF01-AE. The vaccine was sponsored by VaxGen, Inc. (now Global Solutions for Infectious Disease), the Thailand government, and Mahidol University. The selection of the antigen sequences was based on the major clade responsible for the rise in HIV-1 infection in injection drug users (clade B) and the sexually transmitted AIDS epidemic (clade CRF01-AE) in Thailand beginning in the late 1980s. This randomized, double-blind, placebo-controlled efficacy trial of AIDSVAX B/E was conducted in 2546 injection drug users (IDUs) in Bangkok, Thailand.[36] The overall HIV-1 incidence was 3.4 infections/100 person-years (95% CI, 3.0 to 3.9 infections per 100 person-years), and the cumulative incidence was 8.4%. There were no differences between the vaccine and placebo arms. HIV-1 subtype E (83 vaccine and 81 placebo recipients) accounted for 77% of infections. No statistically significant effects of the vaccine on secondary endpoints such as CD counts, viral load, onset of AIDS, and antiretroviral therapy (ART) treatment were observed.

Replication-Defective Ad5 HIV-1 Vaccine

The concept of immune control mediated exclusively by cytotoxic T cells directed at more conserved HIV-1 antigens was tested in a Phase IIB clinical trial (called STEP) by Merck in collaboration with the NIH in 2004.[37] The STEP vaccine is a mixture of three replication-defective (E1-deleted) human adenovirus type 5 viruses which independently express a clade B *gag*, *pol*, and *nef* gene. The vaccine was designed on the basis of several important preclinical and epidemiological studies. Cellular immune responses in 250 HIV-1-infected subjects from various regions of the globe with varying HIV-1 clade distribution were analyzed for reactivities to *gag, pol, nef, rev,* and *tat* peptide pools.[38] The fractions of subjects who responded to clade B antigens were highest with the following hierarchy: *gag > nef, pol > env > rev, tat.* This trend in reactivities is consistent with the level of cross-clade sequence conservation and antigen size. The ratios of the magnitude of the T-cell responses against any *gag* or *nef* sequences from any pair of clades exceeded 0.80. These results support the suggestion that *gag, pol,* and *nef* are the major targets of HIV-1-specific T-cell responses, and a combination of these antigens can provide substantial vaccine coverage.

The second element of the STEP vaccine pertains to the selection of the vector platform. We conducted a systematic screen of multiple live and non-live vector approaches, available at the time, for their property to elicit antigen-specific CD8 and CD4 T-cell responses in non-human primate models or, in certain cases, in clinical studies.[39] These included DNA vectors, poxvirus vectors, alphavirus, bacteria, and multiple human and non-human adenoviruses. The information about the more immunogenic vectors was supplemented by testing their efficacy in simian immunodeficiency virus challenge of vaccinated rhesus macaques. All of these studies led to the selection of the human adenovirus serotype 5 (Ad5) virus (or common cold virus) as a vector system for the STEP vaccine. The replication-defective Ad5 HIV-1 vaccine was shown in early phase studies to be highly immunogenic in HIV-1 negative subjects. The immunogenicity of this vaccine, as expected, is negatively influenced by the level of existing neutralizing Ad5 titers prior to immunization. A Phase IIB study involving HIV-1 seronegative subjects at high risk of HIV-1 infection in predominantly clade B regions (North America, Caribbean, Brazil, Peru, Australia) was initiated in 2004 followed by a second study of the same vaccine in South Africa. The study involved 3000 HIV-1-seronegative participants who receive three injections of Ad5 HIV-1 *gag/pol/nef* vaccine ($n = 1494$) or placebo ($n = 1506$). The study was stopped early because it unexpectedly met the prespecified futility boundaries at the first interim analysis; all but one infections were in men. The vaccine did not reduce the infection rates nor lower the plasma viral HIV RNA relative to those of the placebo control. Most notably, there was an increased trend in HIV-1 infection in Ad5 seropositive men and uncircumcised men.

Several studies have been conducted to understand the outcome (both safety and efficacy) of STEP and inform design of future vaccine approaches. Analyses of T-cell epitope specificities elicited by the Ad5 vaccines suggest that the breadth is highly variable among the subjects yet limited in scope on the average.[40] Furthermore, much like natural infection, the frequencies of recognized epitopes using the rAd5 vaccine are skewed toward the more variable regions of antigens and less toward the most highly conserved epitopes relative to an unbiased sampling across the length of the antigenic sequences.[41] Rolland et al.[42] reported that the vaccine was able to exert immune pressure on the virus during the acute phase of infection. Compared to the original vaccine antigen sequences, the sequences of *gag, pol,* and *nef* in the breakthrough viruses from the vaccine recipients were more divergent than those of the viruses in the placebo subjects. The divergence is only confined to *gag, pol,* and *nef* and not to non-vaccine antigens. The hotspots also mapped to known epitopes based on the patient's HLA alleles, suggesting that an immune pressure was exerted.

The other scientific question arising from STEP is the association between increased infection rates among vaccinees compared to placebo in high Ad5-seropositive subjects. The observation in the STEP study is important to understand in order to assess the utility of this vector class to HIV-1 as well as other vaccine targets, especially those whose demographic footprint overlaps with the global HIV-1 epidemic. One hypothesis pertains to increased levels of HIV-1 cell targets with the induction of activated Ad5-specific CD4 T cells following vaccination in the Ad5-seropositive subjects. However, in an analysis of samples from early stage clinical studies, the baseline Ad5-specific neutralizing antibodies was found not to correlate with Ad5-specific CD4 T-lymphocyte responses and furthermore Ad5-seropositive subjects did not develop higher vector-specific cellular immune responses as compared with Ad5-seronegative subjects after vaccination.[43] The immunological basis for the potential enhanced HIV-1 acquisition especially in Ad5-seropositive subjects remains unclear and to complicate matters mucosal samples were not collected in the STEP study.

DNA Prime, Replication-Defective Ad5 Boost HIV-1 Vaccine

In 2009, a Phase IIB study (HVTN505) was conducted using an investigational HIV vaccine regimen consisting of a primary series of three immunizations with a DNA vaccine expressing antigens HIV-1 *env* (from three major clades) and *gag–pol* fusion, *nef* genes (from clade B) followed by a single boost of a replication-defective Ad5 expressing the matching set of antigens with the exception of the *nef* gene which was excluded.[44] The primary differences from the STEP vaccine reside in the inclusion of *env* antigens for a broader cellular immune response and induction of potential effector antibodies against a surface viral protein.

The 1:1 placebo-controlled study enrolled 2504 U.S. volunteers with high-risk behavior—men who have sex with men and transgender people who have sex with men. In the first interim review, the primary analysis included HIV infections that occurred after 4 weeks following the booster vaccine, and a 27:21 vaccine:placebo case split was reported. Overall, in the study from the day of enrollment through the month-24 study visit, a total of 41 cases of HIV infection occurred in the volunteers who received the investigational vaccine regimen, and 30 cases of HIV infection occurred among the placebo vaccine recipients. These differences in HIV infection rates were not statistically significant. As with the STEP trial, there was no vaccine impact on reducing viral loads following infection.

The lack of any vaccine efficacy in both trials involving a replication-defective Ad5 raises questions about the future utility of adenovirus-vectored vaccines for HIV/AIDS. Although these outcomes may be attributed to the choice of antigens, the HVTN505 vaccine expanded on the antigenic breadth relative to that of the STEP study vaccine. It is unclear whether other antigen choices constitute only incremental improvement over that of these two vaccines or if a combination of these improved immunogens with fully orthogonal vector approaches will result in a positive clinical efficacy outcome.

Poxvirus Prime, Env Protein Boost HIV-1 Vaccine

The lack of efficacy with the original HIV gp120 *env* vaccine in high-risk population prompted the inclusion of a vaccine modality capable of further stimulating a cellular immune response. In 2003, a community-based, randomized, multicenter, double-blind, 1:1 placebo-controlled efficacy trial (called RV144) was initiated in Thailand and designed to evaluate a prime-boost regimen with a recombinant canarypox vector vaccine expressing gp120, *gag*, and *pol* (ALVAC-HIV [vCP1521]) (developed by Sanofi Pasteur) and a recombinant glycoprotein 120-subunit vaccine (AIDSVAX B/E) (developed by Global Solutions for Infectious Disease).[45] Placebo or two injections of the vCP1521 alone followed by two injections with both vCp1521 and the AIDSVAX B/E were given over the course of 6 months to 16,402 healthy subjects, primarily at risk of heterosexual infection.

In contrast to the earlier trials, the study showed a reduction in the rate of HIV-1 infection by 31.2% ($p = 0.039$; 95% CI, 1.1 to 51.1) in modified intent-to-treat analyses, but no impact on viral loads in infected subjects. The outcome was particularly surprising given that the vaccine did not elicit broadly neutralizing antibodies, and apart from detectable anti-HIV1 lymphoproliferative responses also did not induce any measurable cytotoxic T-cell responses.

The RV144 results challenged the field to examine mediators of immune control other than virus neutralization and CTL control. A systematic immune correlate analysis of the RV144 study samples was completed recently. Of the several pre-infection immune variables, IgG antibodies to variable regions 1 and 2 (V1V2) of HIV-1 envelope proteins (Env) and plasma IgA antibodies to Env were found to correlate inversely and directly with the rate of HIV-1 infection, respectively.[46] Additional support for the role of this biomarker originates from an analysis of breakthrough viruses from patients in the RV144 trial which were consistent with immune pressure focused on amino-acid patterns in and flanking the V1V2 region of HIV-1 Env. Additional studies are warranted to establish causality (i.e., the mechanism by which V1V2 antibodies directly mediate vaccine-induced protection from infection) or whether this biomarker is simply associated with the true immune mediator in RV144. The role of non-neutralizing antibodies, including antibody-dependent cellular cytotoxicity (ADCC) and antibody-dependent cell-mediated virus inhibition (ACDVI), was recognized nearly three decades ago by Weinhold and coworkers and is currently being investigated,[47] coupled with the development of more rigorous assays to analyze large sample sets from clinical trials.

New Vaccine Concepts

An effective HIV vaccine will likely require the induction of broadly neutralizing antibodies due to the hypervariability of the virus. There is a growing collection of broadly neutralizing monoclonal antibodies (mAbs) as a result of modern techniques such as single B-cell cloning for isolating mAbs from infected human subjects, deep sequencing, and microneutralization assays. These new monoclonals included a set of molecules that target (1) an epitope preferentially expressed on trimeric HIV Env protein which spans conserved regions of variable loops of gp120 (PG9, PG16, CH01-04); (2) the CD4 binding site (VRC01); and (3) epitopes associated with glycan residues on HIV Env (PGT series) (see Koff[48] for a review). These antibodies in principle represent important tools in the design and screening of HIV Env immunogens that could elicit virus neutralization with a breadth in coverage approaching those observed with these mAbs. However, the natural B-cell pathways that lead to the production of broadly neutralizing antibodies with their unusually long CDR3 involved extensive somatic hypermutations driven by constant antigen stimulation with multiple Env sequences. To mimic these processes using a vaccination approach is particularly challenging. Several approaches are being considered, such as heterologous prime-boost regimens[49] and use of replication-competent viruses[50] expressing minimal Env domains representing the desired epitopes. It is also important to take into consideration how these approaches can induce potent non-neutralizing antibodies that can regulate virus infection as described above.

There are also several recent advances in developing vector systems which include alternative adenoviruses[51] and poxviruses.[52] Picker and coworkers also described the vector use of cytomegalovirus (CMV),[53–55] a herpesvirus capable of establishing latent long-term infection in humans. A rhesus CMV vectored vaccine expressing simian immunodeficiency virus (SIV) *gag*, *rev–tat–nef*, and *env* antigens (RhCMV) was able to establish persistent, high-frequency,

SIV-specific effector memory T-cell (T(EM)) responses in the periphery as well as local sites of SIV replication in rhesus macaques. About 50% of macaques receiving the CMV vaccine manifested early complete control of SIV (undetectable plasma virus) and long-term protection, with only sporadic blips in viremia above the lower limit of detection. More recently, Picker and coworkers showed that this fibroblast-tropic CMV vector elicits a CD8 T-cell response that not only is much broader in epitope specificity than most other vector approaches but is also largely characterized by non-canonical restriction by MHC class II molecules.[55] Although the practical application of this approach for human use remains to be seen given the need to develop a vaccine that would not cause any of the diseases associated with CMV infection[56] while maintaining the immunological potency observed with the rhesus CMV vector, the vector platform produced very remarkable preclinical challenge results, thereby warranting further translational medicine studies.

Summary

Apart from the planned clinical studies to support the RV144 vaccine, there does not appear to be a new vaccine approach with an overwhelmingly strong scientific basis to warrant immediate clinical efficacy testing. Several important scientific advances—understanding of the immunological pathways leading to broadly neutralizing mAbs and development of novel vector systems—signal a new era of HIV R&D. The practical translation of these advances to human vaccine candidates will require continued investments and, if successful, will usher in an exciting new era of HIV vaccine R&D.

DENGUE VACCINES

Dengue vaccine development has been an area of active research and major challenges for over 50 years. However, significant advances have occurred over the last 10 years such that several vaccine candidates are now showing significant promise in clinical studies, with the most advanced candidate having entered Phase III testing. Although our understanding of dengue virus biology and the potential for immunopathogenesis has also progressed, there are still many areas that are unresolved and are the object of significant investigation. Not the least of these is our understanding, or lack thereof, of what constitutes a protective response in humans which is an area of intense investigation.

Disease and Epidemiology of Dengue

Dengue is the most important vectorborne viral disease in terms of morbidity and mortality, with an estimated 4 billion people throughout the tropics and subtropics at risk of infection. Worldwide, an estimated 390 million infections with dengue occur annually, with approximately 96 million symptomatic cases and 20,000 deaths.[57] With increasing urbanization in endemic areas and an expanding area of transmission there is a risk of even more disease in the future.[58,59] Disease caused by dengue virus infection ranges from asymptomatic to severe life-threatening disease. Classical dengue fever is characterized by high fever, headache, rash, eye pain, muscle aches, joint pain, and severe fatigue. In its more severe forms, dengue hemorrhagic fever (DHF) and dengue shock syndrome (DSS), the disease is a plasma leakage syndrome characterized by petechiae, hemoconcentration, and pleural and/or peritoneal effusions that can lead to shock and death if not treated appropriately.

There are changing patterns for the epidemiology of dengue which appear to be multifactorial. The impact of the expansion of the endemic regions of the four dengue viral strains (dengue viruses types 1, 2, 3, and 4, or DENV1, DENV2, DENV3, and DENV4, respectively), and the association between more severe disease and secondary infection has been well documented.[60-63] Differences in circulating viral strains, including viral genotypes, and the sequence of infection has also been suggested to impact the incidence of severe dengue.[64-66] Finally, human factors including genetic makeup, changing patterns of human movement (e.g., movement from rural to urban areas), and longevity appear to be impacting the epidemiology of dengue in different ways in different parts of the world.[67-70] Cumulatively, these factors result in a complex, constantly changing, epidemiologic picture of dengue and present unique challenges for vaccine introduction.

Immunology and Immunopathology

Dengue is caused by any one of the four dengue viruses. Although infection with one type of dengue virus provides life-long immunity against that virus type, it does not provide long-term protection against infection from the other dengue virus types. Furthermore, although the more severe forms of the disease occur at a lower frequency relative to classic dengue fever, the vast majority of DHF cases occur following secondary infection. Several hypotheses exist regarding the mechanisms that result in DHF. The most prominent hypothesis is that non-neutralizing cross-reactive antibodies bind to non-homologous virus and facilitate uptake into Fc receptor-bearing cells which in turn results in greater virus loads and more severe disease (antibody-dependent enhancement, or ADE).[71,72] Cell-mediated immunity presumably triggered by high viral loads is believed to play a key role in severe disease via the release of cytokines and chemokines that mediate plasma leakage.[73] Another hypothesis includes the concept of original antigenic sin (e.g., see Mongkolsapaya et al.[74]) which refers to a phenomenon where the response to sequential infection with related viruses is skewed toward epitopes expressed by the first infecting virus. This phenomenon has been extensively studied in the context of influenza infections and only more recently explored in the context of sequential dengue infections. Although the proposed mechanisms vary, they all postulate that the severe disease manifestation includes an immunopathogenic component. The strategy generally used in vaccine development to mitigate this risk is the development of tetravalent dengue vaccines that attempt to simultaneously induce protective immune responses against all four dengue virus types. Such an approach is widely believed to be the best way to limit both dengue virus-induced disease and to mitigate the risk of exacerbated disease.

Vaccines in Clinical Development

Safe and efficacious vaccines for monotypic flaviviruses such as yellow fever, Japanese encephalitis, and tickborne encephalitis viruses demonstrate the potential for the development of protective vaccines for this family of viruses. However, for dengue the complications posed by the four independent virus targets and the accepted need for simultaneous tetravalent responses have presented challenges that have delayed the field for decades. Clinical testing of classically attenuated vaccine candidates (e.g., passaged through heterologous cell substrates) began in the 1980s. Individual attenuated strains were developed; however, the identification of tetravalent formulations that did not exhibit significant interference between the four viruses was challenging. Two products were able to reach Phase II clinical testing but failed to progress due to issues with interference, stability, and/or formulation.[75–77] However, with the application of molecular techniques over the past decade, significant advances have been made in developing dengue vaccines, with six candidates currently in clinical trials. These vaccines employ a variety of novel approaches, including molecularly defined live-attenuated viruses, adjuvanted inactivated viruses, recombinant subunits, and DNA-based vaccines. In addition, a number of vaccine candidates using other novel approaches are in preclinical evaluation.[78]

The most advanced vaccine candidate is the chimeric yellow fever dengue (CYD) vaccine under development by Sanofi Pasteur. This vaccine is based on the innovative Chimerivax™ technology where the prM-Envelope proteins from the four dengue types are introduced into the YF-17D vaccine strain molecularly cloned backbone resulting in live-attenuated chimeric viruses.[79,80] The novel CYD vaccine has been tested in Phase I and II trials and has demonstrated safety and immunogenicity in flavivirus-naïve and flavivirus-experienced volunteers.[81–84] However, in a Phase IIB efficacy trial conducted in children in Thailand, the CYD vaccine showed mixed results, with evidence of efficacy against DENV1, DENV3, and DENV4 but no efficacy against DENV2.[85] The causes of the vaccine failure for DENV2 are under investigation, and the implications for CYD development and dengue vaccine development in general remain unclear. Phase III studies of the CYD vaccine are ongoing in both Latin American and Asia, with data expected in 2014.[86]

Another live-attenuated, chimeric virus-based approach currently in Phase II testing is DENVax, being developed by Inviragen/Takeda. The candidate is based on DENV2-PDK50 live-attenuated virus that was previously tested in Phase I and II trials.[76,77] DENVax uses a cloned version of DENV2-PDK50 as the backbone and introduces the prM/Envelope proteins of the other DENV types to create chimeras.[87] DENVax has been shown to be safe and immunogenic in a Phase I clinical trial conducted in flavivirus-naïve subjects in Colombia[87] and is currently being tested in Phase II clinical trials in Thailand, Puerto Rico, Colombia, and Singapore.

The U.S. National Institutes of Health (NIH) National Institute of Allergy and Infectious Diseases (NIAID) has conducted preclinical and clinical testing of novel and innovative molecularly defined attenuated-virus vaccine candidates containing defined deletions in the 3' non-coding region as well as additional attenuating mutations in some cases. The NIAID has used a comprehensive and systematic approach whereby unique, potentially attenuated viruses are produced and tested *in vitro* and in animal models to identify appropriate candidates for human clinical testing.[88] Phase I safety and immunogenicity testing of monovalent vaccine candidates was conducted,[89–92] and recently the individual virus strains were combined into tetravalent formulations and tested in healthy adult subjects in the United States. This led to the identification of the TV003 formulation as the lead candidate,[93] and it is now being prepared for Phase II studies in dengue-endemic countries.

In addition, three non-replicating vaccines, each with innovative aspects, are currently being tested in Phase I clinical trials. The non-replicating approaches under evaluation include purified inactivated virus administered with novel adjuvants (PIV),[94] a vaccine comprised of a recombinant-subunit envelope protein expressed in a novel cell substrate,[95,96] and a DNA vaccine candidate being evaluated with and without molecular adjuvants.[97,98] Each of these approaches has applied modern technology to solve critical issues in dengue vaccine development and has shown potential in non-human primate studies and/or monovalent clinical trials and are now being evaluated as tetravalent formulation(s) in Phase I clinical trials.

Challenges

Although progress toward the development of a safe and effective dengue vaccine is significant, the key challenges remain the lack of understanding of protective immune responses in humans as described above and the ability of vaccine candidates to induce long-lasting, balanced, protective responses. The challenges were highlighted again most recently by the mixed results in the CYD Phase IIB efficacy trial.[85]

Conclusions

With several novel and innovative dengue vaccine candidates progressing through clinical trials, several options for controlling this disease appear feasible. This would represent a major achievement and reflect decades of research and development activities. The challenges associated with the limited understanding of protective responses and those factors that determine disease severity remain, but with dengue vaccine efficacy trials ongoing immune responses are being evaluated in the context of protection and severe disease, and these studies are highly likely to provide additional insights. It is important to note that vaccines are registered and approved for use based on their ability to prevent disease, and a detailed understanding of the protective mechanisms is not necessarily required. Thus, we may never completely understand what protects people from disease caused by dengue infection, but with good, careful science and clinical studies we may soon have safe and effective dengue vaccines that will have an important impact on global public health.

STREPTOCOCCUS PNEUMONIAE VACCINES

Streptococcus pneumoniae, or pneumococcus, is the causative agent of both localized and systemic disease in both children and the elderly. In infants and young children, the bacterium causes meningitis, septicemia, pneumonia, sinusitis, and otitis media, whereas in the elderly it is a common cause of both pneumonia and bacteremia. The organism has the been the focus of vaccine development for over a century, and despite the implementation of several effective vaccines it is still the leading cause of vaccine-preventable death in children less than 5 years of age, among whom it causes approximately 800,000 deaths per year.[99] This is primarily the result of inadequate availability of vaccines in regions of the world with high endemic rates of disease, as well as changes in the epidemiology of disease and suboptimal coverage of vaccines in at-risk populations. The development of vaccines with broader serotype coverage, therefore, is highly desirable to increase protection against this pathogen.

Vaccines for pneumococcus have traditionally targeted the polysaccharide capsule that coats this Gram-positive bacterium. This approach, while highly successful, has met with two important barriers for vaccine development. First, the organism is characterized by at least

93 serotypes defined by immunologically distinct polysaccharide structures. Although not all serotypes are equally capable of causing disease, designing vaccines that protect against the majority of serotypes responsible for disease requires multivalent constructs. Furthermore, the serotypes that cause disease in children vary in many cases from those responsible for disease in adults and the representation of serotypes in the developing world often are poorly matched to those causing disease in the industrialized world. Second, polysaccharide vaccines are poorly immunogenic in young children due to their inability to induce T cell help. Because of this immunologic phenomenon, conjugation of polysaccharides to protein carriers was required to generate vaccines with adequate immunogenicity for infants.

Despite the inherent challenges in vaccine development, several highly successful vaccines have been introduced and are currently marketed for the prevention of invasive pneumococcal disease. Among these are the conjugate vaccines Prevnar® and Prevnar13® (Pfizer) and Synflorix® (GlaxoSmithKline), which are licensed for use in infants and children, as well as the polysaccharide vaccine Pneumovax-23® (Merck), which is indicated for use in adults greater than 50 years of age. Recently, Prevnar13® was also approved for use in adults. The development of additional conjugate vaccines with even greater serotype coverage is being investigated by several vaccine organizations; however, a theoretical and practical limit to the number of serotype conjugates will eventually likely be reached, requiring alternative methods for expansion of vaccine coverage.

The introduction of Prevnar® in the United States in the year 2000 led to a rapid reduction in infections caused by the serotypes responsible for disease in the vaccinated population. This vaccine contains polysaccharides from serotypes 4, 6B, 9V, 14, 18C, 19F, and 23F conjugated to the nontoxic mutant version of diphtheria toxin, CRM197, and was shown to be highly efficacious (>97%) for prevention of invasive pneumococcal disease and had 67% efficacy for otitis media for the serotypes contained in the vaccine.[100] The vaccine was rapidly adopted throughout much of the world and has led to a profound decrease in pneumococcal disease in this highly vulnerable population. A second vaccine, Synflorix, which contains the serotypes covered by Prevnar and additionally covers serotypes 1, 5, and 7F, was approved shortly thereafter in much of the world. However, this vaccine is not available in the United States, presumably because it does not include serotype 19A, an important cause of invasive disease that began to increase in prevalence following the introduction of Prevnar. The recently introduced vaccine Prevnar13 includes the serotypes contained in Synflorix and adds serotypes 3, 6A, and 19A. The impact of this vaccine on serotype distribution in regions of the world where it is now widely used remains to be seen; however, preliminary data suggest that this vaccine will also lead to a profound reduction in the prevalence of strains for which it is indicated. Interestingly, introduction of conjugate vaccines into the pediatric marketplace has led to a substantial reduction in disease caused by these same serotypes in the elderly population, indicating that transmission of pneumococci from children to elderly adults is one of the prime mechanisms by which adults become infected.

Polysaccharide vaccines have been the sole vaccines used in the adult population for nearly 30 years. The 23-valent vaccine Pneumovax®, which was licensed in 1983 for the prevention of pneumococcal disease in patients older than 55, contains the serotypes 1, 2, 3, 4, 5, 6B, 7F, 8, 9N, 9V, 10A, 11A, 12F, 14, 15B, 17F, 18C, 19A, 19F, 20, 22F, 23F, and 33F. Although this vaccine has demonstrated modest efficacy against invasive pneumococcal disease, its effectiveness against non-bacteremic pneumonia has been somewhat controversial, and the need for additional vaccines for this indication has been suggested. Recently, Prevnar13 was also approved for use in this target population. Although efficacy data for Prevnar13 in this population are not yet available, the immunogenicity of the polysaccharide conjugate vaccine in the elderly has been well established. However, use of this vaccine in the elderly will continue to be a tradeoff between enhanced immunogenicity and decreased strain coverage afforded by the 13-valent vaccine.

Licensure of Pneumococcal Vaccines

Due to the excellent effectiveness afforded by the pneumococcal conjugate vaccines in the pediatric population for the prevention of invasive pneumococcal disease, efficacy studies are no longer feasible in much of the world for licensure of new pneumococcal conjugate vaccines. Therefore, regulatory bodies have utilized an established correlate of protection for conjugate pneumococcal vaccines that evaluates the percentage of individuals achieving at least a minimum antibody threshold of 0.35 μg/mL for each of the polysaccharide types contained in the vaccine following a primary immunization schedule (three doses in the United States) using a standardized enzyme immunoassay. In addition, manufacturers are required to demonstrate the production of functional antibody responses in a subset of subjects, typically using an assay that establishes the ability of antibodies to coat, or opsonize, bacteria, leading to their uptake and killing by phagocytic cells (opsonophagocytic killing assay, or OPA). These surrogate assays allow for licensure of polysaccharide conjugate vaccines, but do not provide a means for licensure of non-polysaccharide vaccines, an obstacle to novel vaccine development that will be discussed later in this chapter.

Identification of Non-Polysaccharide Vaccines for Pneumococcal Disease

Due to the complex nature of developing polysaccharide conjugate vaccines and the number of serotypes required to fully prevent disease in both the pediatric and adult populations, much effort has been put into the identification of vaccines with broad coverage across the majority of pathogenic strains. Wizemann and coworkers[101] reported in 2001 the use of whole genome screening to identify protective antigens from a serotype 4 pneumococcal strain. They used sequence motifs of proteins to identify 130 open reading frames that likely encoded proteins that were surface accessible on the bacterium. The proteins were expressed recombinantly in *Escherichia coli* and used to immunize mice. Challenge of mice with virulent pneumococcal strains suggested that some of these proteins were broadly protective against several serotypes of pneumococci, and further evaluation suggested that the proteins were indeed surface localized, were expressed during infection in humans, and were conserved across the majority of pneumococcal strains that cause disease in humans.

Using a similar approach, Giefing, et al.[102] utilized a peptide display library to identify antigens that were recognized by sera from individuals who were either exposed to pneumococci and did not become infected or from patients that were convalescing from pneumococcal disease. Of the 140 proteins identified, four were shown to protect mice against pneumococcal sepsis, and two (PcsB and StkP) were found to be highly conserved and protective against multiple pneumococcal strains.

To identify antigens that might protect against pneumococcal infections by inducing a T-cell response that may be important in protection at mucosal surfaces, Moffitt and coworkers[103] utilized a screening strategy whereby recombinant antigen libraries covering the pneumococcal genome were screened utilizing Th17 cells isolated from mice that were immune to colonization by *Streptococcus pneumoniae*. The identified proteins also stimulated Th17 secretion by human PBMCs, and immunization with these antigens reduced pneumococcal colonization in experimentally infected mice. The authors further confirmed that this protection against colonization was dependent upon CD4 or IL17A responses.

Numerous pneumococcal proteins have been evaluated as vaccine candidates, and many have demonstrated robust protection against challenge in animal models of infection. The most promising of these antigens will be discussed in more detail below.

PspA

Among the most highly studied pneumococcal protein antigens, pneumococcal surface protein A (PspA) is a member of the choline-binding protein family. These proteins are secreted from the bacterium and then are non-covalently associated to the cell through interaction of a series of protein-encoded binding domain repeats with phosphoryl choline moieties displayed on the teichoic acid. PspA was initially identified as a protective antigen in the 1980s[104] and was subsequently shown to interfere with the deposition of complement C3b on the surface of the bacterium, thereby leading to an impaired activation of the alternative pathway of complement.[105] The N-terminal portion of this protein, which forms an alpha-helical coiled-coil structure, is highly protective in animal models[106] but is highly diverse in sequence,[107] thereby limiting its usefulness as a vaccine antigen. Nevertheless, PspA has been studied in humans and found to be immunogenic and capable of inducing functional antibodies that passively protected mice from pneumococcal challenge.[108]

CbpA and Other Choline-Binding Proteins

Using affinity chromatographic methods, Rosenow et al.[109] identified additional members of the choline-binding family of proteins in a PspA-deficient strain. The most prominent of these family members was CbpA, and the authors suggested that it was important for binding and colonization by pneumococcus in a mouse model. This protein, which was independently identified by other investigators and named PspC or SpsA, also contains a highly variable N-terminal region and is believed to be important in binding various immune molecules such as secretory IgA as well as complement proteins C3 and factor H.[100] Several of the CBPs have been demonstrated to have protective properties in animal models and to play important roles in adherence as well as cell wall modification.[101,110]

Pht Family Proteins

Adamou et al.[111] identified a family of proteins (the Pht family) from the genomic sequence of a pneumococcal strain based on the presence of a lipoprotein-processing domain. This set of proteins (PhtA, B, D, and E) shared a variable level of sequence identity as well as a defining series of histidine triads. These histidine triad motifs have been implicated in the homeostasis of metal ions, and PhtD binding of Zn^{2+} has been demonstrated.[112] The protective efficacy of several of these proteins has been demonstrated in both mouse models of lethal infection[111] as well as in non-human primates.[113] The safety and immunogenicity of PhtD has been demonstrated, both alone and in combination with the choline-binding protein PcpA in human adults,[114,115] and it appears to be a promising option for future vaccine development.

Pneumolysin

Pneumococcus also produces a thiol-activated cytolysin referred to as pneumolysin which is released upon cell autolysis. This toxin interacts with cholesterol on cell membranes, leading to pore formation and cell lysis.[116] In addition to its cytolytic activity on a broad range of cell types, pneumolysin has been shown to directly activate complement[117] and to interfere with host clearance of bacteria.[116] Use of pneumolysin as a vaccine antigen requires careful detoxification of the protein, and this has been accomplished through the replacement of several key amino acids.[118,119] Detoxified forms of the protein have been shown to be highly protective across multiple serotypes of pneumococci,[120] and a pneumolysoid vaccine was recently evaluated in a clinical study in adult volunteers where it was found to be safe and immunogenic.[121] However, because this protein is not found on the surface of the bacterium but rather is released during cellular lysis, the ability of a vaccine targeting pneumolysin to clear pneumococci from an infected host is not known. Instead, a pneumolysoid vaccine will likely be most efficacious in scenarios where antibody-mediated blockade of toxin activity leads to reduction of pathogenesis.

PsaA

Pneumococcal surface antigen A (PsaA) is a lipoprotein tethered to the bacterial membrane and is therefore surface localized and accessible to antibodies. Like the Pht proteins, PsaA is involved in binding of metals required for survival of the bacterium, although in the case of PsaA the metal bound appears to be Mn^{2+}.[122] PsaA has also been suggested to function as an adhesin and virulence factor, although it is unclear whether its contribution to virulence is independent of its metal-binding activity.[123] Regardless of the function of this protein in bacterial pathogenesis, PsaA is an attractive vaccine candidate due to its surface accessibility and high degree of sequence conservation across strains. The efficacy of this protein as a vaccine has been established in multiple animal models, and it is particularly attractive as it appears to be an important contributor to pneumococcal colonization; therefore, targeting the protein may lead to the reduced carriage that is a necessary prerequisite for disease.

Regardless of the protein or proteins used for next-generation pneumococcal vaccines, a major obstacle for the introduction of a protein vaccine is the lack of an immunological surrogate of protection for protein antigens. Therefore, large efficacy trials may be required to demonstrate the effectiveness of these vaccines. As a consequence, protein antigens likely will be added to existing carbohydrate conjugate vaccines to expand the coverage of these vaccines, rather than as replacements for these conjugate vaccines.

Novel Approaches for Vaccine Development

Whole-Cell Vaccines

A novel approach to developing a vaccine for pneumococcal disease that is both affordable and accessible to the developing world has been suggested by Malley et al.[124] They have used a killed, whole-cell vaccine derived from an unencapsulated strain of pneumococcus and demonstrated protection against both colonization and invasive disease in animal models. The advantages of this vaccine are that it could be manufactured at low cost, presumably by vaccine manufacturers in the developing world, and that protection would likely be serotype independent as it is not dependent upon antibodies to capsular polysaccharides. Further characterization of the immune response indicated that protection against colonization was dependent on IL-17-secreting CD4 cells. This novel method of protection may allow for more feasible vaccine studies as carriage of pneumococci is highly prevalent in children, particularly in the regions of the world where pneumococcal conjugate vaccines are not widely used; it is easily assessed and is a prerequisite for invasive disease and transmission.

Use of Conserved Protein Antigens as Carrier Proteins

Due to a lack of an immunological correlate of protection for protein vaccines for pneumococcus, an alternative approach may be required to demonstrate their benefit for vaccine efficacy. One suggested approach would be to incorporate these proteins as T-cell carriers for pneumococcal polysaccharides. In this scenario, vaccines could be licensed based on the established correlate of protection for polysaccharide conjugates, and the benefit afforded by the conserved protein antigens could be assessed following licensure of the vaccine. This benefit could be enhanced overall efficacy as the result of coverage of additional serotypes whose polysaccharides are not included in the vaccine. A similar approach was undertaken during the development of Synflorix, in which the polysaccharides were conjugated to protein D from *Haemophilus influenzae*, a common cause of ear infections in young children. During the evaluation of this vaccine, the investigators were able to demonstrate efficacy not only against otitis media caused by *Streptococcus pneumoniae* but also against the same disease caused by *H. influenzae*, thereby effectively targeting two important pathogens of children.[125]

An interesting alternative to chemical conjugation of polysaccharides to protein antigens has recently been suggested.[126] In this approach, recombinant *Escherichia coli* strains have been engineered to biosynthetically express heterologous polysaccharides from other vaccine targets and to transfer these polysaccharide subunits directly to endogenously expressed carrier protein molecules. This approach allows for the synthesis of polysaccharide conjugates in a single fermentation and should allow for the production of multiple vaccines in an economical manner.

Recently, several studies have questioned the need for direct conjugation of polysaccharide antigens to protein carriers. Instead, they have suggested that delivery of both the protein and polysaccharide in non-covalent associated mixtures, such as in printed, particulate molds, may be sufficient for antigen uptake and presentation.[127] Although these studies will have to be verified for pneumococcal vaccines, they do provide a potential method for inexpensive development of high-valency conjugate vaccines without the need for expensive and complicated conjugation steps.

Conclusion

Regardless of the method by which new vaccines for *Streptococcus pneumoniae* are developed, any new vaccine will have to have several attributes to be successful:

1. A vaccine will have to provide broad strain coverage equal to or greater than currently available vaccines.
2. The vaccine will have to provide equivalent efficacy against invasive pneumococcal disease while potentially also providing benefit for pneumonia, otitis media, and herd immunity through reduction of carriage.
3. A new vaccine will have to be affordable and available in regions of the world that have, to date, not benefited from currently available vaccines.

Recent technological advances in functional genomics, comparative genomics, molecular and cellular immunology, proteomics, bioinformatics, system biology, and vaccinomics have led to identification of novel modalities of immunogens against evolving pathogens (as described above).[128] As immunogen discovery and design have advanced, the methods to formulate and deliver vaccines have also advanced and new strategies have been created for improving vaccine response rates in the target population. Adjuvant systems and vector delivery technologies (e.g., adenovirus, poxvirus) with improved synergy between delivery and immunostimulants, for example, may provide a new strategy for targeting and tuning response rates even in neonates and the elderly. Similarly, optimizing the delivery route (e.g., injectable versus mucosal) and advanced formulation/stabilization approaches (e.g., particles versus conjugates) may direct and augment the host immune response. A focused review of adjuvants, formulations, and delivery methods is presented below.

The reader is reminded that successful development and commercialization of vaccines against evolving pathogen can be complex, and rationale vaccine design requires a mechanistic understanding of host–pathogen interaction, immune evasion, and immune monitoring, as well as strategies to focus immune response on protective epitopes, elicit broad protective immunity, and induce long-term memory response. Immunogen characteristics (e.g., nature, dose) are key to determining immunogenicity; however, other factors such as adjuvant formulation stability, immunization schedule, animal model, and route of delivery are also undoubtedly critical for successful vaccine development. The following section is not meant to be exhaustive and builds upon the earlier described immunogen characteristics with an emphasis on the trends in adjuvants, formulation, delivery routes, and associated focus examples.

DEVELOPMENT OF NOVEL ADJUVANTS

Vaccine adjuvants are immunogen additives required for boosting potency, longevity or quality of the specific immune response to antigen.[129] In general, an adjuvant causes minimal toxicity, does not confer long-lasting immunity in absence of antigen, and improves the robustness of immune response when formulated with the immunogen.[129] Adjuvants can improve the vaccine product by any combination of factors, such as better targeting of the antigens to immune cells, ultimately leading to dose-sparing by reducing the number of required immunizations or the antigen amount, enhancing phagocytosis, modulating antibody avidity, improving efficacy in immunocompromised individuals, overcoming antigen competition in combination vaccines, improving antigen stability, and providing a competitive advantage.[128,130] Despite a wealth of potent adjuvants proven in experimental animal studies and described in the literature, there is an ever-increasing need for developing better adjuvants for next-generation vaccines, especially for complex pathogens similar to ones described in this chapter. In this section, a historical background of adjuvant classification, currently available adjuvants in licensed human vaccines, and trends and challenges of adjuvant development are described followed by a brief summary.

Adjuvant classification attempts have been historically based on their functionality into delivery systems and immune potentiators by O'Hogan et al.[131] Delivery systems optimally present vaccine antigens to the immune system and include controlled release and depot delivery systems such as alum, virosomes, liposomes, viral vectors, and immune-stimulating complexes (ISCOMs), among others.[128,132] Immunopotentiators, in contrast, exert effects ultimately leading to activation of immune cells and includes TLR agonist, bacterial exotoxins, and cytokines.[128,131,133] Similarly, Schjins[134] categorized adjuvants as signal 1 facilitators or signal 2 facilitators.[134] Signal 1 adjuvants facilitate delivery of antigens, their residence time, and/or spatiotemporal behavior and include all delivery systems mentioned above. Signal 2 adjuvants include inflammatory cytokines as well as danger and stranger molecules, including pattern recognition receptors (PRRs). C-type lectin receptors (CLRs),[135] Nod-like receptors (NLRs),[136] RIG-I-like receptors (RLRs),[137] and Toll-like receptors (TLRs)[138] are four subtypes of PRRs.[139] Additionally, immune polarizing components (IPz) can shift the immunity in a desired direction and are classified as Schjins signal 3 adjuvants.[140] PRRs recognize pathogen-associated molecular patterns (PAMPs) such as lipopolysachharide (LPS), CpG oligodeoxynucleotide (hypomethylated DNA), bacterial flagellin, peptidoglycans, etc., and damage-associated molecular patterns (DAMPs) such as monosodium urate crystals (MSUs).[141,163] LPS or its derivative MPL (3-O-desacyl-4-monophosphoryl lipid A), for example, serves as a ligand for TLR-4 receptor on innate immune cell.[142] This critical finding coupled with an improved appreciation that adaptive immunity is dependent upon and preceded by innate immunity, resulted in the realization of the power of adjuvants, and research focused on developing adjuvants with molecularly and functionally defined activators of innate immune cells for rationally designing vaccine.[141] For the purposes of this discussion, licensed adjuvants are described first to acknowledge learning from current successes followed by a brief description of some relevant adjuvants in various stages of development.

Adjuvants currently used in licensed human vaccines include alum (aluminum salts/compounds containing aluminum phosphate, aluminum hydroxide, aluminum sulfate, etc.), virus-like particles (VLPs), oil-in-water (o/w) emulsions, TLR4 agonist such as MPL (bacterially derived monophosphoryl lipid A) and immunopotentiating reconstituted influenza virosomes (IRIVs). Squalene-containing o/w adjuvant emulsions include AS03 (approved in Europe for H1N1 pandemic), MF59 (approved in Europe for seasonal and pandemic influenza), and AF03 (approved in Spain for H1N1 pandemic influenza).[143] Additionally, AS04 (approved in Europe and the United States for hepatitis B virus and human papillomavirus) is a combination adjuvant containing MPL and alum.[144]

Alum, first used to describe aluminum potassium sulfate in 1926, represents the oldest and most commonly used adjuvant. Manufacturing concerns with aluminum potassium sulfate resulted in its limited use, and most alum-based vaccines today use aluminum hydroxide or aluminum phosphate.[145] Despite the fact that aluminum salts differ in their immunological and pharmacological properties, the observed immune response for alum-based vaccines generally is polarized toward a Th2-biased antibody-mediated immunity.[139] The alum adjuvanticity mechanism, however, is still not clear to date, although various hypothesis have been proposed, including adjuvanticity due to particulate and depot effect, NLRP3 inflammasome activation, release of MSU crystals and nucleic acid as DAMPs (endogenous danger signals), induction of IL-4 (B-cell priming), and stimulation of dendritic cells (DCs) and macrophages to produce IL-18, IL-1β, and PGE-2 by a Syk activation pathway.[139,146] Given the diverse, sometimes contradictory, and enormous database on alum adjuvanticity, it is not possible to reconcile all alum studies, but in general it can be stated that Th-2 response, pleiotropic alum effects, and established safety are hallmarks of alum-based vaccines. Local reactions (induction of granulomas at the injection site), inability to freeze and/or freeze-dry, and lack of proper cytotoxic T-lymphocyte (CTL) priming are some of its potential deficiencies.[140] Additionally, the need for an adjuvant with strong T-cell responses, broader immune response against different serotypes and serogroups, long-term protection and immunological memory, suitable immune response for immune-senescence or immune-suppressed patients, and the need for dose-sparing, especially to stop the spread of a pandemic, has inspired the research for novel potent adjuvants.

GlaxoSmithKline's Adjuvant Systems serve as examples of adjuvant combination that may provide synergistic and/or complementary tailored immune enhancement for a given target population. Vaccination in neonates, for example, produces a Th2 type response, and combination adjuvants may enhance Th1 type responses. Research into adjuvant systems was initiated by GlaxoSmithKline to develop vaccines against complex pathogen such as HIV, HPV, OR malaria that contain a combination of adjuvants facilitating signal 1, signal 2, and signal 3.[147] AS04, the only other licensed adjuvant in the United States besides alum, is a TLR-based adjuvant that contains alum in combination with MPL. Evaluation of an HPV vaccine adjuvanted with AS04 revealed superior anti-HPV antibody responses and memory B-cell responses compared to alum-only formulations.[148] An AS04 mechanistic study suggested that the enhancement of immune responses could be attributed to direct triggering of local cytokine responses, thereby resulting in optimal activation of antigen-presenting cells (APCs).[149] AS04 is currently licensed for use in Cervarix® and Fendrix® (GlaxoSmithKline).

Prominent examples of other adjuvant systems in various phases of development include GlaxoSmithKline's AS01 (combination of liposome, MPL, and QS21 that is used in clinical trials against malaria), AS02 (combination of MPL and QS21 that is used in clinical trials against malaria), and AS15 (combination of CpG, liposome, MPL, and QS21 that is used in clinical trials against prostate cancer).[150] It must be noted that, in general, as the complexity of the combination is increased, the challenges around safety, regulatory issues, manufacturability, and cost increase, and a risk/reward ratio must be assessed for each combination type.

MF59 and AS03 are emulsions consisting of nanometer-size droplets($\sim$ 160 nm) of an oil(squalene)-in-water formulation. There are compositional differences between the two, with the prominent difference being that AS03 contains α-tocopherol (2.5%).[143] An immune potentiator, α-tocopherol is a form of vitamin E and is responsible for enhancing the antibody response through induction of cytokine responses at the local injection site and modulation of cell recruitment, ultimately leading to improved adaptive immunity.[151] Improved efficacy, dose-sparing (3.75 μg HA-MF59 versus 15 μg unadjuvanted for H1N1 or H5N1), and improved breadth of response make both adjuvants attractive options, especially during pandemic outbreaks. A single dose of Focetria® (MF59 adjuvanted H1N1 vaccine by Novartis), for example, was comparably potent to two unadjuvanted vaccine doses in 6-month-old infants as well as in adults.[143] Additionally, it was reported that MF59 could alter the quality of immune responses through epitope spreading, and in an independent study the enhanced avidity of antibodies was also observed.[143,152] Unsubstantiated (now discredited) claims linking "Gulf War syndrome" with the use of squalene and reported incidences of narcolepsy with cataplexy with the use of AS03-adjuvanted vaccine represent some of the safety and tolerability concerns that need to be considered when developing novel adjuvants with a limited track record of safety.[143,153]

Virus-like particles, liposomes, and virosomes are spherical nanoparticle-based vaccine antigen delivery vehicles that rely on the native host's mechanisms to initiate an immune response. VLPs are self-assembled viral proteins/lipid particles, whereas liposomes are phospholipid bi- or multilayered vesicles with an aqueous core. In contrast, virosomes contains viral envelope glycoproteins (influenza HA and NA) intercalated in the phospholipid bilayer to mimic a VLP or a reconstituted enveloped virus membrane known as a reconstituted virosome (IRIV).[154] Inflexal® V (Crucell) for influenza and Epaxal® (Crucell) for hepatitis A are licensed virosomal vaccines approved in some countries.[140] Recombivax HB® (Merck) and Engerix-BTM (GlaxoSmithKline) for hepatitis B and Gardasil® (Merck) and Cervarix® (GlaxoSmithKline) for HPV are examples of VLP-based approved vaccines. In contrast, liposomal adjuvanted vaccines are currently in various phases of clinical trials, and it has been reported that incorporation of PAMPs can enhance their intrinsic adjuvant effect.[153,155]

Combination adjuvants generally contain various combinations of delivery systems and immunostimulatory adjuvants as well as a combination of different subtypes of PRRs, including the (1) use of NLR agonist such as muramyl dipeptide (a NOD-2 agonist) with alum as a delivery system for recombinant antigen *Helicobacter pylori* urease;[156] (2) CLR agonists such as cationic adjuvant formulation 01 consisting of trahalose-6-6-dibehenate with a cationic liposome as a delivery system for a TB vaccine;[157] or (3) a combination of TLR agonists such as poly I:C (TLR-3 agonist) with CpG ODN (TLR-9 agonist) for an HIV Gag vaccine.[158] Recently, a combination of three different TLR agonists (e.g., macrophage-activating TLR-2 agonist with PolyI:C and CpG ODN) with an HIV enveloped peptide was used to enhance the functional avidity of T cells in mice and increase IL-15 production by dendritic cells.[159] The study demonstrated the potent adjuvanticity of the triple combination. Similarly, Finlay adjuvants AFPL1 and AFCo1 proteo-cochleates contain multiple synergistic PAMPs such as lipid-inserted natural LPS, traces of bacterial DNA, and porins. AFPL1TM, a proteoliposome adjuvant, is the main component of VA-MENGOC-BC (a meningococcal BC human vaccine).[160] The reader is guided to a recent in-depth review focused on various adjuvant combinations in development for generating tailored immune responses to vaccines.[147]

Other approaches to adjuvant vaccines rely on using conjugation chemistry, regulating inflammation through RNAi silencing, targeting dendritic cells using vectors, cytokine combinations, using immune-stimulating complexes (ISCOMs), or traditionally using inherent adjuvant mechanisms by using live attenuated or inactivated pathogens.[161] Covalent conjugation allows induction of long-lived thymus-dependent (TD) immune responses for thymus-independent (TI) polysaccharides antigens.[140] Conjugation with carriers such as CRM197 (a nontoxic diphtheria toxin mutant used in Prevnar® from Pfizer), outer membrane proteins OMP NmB from *Neisseria meningitides* serogroup B (used in the *Haemophilus influenzae* B vaccine PedvaxHIB® from Merck), and tetanus toxoid TT (used in the *H. influenzae* B vaccine ActHIB® from Sanofi Pasteur) provides T-cell help in mounting effective antigen specific responses. Various other examples of conjugated vaccines can be viewed in a recent review.[140]

Current Issues in Adjuvants Development

As mentioned above, recent advances in adjuvants stem from the research findings demonstrating that innate immunity (mediated by dendritic cells and macrophages) is essential for eliciting effective induction of adaptive immunity (mediated by B cells, T cells, and memory cells).[162,163] Greater appreciation and understanding of pathogen detection mechanisms by the innate immune system through the uses of pathogen recognition receptors such as toll-like receptors (TLRs), for example, have revolutionized novel vaccine adjuvant development. Despite these advances, few adjuvants are used in commercial settings, underscoring the fact that adjuvant development remains a challenging and difficult endeavor. Some of the challenges associated with adjuvant development are briefly described here. Adjuvant research is not a stand-alone field in vaccinology, and adjuvants are licensed only in the presence of antigens. Given that preventive vaccination is usually given to healthy children in their first year, safety and tolerability are key requirements of successful vaccine. Novel adjuvants with no track record around safety often fail to provide information on adverse events that are rare (<1/1000 doses), found in specific subsets of target population (e.g., infants), and occur with a delayed onset ($\geq$30 days after vaccination).[164] Safety monitoring after licensure is therefore considered critical, and toxicity and unacceptable side effects are still the biggest challenges in developing novel adjuvanted vaccines.

Critical factors that pose a significant barrier in successful development of a new adjuvanted vaccine include the following:

- Limited know-how
- Lack of cross-pollination among vaccine companies with regard to their own adjuvant research programs, underscoring the significance of adjuvant formulation by many vaccinologists
- Complex regulatory pathways and comparability concerns
- Accessibility
- Cost of consumables
- Establishment of new analytical characterization tools
- Difficulty in establishing sustainable and transferable manufacturing processes and documentation (e.g., form/fill, inspection, batch records, standard operating procedures)
- Lack of realization that immune polarization for a desired route of immunization might be essential for induction of protection.

Formulation

Successful vaccine development hinges on multiple factors. Given that antigens, adjuvants, formulations, analyticals, processes, and delivery routes are intimately tied to each other, access to adjuvants is valuable only if it is accompanied by formulation and analytical know-how. For any given modality of vaccine, the end goal of formulation is to deliver a safe, effective, and quality vaccine, which is usually a multistep process beginning with efforts to stabilize the vaccine and improve its immunogenicity. The route of administration significantly impacts the choice of excipients and formulation choices. Vaccine stabilization is essential to maintaining an acceptable shelf-life and involves both chemical and physical stabilization of the vaccine for the intended shelf-life. This section is focused on formulation development of injectables as they are the vaccine delivery benchmark (intramuscular as well as subcutaneous).

Non-adjuvanted formulations, such as certain live attenuated and inactivated vaccines with naturally occurring immunostimulants (e.g., immune polarizers, immune potentiator) have potent antigens and often do not require additional adjuvantation (e.g., Zostavax® from Merck). However, these vaccines are often unstable in an aqueous phase. Additionally, the absence of a structure–function correlation, residual host-cell DNA and protein concentration, lack of appropriate analytical assays when the exact epitope is not well defined, limitation on drug substance availability especially during the early phase of programs, and lack of proper animal models make formulating these vaccines a challenging task. The highly labile nature of vaccines in aqueous states generally prompts their storage and transportation in a frozen or even dried state. Freezing and drying, however, generate various stresses such as formation of ice–solute interfaces, potential pH changes, cold denaturation, and phase separation, which could be detrimental to the vaccine.[165] These issues are often mitigated by proper selection of buffer, pH condition, ionic strength, excipients, and stabilizers as well as by optimization of the drying process.[165] Additionally, time in solution (TIS), including predrying as well as post-reconstitution, and time out of refrigeration (TOR) are critical features to characterize for attaining a scalable process. Drying methods of choice can vary from vaccine to vaccine on a case-by-case basis and may often depend on the route of administration and desired target product profile. Freeze drying, a commonly used approach, for example, has been used to dry smallpox (approved by the U.S. Food and Drug Administration in 1931), MMR®, Zostavax®, and Proquad®, among others. Recent advances in drying technologies have resulted in the use of spray drying, spray freeze drying, atmospheric drying, and supercritical fluid technology.[166] Pulmonary powder influenza vaccine, for example, was recently dried using spray drying or spray freeze drying using oligofructose as the stabilizer.[167]

Adjuvanted formulations, are usually developed for recombinant proteins and DNA vaccines as they are poorly immunogenic due to the absence of many key pathogen features essential for evoking a strong immune response and may requires adjuvants to resemble "actual infection."[168] The choice of adjuvant (as described in the previous section) is critical for successful development of vaccines and depends on antigen properties (e.g., charge, solubility, particulate), type of immunity desired, stability, route of delivery, and known side effects. Four recombinant dengue subunit proteins, for example, when formulated with various novel and licensed adjuvants (e.g., MF59, alum, MF75 with threonyl-MDP, ISCOMATRIX™) revealed the most potent virus-neutralizing titers in ISCOMATRIX adjuvant in both mouse and non-human primate models.[96] During these studies no signs of immunological or pharmaceutical interference or competition was evident between the four antigen studied. Similarly, formulating DNA vaccines in microparticle or liposomal vesicles has been reported to increase their uptake by cells.[169] Formulation of an influenza DNA vaccine in Vaxfectin® adjuvant (Vical), for example, induced T-cell responses and protective antibody titers in patients. Additionally, DNA vaccines allow modulating the immune response through coimmunization with molecular adjuvants (cytokine genes).[170] Codelivery of granulocyte–macrophage colony-stimulating factor (GM-CSF) as molecular adjuvant, for example, induced higher HIV-1 antibody avidity and resulted in improved neutralizing antibody production in non-human primates (NHPs).[171] These examples illustrate the impact of choosing the right formulation to improve the breadth, durability, and magnitude of immune response.

Viral vector platforms, such as adenovirus (Ad) or vaccinia virus (VV), can induce strong cellular immune responses but their production can be unstable, complex, and expensive. Although effective in prime-boost regimens, these vectors generate antivector immunity and can be pathogenic in immunocompromised individuals, especially upon repeated administration.[170]

III. NOVEL APPROACHES FOR VACCINES

Use of a rare serotype vector may overcome this issue and help development of vaccines against pathogens as complex as HIV due to strong induction of cellular immunity. Additionally, characterizing the adjuvant and antigen–adjuvant interaction is important to optimize formulation development for maximum stabilization. Aluminum hydroxide adjuvant has a positive charge (point of zero charge is 11.4), while aluminum phosphate has a negative surface charge at physiological pH (point of zero charge is ~5.5).[172] Adsorption studies and chemical (e.g., chromatography) and physical (e.g., light-scattering) characterization must be used to characterize the vaccine wherever possible. Correlation (if proven) of biological assays (e.g., cell-based potency assay) to structural characterization may result in expedited development of a stable, quality product (provided a structure–function correlation exists). Some of the other factors to consider while developing a suitable particle formulation include the following:[168]

- Antimicrobial effectiveness for multivalent products (e.g., 2-phenoxyenthanol for Prevnar13[173])
- Non-ionic surfactants to prevent loss of antigen due to adsorption on glass or to prevent aggregation
- Size, surface charge, and hydrophobicity for microparticles
- Lamellarity, surface charge, fluidity, and fusogenicity for liposomes
- Covalent conjugation, adsorption, and encapsulation.

For phagocytosis, for example, the optimal particle size suggested is between 200 nm to 1 μm; thus, it essential that the selected formulation be viewed not only for stability but also from the standpoint of a desired immune response.[139]

Route of Delivery

Defining the most appropriate route of immunization requires an enhanced understanding of the local factors, at the site of infection, that regulate immunity. There is a general consensus among scientists that the efficacy of even the best vaccine candidate can be compromised by a poor selection of delivery route. Pathogens responsible for gastrointestinal, respiratory, and sexually transmitted diseases, for example, initiate local infection at the mucosal surface, and it is likely that mucosal immunity may be essential for their control and prevention.[174]

As mentioned in the above section, most vaccines are delivered intramuscularly or subcutaneously, and these injectables routes have been the benchmark for vaccine delivery. Although their use is common, syringes and needles have several disadvantages, such as the risk of needle-related injuries, bloodborne disease transmission, need for trained medical professionals, needle phobia, and inefficient immunological responses. Therefore, to overcome the current limitations of injectable vaccines, improve patient compliance, develop easy-to-use worldwide mass vaccination for avoiding pandemics, and target desired immune responses several alternatives to injectables are currently in use or are being explored, as described below. This section focuses on recent trends and strategies used in developing effective transcutaneous and mucosal vaccines.

Transcutaneous vaccination serves as an appealing alternative to intramuscular (i.m.) or subcutaneous (s.c.) injections due to the presence of various immunocompetent cells (e.g., Langerhans cells, dermal dendritic cells, macrophages, keratinocytes, mast cells, T cells) in the skin. The reader is reminded that skin is composed of stratum corneum (20 μm thick), epidermis (200 μm thick), and dermis (2 mm thick).[175] Due to the presence of complementary antigen-presenting cells, delivery in the transcutaneous space induces strong, broad, and potent immune responses. Transcutaneous vaccination requires antigen delivery through the stratum corneum, often achieved either by promoting antigen permeation or through physical delivery of antigen into the skin. Partial stripping of the stratum corneum (i.e., skin abrasion), followed by application of Intercell's vaccine patch (Phase II clinical trial) showed promising transcutaneous immunostimulation and induced mucosal immunity against traveler's diarrhea; however, the approach failed to meet its efficacy endpoint in a Phase III trial.[176] Delivery of a trivalent seasonal influenza vaccine using the BD Soluvia™ device (1.5-mm-long, 30g needle) underlines the effectiveness of skin immunization protocols.[177] Microneedles (which provide targeted delivery in dermis and epidermis) for intradermal injection are an attractive alternative to overcome the skin barrier for delivery of an antigen. The Nanopatch™ device, for example, is a vaccine-coated microprojection array (1 cm^2 surface with ~20,000 projections) for intradermal delivery that targets immune cells in the dermis and epidermis.[178] Preclinical studies in a mouse model using Fluvax® and Gardasil® demonstrated improved efficacy compared to conventional i.m. injections. Development and evaluation of various delivery strategies using microneedles (e.g., solid, hollow, coated, or dissolving microneedles) are underway. Intradermal delivery for influenza vaccine (3.3 μg of hemagglutinin) to human volunteers using MicronJet™ (a 4 × 1 hollow microneedle with 450-μm-long needle, developed by NanoPass), for example, induced immune responses comparable to 3.3 μg of a hemagglutinin i.m. injection.[179] Physical techniques such as ultrasound, eltroporation, and jet injectors have also been used to overcome delivery issues across the stratum corneum.[175] The use of these specialized devices has shown early promise. Optimization of delivery device parameters such as microneedle size, diameter, tip geometry, and density; choice of adjuvants (if required) such as bacterial enterotoxins and TLR ligands; and selection of the excipient and drying/coating approach are essential for developing a successful formulation for transcutaneous delivery.

Mucosal vaccination (i.e., oral, intranasal, sublingual, rectal, and intravaginal) is an attractive alternative because it offers improved patient compliance, ease of administration for mass vaccinations, reduced risk of spreading bloodborne infections, and, from a regulatory and manufacturing perspective, low endotoxin concerns in comparison to parenterally injected vaccines.[180] Furthermore, mucosal immunization can trigger both humoral and cell-mediated immune protection not only at the site of delivery but also systemically with induction of long-term B-cell and T-cell memory.[180]

Despite the success of the oral polio vaccine (live attenuated) only a few mucosal vaccines exist commercially. Mucosal vaccination is a challenging task for the following reasons:

- Risk of mucosal tolerance in contrast to protective immunity
- Poor stability of live attenuated vaccines
- Higher dose and prolonged antigen exposure requirements
- Need for repeated immunization, which requires balancing attenuation of live virus with vaccine immunogenicity
- Differences in efficacy in developed versus developing countries (the tropical barrier)
- Imprecise protection correlates
- Sophisticated formulation requirements for exploiting the interaction of mucosal inductive sites and effector sites.

Vaccination to stimulate immunity within specific subcompartments—bronchus-associated lymphoid tissue (BALT), nasopharynx-associated lymphoid tissue (NALT), gut-associated lymphoid tissue (GALT), genital tract-associated lymphoid tissue, and closely located subcompartments of mucosa-associated lymphoid tissue (MALT)—is essential for developing suitable mucosal vaccines against complex pathogens.[180] Intranasal immunity, for example, stimulates protective immunity not only at upper and lower respiratory tracts but also at gastric mucosa and the genital tract mucosa. FluMist®, an example of a live attenuated influenza vaccine from MedImmune, not only has proven to be effective against seasonal infection but also provides cross-protection against antigenically drifted influenza strains.[181]

Oral vaccines, in contrast, prime the gut by infecting the host at microfold cells (M cells) present in the follicle-associated epithelium (FAE) which overlies Peyer's patches and by increasing antigen uptake in interstitially located dendritic intestinal cells. Examples of licensed oral vaccines include RotaTeq® (live attenuated multivalent rotavirus vaccine), Vivotif® (live attenuated *Salmonella typhi*), and Dukoral® and Shanchol® (whole killed *Vibrio cholerae* bacteria with and without recombinant cholera toxin). It should be noted that oral vaccines are stable in acidic conditions and are often formulated in bicarbonate buffers to protect antigens from harsh gastric conditions.[166] Sublingual vaccines induce strong protective IgA, systemic IgG antibody, and cytotoxic CD8+ T-cell immunity.[180] Additionally, it was demonstrated that sublingual administration of influenza (inactivated or live) virus in mice avoids any perturbation of central nervous function.[182] Besides safety, dose-sparing compared to oral vaccines and ease of administration even for children are some of the key advantages of a sublingual vaccination route. Mucosal formulations (soluble or particulate), in general, can be formulated with muco(bio)adhesives (e.g., chitosan, lectins, antibodies specific for M cells) and immunomodulating properties (e.g., TLR ligands, cholera toxin subunit B).

Recommendations

Recent advances in adjuvanted vaccines open new avenues to rationally direct innate immunity sensors to alter the quality and quantity of adaptive immune responses. Optimization of delivery systems and immunopotentiators, PAMP-/DAMP-based adjuvants, targeting moieties through conjugation or non-specific methods, combination adjuvants, and development of synthetic analogs present an exciting opportunity to develop successful vaccination against difficult targets such as HIV. Given the established safety track record of alum, its wide acceptance and approval, and its low cost, alum must be used if the adjuvant effect is clear. For potent antigens, no adjuvant may be required. In addition to alum, licensed adjuvants of known safety (by themselves as well as in combination with the antigen *in vivo*, *in vitro*, and *in silico*), mechanisms of action for the target populations, accessibility, and minimal side effects must be used. Vaccine development can be approached rationally if the adjuvanticity mechanism and immunological correlates of protection are known. In addition to suitable antigen–adjuvant combinations (e.g., antigens capable of inducing BnAbs for HIV-1 and influenza with vectored delivery), the formulation (for stability as well as immunogenicity improvement), route of delivery, and immunization regimen for the targeted response (e.g., intranasal priming with intravaginal boosting to elicit strong immune responses in the genital tract) are critical to winning the race against evolving pathogens. Improved vector delivery technologies targeted for systemic and mucosal immunity such as paramyxovirus, adenovirus, and bacterial vectors, for example, may be beneficial (even necessary) for the control and prevention of emerging and reemerging pathogens. In all considerations, an up-front risk/reward ratio needs to be assessed, and mechanistic approaches (e.g., immune correlates, disease evasion mechanisms, immunization strategies) must be used to evaluate the success and/or failure to better design the next-generation adjuvant. Additionally, if feasible, small human clinical experimental studies must be performed to expedite an early go/no-go decision and better quantify the risk/reward ratio with greater emphasis on safety in comparison to efficacy.

References

1. Lam TT, Wang J, Shen Y, Zhou B, Duan L, Cheung CL, et al. The genesis and source of the H7N9 influenza viruses causing human infections in China. Nature 2013;502:241–4.
2. Russell CA, Jones TC, Barr IG, Cox NJ, Garten RJ, Gregory V, et al. The global circulation of seasonal influenza A (H3N2) viruses. Science 2008;320:340–6.
3. DiazGranados CA, Denis M, Plotkin S. Seasonal influenza vaccine efficacy and its determinants in children and non-elderly adults: a systematic review with meta-analyses of controlled trials. Vaccine 2012;31:49–57.
4. Beyer WE, McElhaney J, Smith DJ, Monto AS, Nguyen-Van-Tam JS, Osterhaus AD. Cochrane re-arranged: Support for policies to vaccinate elderly people against influenza. Vaccine 2013;31:6030–3.
5. Sridhar S, Begom S, Bermingham A, Hoschler K, Adamson W, Carman W, et al. Cellular immune correlates of protection against symptomatic pandemic influenza. Nat. Med. 2013;19:1305–12.
6. Li CK, Rappuoli R, Xu XN. Correlates of protection against influenza infection in humans-on the path to a universal vaccine? Curr. Opin. Immunol. 2013;25:470–6.
7. Pépin S, Donazzolo Y, Jambrecina A, Salamand C, Saville M. Safety and immunogenicity of a quadrivalent inactivated influenza vaccine in adults. Vaccine 2013;31:5572–8.
8. Haaheim LR, Katz JM. Immune correlates of protection against influenza - challenges for licensure of seasonal and pandemic influenza vaccines, Miami, FL, USA, March 1-3, 2010. Influenza Other Resp. Viruses 2011;5:288–95.
9. Schwarz TF, Horacek T, Knuf M, Damman HG, Roman F, Dramé M, et al. Single dose vaccination with AS03–adjuvanted H5N1 vaccines in a randomized trial induces strong and broad immune responsiveness to booster vaccination in adults. Vaccine 2009;27:6284–90.
10. Leroux-Roels I, Roman F, Forgus S, Maes C, De Boever F, Dramé M, et al. Priming with AS03 A-adjuvanted H5N1 influenza vaccine improves the kinetics, magnitude and durability of the immune response after a heterologous booster vaccination: an open non-randomised extension of a double-blind randomised primary study. Vaccine 2010;28:849–57.
11. Vesikari T, Knuf M, Wutzler P, Karvonen A, Kieninger-Baum D, Schmitt HJ, et al. Oil-in-water emulsion adjuvant with influenza vaccine in young children. N. Engl. J. Med. 2011;365:1406–16.
12. Banzhoff A, Stoddard JJ. Effective influenza vaccines for children: critical unmet medical need and a public health priority. Hum. Vaccin. Immunother. 2012;8:398–402.
13. McElhaney JE, Beran J, Devaster JM, Esen M, Launay O, Leroux-Roels G, et al. AS03-adjuvanted versus non-adjuvanted inactivated trivalent influenza vaccine against seasonal influenza in elderly people: a phase 3 randomised trial. Lancet Infect Dis. 2013;13:485–96.
14. Galli G, Medini D, Borgogni E, Zedda L, Bardelli M, Malzone C, et al. Adjuvanted H5N1 vaccine induces early CD4+ T cell response that predicts long-term persistence of protective antibody levels. Proc. Natl. Acad. Sci. U.S.A. 2009;106:3877–82.
15. O'Hagan DT, Ott GS, De Gregorio E, Seubert A. The mechanism of action of MF59 - an innately attractive adjuvant formulation. Vaccine 2012;30:4341–8.
16. Khurana S, Verma N, Yewdell JW, Hilbert AK, Castellino F, Lattanzi M, et al. MF59 adjuvant enhances diversity and affinity of antibody-mediated immune response to pandemic influenza vaccines. Sci. Transl. Med. 2011;3:85ra48.

17. Partinen M, Saarenpää-Heikkilä O, Ilveskoski I, Hublin C, Linna M, Olsén P, et al. Increased incidence and clinical picture of childhood narcolepsy following the 2009 H1N1 pandemic vaccination campaign in Finland. PLoS ONE 2012;7:e33723.

18. Miller E, Andrews N, Stellitano L, Stowe J, Winstone AM, Shneerson J, et al. Risk of narcolepsy in children receiving an AS03 adjuvanted AH1N1 (2009) influenza vaccine in England. BMJ 2013;346:f794.

19. Clegg CH, Roque R, Van Hoeven N, Perrone L, Baldwin SL, Rininger JA, et al. Adjuvant solution for pandemic influenza vaccine production. Proc. Natl. Acad. Sci. U.S.A. 2012;109:17585–90.

20. Yang LP. Recombinant trivalent influenza vaccine (Flublok®): a review of its use in the prevention of seasonal influenza in adults. Drugs 2013;73:1357–66.

21. DuBois RM, Aguilar-Yañez JM, Mendoza-Ochoa GI, Oropeza-Almazán Y, Schultz-Cherry S, Alvarez MM, et al. The receptor-binding domain of influenza virus hemagglutinin produced in *Escherichia coli* folds into its native, immunogenic structure. J. Virol. 2011;85:865–72.

22. Taylor DN, Treanor JJ, Strout C, Johnson C, Fitzgerald T, Kavita U, et al. Induction of a potent immune response in the elderly using the TLR-5 agonist, flagellin, with a recombinant hemagglutinin influenza–flagellin fusion vaccine (VAX125, STF2. HA1 SI). Vaccine 2011;29:4897–902.

23. Corti D, Voss J, Gamblin SJ, Codoni G, Macagno A, Jarrossay D, et al. A neutralizing antibody selected from plasma cells that binds to group 1 and group 2 influenza A hemagglutinins. Science 2011;333: 850–6.

24. Bommakanti G, Lu X, Citron MP, Najar TA, Heidecker GJ, ter Meulen J, et al. Design of *Escherichia coli*-expressed stalk domain immunogens of H1N1 hemagglutinin that protect mice from lethal challenge. J. Virol. 2012;86:13434–44.

25. Margine I, Krammer F, Hai R, Heaton NS, Tan GS, Andrews SA, et al. Hemagglutinin stalk-based universal vaccine constructs protect against group 2 influenza A viruses. J. Virol. 2013;87:10435–46.

26. Kanekiyo M, Wei CJ, Yassine HM, McTamney PM, Boyington JC, Whittle JR, et al. Self-assembling influenza nanoparticle vaccines elicit broadly neutralizing H1N1 antibodies. Nature 2013;499:102–6.

27. Khurana S, Loving CL, Manischewitz J, King LR, Gauger PC, Henningson J, et al. Vaccine-induced anti-HA2 antibodies promote virus fusion and enhance influenza virus respiratory disease. Sci. Transl. Med. 2013;5:200ra114.

28. UNAIDS. *Global Report: UNAIDS Report on the Global AIDS Epidemic*. Geneva, Switzerland: Joint United Nations Programme on HIV/AIDS (UNAIDS), 2013.

29. Wonderlich ER, Leonard JA, Collins KL. HIV immune evasion: disruption of antigen presentation by the HIV nef protein. Adv. Virus Res. 2011;80:103–27.

30. Goulder PJ, Walker BD. The great escape—AIDS viruses and immune control. Nat. Med. 1999;5:1233–5.

31. Frost SD, Trkola A, Günthard HF, Richman DD. Antibody responses in primary HIV-1 infection. Curr. Opin. HIV AIDS 2008;3:45–51.

32. Lyerly HK, Reed DL, Matthews TJ, Langlois AJ, Ahearne PA, Petteway SR, et al. Anti-gp-120 antibodies from HIV seropositive individuals mediate broadly reactive anti-HIV ADCC. AIDS Res. Hum. Retroviruses 1987;3:409–22.

33. Evans CM, Kudesia G, McKendrick M. Management of herpesvirus infections. Int. J. Antimicrob. Agents 2013;42:119–28.

34. Baker BM, Block BL, Rothchild AC, Walker BD. Elite control of HIV infection: implications for vaccine design. Exp. Opin. Biol. Ther. 2009;9:55–69.

35. Kiepela P, Ngumbela K, Thobakgale C, Rambuth D, Honeyborne I, Moodley E, et al. CD8+ T-cell responses to different HIV proteins have discordant associations with viral load. Nat. Med. 2007;13:46–53.

36. Pitisuttithum P, Gilbert P, Gurwith M, Heyward W, Martin M, van Griensven F, et al. Bangkok Vaccine Evaluation Group. Randomized, double-blind, placebo-controlled efficacy trial of a bivalent recombinant glycoprotein 120 HIV-1 vaccine among injection drug users in Bangkok, Thailand. J. Infect. Dis. 2006;194:1661–71.

37. Buchbinder SP, Mehrotra DV, Duerr A, Fitzgerald DW, Mogg R, Li D, et al. Step Study Protocol Team. Efficacy assessment of a cell-mediated immunity HIV-1 vaccine (the Step Study): a double-blind, randomised, placebo-controlled, test-of-concept trial. Lancet 2008;372:1881–93.

38. Coplan PM, Gupta S, Dubey SA, Pitisuttithum P, Nikas A, Mbewe B, et al. Cross-reactivity of anti-HIV1 T cell immune response among the major HIV-1 clades in HIV-1-positive individuals from 4 continents. J. Infect. Dis. 2005;191:1427–34.

39. Bett AJ, Dubey SA, Mehrotra DV, Guan L, Long R, Anderson K, et al. Comparison of T cell immune responses induced by vectored HIV vaccines in non-human primates and humans. Vaccine 2010;28: 7881–9.

40. Hertz T, Ahmed H, Friedrich DP, Casimiro DR, Self SG, Corey L, et al. HIV-1 vaccine-induced T-cell responses cluster in epitope hotspots that differ from those induced in natural infection with HIV-1. PLoS Pathog. 2013;9:e1003404.

41. Li F, Finnefrock AC, Dubey SA, Korber BT, Szinger J, Cole S, et al. Mapping HIV-1 vaccine induced T cell-responses: bias towards less-conserved regions and potential impact on vaccine efficacy in the Step Study. PLoS ONE 2011;6:e20479.

42. Rolland M, Tovanabutra S, deCamp AC, Frahm N, Gilbert PB, Sanders-Buell E, et al. Genetic impact of vaccination on breakthrough HIV-1 sequences from the STEP trial. Nat. Med. 2011;17:366–71.

43. O'Brien KL, Liu J, King SL, Sun YH, Schmitz JE, Lifton MA, et al. Adenovirus-specific immunity after immunization with an Ad5 HIV-1 vaccine candidate in humans. Nat. Med. 2009;15:873–5.

44. Hammer SM, Sobieszczyk ME, Janes H, Karuna ST, Mulligan MJ, Grove D, et al. Efficacy trial of a DNA/rAd5 HIV-1 preventive vaccine. N. Engl. J Med. 2013;69:2083–92.

45. Rerks-Ngarm S, Pitisuttithum P, Nitayaphan S, Kaewkungwal J, Chiu J, Paris R, et al. Vaccination with ALVAC and AIDSVAX to prevent HIV-1 infection in Thailand. N. Engl. J. Med. 2009;361(23): 2209–20.

46. Haynes BF, Gilbert PB, McElrath MJ, Zolla-Pazner S, Tomaras GD, Alam SM, et al. Immune-correlates analysis of an HIV-1 vaccine efficacy trial. N. Engl. J. Med. 2012;366:1275–86.

47. Forthal D, Hope TJ, Alter G. New paradigms for functional HIV-specific nonneutralizing antibodies. Curr. Opin. HIV AIDS 2013;8:393–401.

48. Koff W. HIV vaccine development: challenges and opportunities towards solving the HIV vaccine-neutralizing antibody problem. Vaccine 2012;30:4310–5.

49. Barouch DH, Liu J, Li H, Maxfield LF, Abbink P, Lynch DM, et al. Vaccine protection against acquisition of neutralization-resistant SIV challenges in rhesus monkeys. Nature 2012;482:89–93.

50. Parks CL, Picker LJ, King CR. Development of replication-competent viral vectors for HIV vaccine delivery. Curr. Opin. HIV AIDS 2013;8:402–11.

51. Barouch DH, O'Brien KL, Simmons NL, King SL, Abbink P, Maxfield LF, et al. Mosaic HIV-1 vaccines expand the breadth and depth of cellular immune responses in rhesus monkeys. Nat. Med. 2010;16: 319–23.

52. Kibler KV, Gomez CE, Perdiguero B, Wong S, Huynh T, Holechek S, et al. Improved NYVAC-based vaccine vectors. PLoS ONE 2011;6:e25674.

53. Hansen SG, Vieville C, Whizin N, Coyne-Johnson L, Siess DC, Drummond DD, et al. Effector memory T cell responses are associated with protection of rhesus monkeys from mucosal simian immunodeficiency virus challenge. Nat. Med. 2009;15:293–9.

54. Hansen SG, Ford JC, Lewis MS, Ventura AB, Hughes CM, Coyne-Johnson L, et al. Profound early control of highly pathogenic SIV by an effector memory T-cell vaccine. Nature 2011;473:523–7.

55. Hansen SG, Sacha JB, Hughes CM, Ford JC, Burwitz BJ, Scholz I, et al. Cytomegalovirus vectors violate CD8+ T cell epitope recognition paradigms. Science 2013;340:1237874.

56. Burny W, Liesnard C, Donner C, Marchant A. Epidemiology, pathogenesis and prevention of congenital cytomegalovirus infection. Exp. Rev. Anti-Infect. Ther. 2004;2:881–94.

57. Bhatt S, Gething PW, Brady OJ, Messina JP, Farlow AW, Moyes CL, et al. The global distribution and burden of dengue. Nature 2013;496:504.

58. Gubler DJ. Dengue, urbanization, and globalization: the unholy trinity of the 21st century. Trop. Med. Health. 2011;39(Suppl.):3–11.

59. Simmons CP, Farrar JJ, Vinh Chau N, Wills B. Current concepts: dengue. N. Engl. J. Med. 2012;366:75.

60. Guzman MG, Halstead SB, Artsob H, Buchy P, Farrar J, Gubler DJ, et al. Dengue: a continuing global threat. Nat. Rev. Microbiol. 2010;8(12, Suppl.):S7.

61. Guzman A, Istúriz RE. Update on the global spread of dengue. Int. J. Antimicrob Agents 2010;36(Suppl. 1):S40.

62. Halstead SB. Dengue. Lancet 2007;370:1644.

63. Tapia-Conyer R, Méndez-Galván JF, Gallardo-Rincón H. The growing burden of dengue in Latin America. J. Clin. Virol. 2009;46(Suppl. 2):S3–6.

III. NOVEL APPROACHES FOR VACCINES

64. Fried JR, Gibbons RV, Kalayanarooj S, Thomas SJ, Srikiatkhachorn A, Yoon IK, et al. Serotype-specific differences in the risk of dengue hemorrhagic fever: an analysis of data collected in Bangkok, Thailand from 1994 to 2006. PLoS Negl. Trop. Dis. 2010;4:e617.

65. Recker M, Blyuss KB, Simmons CP, Hien TT, Wills B, Farrar J, et al. Immunological serotype interactions and their effect on the epidemiological pattern of dengue. Proc. Biol. Sci. 2009;276:2541.

66. Vu TT, Holmes EC, Duong V, Nguyen TQ, Tran TH, Quail M, et al. Emergence of the Asian 1 genotype of dengue virus serotype 2 in Viet Nam: *in vivo* fitness advantage and lineage replacement in South-East Asia. PLoS Negl. Trop. Dis. 2010;4:e757.

67. Simmons CP, Farrar J. Changing patterns of dengue epidemiology and implications for clinical management and vaccines. PLoS Med. 2009;9:e1000129.

68. Cummings DAT, Iamsirithaworn S, Lessler JT, McDermott A, Prasanthong R, Nisalak A, et al. The impact of the demographic transition on dengue in Thailand: insights from a statistical analysis and mathematical modeling. PLoS Med. 2009;6:e1000139.

69. Halstead SB. Dengue in the Americas and Southeast Asia: do they differ? Pan Am. J. Public Health 2006; 20:407.

70. Halstead SB, Streit TG, LaFontant JG, Putvatana R, Russell K, Sun W, et al. Haiti: Absence of dengue hemorrhagic fever despite hyperendemic dengue virus transmission. Am. J. Trop. Med. Hyg. 2001;65:180.

71. Halstead SB. Antibodies determine virulence in dengue. Ann. N.Y. Acad. Sci. 2009;1171(Suppl. 1):E48.

72. Balsitis SJ, Williams KL, Lachica R, Flores D, Kyle JL, Mehlhop E, et al. Lethal antibody enhancement of dengue disease in mice is prevented by Fc modification. PLoS Pathogens 2010;6:e1000790.

73. Mathew A, Rothman AL. Understanding the contribution of cellular immunity to dengue disease pathogenesis. Immunol Rev. 2008;225:300.

74. Mongkolsapaya J, Dejnirattisai W, Xu X-N, Vasanawathana S, Tangthawornchaikul N, Chairunsri A, et al. Original antigenic sin and apoptosis in the pathogenesis of dengue hemorrhagic fever. Nat. Med. 2003;9:921.

75. Thomas SJ, Eckels JH, Carletti I, De La Barrera R, Dessy F, Fernandez S, et al. A phase II., randomized, safety and immunogenicity study of a re-derived, live-attenuated dengue virus vaccine in healthy adults. Am. J. Trop. Med. Hyg. 2013;88:73.

76. Chanthavanich P, Luxemburger C, Sirivichayakul C, Lapphra K, Pengsaa K, Yoksan S, et al. Short report: Immune response and occurrence of dengue infection in Thai children three to eight years after vaccination with live attenuated tetravalent dengue vaccine. Am. J. Trop. Med. Hyg. 2006;75:26.

77. Kitchener S, Nissen M, Nasveld P, Forrat R, Yoksan S, Lang J, et al. Immunogenicity and safety of two live-attenuated tetravalent dengue vaccine formulations in healthy Australian adults. Vaccine 2006; 24:1238.

78. Schmitz J, Roehrig J, Barrett A, Hombach J. Next generation dengue vaccines: A review of candidates in pre-clinical development. Vaccine 2011;29:7276.

79. Guy B, Saville M, Lang J. Development of Sanofi Pasteur tetravalent dengue vaccine. Hum. Vaccin. 2010;6:696.

80. Guy B, Guirakhoo F, Barban V, Higgs S, Monath TP, Lang J. Preclinical and clinical development of YFV 17D-based chimeric vaccines against dengue, West Nile and Japanese encephalitis viruses. Vaccine 2010;28:632.

81. Morrison D, Legg TJ, Billings CW, Forrat R, Yoksan S, Lang J. A novel tetravalent dengue vaccine is well tolerated and immunogenic against all 4 serotypes in flavivirus-naïve adults. J. Infect. Dis. 2010;201:370.

82. Poo J, Galan F, Forrat R, Zambrano B, Lang J, Dayan GH. Live-attenuated tetravalent dengue vaccine in dengue naïve children, adolescents, and adults in Mexico City. Ped. Infect. Dis. J. 2011;30:e9.

83. Capeding RZ, Luna IA, Bomasang E, Lupisan S, Lang J, Forrat R, et al. Live-attenuated, tetravalent dengue vaccine in children, adolescents and adults in a dengue endemic country: Randomized controlled phase I trial in the Philippines. Vaccine 2011;29:3863.

84. Leo YS, Wilder-Smith A, Archuleta S, Shek LP, Chong CY, et al. Immunogenicity and safety of recombinant tetravalent dengue vaccine (CYD-TDV) in individuals 2-45 years. Hum. Vaccin. Immunother. 2012;8:1259.

85. Sabchareon A, Wallace D, Sirivichayakul C, Limkittikul K, Chanthavanich P, Suvannadabba S, et al. Protective efficacy of the recombinant, live-attenuated, CYD tetravalent dengue vaccine in Thai schoolchildren: a randomized, controlled phase 2b trial. Lancet 2012;380:1559.

86. Guy B, Barrere B, Malinowski C, Saville M, Teyssou R, Lang J. From research to phase III: preclinical, industrial and clinical development of the Sanofi Pasteur tetravalent dengue vaccine. Vaccine 2011;29:7229.

87. Osorio JE, Huang CY-H, Kinney RM, Stinchcomb DT. Development of DENVax: a chimeric dengue-2 PDK-53-based tetravalent vaccine for protection against dengue fever. Vaccine 2011;29:7251.

88. Durbin AP, Kirkpatrick BD, Pierce KK, Schmidt AC, Whitehead SS. Development and clinical evaluation of multiple investigational monovalent DENV vaccines to identify components for inclusion in a live attenuated tetravalent DENV vaccine. Vaccine 2011;29:7242.

89. Durbin AP, McArthur JH, Marron JA, Blaney JE, Thumar B, Wanionek K, et al. rDEN2/4Δ30(ME), A live attenuated chimeric dengue serotype 2 vaccine is safe and highly immunogenic in healthy dengue-naïve adults. Hum. Vaccin. 2006;2:255–60.

90. McArthur JH, Durbin AP, Marron JA, Wanionek KA, Thumar B, Pierro DJ, et al. Phase I clinical evaluation of rDEN4Δ30-200,201: a live attenuated dengue 4 vaccine candidate designed for decreased hepatotoxicity. Am. J. Trop. Med. Hyg. 2008;79:678–84.

91. Wright PF, Durbin AP, Whitehead SS, Ikizler MR, Henderson S, Blaney JE, et al. Phase 1 trial of the dengue virus type 4 vaccine candidate rDEN4Δ30-4995 in healthy adult volunteers. Am. J. Trop. Med. Hyg. 2009;81:834–41.

92. Durbin AP, McArthur J, Marron JA, Blaney JE, Thumar B, Wanionek K, et al. The live attenuated dengue serotype 1 vaccine rDEN1Δ30 is safe and highly immunogenic in healthy adult volunteers. Hum. Vaccin. 2006;2:167–73.

93. Durbin AP, Kirkpatrick BD, Pierce KK, Elwood D, Larsson CH, Lindow JC, et al. A single dose of any of four different live attenuated tetravalent dengue vaccines is safe and immunogenic in flavivirus-naïve adults: a randomized, double-blind clinical trial. J. Inf. Dis. 2013;207:957.

94. Putnak JR, Coller BA, Voss G, Vaughn DW, Clements D, Peters I, et al. An evaluation of dengue type-2 inactivated, recombinant subunit and live attenuated vaccine candidates in the rhesus macaque model. Vaccine 2005;23:4442.

95. Clements D, Coller BAG, Lieberman MM, Ogata S, Wang G, Harada KE, et al. Development of a recombinant tetravalent dengue virus vaccine: immunogenicity and efficacy studies in mice and monkeys. Vaccine 2010;28:2705.

96. Coller BAG, Clements DE, Bett AJ, Sagar SL, ter Meulen JH. The development of recombinant subunit envelope-based vaccines to protect against dengue virus induced disease. Vaccine 2011;29:7267.

97. Beckett CG, Tjaden J, Burgess T, Danko JR, Tamminga C, Simmons M, et al. Evaluation of a prototype dengue-1 DNA vaccine in a Phase 1 clinical trial. Vaccine 2011;29:960.

98. Danko JR, Beckett CG, Porter KR. Development of dengue DNA vaccines. Vaccine 2011;29:7261.

99. O'Brien KL, Wolfson LJ, Watt JP, Henkle E, Deloria-Knoll M, McCall N, et al. Burden of disease caused by *Streptococcus pneumoniae* in children younger than 5 years: global estimates. Lancet 2009;374: 893–902.

100. Black S, Shinefield H, Fireman B, Lewis E, Ray P, Hansen JR, et al. Efficacy, safety and immunogenicity of heptavalent pneumococcal conjugate vaccine in children. Northern California Kaiser Permanente Vaccine Study Center Group. Pediatr. Infect. Dis. J. 2000;19:187–95.

101. Wizemann TM, Heinrichs JH, Adamou JE, Erwin AL, Kunsch C, Choi GH, et al. Use of a whole genome approach to identify vaccine molecules affording protection against *Streptococcus pneumoniae* infection. Infect. Immun. 2001;69:1593–8.

102. Giefing C, Meinke AL, Hanner M, Henics T, Bui MD, Gelbmann D, et al. Discovery of a novel class of highly conserved vaccine antigens using genomic scale antigenic fingerprinting of pneumococcus with human antibodies. J. Exp. Med. 2008;205:117–31.

103. Moffitt KL, Gierahn TM, Lu YJ, Gouveia P, Alderson M, Flechtner JB, et al. T(H)17-based vaccine design for prevention of *Streptococcus pneumoniae* colonization. Cell Host Microbe. 2011;9:158–65.

104. Briles DE, Yother J, McDaniel LS. Role of pneumococcal surface protein A in the virulence of *Streptococcus pneumoniae*. Rev. Infect. Dis. 1988;10(Suppl. 2):S372–4.

105. Tu AH, Fulgham RL, McCrory MA, Briles DE, Szalai AJ. Pneumococcal surface protein A inhibits complement activation by *Streptococcus pneumoniae*. Infect. Immun. 1999;67:4720–4.

106. Talkington DF, Crimmins DL, Voellinger DC, Yother J, Briles DE. A 43-kilodalton pneumococcal surface protein, PspA: isolation, protective abilities, and structural analysis of the amino-terminal sequence. Infect. Immun. 1991;59:1285–9.

III. NOVEL APPROACHES FOR VACCINES

107. Hollingshead SK, Becker R, Briles DE. Diversity of PspA: mosaic genes and evidence for past recombination in *Streptococcus pneumoniae*. Infect. Immun. 2000;68:5889–900.

108. Briles DE, Hollingshead SK, King J, Swift A, Braun PA, Park MK, et al. Immunization of humans with recombinant pneumococcal surface protein A (rPspA) elicits antibodies that passively protect mice from fatal infection with *Streptococcus pneumoniae* bearing heterologous PspA. J. Infect. Dis. 2000;182: 1694–701.

109. Rosenow C, Ryan P, Weiser JN, Johnson S, Fontan P, Ortqvist A, et al. Contribution of novel choline-binding proteins to adherence, colonization and immunogenicity of *Streptococcus pneumoniae*. Mol. Microbiol. 1997;25:819–29.

110. Hakenbeck R, Madhour A, Denapaite D, Bruckner R. Versatility of choline metabolism and choline-binding proteins in *Streptococcus pneumoniae* and commensal streptococci. FEMS Microbiol. Rev. 2009;33: 572–86.

111. Adamou JE, Heinrichs JH, Erwin AL, Walsh W, Gayle T, Dormitzer M, et al. Identification and characterization of a novel family of pneumococcal proteins that are protective against sepsis. Infect. Immun. 2001; 69:949–58.

112. Loisel E, Chimalapati S, Bougault C, Imberty A, Gallet B, Di Guilmi AM, et al. Biochemical characterization of the histidine triad protein PhtD as a cell surface zinc-binding protein of pneumococcus. Biochemistry 2011;50:3551–8.

113. Denoel P, Philipp MT, Doyle L, Martin D, Carletti G, Poolman JT. A protein-based pneumococcal vaccine protects rhesus macaques from pneumonia after experimental infection with *Streptococcus pneumoniae*. Vaccine. 2011;29:5495–501.

114. Seiberling M, Bologa M, Brookes R, Ochs M, Go K, Neveu D, et al. Safety and immunogenicity of a pneumococcal histidine triad protein D vaccine candidate in adults. Vaccine. 2012;30:7455–60.

115. Bologa M, Kamtchoua T, Hopfer R, Sheng X, Hicks B, Bixler G, et al. Safety and immunogenicity of pneumococcal protein vaccine candidates: monovalent choline-binding protein A (PcpA) vaccine and bivalent PcpA-pneumococcal histidine triad protein D vaccine. Vaccine. 2012;30:7461-8.

116. Paton JC. The contribution of pneumolysin to the pathogenicity of *Streptococcus pneumoniae*. Trends Microbiol. 1996;4:103–6.

117. Paton JC, Rowan-Kelly B, Ferrante A. Activation of human complement by the pneumococcal toxin pneumolysin. Infect. Immun. 1984;43:1085–7.

118. Boulnois GJ, Paton JC, Mitchell TJ, Andrew PW. Structure and function of pneumolysin, the multifunctional, thiol-activated toxin of *Streptococcus pneumoniae*. Mol. Microbiol. 1991;5:2611–6.

119. Kirkham LA, Kerr AR, Douce GR, Paterson GK, Dilts DA, Liu DF, et al. Construction and immunological characterization of a novel nontoxic protective pneumolysin mutant for use in future pneumococcal vaccines. Infect. Immun. 2006;74:586–93.

120. Alexander JE, Lock RA, Peeters CC, Poolman JT, Andrew PW, Mitchell TJ, et al. Immunization of mice with pneumolysin toxoid confers a significant degree of protection against at least nine serotypes of *Streptococcus pneumoniae*. Infect. Immun. 1994;62:5683–8.

121. Kamtchoua T, Bologa M, Hopfer R, Neveu D, Hu B, Sheng X, et al. Safety and immunogenicity of the pneumococcal pneumolysin derivative PlyD1 in a single-antigen protein vaccine candidate in adults. Vaccine 2012;31:327–33.

122. Dintilhac A, Alloing G, Granadel C, Claverys JP. Competence and virulence of *Streptococcus pneumoniae*: Adc and PsaA mutants exhibit a requirement for Zn and Mn resulting from inactivation of putative ABC metal permeases. Mol. Microbiol. 1997;25:727–39.

123. Rajam G, Anderton JM, Carlone GM, Sampson JS, Ades EW. Pneumococcal surface adhesin A (PsaA): a review. Crit. Rev. Microbiol. 2008;34:131–42.

124. Malley R, Lipsitch M, Stack A, Saladino R, Fleisher G, Pelton S, et al. Intranasal immunization with killed unencapsulated whole cells prevents colonization and invasive disease by capsulated pneumococci. Infect. Immun. 2001;69:4870–3.

125. Prymula R, Peeters P, Chrobok V, Kriz P, Novakova E, Kaliskova E, et al. Pneumococcal capsular polysaccharides conjugated to protein D for prevention of acute otitis media caused by both *Streptococcus pneumoniae* and non-typable *Haemophilus influenzae*: a randomised double-blind efficacy study. Lancet 2006; 367:740–8.

126. Ihssen J, Kowarik M, Dilettoso S, Tanner C, Wacker M, Thony-Meyer L. Production of glycoprotein vaccines in *Escherichia coli*. Microb. Cell Fact. 2010;9:61.

127. Galloway AL, Murphy A, DeSimone JM, Di J, Herrmann JP, Hunter ME, et al. Development of a nanoparticle-based influenza vaccine using the PRINT technology. Nanomedicine 2013;9:523–31.

128. Bagnoli F, Baudner B, Mishra RPN, Bartolini E, Fiaschi L, Mariotti P, et al. Designing of next generation of vaccines for global public health. OMICS 2011;15(9):545–66.

129. Vogel FR, Powell MF. A compendium of vaccine adjuvants and excipients. In: Powell MF, Newman MJ, editors. Vaccine Design: The Subunit and Adjuvant Approach. New York: Plenum Press; 1995. p. 141–228.

130. Reddy ST, Swartz MA, Hubbell JA. Targeting dendritic cells with biomaterials, developing the next generation of vaccines. Trends Immunol. 2006;27:573–9.

131. O'Hogan DT, Valiante NM. Recent advances in the discovery and delivery of vaccine adjuvants. Nat. Rev. Drug Discov. 2003;2:727–35.

132. Cavanagh DR, Remarque EJ, Sauerwein RW, Hermsen CC, Luty AJ. Influenza virosomes: a flu jab for malaria? Trends Parasitol. 2008;24:382–5.

133. Garcon N, Van Mechelen M, Wettendorff M. Development and evaluation of AS04, a novel and improved adjuvant system containing MPL and aluminum salt. In: Schijns VEJC, O'Hagan DT, editors. Immunopotentiators in Modern Vaccines. Burlington, MA: Academic Press; 2006. p. 161–78.

134. Schjins VE. Immunological concepts of vaccine adjuvant activity. Curr. Opin. Immunol. 2000;12:456–63.

135. Osorio F, Reise SC. Myeloid C-type lectin receptors in pathogen recognition and host defense. Immunity 2011;34:651–4.

136. Elinav E, Strowig T, Henao-Mejia J, Flavell RJ. Regulation of the antimicrobial response by NLR proteins. Immunity 2011;34:665–79.

137. Loo YM, Gale M. Immune signaling by RIG-I-like receptors. Immunity 2011;34:680–92.

138. Kawai T, Akira S. Toll-like receptors and their crosstalk with other innate receptors in infection and immunity. Immunity 2011;34:637–50.

139. Kuroda E, Coban C, Ishii KJ. Particulate adjuvant and innate immunity: past achievements, present findings, and future prospects. Int. Rev. Immunol. 2013;32:209–20.

140. Perez O, Batista-Duharte A, Gonzalez E, Zayas C, Balboa J, Cuello M, et al. Human prophylactic vaccine adjuvants and their determinant role in new vaccine formulations. Braz. J. Med. Biol. Res. 2012;45(8):681–92.

141. Desmet CJ, Ishii KJ. Nucleic acid sensing at the interface between innate and adaptive immunity in vaccination. Nat. Rev. Immunol. 2012;21:23–9.

142. Poltorak A, He X, Smirnova I, Liu MY, Van Huffel C, Du X, et al. Defective LPS signaling in C3H/HeJ and C57BL/10ScCr mice: mutations in TLR4 gene. Science 1998;282:2085–8.

143. O'Hagan DT, Ott GS, Nest GV, Rappoulli R, Giudice GD. The history of MF59® adjuvant: a phoenix that arose from the ashes. Expert Rev. Vaccines 2013;12(1):13–30.

144. Montomoli E, Piccirella S, Khadang B, Mennitto E, Camerini R, Rosa AD. Current adjuvants and new perspectives in vaccine formulation. Expert Rev. Vaccines 2011;10(7):1053–61.

145. Marrack P, McKee AS, Munks MW. Towards an understanding of the adjuvant action of aluminum. Nat. Rev. Immunol. 2009;9:287–93.

146. Levitz SM, Gloenbock DT. Beyond empiricism: informing vaccine development through through innate immunity research. Cells 2012;148(16):1284–92.

147. Mutwiri G, Gerdts V, Drunen SV, Hurk LD, Auray G, Eng N, et al. Combination adjuvants: the next generation of adjuvants? Expert Rev. Vaccines 2011;10(1):95–107.

148. Giannini SL, Hanon E, Moris P, Van Mechelen M, Morel S, Dessy F, et al. Enhanced humoral and memory B cellular immunity using HPV16/18 L1 VLP vaccine formulated with the MPL/aluminum salt combination (AS04) compared to aluminum salt only. Vaccine 2006;24:5937–49.

149. Didierlaurent AM, Morel S, Lockman L, Giannini SL, Bisteau M, Carlsen H, et al. AS04, an aluminum salt- and TLR4 agonist-based adjuvant system, induces a transient localized innate immune response leading to enhanced adaptive immunity. J. Immunol. 2009;183:6186–97.

150. Garcon N, Chomez P, Van Mechelen M. GlaxoSmithKline adjuvant systems in vaccines: concepts, achievements and perspectives. Expert Rev. Vaccines 2007;6(5):723–39.

III. NOVEL APPROACHES FOR VACCINES

151. Morel S, Didierlaurent A, Bourguignon P, Delhaye S, Baras B, Jacob V, et al. Adjuvant System AS03 containing α-tocopherol modulates innate immune response and leads to improved adaptive immunity. Vaccine 2011;29:2461–73.

152. Khurana A, Verma N, Yewdell JW, Hilbert AK, Castellino F, Lattanzi M, et al. MF59 adjuvant enhances diversity and affinity of antibody-mediated immune response to pandemic influenza vaccines. Sci. Transl. Med. 2011;3(85):85ra48.

153. Del Guidice G, Fragapane E, Burgarini R, Hora M, Henriksson T, Palla E, et al. Vaccines with the MF59 adjuvant do not stimulate antibody responses against squalene. Clin. Vaccine Immunol. 2006;13(9):1010–3.

154. Gluck R, Burri KG, Metcalfe I. Adjuvant and antigen delivery properties of virosomes. Curr. Drug Deliv. 2005;2:395–400.

155. Demento SL, Siefert AL, Bandyopathyay A, Sharp FA, Fahmy TM. Pathogen-associated molecular patterns on biomaterials: a paradigm for engineering new vaccines. Trends Biotechnol. 2011;29:294–306.

156. Moschos SA, Bramwell VW, Somavarapu S, Alpar HO. Modulating the adjuvanticity of alum by co-administration of muramyl di-peptide (MDP) or Quil-A. Vaccine 2006;24(8):1081–6.

157. Lindenstrom T, Agger EM, Korsholm KS, Darrah PA, Aagaard C, Seder RA, et al. Tuberculosis subunit vaccination provides long-term protective immunity characterized by multifunctional CD4 memory T cells. J. Immunol. 2009;182(12):8047–55.

158. Grossman C, Tenbusch M, Nchinda G, Temchura V, Nabi G, Stone GW, et al. Enhancement of the priming efficacy of DNA vaccines encoding dendritic cell-targeted antigens by synergistic Toll-like receptor ligands. BMC Immunol. 2009;10:43.

159. Zhu Q, Egelston C, Gagnon S, Sui Y, Belyakov IM, Klinman DM, et al. Using 3 TLR ligands as a combination adjuvant induces qualitative changes in T cell responses needed for antiviral protection in mice. J. Clin. Invest. 2010;120(2):607–16.

160. Sierra GV, Campa HC, Varcacel NM, Garcia IL, Izquierda PL, Sotolongo PF, et al. Vaccine against group B *Neisseria meningitides*: protection trial and mass vaccination results in Cuba. NIPH Ann. 1991;14:195–207.

161. Koff WC, Burton DR, Johnson PR, Walker BD, King CR, Nabel GJ, et al. Accelerating next-generation vaccine development for global disease prevention. Science 2013;340:1232910–1232917.

162. Coquerelle C, Moser M. DC subsets in positive and negative regulation of immunity. Immunol. Rev. 2010;234:317–34.

163. Akira S. Innate immunity and adjuvants. Phil. Trans. R. Soc. B. 2011;366:2748–55.

164. Chen RT, Pless R, Destefano F. Epidemiology of autoimmune reactions induced by vaccination. J. Autoimmun. 2001;16:309–18.

165. Bhambhani A, Blue JT. Lyophilization strategies for development of a high-concentration monoclonal antibody formulation: benefits and pitfalls. Am. Pharmaceut. Rev. 2009;16–21.

166. Amorij JP, Kersten GFA, Saluja V, Tonnis WF, Hinrich WLJ, Slutter B, et al. Towards tailored vaccine delivery: needs, challenge and perspective. J. Control. Release 2012;161:363–76.

167. Saluja V, Amorij JP, Kapteyn JC, De Boer AH, Frijlink HW, Hinrich WL. A comparison between spray drying and spray freeze drying to produce an influenza subunit vaccine powder by inhalation. J. Control. Release 2010;144(2):127–33.

168. Dey A, Srivastava IK. Novel adjuvants and delivery systems for enhancing immune responses induced by immunogens. Expert Rev. Vaccines 2011;10(2):227–51.

169. Smith LR, Wloch MK, Ye M, Reyes LR, Boutsaboualoy S, Dunne CE, et al. Phase I clinical trials of the safety and immunogenicity of adjuvanted plasmid DNA vaccines encoding influenza A virus H5 hemagglutinin. Vaccine 2010;28:2565–72.

170. Villarreal DO, Talbott KT, Choo DK, Shedlock DJ, Weiner DJ. Synthetic DNA vaccine strategies against persistent viral infections. Expert Rev. Vaccines 2013;12(5):537–54.

171. Lai L, Vodros D, Kozlowski PA, Montefiori DC, Wilson RL, Akerstrom VL, et al. GM-CSF DNA: an adjuvant for higher avidity IgG, rectal IgA, and increased protection against the acute phase of a SHIV-89.6P challenge by a DNA/MVA immunodeficiency virus vaccine. Virology 2007;369:153–67.

172. Iyer S, HogenEsch H, Hem SL. Effect of the degree of phosphate substitution in aluminum hydroxide adjuvant on the adsorption of phohsphorylated proteins. Pharm. Dev. Technol. 2003;8:81–6.

173. Khandke L, Yang C, Krylova K, Jansen K, Rashidbaigi A. Preservative of choice for Prev(e)nar 13TM in a multi dose formulation. Vaccine 2011;29(41):7144–53.

174. Chen K, Cerutti A. Vaccination strategies to promote mucosal antibody responses. Immunity 2010;33:479.

175. Hirobe S, Okada N, Nakagawa S. Transcutaneous vaccines-current and emerging strategies. Expert Opin. Drug Deliv. 2013;10(4):485–98.

176. Frech SA, Dupont HL, Bourgeois AL, Mckenzie R, Belkind-Gerson J, Fiquero JF, et al. Use of a patch containing heat-labile toxin from Escheria coli against traveller's diarrhea: a phase II, randomized, double-blind, placebo-controlled field trial. Lancet 2008;371:2019–25.

177. Prymula R, Usluer G, Altinel S, Sichova R, Weber F. Acceptance and opinions of Intanza/IDflu intradermal influenza vaccine in the Czech Republic and Turkey. Adv. Ther. 2012;29:41–52.

178. Corbett HJ, Germain JP, Fernando JP, Chen X, Frazer IH, Kendall MAF. Skin vaccination against cervical cancer associated human papillomavirus with a novel micro-projection array in a mouse model. PLoS ONE 2010;5(10):e13460.

179. Van Damme P, Oosterhuis-Kafeja F, Van der Wielen M. Safety and efficacy of a novel microneedle device for dose sparing intradermal influenza vaccination in healthy adults. Vaccine 2009;27:454–9.

180. Lycke N. Recent progress in mucosal vaccine development: potential and limitations. Nat. Rev. Immunol. 2012;12:592–605.

181. Carter NJ, Curran MP. Live attenuated influenza vaccine (FluMist: Fluenz): a review of its use in prevention of seasonal influenza in children and adults. Drugs 2011;71:1591–622.

182. Song JH, Nguyen HH, Cuburu N, Horimoto T, Ko SY, Park SH, et al. Sublingual vaccination with influenza virus protects mice against lethal viral infection. Proc. Natl. Acad. Sci. U.S.A. 2008;105(5):1644–9.

Prime-Boost Vaccination: Impact on the HIV-1 Vaccine Field

Robert De Rose[1], Stephen J. Kent[1], Charani Ranasinghe[2]

[1]Department of Microbiology and Immunology, The University of Melbourne, at the Peter Doherty Institute for Infection and Immunity, University of Melbourne, Melbourne, Australia
[2]John Curtin School of Medical Research, Australian National University, Canberra, Australia

INTRODUCTION

The development of high-efficacy vaccines for globally important chronic infections such as human immunodeficiency virus (HIV)-1/acquired immunodeficiency syndrome (AIDS), malaria, tuberculosis, and hepatitis C has been slow and difficult. Over 35 million people are living with HIV-1, and over 2 million new infections occur each year. Although anti-HIV-1 drug therapies are very effective at suppressing the virus, they do not cure the infection and the drugs must be taken life-long. This is unsustainably expensive at a global level. Further,

Novel Approaches and Strategies for Biologics, Vaccines and Cancer Therapies. DOI: 10.1016/B978-0-12-416603-5.00012-2

long-term treatment can lead to both multiple side-effects and the risk of developing drug-resistant strains. Intensified efforts at preventing HIV-1 infection are needed. Several biomedical prevention technologies are emerging, including pre-exposure prophylaxis with anti-HIV drugs and vaginal microbicides. Although these have been effective in some studies, other studies have not confirmed their efficacy.[1–3] This is at least in part due to the high level of compliance required to regularly adhere to many of these methods.[4] A safe and effective vaccine is widely viewed as a necessary component to making important headway in reducing new HIV-1 infections. Heterologous prime-boost vaccine techniques, where one vaccine modality is administered first and then some time later a second different vaccine modality is administered, can induce potent immune responses. Targeting the most effective anti-HIV-1 immune response through this strategy remains a challenge but may eventually form the basis of a successful HIV-1 vaccine strategy. This review focuses on the development of prime-boost vaccines for the prevention of HIV-1.

IMMUNITY TO HIV-1

Human immunodeficiency virus is a lentivirus capable of existing in a latent state when integrated in the host genome. As such, there is likely no true natural immunity such that the infection is completely cleared. Further, there have been no highly protective vaccine studies conducted in humans, so the correlates of vaccine-induced immunity to HIV-1 in humans are largely unknown. Nonetheless, subgroups of humans appear to control HIV-1 very effectively and much can be learned from the immune responses they make that assist in control of HIV-1.[5] Further, macaque models of the closely related lentivirus simian immunodeficiency virus (SIV) have proven very useful in dissecting vaccine-induced immunity. This section highlights aspects of immune responses to HIV-1 and SIV that are relevant to the induction of immunity by prime-boost vaccine techniques.

Humoral Immunity to HIV-1

Neutralizing antibodies to HIV-1 Envelope are highly effective in preventing infection with chimeric SIV–HIV (SHIV) viruses in macaques.[6] A growing series of monoclonal antibodies that potently neutralize HIV-1 have been isolated from patients with HIV-1.[7] However, such neutralizing antibodies appear to evolve over many months during ongoing HIV-1 infection and have high levels of somatic mutations in the immunoglobulin genes.[8] Vaccine strategies have to date not been able to induce broadly reactive neutralizing antibodies, perhaps in part because of the extensive evolution of the antibody genes that appears to be required. Neutralizing antibodies that recognize at least a limited number of HIV-1 strains can be induced by vaccination, and there is evidence that prime-boost strategies using protein antigens as the boost can substantially increase the antibody titer. It is notable that the titer of neutralizing antibodies needed to protect macaques from SHIV is important but does not need to be unobtainably high.[9,10] However, given the massive diversity of circulating HIV-1 strains, vaccines that induce only a modest breadth of neutralizing antibodies may not be highly efficacious in the field. Novel antigen preparations that induce broadly reactive antibodies, rather than innovations in prime-boost immunization strategies, are likely to be needed to realize the potential of neutralizing antibodies in protecting against HIV-1.

Non-neutralizing antibodies with Fc-mediated functions, such as antibody-dependent cellular cytotoxicity (ADCC), are of increasing interest in HIV-1 vaccine design. There is evidence that HIV-specific ADCC antibody responses are associated with slower HIV-1 progression.[11] Further, ADCC responses can force immune escape, implying they impart significant pressure on virus replication.[12] Macaque studies suggest that ADCC functions of antibodies can assist in protection from SHIV acquisition.[13] The partially successful RV144 Thai HIV-1 vaccine efficacy trial utilized a prime-boost regimen of a canarypox vector followed by a protein boost and induced robust ADCC responses.[14,15] Interestingly, non-neutralizing antibody responses to specific Env regions were associated with protection from HIV-1 acquisition.[14]

Cellular Immunity to HIV-1

CD4 and CD8 T-cell responses to HIV-1 are closely linked to control of natural HIV-1 infection. Preservation of HIV-specific CD4 T-cell responses, particularly to the conserved Gag protein, is common in subjects with slowly progressive HIV-1.[16] Indeed, loss and dysfunction of HIV-specific CD4 T-cell helper functions are likely responsible for an array of HIV-mediated immune deficits.[17,18] Unfortunately, HIV-1 replicates most efficiently in activated CD4 T cells and preferentially targets and destroys HIV-specific CD4 T-cell responses.[19] HIV-specific CD4 T cells are a desirable, and probably necessary, immune response to induce by vaccination. However, excessively activated HIV-specific CD4 T cells, particularly if located at mucosal sites of transmission, may provide target cells for HIV-1 that facilitate initial infection. Prime-boost regimens usually enhance the magnitude and durability of HIV-specific CD4 T-cell responses. The induction of CD4 T-helper responses is likely to be one mechanism behind their immunogenicity and efficacy.

Particular CD8 T-cell responses (cytotoxic T cells, or CTLs) to HIV-1 are among the strongest responses linked to control HIV-1. However, as with many immune responses, the specificity and quality of the response are critically important in governing their effectiveness. The HLA class I B alleles B*27 and B*57 present CTL epitopes in the conserved part of the Gag protein, and people expressing these alleles have substantially slower HIV-1 progression.[20–22] Further, the number of Gag CTL epitopes targeted is also linked to slow HIV-1 progression, whereas the presence of CTL responses to epitopes in other proteins is not closely linked to slow HIV-1 progression.[23] Macaques that present conserved SIV epitopes, frequently in the Gag protein, also have slower progression to AIDS.[24] The presence of functional HIV-specific CD4 T-helper cell responses is strongly linked to preserved CD8 T cell responses.[17,18] CTL responses reliably and predictably force immune escape mutations in HIV and SIV, and some of these mutations, particularly in conserved regions of important proteins (such as Gag), result in much lower levels of viral replicative capacity (lower fitness).[25] The fitness cost of CTL-induced escape mutations may underlie some of the effectiveness of CTL responses in controlling viral replication.

The generation of CTL responses to HIV-1 has long been sought as a vaccine-induced immune response. Induction of CTL responses usually requires generation of immunogenic peptides within cells and thus DNA or viral vector vaccines (rather than protein-based vaccines) have been studied most intensively. Although murine studies commonly induce CTL responses using a single vaccine strategy, initial approaches using poxvirus vectors and DNA vaccines on their own were usually poorly immunogenic in macaques and humans. Research groups in Australia, the United Kingdom, and the United States all showed in the late 1990s that prime-boost approaches using DNA vaccine primes and viral vector boosts can induce high levels of CTL responses in both mice and macaques and such responses could partially control SHIV challenge of macaques.[26–30] These tools led to an explosion of studies on HIV-1 vaccine prime-boost vaccination approaches.

LANDSCAPE OF HIV-1 VACCINES

There is no licensed HIV-1 vaccine, and none is likely to emerge at least for the next 5 years. There have been six efficacy trials conducted in humans (Table 12.1); five of these have been reported in the literature, but the sixth one was stopped recently by the Data Safety and Monitoring Board (DSMB). The first three trials used single modality approaches and the last two used prime-boost approaches. The first two Envelope protein-only approaches (VaxGen trials) induced some antibody responses but were unsuccessful,[31] although *post hoc* subgroup analyses did point to a possible association of protection with ADCC antibodies.[32] The third and fourth trials (STEP and Phambili) used an adenovirus type 5 (Ad5) vector-only regimen and induced modest T-cell immunity, but the trials were stopped early when the vaccine arm of the STEP trial had a higher incidence of infection than the placebo arm.[33,34] This appeared linked to uncircumcised men with high preexisting adenovirus-specific antibodies. The HIV-specific CTL responses induced by the Ad5 vaccines were not particularly broad or of high magnitude. Analyses on viruses that caused infection in the study did however suggest that the CTL responses induced by the vaccine did result in transiently lower levels of virus replication, and the CTL responses did force immune escape.[35] This raises the possibility that more potent prime-boost regimens that induce higher, broader, or more functional CTL responses may lead to some efficacy.

The fifth large-scale HIV-1 vaccine study used a canarypox vector prime with an Envelope protein vaccine boost (the RV144 trial). This has been the only study to show any efficacy, albeit marginal (31.2% efficacy, $p = 0.04$).[36] The efficacy of this approach was initially surprising and controversial. Indeed, the conduct of the trial was questioned by many because the vaccines induced neither CTL responses nor broad neutralizing antibody responses.[37] Correlates of protection analyses have shown that non-neutralizing antibody responses to parts of Env were associated with protection.[14] This was supported by sieve analyses of breakthrough virus infections.[38] Further analyses also showed that the Env antibody responses to the regimen declined substantially within 6 months of the last vaccination and this was associated with a waning of vaccine efficacy.[36] Detailed work is now ongoing studying immune responses more precisely and re-studying similar regimens in macaques.[39] Additional human trials of this, or related, poxvirus prime-protein boost approaches are now in the planning phase, due to start in 2014/2015. There is a significant opportunity to improve the titer and durability of the immune responses induced by this regimen, or similar ones, through the use of improved, more replication-competent poxviruses and the use of alternative adjuvants with the protein boost.

An important aspect of this RV144 trial, unlike the other five efficacy trials, was that it was conducted in a lower risk setting of predominantly heterosexual HIV-1 transmission.[36] All other efficacy trials were conducted in higher risk gay men or injecting drug users. The male-to-female mucosal transmission in the RV144 trial may have been a "lower bar" to protect

TABLE 12.1   Efficacy of Human HIV-1 Vaccine Trials

Trial	Type of Vaccine	Total No.	No. Vaccinated	No. Given Placebo	No. of Infections in Vaccine Group	No. of Infections in Placebo Group	Efficacy (%)	Comment	Refs.
Vaxgen B/E	Gp120 protein (two strains: one subtype, B, one subtype E) in alum	2527	1267	1260	106	105	None	Thai study	Pitisuttithum et al.[136]
Vaxgen B/B	Gp120 protein (two strains, both subtype B) in alum	5403	3598	1805	241	127	None	Primarily U.S. based	Flynn et al.[137]
STEP	Adenovirus type 5 vector (three vectors: one expressing Gag, one Nef, and one Pol)	3000	1494	1506	19	11	None	Primarily U.S. based; stopped early when more recipients in vaccine arm acquired HIV than those in placebo arm	Buchbinder et al.[34]
Phambili	Adenovirus type 5 vector (three vectors: one expressing Gag, one Nef, and one Pol)	801	400	401	34	28	None	Primarily South Africa; stopped early when STEP study results announced	Gray et al.[138]
RV144	(1) Canarypox vector prime (expressing Gag–Pol–Env) (2) Gp120 protein boost (two strains: one subtype B, one subtype E) in alum	16395	8197	8198	51	74	31.2	Thai study; efficacy correlated with non-neutralizing Ab responses	Rerks-Ngarm et al.[36]
HVTN 505	(1) DNA vaccine prime (six plasmids: three expressing Gag, Pol, and Nef and three expressing Env strains) (2) Adenovirus type 5 vector boost (four vectors: one expressing Gag–Pol and three expressing Env)	2494	1250	1244	41	30	None	Stopped early for futility; full results not yet published	Cohen[139]

against. This highlights the interest in mucosal immunity induced by prime-boost regimens. Nonetheless, robust long-term efficacy of HIV-1 vaccines is likely to require protection against multiple routes of HIV-1 transmission. There is currently discussion on future efficacy trials based around the RV144 approach with the goal of improving the efficacy of this approach toward a licensable vaccine. These potential improvements include the use of improved adjuvants in the protein boost, longer duration of protein boosts, and alternative vaccinia-based poxvirus vectors for use as the priming vaccine.

The sixth HIV-1 vaccine efficacy study used a DNA prime, Ad5 boost approach. This trial focused in part on the use of multiple Envelope strains in an attempt to induce both cellular and humoral immunity. The DSMB recently halted this trial when it was clear the vaccines used were not efficacious.[40] Final evaluation showed that the vaccine did not reduce the rate of HIV-1 acquisition or the viral load set point.[40a] The reasons for the lack of efficacy are not yet clear. DNA prime–Ad5 boost regimens have induced potent CTL responses in macaques.[41] However, Env-specific CTLs have been reported to be less efficacious than CTLs to Gag in controlling virus replication.[42,43]

Overall, there is considerable scope for novel approaches to improve the immunogenicity and protective efficacy of HIV-1 vaccines. Focusing immunity on important epitopes (both humoral: CD4 and CTL), on the quality of the immune response induced, and on immunity at mucosal levels are among the aspects that can be manipulated by future prime-boost HIV vaccine strategies.

PRINCIPLES OF PRIME-BOOST VACCINATION

Prime-boost vaccination for HIV-1 typically utilizes an initial vaccination (usually a DNA vaccine or a recombinant viral vector) that expresses HIV-1 antigens and initiates a detectable but low-level immune response. HIV-1 DNA vaccines are plasmids that express inserted HIV-1 genes off a promoter; when injected into the body, these vaccines express the HIV-1 antigens encoded by the HIV-1 gene. Recombinant viral vectors are viruses that cause minimal or no disease in the host but are genetically manipulated in the laboratory to contain HIV-1 genes behind a promoter and the genes are expressed during the viral lifecycle.

After the prime vaccine is given, the boost vaccination is usually given some weeks or months later. It is usually either a recombinant viral vector (different to the one utilized in the prime) or a protein vaccine that contains or expresses the same or a similar set of HIV-1 antigens expressed by the priming vaccine (Figure 12.1). The "primed" immune responses induced by the priming vaccine are usually substantially boosted in magnitude after the boosting vaccine. A key advantage of this strategy, compared to giving the same vaccine twice, is that the immune system recognizes the expressed HIV-1 antigens in the boost more strongly than other antigens expressed by the viral vector. Thus, the immune response is focused on the inserted HIV-1 antigens within the vaccines, rather than antigens expressed by the carrier viruses. By using different vectors for prime and booster vaccines, anti-vector immunity, which would limit expression of the encoded HIV-1 gene(s), is avoided.[44]

A key advantage of prime-boost strategies using DNA and viral vector vaccines is that both of these vaccines express HIV-1 antigens from within cells and thus present HIV-1 epitopes to CD8+ CTLs. Most prior vaccine strategies for other pathogens have focused on generating antibody responses. Given the failure of initial antibody-based HIV-1 vaccine strategies (VaxGen trials; see Table 12.1) and the continued difficulty in inducing broad neutralizing antibodies,

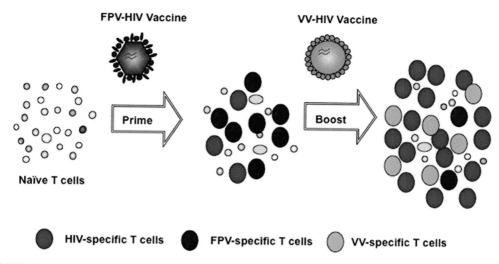

FIGURE 12.1 **Principles of prime–boost vaccination.**

approaches that induce CTL responses or induce both CTL and antibodies were also pursued. Prime-boost strategies are thus a prominent technique to induce robust CTL responses.

Several general refinements to prime-boost immunization techniques have been made since the first utilization of this vaccine approach (Table 12.2). Manipulating the cytokine milieu at the site of vaccination to generate more targeted and robust immune responses as well as improving mucosal immunity have been intensively studied in the recent years (see discussion on mucosal immunity and novel approaches below).

TABLE 12.2   Important Factors That Modulate Immune Outcomes Following Prime-Boost Vaccination

Factors	Outcome/ Findings	Refs.
Vaccine route	Systemic immunization provides robust systemic immunity but short-lived mucosal immunity. Mucosal vaccination induces robust high-avidity mucosal immunity. Routes that mimic natural infection are desirable for achieving optimal protection against mucosal pathogens	Ranasinghe et al.,[62] Belyakov et al.,[94] Corbett et al.,[98] Kent et al.,[102] Perrone et al.[140]
Vaccine vectors	Recombinant DNA is normally used in the priming vaccination and, due to reduced uptake, induces a low level of immunity compared to viral vector delivery. Recombinant live attenuated viral vectors are able to express higher levels of vaccine antigens and induce better vaccine efficacy. The vaccine vector combination plays a critical role in modulating the final immune efficacy of a vaccine (which vector is used in the priming or the booster phase). Viral vector prime/protein booster strategies can induce good humoral immunity.	Rerks-Ngarm et al.,[36] Pillai et al.,[60] Ranasinghe et al.,[61,64] Kent et al.,[102] Ramsay et al.,[141] Wijesundara et al.[152]

(Continued)

TABLE 12.2   Important Factors That Modulate Immune Outcomes Following Prime-Boost Vaccination (*cont.*)

Factors	Outcome/ Findings	Refs.
Vaccine antigens	Antigens that are immunogenic, have lesser ability to mutate, and have a fitness cost to the pathogen are best suited to induce CTL immunity (e.g., Gag–Pol). Immunodominant epitopes may be incorporated into vaccine vectors to augment the development of high-avidity CTLs. Antigens that are on the outer membrane (e.g., Env) are best suited to induce effective humoral immunity.	Borrow et al.,[142] Reece et al.,[143] Dzutsev et al.,[144] Klein et al.,[145] Center et al.[146]
Molecular adjuvants	Molecular adjuvants can enhance immunity and have the ability to modulate T_H1 and T_H1 immunity. Coexpression of adjuvants such as unmethylated CpG and cytokines/chemokines (IL-12, IL-15, CCL5 4-1BBL) can enhance T_H1 immune responses. Cytokines such as novel type I interferon epsilon (IFN-ε) can enhance mucosal immunity and homing. Co-expression of cytokine inhibitors such as IL-13R2 can enhance CD8 T cell avidity, mucosal immunity, and protective efficacy.	Ranasinghe et al.,[61,127] Harrison et al.,[116] Boyer et al.,[147] Tapia et al.,[148] Gomez et al.,[149] Xi et al.[150]
Cytokine milieu	Transient inhibition of cytokines such as IL-4 and IL-13 can enhance avidity of HIV-specific CD8+ T cells	Ranasinghe et al.,[62,127] Ranasinghe and Ramshaw[118]

DNA PRIME-BOOST STRATEGIES

Heterologous prime-boost vaccination induces an immune response that is with few exceptions better in magnitude and quality compared with sequential homologous vaccinations. The complementary nature of prime-boost vaccines is best exemplified by the RV144 HIV-1 vaccine efficacy study, which combined two vaccines that were ineffective or modestly immunogenic when used alone, yet provided significant levels of protection in combination.[36]

By far the most common component in prime-boost vaccines for HIV-1 is the DNA vaccine, which is almost always used as the first, or priming component. DNA vaccines are generally considered to be poorly immunogenic in higher mammals, although recent improvements in design and methods of delivery are making progress toward a more effective vaccine.[45] DNA vaccines are the simplest of all vaccines, relatively inexpensive to manufacture, and chemically identical, so DNA vaccines pose fewer regulatory hurdles than other types of vaccines. Expression is limited to one or a few encoded antigens with no competition from other vector-encoded antigens, as occurs in recombinant viral vector systems. Stimulation of the innate immune system is provided by DNA ligation to TLR9, and the result is an elevation of the precursor frequency of antigen-specific cells with a memory phenotype. These T cells are primed to expand upon subsequent vaccination, particularly in the context of vaccines that strongly stimulate the innate immune response, such as viral vectors or protein vaccines with synthetic adjuvants.

The development of vaccine strategies with a DNA priming component and their evaluation in preclinical studies constitute a large body of literature. There has been a wide assortment of DNA prime/heterologous boost vaccine combinations studied. The most common booster vaccines used in combination with DNA vaccines have been whole proteins, adenovirus (Ad) vectors, and four poxvirus vectors: vaccinia virus (VV), modified vaccinia virus Ankara (MVA), New York vaccinia (NYVAC, a highly attenuated strain of VV), and fowlpoxvirus (FPV). Each vaccine type is disposed toward generating a particular type of immune response. Early HIV-1 vaccine studies recognized the importance of inducing both a T cell and neutralizing antibody (NAb) response.[46] This drove the development of DNA and protein vaccine combinations, in particular because the CD4 T cell helper response that is primed by a DNA vaccine can assist the humoral response generated by an adjuvanted protein vaccine. Combining vaccines also provided unexpected synergies such as a broadening of the antibody response. The breadth of the antibody response to HIV-1 is improved with DNA prime-protein-boost approaches compared to homologous protein vaccination alone.[47] Early vaccine studies incorporated Env predominantly with the aim of inducing NAb, as passive transfer of NAb can prevent SHIV infection in monkeys.[48] However, it was soon recognized that generating antibodies that could neutralize a wide gamut of primary isolates was not achievable, even with DNA prime/protein boost approaches. There was therefore a switch in focus to DNA/viral-vectored vaccines designed to generate T-cell immunity. Later studies, including the RV144 efficacy trial, rediscovered the additive value of Env antibodies in protective efficacy even when broad neutralizing antibodies were not induced.

Viral vector vaccines benefit from combination with a DNA vaccine because the benefits of multiple vaccinations are provided without interference from immune responses against the viral vector, as only a single application of the vector is used. A number of studies in nonhuman primates (NHPs) with DNA/MVA, DNA/FPV, DNA/NYVAC, and DNA/Ad were deemed successful according to the definition of protection that was accepted at the time and underwent clinical trial evaluation.

Around the year 2000, enthusiasm for DNA-primed HIV-1 vaccines was high because the safety profile, immunogenicity, and protective efficacy data evidenced in NHP studies would, if replicated in humans, be suitable as first generation HIV-1 vaccines that would partially control HIV-1 replication.[49] Although sterilizing immunity was rarely achieved in NHP studies, reductions in viral load and CD4 T-cell loss were observed that could protect from disease and lower forward transmission rates. Early highlights were evidenced for each of the main DNA-primed heterologous vaccines (Table 12.3). In a DNA-primed, protein-boost vaccine insert, four of six NHPs were protected from viral challenge in contrast to one of six that were administered two doses of DNA vaccine.[50] A DNA-primed, adenoviral boost vaccine expressing Gag alone showed great promise in NHP challenge trials by dramatically reducing viral loads and preserving CD4 T cells.[51] The absence of Env antigens in these vaccines showed the immunity was mediated primarily by T cells. Similarly, a DNA/MVA vaccine induced T cell responses that controlled viral replication to very low levels in macaques ($\sim 10^3$ copies/mL of plasma).[52] Such viral replication levels are associated with very slow disease progression and reduced transmission of HIV-1 in humans. Early successes were also evidenced from DNA/FPV vaccines, which significantly lowered the viral burden after challenge,[53] and for a DNA/VV vaccine that reduced CD4 T cell loss and delayed the onset of disease.[54] However, many of the pathogenic challenge strains that were used in this

TABLE 12.3   DNA Prime-Boost Vaccine Strategies

Year	Strategy	Immunogenicity and Protective Efficacy	Comment	Refs.
2000	DNA/protein	Sterile immunity in 4/6 animals challenged with non-pathogenic SHIV89.6	Demonstrated that protection from mucosal challenge was possible	Habel et al.[50]
2002	DNA/Ad	Strong T-cell responses; maintenance of CD4 T cells during chronic infection; containment of viral loads to 10^3/mL	Showed that a CTL response to Gag could mediate effective long-term-control of SHIV89.6P replication	Shiver et al.[51]
2001	DNA/MVA	Strong T-cell responses; antibody to Env and Gag; long-term memory induced; control of SHIV89.6P replication to 10^3/mL following mucosal challenge	Long interval between vaccination and challenge showed that immunological memory generated by vaccination was protective	Amara et al.[28]
2004	DNA/FPV	CD4 and CD8 T cell responses; p24 positive on western blot; 1 log reduction in chronic viral load; significant preservation of CD4 T cells	Led to Phase I clinical evaluation of a subtype B vaccine in Sydney, Australia	Dale et al.[53]
2003	DNA/VV	DNA vaccine highly effective prime for VV; strong T cell and antibody responses; maintenance of CD4 T cell count in 6/6 animals and protection from disease	Order of vaccinations was not important for vaccine efficacy; protection from SHIV89.6 challenge was as good as any other vaccine at the time	Doria-Rose et al.,[54,151]
2002	DNA/NYVAC	Long-term suppression of viremia in most macaques that was inversely associated with the SIV-specific CD4 T cell response at the peak viremia, the Gag-specific proliferative response, and an immunodominant Gag CM9 epitope response	One of the first studies to use the rigorous SIVmac251 challenge model; suggested that the CD4 T-cell response is also important in protection; promising findings augured well for translation in clinical studies	Hel et al.[55]
2012	DNA/MVA	T-cell responses recognized multiple epitopes; protection correlated with Env-binding antibody responses and tier 1 NAb; virological control correlated with the breadth and magnitude of the T cell response to Gag	Demonstrated protection against infection in a more rigorous challenge model using heterologous virus	Barouch et al.[56]

period, commonly CXCR4-tropic chimeric SHIV viruses, were subsequently identified to be easily neutralized and poorly representative of the CCR5-tropic stains of HIV-1 that typically infect humans. More recently, preclinical evaluation in NHPs has shifted to challenge with neutralization-resistant, heterologous SIV swarm viruses such as SIV_{mac251} or SIV_{smE660}. A promising early candidate was a DNA/NYVAC vaccine combination that was able to manifest significant long-term suppression of viremia following mucosal challenge with SIV_{mac251}, which correlated with the total SIV-specific CD4 T-cell response at peak viremia and Gag-specific proliferation.[55] Subsequent challenge models also incorporated low-dose challenges that are repeated multiple times to better mimic a natural exposure to HIV-1 that results in infection. In this setting, there has been one standout vaccine. A DNA/MVA combination encoding Gag, Pol, and Env reduced the per-exposure risk of infection with heterologous neutralization-resistant SIV_{mac239} by 73%,[56] although when infection did occur there was no reduction in viral load in comparison to infected naïve controls.

The investment in DNA-primed HIV-1 vaccines has been enormous, yet there has been poor translation into clinical findings. One exception appears to be a DNA/NYVAC vaccine combination that is highly immunogenic in subjects and reflects earlier results demonstrated in NHP studies.[57] Durable T-cell responses were detected in 90% of subjects, and these were shown to be polyfunctional in nature, expressing multiple effector functions and proliferative capability. The response was CD4 dominant, which was shown in a prior DNA/NYVAC study in macaques to correlate with containment of viral replication.[55] DNA-primed heterologous vaccines studies have also informed us about the type of immune response that is important for controlling HIV-1 replication. We have learned that neutralizing and binding antibodies and T-cell responses contribute to viral control, and both arms of the adaptive immune system would ideally be activated by a HIV-1 vaccine strategy.[46]

Improvements are required if heterologous DNA vaccine combinations are to realize their potential for use as an HIV-1 vaccine. Future efforts are focusing on improving the DNA vaccine itself and alternative methods of vaccine delivery that promise to improve vaccine performance in primates.[45,58]

POX VIRAL PRIME-BOOST STRATEGIES

Prime-boost strategies using DNA as a priming vaccine have been disappointing in clinical trials (including the recent HVTN505 trial; see Table 12.1). Attention has focused on using poxvirus-based strategies, and a number of vectors have been developed against HIV-1. Researchers have generated and studied several recombinant poxvirus vectors, including FPV, NYVAC, canarypox, and MVA. Studies in mice and macaques have demonstrated that combinations of these pox viral vectors can induce significantly better immune outcomes compared to the other delivery strategies. Good testimony is the partially successful RV144 Thai HIV-1 vaccine efficacy trial, which utilized a canarypox virus prime/protein booster vaccination strategy and elicited 31.2% protective efficacy in humans (Table 12.1).[36] The vaccination regime predominantly induced a non-neutralizing antibody response to specific Env regions that were associated with protection from HIV-1 acquisition.[14,15] The trial demonstrated that prime-boost regimens using protein booster strategies have greater potential to induce ADCC antibody responses compared to non-prime-boost strategies. It is not known whether the quality or antigen specificity of ADCC immunity induced by various prime-boost regimens can be improved to yield higher efficacy. This is currently an active area of research.

Studies also have demonstrated that a rAd35 prime and rMVA booster HIV-1 vaccine strategy can induce stronger cellular immune responses to encoded vaccine antigens.[59] A recent study has elegantly demonstrated that, with the use of Ad5 and rMVA in prime-boost vaccination, the vector combination plays a significant role in modulating HIV-specific memory T-cell differentiation. rMVA primed animals were shown to mount mainly a CD62L-positive central memory response, while Ad5 prime induced a CD62L-negative CD8 T-cell subset. Moreover, the Ad5 booster was shown to alter the quality of these MVA-primed CD8 T cells compared to the Ad5/rMAV booster strategy.[60] These studies highlight the importance of understanding the immune regulatory mechanisms of these vectors as they progress toward human trials.

Similarly, studies in mice in our laboratory have shown that an intranasal (i.n.) or intramuscular (i.m.) FPV-HIV prime followed by i.m VV-HIV boost immunization can induce robust long-term CD4+ and CD8+ systemic T-cell responses to HIV Gag antigen in BALB/c mice.[61,62] Unlike a vaccination strategy using only i.m. delivery, the i.n. FPV-HIV/i.m. VV-HIV strategy induced sustained HIV-1 Gag-specific mucosal CD8 T-cell immunity. Interestingly, mucosal or systemic administration of VV-HIV prime followed by FPV-HIV booster vaccination did not generate good HIV-specific CTLs.[61] We have also found that the rVV and rMVA behave in a similar manner. This may explain the poor immune responses observed in the recent rMVA/rFPV Phase I HIV-1 clinical trial.[63]

Our studies in mice have shown that poxvirus prime-boost vaccine approaches can induce much better immune outcomes compared to rDNA/pox viral prime-boost strategies. This improvement is evidenced in terms of the induction of polyfunctional, high-avidity CTLs with better protective efficacy.[64] The vector choice and the combination (which vector is used in the prime or the booster) play key roles in determining the immunogenicity of a vaccine in terms of T cell avidity, mucosal T cell immunity, and protective immunity. The above examples suggest that pox viral vectors such as FPV, canarypox, and various attenuated vaccinia virus vectors (e.g., MVA, NYVAC, Tiantan strains) still offer promise for the future. These vectors have been shown to be safe in humans and can package large amounts of pathogen-specific genetic material of interest for intracellular expression. For example, we have shown that rFPV can express 65% of the HIV-1 genome.[65–67]

OTHER VIRAL VECTOR PRIME-BOOST VACCINATION STRATEGIES

In addition to DNA vaccines and poxvirus vectors, a diverse range of other viral vectors have been used in HIV-1 vaccine development (Table 12.4). This list is large and includes vesicular stomatitis virus, Semliki Forest virus, alphavirus, poliovirus, influenza virus, rabies virus, bluetongue virus, Sendai virus, and yellow fever virus. Many of these concepts did not go beyond immunogenicity studies in mice, and only a few were tested in NHP studies. The most advanced of these technologies has been adenovirus, which has been evaluated in clinical trials. More recently, CMV vectors have yielded some surprising results in NHP studies.

Adenovirus vectors first came to prominence in studies in chimpanzees because infection at mucosal surfaces in the upper respiratory tract and intestinal tract offered the possibility

TABLE 12.4 Significant Developments in Other Non-Poxvirus Viral Vectored Vaccines for HIV-1

Year	Strategy	Immunogenicity and Efficacy	Comment	Ref.
1998	Ad/protein	NAb and CTL; sterilizing immunity in 4 out of 5 vaccinees in a low-stringency HIV-1 challenge model	Demonstrated for the first time induction of NAb to homologous and heterologous isolates of HIV-1	Zolla-Pazner et al.[68]
2009	Ad26/Ad5	More immunogenic than homologous Ad5/Ad5; T cell response increased 8.7-fold in magnitude, 3.9-fold better breadth, and a greater proportion of polyfunctional T cells; significantly reduced mortality	Demonstrated how much more effective heterologous vaccination with different Ad serotypes is compared with homologous vaccination with Ad5	Liu et al.[69]
2009 2011 2013	CMV/Ad5 CMV/Ad5 CMV/Ad5	Induction and maintenance of long-term CD4 and CD8 T_{EM} cells with a polyfunctional phenotype; little or no NAb to Env; no loss of CD4 T cells and control of viremia to the limit of detection in approximately 50% of macaques; protection correlated with magnitude of vaccine-induced peak; further investigation demonstrated clearance of virus	A series of three studies that demonstrated profound control of viral replication in approximately 50% of macaques; for the first time, clearance of an established SIV infection was demonstrated; vaccine was also effective in the setting of preexisting immunity to CMV	Hansen et al.[71-73]

of inducing responses in the gut where the vast majority of CCR5 and CD4 T cells, the prime target for HIV-1 infection, are present. An early adenoviral vaccine encoding gp160, followed by a gp120 protein booster, induced NAb in three out of five chimpanzees and a CTL response in a fourth animal.[68] All four animals with a response to the vaccine were protected from a low-dose i.v. challenge with heterologous HIV-1$_{SF2}$ in this low-virulence challenge model of HIV-1 infection, and the three animals that induced NAb were protected from a second higher dose challenge. This study demonstrated for the first time the induction of NAb to homologous and heterologous HIV-1 isolates. As NAb-inducing vaccines fell out of favor adenovirus vaccine studies focused on inducing T cell responses.

For many years, a replication-incompetent adenovirus vector based on adenovirus serotype 5 (Ad5) was the leading T cell HIV-1 vaccine candidate (Table 12.4). However, the unexpected failure of the STEP Phase IIB efficacy study forced a reevaluation of adenovirus vaccine development and research priorities for T cell based HIV-1 vaccines in general. There was an obvious shift in focus away from Ad5 to other serotypes that have much lower seroprevalence in the general population. Heterologous adenoviral prime-boost combinations were tested, and one example highlighted how much more effective heterologous prime-boost adenoviral vaccines could be relative to homologous vaccination. A study in macaques used a rAd26/rAd5 regimen that expressed SIV Gag only. The regimen induced T cell responses with superior magnitude, breadth, and quality compared to homologous Ad5 vaccination and provided superior partial protection following challenge with pathogenic SIV_{mac251} compared to homologous Ad5 vaccination.[69] Peak viral load was reduced by 1.4 $\log_{10}$ copies/mL, and there was a 2.4-$\log_{10}$ copies/mL reduction in chronic levels of viremia. The reduction in viremia correlated with the magnitude and breadth of the T cell response at the time of challenge. Vaccination resulted in an overall significantly decreased mortality from AIDS over the 500-day study period. This work has reinvigorated the development of alternate adenovirus vaccines, which are again poised for further clinical evaluation. The study also demonstrated deficiencies in the SHIV challenge models used to evaluate the preclinical efficacy of Ad5 vaccines, which were poor predictors of vaccine efficacy in humans in comparison to SIV challenge models.[70] Somewhat paradoxically, the investigations that followed the failure of the STEP trial have provided an impetus for better HIV-1 vaccines. Future studies will evaluate prime-boost combinations of serologically distinct serotypes as well as adenovirus of simian origin and use more rigorous SIV challenge models.

Arguably the greatest recent advance in HIV-1 vaccine research has been the use of replication-competent attenuated CMV vectors.[71] These vectors have established a new paradigm for HIV-1 vaccines—that a persistent effector memory T cell (T_{EM}) response can provide long-term control over viral replication and eventual clearance of the infection, a functional cure. Two related efficacy trials in an NHP model (and a follow-up study to investigate the nature of the infection) evaluated a CMV vaccine expressing Gag, a Rev–Tat–Nef polyprotein, Pol and Env, either alone or in combination with an Ad5 booster vaccine. This vaccine provided durable and stringent control of viral replication in the absence of NAb to Env. In the first efficacy study, 4 out of 12 macaques demonstrated robust control of viral infection, and a second study was even more successful, with 12/24 macaques protected for one year with no reduction in CD4 T cell count and SIV viremia that was below the limit of detection at most timepoints with occasional blips above baseline that diminished over time.[71,72] All of the vaccinated animals were shown to be infected after a series of low-dose challenges with pathogenic SIV_{mac239}, but there was a dichotomy with regard to protection; about half of the macaques maintained stringent control over viral replication, while the remainder failed to prevent systemic dissemination of virus. A third study demonstrated hemotogenous viral dissemination prior to clearance of virus. This was unexpected because it was assumed that the vaccine contained the infection to the local mucosa and draining lymphoid tissues. Protection was associated with a polyfunctional T_{EM} cell response, with IFN-γ, TNF-α, and IL-2 expression by CD4 T cells and IFN-γ, TNF-α, and CD107 by CD8 T cells. Investigation of these modified CMV vectors identified immunoregulation of the T cell response. In comparison to other T cell-inducing vaccines, CMV vectors induced a much broader CD8 T cell response by interfering with canonical forms of epitope processing and presentation.[73] In combination with an Ad5 booster, the peak VL was significantly reduced in animals that were infected systemically, in contrast with a CMV-only vaccine regimen, but it did not alter the long-term outcome of infection compared with controls. A DNA/Ad5 vaccine that was used as a comparator T_{CM}-inducing vaccine and challenged in the same way did not protect. Surprisingly, depletion of CD4 or CD8 T cells in protected animals did not result in viral recrudescence, suggesting that viral reservoirs were minimal or absent. The early T_{EM} response at the mucosa thus appears to have limited systemic dissemination of virus, and a sustained T_{EM} response deleted remaining reservoirs of infection over time. Early control was crucial; in animals that were not protected, viral loads and CD4 T cell loss were equivalent to the naïve controls. The CMV vaccine induced a highly durable and almost exclusive T_{EM} response in CD8 T cells and a mixed T_{EM} and T_{CM} response in CD4 T cells. An Ad5 booster improved the T_{CM} response, and this reduced peak VL in this group but failed to provide long-term protection. Supplementation of a CMV vaccine with alternative booster vaccines that induce robust T_{CM} and/or NAb may benefit poor responders by providing a degree of "backup" systemic immunity when there is failure to control early viral replication and thus reduce the long-term consequences of HIV-1 infection.

Despite the success of these CMV efficacy trials, translation into clinical trials will be challenging. CMV vectors for human studies will have to be sufficiently attenuated for safety reasons but must still retain similar immunogenicity to the vectors used in NHP studies and be capable of overcoming preexisting immunity to human CMV, which is common in many parts of the world and is particularly high in high-risk groups for HIV-1 (e.g., men who have sex with men).[74,75]

MUCOSAL IMMUNITY AND PRIME-BOOST VACCINATION APPROACHES

Mucosal-associated lymphoid tissue is linked with what is now known as the "common mucosal immune system" such that antigenic stimulation at one site results in both local immune responses and reactivity at distant mucosal sites.[76] Exploitation of this system can be critically important for the development of effective mucosal vaccines.[77] In general, the systemic delivery of vaccine antigens rarely induces optimal or durable mucosal immunity, while delivery of a vaccine at a mucosal surface can trigger immunity at both local and distant mucosae.[64,78–81] Compared to the systemic immune compartment, microfold (M) cells, which are present on the mucosal epithelial layer, possess a unique ability to process/present antigens, neutralize pathogens, and activate T cells within the mucosal environment.[82,83] During cognate antigen encounters, mucosal dendritic cells have a distinctive ability to imprint T cells with tissue-specific mucosal-homing markers, enabling them to migrate to specific mucosal sites.[84,85] These unique features of the common immune system account for the reasons why the majority of the systemic vaccinations tested do not induce strong or sustained mucosal immunity, specifically against chronic mucosal pathogens. Thus, to induce effective sustained mucosal immunity, a vaccine must be delivered to the mucosae (e.g., nasal, oral, rectal, vaginal tissues) (Figure 12.2).[86–88] HIV-1 is first encountered at the genitorectal or vaginal mucosa, and the gastrointestinal tract is a primary site of HIV-1 replication and CD4 T cell depletion.[89–93] Designing vaccine strategies that can induce good mucosal immunity at the first line of defense would be of great importance.[94,95]

The immune responses induced by a given vaccine are dependent on the route of vaccine delivery, the order in which each vaccine vector is delivered (in the prime or the booster vaccination), the cytokine milieu at the vaccination site, and the molecular adjuvants used (Table 12.2). Studies have now clearly established that, even though recombinant pDNA-based vaccines can be successfully delivered systemically (e.g., gene gun, i.m. or i.d. delivery, electroporation), uptake of these vaccines via the mucosae has been ineffective.[64] Interestingly,

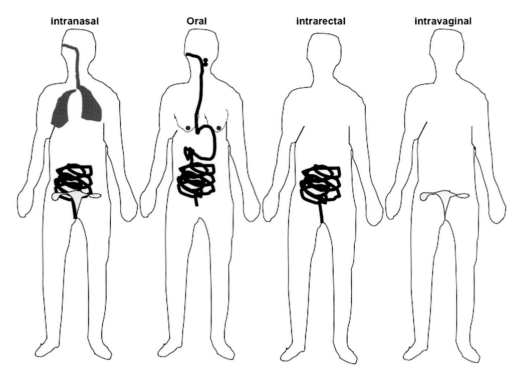

FIGURE 12.2   **Immunity induced according to the route of vaccine delivery.**

unlike recombinant pDNA vectors, several pox viral vectors (e.g., rFPV, rMVA, NYVAC, TiantanVV[52,61,64,96–99]), recombinant influenza viral vectors,[100] and recombinant polio virus vectors[101] have been shown to induce good mucosal immunity to HIV vaccine antigens. Our group has demonstrated that mice or macaques primed i.n. followed by i.m. FPV-HIV vaccination yielded poor protective efficacy, but i.m. pDNA-HIV prime, followed by a mucosal HIV-fowlpox virus (FPV) booster, yielded enhanced T cell immunity in the rectal and endocervical tissue and protection against a mucosal SHIV challenge.[64,102] Similarly, Belyakov and coworkers[103] have demonstrated that i.m. rDNA followed by intrarectal (i.r.) rMVA booster vaccinations in NHPs can induce better SIV-specific mucosal immune responses (gut-specific immunity), compared to i.m. rDNA/i.m. rMVA immunization. Further, i.m. pDNA-HIV-Clade C prime followed by aerosol NYVAC-C delivery was reported to induce long-lasting HIV-specific immune response in the genitorectal tract.[98] This study also confirmed that that the aerosol delivery of both NYVAC and rMVA was safe in NHPs and had no vaccine-associated pathology in the brain or lungs. Similar safety data were also reported in mice following i.n. rMVA delivery.[104] Recently, in rhesus macaques, an i.n. Tiantan vaccinia SIV–*gag–pol–env* followed by i.m. rAd5 SIV–*gag–pol–env* booster strategy was shown to induce good T cell immunity, neutralizing antibodies to $SIV_{mac1A11}$ and providing protection against a high-dose i.r. SIV_{mac239} challenge.[99] Moreover, our murine studies have now clearly established that compared to an i.m. pDNA-HIV/ i.n. FPV-HIV immunization regime, the i.n. FPV-HIV/i.m.

VV-HIV immunization strategy induced strong sustained systemic and mucosal HIV-specific CTLs of higher avidity with better protective efficacy.[62,64]

Due to the ease of administration and their safety, oral vaccines have been an attractive alternative to i.n. delivery. Several bacterial vectors and viral vectors have been evaluated as candidates to induce good gut- and genitorectal tract-specific CD8 T-cell and IgA immunity. Rhesus macaques immunized with DNA-SIV–Gag prime/oral *Listeria*-SIV–Gag booster strategy was shown to induce elevated numbers of SIV-specific mucosal CD8+α4β7+ T cells that were capable of migrating to the gut mucosae.[105] Similarly, oral *Clostridium perfringens* expressing SIV p27 followed by an i.m. Ad5 boost also elicited robust multifunctional CD8+ T cells in the gut mucosae.[106] Our studies have shown that oral FPV-HIV followed by i.m. VV-HIV can induce systemic CD8 T cell responses to not only HIV-1 Gag but also Pol antigens, demonstrating that in some instances the route of vaccine delivery can also alter the immune-dominant hierarchy to vaccine antigens. However, despite the use of high doses of purified vaccines, oral rFPV delivery was unable to induce any immunity in the genitorectal mucosa.[61] In a recent oral versus ileum Ad5–HIVgp140 prime followed by an i.m. booster vaccination study, Wang et al.[107] elegantly demonstrated that in a low-pH environment the presence of proteases and mucosal glycocalyx in the gastrointestinal tract can have major implications when designing effective oral vaccines.

Collectively, all of the above examples highlight the importance of the careful selection of the route of vaccine delivery and the correct vaccine vector combinations for the induction optimal mucosal and systemic immunity against HIV-1.

IMPORTANCE OF HIV-SPECIFIC T- AND B-CELL AVIDITY AND NOVEL HIV-1 PRIME-BOOST VACCINATION STRATEGIES

Co-expression of cytokines, chemokines, and other immune modulators together with HIV-1 vaccine antigens have been utilized in prime or booster vaccinations to enhance the magnitude of immunity to vaccine antigens. For example, danger signals such as unmethylated CpG motifs; the cytokines IFN-α/β, IFN-γ, IL-12, IL-15, and IL-18;[62,108–112] the chemokine granulocyte-macrophage colony-stimulating factor (GM-CSF);[113] the costimulatory molecules CD40L, B7-1, ICAM-1, and LFA-3;[114,115] and molecules such as 41BBL have been used to enhance the magnitude of CD8 T-cell immunity.[116,117] Although many costimulatory molecules enhance the magnitude of immunity measured by IFN-γ production, many of them have been incapable of enhancing the quality or avidity of T-cell immunity.[116,118]

It is now becoming increasingly evident that enhancing not only the magnitude but also the avidity of T cell immunity may be important in protecting against pathogenic organisms, particularly those proven to be resistant to existing immunization strategies. The quality of the T cell response is reflected in the functional avidity of T cells toward the MHC–peptide complex on target cells. High-avidity CTLs recognize low concentrations of antigen, but low-avidity CTLs are ineffective in effector function at low concentrations of antigen.[119] Moreover, high-avidity CTLs are typically polyfunctional in nature and have the ability to produce a range of cytokines and chemokines, such as IFN-γ, TNF-α, IL-2, CCL3, and CCL5. Such T cells have a greater capacity to clear an infection compared to low-avidity T cells.[120–124] Because high-avidity CTLs can recognize target cells expressing very low levels of viral antigen (e.g., early after infection of a cell) and initiate more rapid target cell lysis at low concentrations of target antigen, vaccine strategies that can induce high-avidity CTLs at sites of initial exposure to HIV-1 will have greater potential for local control of virus infection. Interestingly, several studies have now established that mucosal HIV-1 vaccines that can induce high-avidity mucosal HIV-specific CTLs are more effective in controlling systemic dissemination of SIV compared to systemic immunization.[125] Belyakov et al.[126] demonstrated that a vaccine delivered to mucosa induced a higher percentage of functional Ag-specific CTL cells in the gut mucosa, whereas systemic immunization induced higher avidity HIV-specific CTLs in the draining lymph nodes but offered no protection against mucosal CD4+ T cell depletion.

Using a pox-viral prime-boost model we have demonstrated that purely mucosal (i.n./i.n.) or combined mucosal/systemic (i.n./i.m.) FPV HIV/VV HIV prime-boost immunization induced HIV-specific CTLs of higher avidity with better protective efficacy against a surrogate mucosal HIV-1 challenge compared to purely systemic (i.m./i.m.) immunization.[62] We have attributed this mainly to the route-dependent hierarchical expression of Th2 cytokines IL-4 and IL-13, where the expression profiles were i.n./i.n. < i.n./i.m. < i.m./i.m. (Table 12.5).[118] Moreover, by using animals lacking the IL-4 or IL-13 cytokine, we have demonstrated that, compared to IL-4, IL-13 plays a more critical role in modulating the induction and expansion of effector and memory CD8 T-cell avidity in a murine setting.[118]

Thus, we have now designed novel recombinant HIV-1 poxvirus-based vaccines that co-express soluble and/or membrane-bound forms of IL-13R2 that have the ability to transiently inhibit IL-13 activity at the vaccination site. These vaccines, delivered using a combined mucosal–systemic prime-boost strategy (i.n. FPV-HIV-IL-13R2/ i.n. VV-HIV-IL-13R2), have been shown to induce robust mucosal and systemic HIV-specific effector/memory T cells with enhanced magnitude, avidity, and broader cytokine and chemokine profiles, as well as excellent protective efficacy following a surrogate mucosal HIV-1 challenge. Importantly, these vaccines have been shown to induce excellent long-lived, HIV-specific CD8 T cells in the gut mucosae, which is an exciting prospect for an HIV-1 vaccine.[127] More interestingly, these

TABLE 12.5   Route of Immunization, IL-4/IL-13 Cytokine Expression, and HIV-Specific CTL Avidity Following HIV-1 Prime-Boost Vaccination

Route of Delivery	Mice	Magnitude of CTL Immunity	IL-4/IL-13 Expression by CTL	Avidity	Protection
Pure mucosal i.n./i.n.	BALB/c	+	—	High	+++
	IL-13$^{-/-}$	+	–	High	+++++
Combined i.n./i.m.	BALB/c	+++	++	Medium	+++
	IL-13$^{-/-}$	+++	–	High	+++++
Pure systemic i.m./i.m.	BALB/c	+++	+++	Low	++
	IL-13$^{-/-}$	+++	–	Medium/high	++++

Note: Mice (H-2^d) were primed with rFPV encoding HIV-1 genes *gag*, *pol*, *env*, *rev*, and *tet* and boosted two weeks later with rVV encoding *gag–pol* antigens. i.n. = intranasal, i.m. = intramuscular. Two weeks after booster vaccination, the magnitude of response was measured by IFN-γ ELISpot or intracellular cytokine staining, and HIV-specific T-cell avidity was measured by tetramer dissociation. Eight weeks after booster vaccination, protection was evaluated using an i.n. K^{d}Gag$_{197-205}$-influenza surrogate mucosal challenge.

studies have highlighted that the quality of a vaccine, specifically CD8 T-cell avidity, is determined within the first 24 hours according to the unique antigen-presenting cell (APC) subsets they induce or recruit to the priming vaccination site (i.e., lung mucosae).[127] Our studies into the mechanisms by which these vaccines induce high-avidity CD8 T cells have established that downregulation of IL-4R and upregulation of CD8 coreceptors following vaccination play an important role in modulating the quality of CD8 T cell immunity.[124,128]

The partial success of the RV144 trial suggests that improving vector efficacy and designing robust protein adjuvants may be of great importance when developing more efficacious HIV-1 vaccines. Recent studies have shown that removal of the IL-18 binding protein from MVA vectors can improve vaccine efficacy.[129] Also, improved NYVAC-based vaccine vectors have been reported to (1) induce higher levels of antigen expression, (2) replicate better in human keratinocytes and dermal fibroblasts, and (3) activate selective host cell signal pathways limiting virus spread.[130] Similarly, compared to conventional adjuvants, some APC-targeted protein adjuvants have been shown to induce better vaccine-specific mucosal and/or systemic immunity.[131–135] These novel approaches offer promise for the future.

CONCLUSIONS

Human immunodeficiency virus has proven to be a difficult pathogen to vaccinate against, with only one of the first six efficacy trials showing any promise. The RV144 trial used a poxvirus prime- and protein-booster approach and showed 31% efficacy. It is widely hoped that future refinements in this approach may improve this efficacy to yield a viable HIV-1 vaccine. Such refinements could include (1) improving the current pox viral vaccine vectors to induce effective immunity, (2) understanding how these vaccine vectors actually work, (3) designing more potent vaccine adjuvants, (4) understanding the fundamental mechanisms regarding how some chronic pathogens evade the host immune system, and (5) designing strategies to induce strong sustained mucosal immunity at the viral entry sites, which may help design more effective vaccines not only for HIV-1 but also for many other chronic mucosal pathogens in the future. Prime-boost approaches to HIV-1 vaccines hold substantial promise for the eventual control of the HIV-1 epidemic.

References

1. Abdool Karim Q, Abdool Karim SS, Frohlich JA, et al. Effectiveness and safety of tenofovir gel, an antiretroviral microbicide, for the prevention of HIV infection in women. Science 2010;329(5996):1168–74.
2. van der Straten A, Van Damme L, Haberer JE, Bangsberg DR. Unraveling the divergent results of pre-exposure prophylaxis trials for HIV prevention. AIDS 2012;26(7):F13–9.
3. Van Damme L, Corneli A, Ahmed K, et al. Preexposure prophylaxis for HIV infection among African women. N. Engl. J. Med. 2012;367(5):411–22.
4. Anderson PL, Glidden DV, Liu A, et al. Emtricitabine-tenofovir concentrations and pre-exposure prophylaxis efficacy in men who have sex with men. Sci. Transl. Med. 2012;4(151):151ra25.
5. Walker BD. Elite control of HIV Infection: implications for vaccines and treatment. Top. HIV Med. 2007;15(4):134–6.
6. Shibata R, Igarashi T, Haigwood N, et al. Neutralizing antibody directed against the HIV-1 envelope glycoprotein can completely block HIV-1/SIV chimeric virus infections of macaque monkeys. Nat. Med. 1999;5(2):204–10.

7. Burton DR, Poignard P, Stanfield RL, Wilson IA. Broadly neutralizing antibodies present new prospects to counter highly antigenically diverse viruses. Science 2012;337(6091):183–6.

8. Wu X, Zhou T, Zhu J, et al. Focused evolution of HIV-1 neutralizing antibodies revealed by structures and deep sequencing. Science 2011;333(6049):1593–602.

9. Nishimura Y, Igarashi T, Haigwood N, et al. Determination of a statistically valid neutralization titer in plasma that confers protection against simian-human immunodeficiency virus challenge following passive transfer of high-titered neutralizing antibodies. J. Virol. 2002;76(5):2123–30.

10. Hessell AJ, Rakasz EG, Poignard P, et al. Broadly neutralizing human anti-HIV antibody 2G12 is effective in protection against mucosal SHIV challenge even at low serum neutralizing titers. PLoS Pathog. 2009;5(5):e1000433.

11. Wren LH, Chung AW, Isitman G, et al. Specific antibody-dependent cellular cytotoxicity responses associated with slow progression of HIV infection. Immunology 2013;138(2):116–23.

12. Chung AW, Isitman G, Navis M, et al. Immune escape from HIV-specific antibody-dependent cellular cytotoxicity (ADCC) pressure. Proc. Natl. Acad. Sci. U.S.A. 2011;108(18):7505–10.

13. Hessell AJ, Hangartner L, Hunter M, et al. Fc receptor but not complement binding is important in antibody protection against HIV. Nature 2007;449(7158):101–4.

14. Haynes BF, Gilbert PB, McElrath MJ, et al. Immune-correlates analysis of an HIV-1 vaccine efficacy trial. N. Engl. J. Med. 2012;366(14):1275–86.

15. Karnasuta C, Paris RM, Cox JH, et al. Antibody-dependent cell-mediated cytotoxic responses in participants enrolled in a phase I/II ALVAC-HIV/AIDSVAX B/E prime-boost HIV-1 vaccine trial in Thailand. Vaccine 2005;23(19):2522–9.

16. Rosenberg ES, Billingsley JM, Caliendo AM, et al. Vigorous HIV-1-specific CD4+ T cell responses associated with control of viremia. Science 1997;278(5342):1447–50.

17. Kalams SA, Buchbinder SP, Rosenberg ES, et al. Association between virus-specific cytotoxic T-lymphocyte and helper responses in human immunodeficiency virus type 1 infection. J. Virol. 1999;73(8):6715–20.

18. Lichterfeld M, Kaufmann DE, Yu XG, et al. Loss of HIV-1-specific CD8+ T cell proliferation after acute HIV-1 infection and restoration by vaccine-induced HIV-1-specific CD4+ T cells. J. Exp. Med. 2004;200(6):701–12.

19. Douek DC, Brenchley JM, Betts MR, et al. HIV preferentially infects HIV-specific CD4+ T cells. Nature 2002;417(6884):95–8.

20. Pereyra F, Jia X, McLaren PJ, et al. The major genetic determinants of HIV-1 control affect HLA class I peptide presentation. Science 2010;330(6010):1551–7.

21. Kosmrlj A, Read EL, Qi Y, et al. Effects of thymic selection of the T-cell repertoire on HLA class I-associated control of HIV infection. Nature 2010;465(7296):350–4.

22. Miura T, Brockman MA, Schneidewind A, et al. HLA-B57/B*5801 human immunodeficiency virus type 1 elite controllers select for rare gag variants associated with reduced viral replication capacity and strong cytotoxic T-lymphocyte [corrected] recognition. J. Virol. 2009;83(6):2743–55.

23. Kiepiela P, Ngumbela K, Thobakgale C, et al. CD8+ T-cell responses to different HIV proteins have discordant associations with viral load. Nat. Med. 2007;13(1):46–53.

24. Smith MZ, Dale CJ, De Rose R, et al. Analysis of pigtail macaque major histocompatibility complex class I molecules presenting immunodominant simian immunodeficiency virus epitopes. J. Virol. 2005;79(2):684–95.

25. Fernandez CS, Stratov I, De Rose R, et al. Rapid viral escape at an immunodominant simian-human immunodeficiency virus cytotoxic T-lymphocyte epitope exacts a dramatic fitness cost. J. Virol. 2005;79(9):5721–31.

26. Leong KH, Ramsay AJ, Morin MJ, Robinson HL, Boyle DB, Ramshaw IA. Generation of enhanced immune responses by consecutive immunisation with DNA and recombinant fowlpox viruses. In: Brown F, Chanock H, Norrby E, editors. Vaccines 95. Cold Spring Harbor, NY: Cold Spring Harbor Laboratory Press; 1995. p. 327–31.

27. Kent SJ, Zhao A, Best S, Chandler JD, Boyle DB, Ramshaw IA. Enhanced T cell immunogenicity and protective efficacy from a HIV-1 vaccine regimen consisting of consecutive priming with DNA and boosting with recombinant fowlpoxvirus. J. Virol. 1998;72:10180–8.

28. Amara RR, Villinger F, Altman JD, et al. Control of a mucosal challenge and prevention of AIDS by a multiprotein DNA/MVA vaccine. Science 2001;292:69–74.

29. Schneider J, Gilbert SC, Blanchard TJ, et al. Enhanced immunogenicity for CD8+ T cell induction and complete protective efficacy of malaria DNA vaccination by boosting with modified vaccinia virus Ankara. Nat. Med. 1998;4(4):397–402.

30. Allen TM, Vogel TU, Fuller DH, et al. Induction of AIDS virus-specific CTL activity in fresh, unstimulated peripheral blood lymphocytes from rhesus macaques vaccinated with a DNA prime/modified vaccinia virus Ankara boost regimen. J. Immunol. 2000;164(9):4968–78.

31. Pitisuttithum P, Gilbert P, Gurwith M, et al. Randomized, double-blind, placebo-controlled efficacy trial of a bivalent recombinant glycoprotein 120 HIV-1 vaccine among injection drug users in Bangkok, Thailand. J. Infect. Dis. 2006;194(12):1661–71.

32. Gilbert PB, Peterson ML, Follmann D, et al. Correlation between immunologic responses to a recombinant glycoprotein 120 vaccine and incidence of HIV-1 infection in a phase 3 HIV-1 preventive vaccine trial. J. Infect. Dis. 2005;191(5):666–77.

33. McElrath MJ, De Rosa SC, Moodie Z, et al. HIV-1 vaccine-induced immunity in the test-of-concept STEP study: a case-cohort analysis. Lancet 2008;372(9653):1894–905.

34. Buchbinder SP, Mehrotra DV, Duerr A, et al. Efficacy assessment of a cell-mediated immunity HIV-1 vaccine (the STEP study): a double-blind, randomised, placebo-controlled, test-of-concept trial. Lancet 2008;372(9653):1881–93.

35. Rolland M, Tovanabutra S, deCamp AC, et al. Genetic impact of vaccination on breakthrough HIV-1 sequences from the STEP trial. Nat. Med. 2011;17(3):366–71.

36. Rerks-Ngarm S, Pitisuttithum P, Nitayaphan S, et al. Vaccination with ALVAC and AIDSVAX to prevent HIV-1 infection in Thailand. N. Engl. J. Med. 2009;361(23):2209–20.

37. Binley JM, Wrin T, Korber B, et al. Comprehensive cross-clade neutralization analysis of a panel of anti-human immunodeficiency virus type 1 monoclonal antibodies. J. Virol. 2004;78(23):13232–52.

38. Rolland M, Edlefsen PT, Larsen BB, et al. Increased HIV-1 vaccine efficacy against viruses with genetic signatures in Env V2. Nature 2012;490(7420):417–20.

39. Pegu P, Vaccari M, Gordon S, et al. Antibodies with high avidity to the gp120 envelope protein in protection from simian immunodeficiency virus SIV(mac251) acquisition in an immunization regimen that mimics the RV-144 Thai trial. J. Virol. 2013;87(3):1708–19.

40. Cohen J. AIDS clinical trials. More woes for novel HIV prevention approach. Science 2005;307(5716):1708.

40a. Hammer SM, Sobieszcayk ME, Janes H, et al. Efficacy trial of a DNA/rAd5 HIV-1 preventative vaccine. N Engl J Med 2013;369(22):2083–92.

41. Letvin NL, Mascola JR, Sun Y, et al. Preserved CD4+ central memory T cells and survival in vaccinated SIV-challenged monkeys. Science 2006;312(5779):1530–3.

42. Peut V, Kent SJ. Utility of human immunodeficiency virus type 1 envelope as a T-cell immunogen. J. Virol. 2007;81(23):13125–34.

43. Peut V, Kent SJ. Substantial envelope-specific CD8 T-cell immunity fails to control SIV disease. Virology 2009;384(1):21–7.

44. Frahm N, DeCamp AC, Friedrich DP, et al. Human adenovirus-specific T cells modulate HIV-specific T cell responses to an Ad5-vectored HIV-1 vaccine. J. Clin. Invest. 2012;122(1):359–67.

45. Ramirez LA, Arango T, Boyer J. Therapeutic and prophylactic DNA vaccines for HIV-1. Expert Opin. Biol. Ther. 2013;13(4):563–73.

46. Rasmussen RA, Hofmann-Lehmann R, Li PL, et al. Neutralizing antibodies as a potential secondary protective mechanism during chronic SHIV infection in CD8+ T-cell-depleted macaques. Aids 2002;16(6):829–38.

47. Vaine M, Wang S, Hackett A, Arthos J, Lu S. Antibody responses elicited through homologous or heterologous prime-boost DNA and protein vaccinations differ in functional activity and avidity. Vaccine 2010;28(17):2999–3007.

48. Mascola JR, Stiegler G, VanCott TC, et al. Protection of macaques against vaginal transmission of a pathogenic HIV-1/SIV chimeric virus by passive infusion of neutralizing antibodies. Nat. Med. 2000;6(2):207–10.

49. Robinson HL. New hope for an AIDS vaccine. Nat. Rev. Immunol. 2002;2(4):239–50.

50. Habel A, Chanel C, Le Grand R, et al. DNA vaccine protection against challenge with simian/human immunodeficiency virus 89.6 in rhesus macaques. Dev. Biol. (Basel) 2000;104:101–5.

51. Shiver JW, Fu TM, Chen L, et al. Replication-incompetent adenoviral vaccine vector elicits effective anti-immunodeficiency-virus immunity. Nature 2002;415(6869):331–5.

52. Amara RR, Villinger F, Altman JD, et al. Control of a mucosal challenge and prevention of AIDS by a multiprotein DNA/MVA vaccine. Science 2001;292(5514):69–74.

53. Dale CJ, De Rose R, Stratov I, et al. Efficacy of DNA and fowlpox virus priming/boosting vaccines for simian/human immunodeficiency virus. J. Virol. 2004;78(24):13819–28.

54. Doria-Rose NA, Pierce CC, Hensel MT, et al. Multigene DNA prime-boost vaccines for SHIV89.6P. J. Med. Primatol. 2003;32(4-5):218–28.

55. Hel Z, Nacsa J, Tryniszewska E, et al. Containment of simian immunodeficiency virus infection in vaccinated macaques: correlation with the magnitude of virus-specific pre- and postchallenge CD4+ and CD8+ T cell responses. J. Immunol. 2002;169(9):4778–87.

56. Barouch DH, Liu J, Li H, et al. Vaccine protection against acquisition of neutralization-resistant SIV challenges in rhesus monkeys. Nature 2012;482(7383):89–93.

57. Harari A, Bart PA, Stohr W, et al. An HIV-1 clade C DNA prime, NYVAC boost vaccine regimen induces reliable, polyfunctional, and long-lasting T cell responses. J. Exp. Med. 2008;205(1):63–77.

58. Verstrepen BE, Bins AD, Rollier CS, et al. Improved HIV-1 specific T-cell responses by short-interval DNA tattooing as compared to intramuscular immunization in non-human primates. Vaccine 2008;26(26):3346–51.

59. Ratto-Kim S, Currier JR, Cox JH, et al. Heterologous prime-boost regimens using rAd35 and rMVA vectors elicit stronger cellular immune responses to HIV proteins than homologous regimens. PLoS ONE 2012;7(9):e45840.

60. Pillai VK, Kannanganat S, Penaloza-Macmaster P, et al. Different patterns of expansion, contraction and memory differentiation of HIV-1 Gag-specific CD8 T cells elicited by adenovirus type 5 and modified vaccinia Ankara vaccines. Vaccine 2011;29(33):5399–406.

61. Ranasinghe C, Medveczky JC, Woltring D, et al. Evaluation of fowlpox-vaccinia virus prime-boost vaccine strategies for high-level mucosal and systemic immunity against HIV-1. Vaccine 2006;24:5881–95.

62. Ranasinghe C, Turner SJ, McArthur C, et al. Mucosal HIV-1 pox virus prime-boost immunization induces high-avidity CD8+ T cells with regime-dependent cytokine/granzyme B profiles. J. Immunol. 2007;178(4):2370–9.

63. Keefer MC, Frey SE, Elizaga M, et al. A phase I trial of preventive HIV vaccination with heterologous poxviral-vectors containing matching HIV-1 inserts in healthy HIV-uninfected subjects. Vaccine 2011;29(10):1948–58.

64. Ranasinghe C, Eyers F, Stambas J, Boyle DB, Ramshaw IA, Ramsay AJ. A comparative analysis of HIV-specific mucosal/systemic T cell immunity and avidity following rDNA/rFPV and poxvirus-poxvirus prime boost immunisations. Vaccine 2011;29(16):3008–20.

65. Coupar BEH, Purcell DFJ, Thomson SA, Ramshaw IA, Kent SJ, Boyle DB. Fowlpox virus vaccines for HIV and SIV clinical and pre-clinical trials. Vaccine 2006;24(9):1378–88.

66. Hemachandra A, Puls RL, Sirivichayakul S, et al. An HIV-1 clade A/E DNA prime, recombinant fowlpox virus boost vaccine is safe, but non-immunogenic in a randomized phase I/IIa trial in Thai volunteers at low risk of HIV infection. Hum. Vaccin. 2010;6(10):835–40.

67. Kelleher AD, Puls RL, Bebbington M, et al. A randomised, placebo-controlled phase I trial of DNA prime, recombinant fowlpox virus boost prophylactic vaccine for HIV-1. AIDS 2006;20(2):294–7.

68. Zolla-Pazner S, Lubeck M, Xu S, et al. Induction of neutralizing antibodies to T-cell line-adapted and primary human immunodeficiency virus type 1 isolates with a prime-boost vaccine regimen in chimpanzees. J. Virol. 1998;72(2):1052–9.

69. Liu J, O'Brien KL, Lynch DM, et al. Immune control of an SIV challenge by a T-cell-based vaccine in rhesus monkeys. Nature 2009;457(7225):87–91.

70. Watkins DI, Burton DR, Kallas EG, Moore JP, Koff WC. Nonhuman primate models and the failure of the Merck HIV-1 vaccine in humans. Nat Med. 2008;14(6):617–21.

71. Hansen SG, Ford JC, Lewis MS, et al. Profound early control of highly pathogenic SIV by an effector memory T-cell vaccine. Nature 2011;473(7348):523–7.

72. Hansen SG, Vieville C, Whizin N, et al. Effector memory T cell responses are associated with protection of rhesus monkeys from mucosal simian immunodeficiency virus challenge. Nat. Med. 2009;15(3):293–9.

73. Hansen SG, Sacha JB, Hughes CM, et al. Cytomegalovirus vectors violate CD8+ T cell epitope recognition paradigms. Science 2013;340(6135):1237874.

74. Staras SA, Dollard SC, Radford KW, Flanders WD, Pass RF, Cannon MJ. Seroprevalence of cytomegalovirus infection in the United States, 1988-1994. Clin. Infect. Dis. 2006;43(9):1143–51.

75. Jackson JB, Erice A, Englund JA, Edson JR, Balfour HH Jr. Prevalence of cytomegalovirus antibody in hemophiliacs and homosexuals infected with human immunodeficiency virus type 1. Transfusion 1988;28(2):187–9.

76. Ogra PL, Faden H, Welliver RC. Vaccination strategies for mucosal immune responses. Clin. Microbiol. Rev. 2001;14(2):430–45.

77. Sato S, Kiyono H. The mucosal immune system of the respiratory tract. Curr. Opin. Virol. 2012;2(3):225–32.

78. Belyakov IM, Derby MA, Ahlers JD, et al. Mucosal immunization with HIV-1 peptide vaccine induces mucosal and systemic cytotoxic T lymphocytes and protective immunity in mice against intrarectal recombinant HIV-vaccinia challenge. Proc. Natl. Acad. Sci. U.S.A. 1998;95(4):1709–14.

79. Belyakov IM, Ahlers JD. Comment on "trafficking of antigen-specific CD8+ T lymphocytes to mucosal surfaces following intramuscular vaccination.". J. Immunol. 2009;182(4):1779. author reply, 1780.

80. Mitchell EA, Bergmeier LA, Doyle C, et al. Homing of mononuclear cells from iliac lymph nodes to the genital and rectal mucosa in non-human primates. Eur. J. Immunol. 1998;28(10):3066–74.

III. NOVEL APPROACHES FOR VACCINES

81. Kozlowski PA, Neutra MR. The role of mucosal immunity in prevention of HIV transmission. Curr. Mol. Med. 2003;3(3):217–28.

82. Hathaway LJ, Kraehenbuhl JP. The role of M cells in mucosal immunity. Cell. Mol. Life Sci. 2000;57(2):323–32.

83. Neutra MR, Frey A, Kraehenbuhl JP. Epithelial M cells: gateways for mucosal infection and immunization. Cell 1996;86(3):345–8.

84. Brandtzaeg P. Mucosal immunity: induction, dissemination, and effector functions. Scand. J. Immunol. 2009;70(6):505–15.

85. Czerkinsky C, Holmgren J. Mucosal delivery routes for optimal immunization: targeting immunity to the right tissues. Curr. Top. Microbiol. Immunol. 2012;354:1–18.

86. Neutra MR, Kozlowski PA. Mucosal vaccines: the promise and the challenge. Nat. Rev. Immunol. 2006;6(2):148–58.

87. Belyakov IM, Ahlers JD. What role does the route of immunization play in the generation of protective immunity against mucosal pathogens? J. Immunol. 2009;183(11):6883–92.

88. Lycke N. Recent progress in mucosal vaccine development: potential and limitations. Nat. Rev. Immunol. 2012;12(8):592–605.

89. Veazey RS, DeMaria M, Chalifoux LV, et al. Gastrointestinal tract as a major site of CD4+ T cell depletion and viral replication in SIV infection. Science 1998;280(5362):427–31.

90. Brenchley JM, Douek DC. HIV infection and the gastrointestinal immune system. Mucosal Immunol. 2008;1(1):23–30.

91. Brenchley JM, Douek DC. The mucosal barrier and immune activation in HIV pathogenesis. Curr. Opin. HIV AIDS 2008;3(3):356–61.

92. Li Q, Duan L, Estes JD, et al. Peak SIV replication in resting memory CD4+ T cells depletes gut lamina propria CD4+ T cells. Nature 2005;434(7037):1148–52.

93. Guadalupe M, Reay E, Sankaran S, et al. Severe CD4+ T-cell depletion in gut lymphoid tissue during primary human immunodeficiency virus type 1 infection and substantial delay in restoration following highly active antiretroviral therapy. J. Virol. 2003;77(21):11708–17.

94. Belyakov IM, Hel Z, Kelsall B, et al. Mucosal AIDS vaccine reduces disease and viral load in gut reservoir and blood after mucosal infection of macaques. Nat. Med. 2001;7(12):1320–6.

95. Freihorst J, Ogra PL. Mucosal immunity and viral infections. Ann. Med. 2001;33(3):172–7.

96. Huang X, Liu L, Ren L, Qiu C, Wan Y, Xu J. Mucosal priming with replicative Tiantan vaccinia and systemic boosting with DNA vaccine raised strong mucosal and systemic HIV-specific immune responses. Vaccine 2007;25(52):8874–84.

97. Gherardi MM, Esteban M. Recombinant poxviruses and mucosal vaccine vectors. J. Gen. Virol. 2005;86:2925–36.

98. Corbett M, Bogers WM, Heeney JL, et al. Aerosol immunization with NYVAC and MVA vectored vaccines is safe, simple, and immunogenic. Proc. Natl. Acad. Sci. U.S.A. 2008;105(6):2046–51.

99. Sun C, Chen Z, Tang X, et al. Mucosal priming with a replicating-vaccinia virus-based vaccine elicits protective immunity to simian immunodeficiency virus challenge in rhesus monkeys. J. Virol. 2013;87(10):5669–77.

100. Sexton A, De Rose R, Reece JC, et al. Evaluation of recombinant influenza virus-simian immunodeficiency virus vaccines in macaques. J. Virol. 2009;83(15):7619–28.

101. Crotty S, Andino R. Poliovirus vaccine strains as mucosal vaccine vectors and their potential use to develop an AIDS vaccine. Adv. Drug Deliv. Rev. 2004;56(6):835–52.

102. Kent SJ, Dale CJ, Ranasinghe C, et al. Mucosally-administered human-simian immunodeficiency virus DNA and fowlpoxvirus-based recombinant vaccines reduce acute phase viral replication in macaques following vaginal challenge with CCR5-tropic SHIV(SF162P3). Vaccine 2005;23:5009–21.

103. Belyakov IM, Ahlers JD, Nabel GJ, Moss B, Berzofsky JA. Generation of functionally active HIV-1 specific CD8+ CTL in intestinal mucosa following mucosal, systemic or mixed prime-boost immunization. Virology 2008;381(1):106–15.

104. Ramirez JC, Finke D, Esteban M, Kraehenbuhl JP, Acha-Orbea H. Tissue distribution of the Ankara strain of vaccinia virus (MVA) after mucosal or systemic administration. Arch. Virol. 2003;148(5):827–39.

105. Neeson P, Boyer J, Kumar S, et al. A DNA prime-oral Listeria boost vaccine in rhesus macaques induces a SIV-specific CD8 T cell mucosal response characterized by high levels of alpha4beta7 integrin and an effector memory phenotype. Virology 2006;354(2):299–315.

106. Helmus RA, Poonam P, Caruso L, Gupta P, Chen Y. Induction of SIV p27-specific multifunctional T cells in the gut following prime-boost immunization with Clostridium perfringens and adenovirus vaccines expressing SIV p27. Curr. HIV Res. 2010;8(2):101–12.

III. NOVEL APPROACHES FOR VACCINES

107. Wang L, Cheng C, Ko SY, et al. Delivery of human immunodeficiency virus vaccine vectors to the intestine induces enhanced mucosal cellular immunity. J Virol. 2009;83(14):7166–75.

108. Gherardi MM, Ramirez JC, Esteban M. Interleukin-12 (IL-12) enhancement of the cellular immune response against human immunodeficiency virus type 1 Env antigen in a DNA prime/vaccinia virus boost vaccine regimen is time and dose dependent: suppressive effects of IL-12 boost are mediated by nitric oxide. J. Virol. 2000;74(14):6278–86.

109. Dale CJ, De Rose R, Wilson KM, et al. Evaluation in macaques of HIV-1 DNA vaccines containing primate CpG motifs and fowlpoxvirus vaccines co-expressing IFNgamma or IL-12. Vaccine 2004;23(2):188–97.

110. Boyer JD, Robinson TM, Kutzler MA, et al. SIV DNA vaccine co-administered with IL-12 expression plasmid enhances CD8 SIV cellular immune responses in cynomolgus macaques. J. Med. Primatol. 2005;34(5-6):262–70.

111. Kutzler MA, Robinson TM, Chattergoon MA, et al. Coimmunization with an optimized IL-15 plasmid results in enhanced function and longevity of CD8 T cells that are partially independent of CD4 T cell help. J. Immunol. 2005;175(1):112–23.

112. Day SL, Ramshaw IA, Ramsay AJ, Ranasinghe C. Differential effects of the type I interferons alpha4, beta, and epsilon on antiviral activity and vaccine efficacy. J. Immunol. 2008;180(11):7158–66.

113. Ahlers JD, Belyakov IM, Terabe M, et al. A push-pull approach to maximize vaccine efficacy: abrogating suppression with an IL-13 inhibitor while augmenting help with granulocyte/macrophage colony-stimulating factor and CD40L. Proc. Natl. Acad. Sci. U.S.A. 2002;99(20):13020–5.

114. Liu J, Yu Q, Stone GW, et al. CD40L expressed from the canarypox vector, ALVAC, can boost immunogenicity of HIV-1 canarypox vaccine in mice and enhance the in vitro expansion of viral specific CD8+ T cell memory responses from HIV-1-infected and HIV-1-uninfected individuals. Vaccine 2008;26(32):4062–72.

115. Oh S, Hodge JW, Ahlers JD, Burke DS, Schlom J, Berzofsky JA. Selective induction of high avidity CTL by altering the balance of signals from APC. J. Immunol. 2003;170(5):2523–30.

116. Harrison JM, Bertram EM, Boyle DB, Coupar BE, Ranasinghe C, Ramshaw IA. 4-1BBL coexpression enhances HIV-specific CD8 T cell memory in a poxvirus prime-boost vaccine. Vaccine 2006;24(47-48):6867–74.

117. Ganguly S, Liu J, Pillai VB, Mittler RS, Amara RR. Adjuvantive effects of anti-4-1BB agonist Ab and 4-1BBL DNA for a HIV-1 Gag DNA vaccine: different effects on cellular and humoral immunity. Vaccine 2010;28(5):1300–9.

118. Ranasinghe C, Ramshaw IA. Immunisation route-dependent expression of IL-4/IL-13 can modulate HIV-specific CD8+ CTL avidity. Eur. J. Immunol. 2009;39(7):1819–30.

119. Alexander-Miller MA, Leggatt GR, Sarin A, Berzofsky JA. Role of antigen, CD8, and cytotoxic T lymphocyte (CTL) avidity in high dose antigen induction of apoptosis of effector CTL. J. Exp. Med. 1996;184(2):485–92.

120. Alexander-Miller MA. High-avidity CD8+ T cells: optimal soldiers in the war against viruses and tumors. Immunol. Res. 2005;31(1):13–24.

121. Almeida JR, Price DA, Papagno L, et al. Superior control of HIV-1 replication by CD8+ T cells is reflected by their avidity, polyfunctionality, and clonal turnover. J. Exp. Med. 2007;204(10):2473–85.

122. McCormack S, Stohr W, Barber T, et al. EV02: a Phase I trial to compare the safety and immunogenicity of HIV DNA-C prime-NYVAC-C boost to NYVAC-C alone. Vaccine 2008;26(25):3162–74.

123. Sekaly RP. The failed HIV Merck vaccine study: a step back or a launching point for future vaccine development? J. Exp. Med. 2008;205(1):7–12.

124. Wijesundara DK, Jackson RJ, Tscharke DC, Ranasinghe C. IL-4 and IL-13 mediated down-regulation of CD8 expression levels can dampen anti-viral CD8 T cell avidity following HIV-1 recombinant pox viral vaccination. Vaccine 2013;31(41):4548–55.

125. Belyakov IM, Kuznetsov VA, Kelsall B, et al. Impact of vaccine-induced mucosal high-avidity CD8+ CTLs in delay of AIDS viral dissemination from mucosa. Blood 2006;107(8):3258–64.

126. Belyakov IM, Isakov D, Zhu Q, Dzutsev A, Berzofsky JA. A novel functional CTL avidity/activity compartmentalization to the site of mucosal immunization contributes to protection of macaques against simian/human immunodeficiency viral depletion of mucosal CD4+ T cells. J. Immunol. 2007;178(11):7211–21.

127. Ranasinghe C, Trivedi S, Stambas J, Jackson RJ. Unique IL-13Rα2 based HIV-1 vaccine strategy to enhance mucosal immunity, CD8+ T cell avidity and protective immunity. Mucosal Immunol. 2013;6(6):1068–80.

128. Wijesundara DK, Tscharke DC, Jackson RJ, Ranasinghe C. Reduced interleukin-4 receptor alpha expression on CD8+ T cells correlates with higher quality anti-viral immunity. PLoS ONE 2013;8(1):e55788.

129. Falivene J, Del Medico Zajac MP, Pascutti MF, et al. Improving the MVA vaccine potential by deleting the viral gene coding for the IL-18 binding protein. PLoS ONE 2012;7(2):e32220.

III. NOVEL APPROACHES FOR VACCINES

130. Kibler KV, Gomez CE, Perdiguero B, et al. Improved NYVAC-based vaccine vectors. PLoS ONE 2011;6(11):e25674.

131. Gamvrellis A, Leong D, Hanley JC, Xiang SD, Mottram P, Plebanski M. Vaccines that facilitate antigen entry into dendritic cells. Immunol. Cell Biol. 2004;82(5):506–16.

132. Lori F, Kelly LM, Lisziewicz J. APC-targeted immunization for the treatment of HIV-1. Expert Rev. Vaccines 2004;3(4, Suppl.):S189–98.

133. Lycke N. From toxin to adjuvant: basic mechanisms for the control of mucosal IgA immunity and tolerance. Immunol. Lett. 2005;97(2):193–8.

134. Chavez-Santoscoy AV, Roychoudhury R, Pohl NL, Wannemuehler MJ, Narasimhan B, Ramer-Tait AE. Tailoring the immune response by targeting C-type lectin receptors on alveolar macrophages using "pathogen-like" amphiphilic polyanhydride nanoparticles. Biomaterials 2012;33(18):4762–72.

135. Trumpfheller C, Caskey M, Nchinda G, et al. The microbial mimic poly IC induces durable and protective CD4+ T cell immunity together with a dendritic cell targeted vaccine. Proc. Natl. Acad. Sci. U.S.A. 2008;105(7):2574–9.

136. Pitisuttithum P, Gilbert P, Gurwith M, et al. Randomized, double-blind, placebo-controlled efficacy trial of a bivalent recombinant glycoprotein 120 HIV-1 vaccine among injection drug users in Bangkok, Thailand. J. Infect. Dis. 2006;194(12):1661–71.

137. Flynn NM, Forthal DN, Harro CD, Judson FN, Mayer KH, Para MF. Placebo-controlled phase 3 trial of a recombinant glycoprotein 120 vaccine to prevent HIV-1 infection. J. Infect. Dis. 2005;191(5):654–65.

138. Gray GE, Allen M, Moodie Z, et al. Safety and efficacy of the HVTN 503/Phambili study of a clade-B-based HIV-1 vaccine in South Africa: a double-blind, randomised, placebo-controlled test-of-concept phase 2b study. Lancet Infect. Dis. 2011;11(7):507–15.

139. Cohen J. AIDS research: more woes for struggling HIV vaccine field. Science 2013;340(6133):667.

140. Perrone LA, Ahmad A, Veguilla V, et al. Intranasal vaccination with 1918 influenza virus-like particles protects mice and ferrets from lethal 1918 and H5N1 influenza virus challenge. J. Virol. 2009;83(11):5726–34.

141. Ramsay AJ, Leong KH, Ramshaw IA. DNA vaccination against virus infection and enhancement of antiviral immunity following consecutive immunization with DNA and viral vectors. Immunol. Cell Biol. 1997;75(4):382–8.

142. Borrow P, Lewicki H, Wei X, et al. Antiviral pressure exerted by HIV-1-specific cytotoxic T lymphocytes (CTLs) during primary infection demonstrated by rapid selection of CTL escape virus. Nat. Med. 1997;3(2):205–11.

143. Reece JC, Alcantara S, Gooneratne S, et al. Trivalent live attenuated influenza-SIV vaccines: efficacy and evolution of CTL escape in macaques. J. Virol. 2013;98(9):4146–70.

144. Dzutsev AH, Belyakov IM, Isakov DV, Margulies DH, Berzofsky JA. Avidity of CD8 T cells sharpens immunodominance. Int. Immunol. 2007;19(4):497–507.

145. Klein F, Gaebler C, Mouquet H, et al. Broad neutralization by a combination of antibodies recognizing the CD4 binding site and a new conformational epitope on the HIV-1 envelope protein. J. Exp. Med. 2012;209(8):1469–79.

146. Center RJ, Wheatley AK, Campbell SM, et al. Induction of HIV-1 subtype B and AE-specific neutralizing antibodies in mice and macaques with DNA prime and recombinant gp140 protein boost regimens. Vaccine 2009;27(47):6605–12.

147. Boyer JD, Kim J, Ugen K, et al. HIV-1 DNA vaccines and chemokines. Vaccine 1999;17(Suppl. 2):S53–64.

148. Tapia E, Perez-Jimenez E, Lopez-Fuertes L, Gonzalo R, Gherardi MM, Esteban M. The combination of DNA vectors expressing IL-12 + IL-18 elicits high protective immune response against cutaneous leishmaniasis after priming with DNA-p36/LACK and the cytokines, followed by a booster with a vaccinia virus recombinant expressing p36/LACK. Microbes Infect. 2003;5(2):73–84.

149. Gomez CE, Najera JL, Sanchez R, Jimenez V, Esteban M. Multimeric soluble CD40 ligand (sCD40L) efficiently enhances HIV specific cellular immune responses during DNA prime and boost with attenuated poxvirus vectors MVA and NYVAC expressing HIV antigens. Vaccine 2009;27(24):3165–74.

150. Xi Y, Day SL, Jackson RJ, Ranasinghe C. Role of novel type I interferon epsilon in viral infection and mucosal immunity. Mucosal Immunol. 2012;5(6):610–22.

151. Doria-Rose NA, Ohlen C, Polacino P, et al. Multigene DNA priming-boosting vaccines protect macaques from acute CD4+-T-cell depletion after simian-human immunodeficiency virus SHIV89.6P mucosal challenge. J. Virol. 2003;77(21):11563–77.

152. Wijesundara DK, Ranasinghe C, Jackson RJ, et al. Use of an in vivo FTA assay to assess the magnitude, functional avidity and epitope variant cross-reactivity of T cell responses following HIV-1 recombinant poxvirus vaccination. PlosOne. In press.

Personalized Therapies for Cancer Treatment

Lakshmy Nair, Ana Maria Gonzalez-Angulo

Department of Breast Medical Oncology, Department of Systems Biology,
The University of Texas M.D. Anderson Cancer Center, Houston, TX, USA

INTRODUCTION

Personalized medicine is a broad and rapidly advancing field of health care that is informed by each person's unique clinical, genetic, genomic, and environmental information.[1] Our understanding of the molecular basis of a disease helps to enhance preventative healthcare strategies and allows for therapeutic intervention at the earliest stage of the disease. The overarching goal of personalized medicine is to optimize medical care and outcomes for each individual, resulting in an unprecedented customization of patient care.[1] Research has unraveled hundreds of genes associated with human diseases, correlated treatment response

Novel Approaches and Strategies for Biologics, Vaccines and Cancer Therapies. DOI: 10.1016/B978-0-12-416603-5.00013-4

to genetic variability, and has begun targeted molecular therapy. The use of diagnostic tests based on genetics or other molecular mechanisms, to better predict patients' responses to targeted therapy, is in vogue. Diagnosis, prognosis, treatment, and prevention are being tailored to an individual's genetic and phenotypic information. The interpretation of the human genome gave birth to personalized medicine, which will revolutionize health care.

Developments in genomics, including low-cost, next-generation sequencing technologies, and high-throughput proteomics are expected to enable a more personalized approach to clinical care, with improved risk stratification and treatment selection.[1–3] In oncology, personalized medicine is particularly advanced, with increased use of genomic testing technologies to identify those oncogenic variants in tumor tissue that predict responsiveness to specific drugs.[2,4–6] This will bring us closer to the development of efficacious and less toxic tumor-specific agents and immunotherapeutic approaches. The clinical management of cancer may be suited to a form of personalized medicine in which the mutational landscape of an individual's cancer informs clinical decision making, particularly the selection of targeted therapies.[5,7–9]

Despite improvements in technology, complex mechanisms driving cancer evolution continue to present challenges for the use of genomic approaches to better understand breast and other cancers.[10] There are many technical and regulatory challenges that remain to be resolved prior to widespread implementation of personalized therapy. The following chapter reviews the strategies and challenges associated with the development of high-throughput technologies and targeted therapies against cancer.

THE CANCER GENOME ATLAS

There are at least 200 forms of cancer, and many more subtypes. Each of these is caused by errors in DNA that cause cells to grow uncontrolled. Identifying the changes in each cancer's complete set of DNA—its genome—and understanding how such changes interact to drive the disease will lay the foundation for improving cancer prevention, early detection, and treatment.[11] It is widely accepted that many germline genetic loci contribute a small amount to the heritability of cancer,[12–14] but it is unclear how many of these disease susceptibility loci have prognostic importance.[14] The Cancer Genome Atlas (TCGA), a joint program of the National Cancer Institute (NCI) and the National Human Genome Research Institute, is an effort to accelerate the understanding of the molecular basis of cancer through genome analysis, including large-scale genome sequencing, analysis of DNA copy number, methylation, transcriptional profiling, and assessment of splicing aberrations.[15] The goal of TCGA is to provide the molecular and physical map of cancer aberrations to improve our ability to diagnose, treat, and prevent cancer. The TCGA report on breast cancer provides key insights into previously defined gene expression subtypes and demonstrates the existence of four main breast cancer classes when combining data from five platforms, each of which shows significant molecular heterogeneity.[16] The novel observation in their study is that diverse genetic and epigenetic alterations converge phenotypically into four main breast cancer classes.[16] This is consistent not only with convergent evolution of gene circuits, as seen across multiple organisms, but also with models of breast cancer clonal expansion and *in vivo* cell selection proposed to explain the phenotypic heterogeneity observed within defined breast cancer subtypes.[16] TCGA is a large effort to categorize somatic mutation, expression, copy number, and epigenetic modification within various tumor types.[17] However, the challenge is to determine the role of each aberration as a biomarker and as a therapeutic target.

HIGH-THROUGHPUT TECHNOLOGIES

DNA Copy Number Aberrations

Copy number aberrations (CNAs) are commonly found in tumor tissue and can range from losses (deletions) of one or both copies of chromosomal regions to gains of numerous additional copies (amplifications).[18] These aberrations could be as large as the entire chromosome's arm, and the smaller aberrations could be less than 100 kb. DNA copy number aberrations alter the amount and organization of genomic material, which can increase or decrease the transcriptional activity of critical genes or regulatory RNAs.[15] CNAs can be a small altering function of a single gene or potentially affect a large chromosomal region, and are inherited or caused by deletions, duplications, inversions, or translocations. High-throughput technologies, including comparative genomic hybridization, digital karyotyping, representational oligonucleotide microarray (ROMA), single-nucleotide polymorphism arrays, molecular inversion probes, and next-generation sequencing, are now capable of rapidly and efficiently profiling copy number changes across entire cancer genomes.[15,19–21]

Curtis et al.[22] subjected approximately 2000 clinically annotated primary breast cancer samples to DNA copy number and gene expression analysis using single-nucleotide polymorphism (SNP) arrays and microarrays, respectively. They assessed the influence of SNPs, copy number variants (CNVs), and copy number aberrations on gene expression and found that somatically acquired tumor CNAs had the most influence on genome-wide expression variation on a per-gene basis, affecting roughly equal numbers of genes in *cis* or *trans*.[22] Furthermore, clustering of a discovery set of 997 breast cancers by the 1000 most *cis*-regulated genes suggested 10 subgroups with distinct clinical outcomes and was reproduced by a validation set of 995 tumors.[22] Collectively, these findings demonstrate the power of integrated genomic analyses of large numbers of tumors to reveal recurring genetic lesions and refine patient stratification.[22]

Comparative Genomic Hybridization

Comparative genomic hybridization (CGH) technology is used for the assessment of genome copy number. Typically, analysis proceeds by hybridizing differentially labeled tumor and normal DNA to a representation of the normal genome, although some platforms perform tumor and normal reference hybridization in separate representations.[23] The ratio of tumor label to normal label, hybridized to each locus on the representation, is then measured as an estimate of relative copy number at that locus. Array CGH or aCGH uses slides arrayed with small segments of DNA as the targets for analysis.[24] These microarrays are created by depositing and immobilizing DNA probes on a solid support, such as a glass slide, in an ordered fashion. Commercial vendors, such as Affymetrix, Agilent, Illumina, and NimbleGen, have begun offering oligonucleotide-based arrays with which to study genome-wide CNAs.[23,25–27] The Illumina arrays are unique in that the oligonucleotide probes are attached to microbeads,[23,28] while the NimbleGen arrays are synthesized on demand and so can be easily customized.[23,29] Although the smaller target sequences (25 to 85 bp), used in commercial oligonucleotide arrays, offer the possibility of higher resolution, they also present some disadvantages. Foremost among these is the low signal-to-noise ratio generated during hybridization.

MIP Array

The most recent array CGH analysis platform does not operate through hybridization of tumor and normal DNA to a normal representation. Instead, it utilizes a molecular inversion probe (MIP) interrogation strategy to perform allele-specific copy number analysis.[23,30] MIP assay is an efficient technology for large-scale single-nucleotide polymorphism analysis. It is used for SNP discovery and genotyping. This technique produces "inverted" probes in which SNPs are introduced into tag sequences that could be analyzed using a universal sequence tag. This technology allows multiplex analysis of more than 10,000 probes in a single tube.

Studies of breast tumors by conventional karyotyping, fluorescent *in situ* hybridization (FISH), spectral karyotyping, chromosomal CGH, and array CGH have found a wide range in the number and variety of types of chromosome-level alterations in different breast cancer cell lines and tumors. Often net gain or loss of whole chromosomes or parts of chromosomes is observed, but more focal aberrations including gene amplifications, increases of a restricted region of a chromosome arm, or deletions are also seen.[31] Further, a number of highly frequent genomic aberrations that may act as "drivers" of tumor progression in breast cancer have been discovered and compared with the genomic profiles of "normal" breast tissue samples at least 2 cm away from the primary tumor sites. Interestingly, the normal adjacent tissue was also found to have some genomic aberrations that occurred with high frequency in the primary tumors. This may have important implications for clinical therapy.[20] Additionally, when looking at class comparison and class prediction for clinicopathological parameters, a series of characteristic genomic aberrations associated with different breast cancer subtypes have been described.[20,32,33] These studies provide important information for subsequent research of the underlying mechanisms of breast carcinogenesis.

DNA Mutation Detection

It appears that the strongest predictors of risk of developing breast cancer and of response to therapy are at the DNA level (i.e., HER2/neu). What remains to be solved is if these are readily assessed dichotomous variables (i.e., presence or absence of a mutation versus changes in levels of RNA or protein) or if it reflects a greater effect on underlying biology. In terms of identifying indicators of increased risk of developing cancer, efforts have now moved from positional cloning of rare, high-risk alleles such as BRCA1 and BRCA2 to the identification of common low-risk variants through candidate gene analysis or genome-wide association studies (GWAS). Although these latter approaches have served to identify genes of functional importance in cancer, the low risk associated with the candidate variants has resulted in a challenge in determining how to capitalize on the data clinically. The *BRCA1* and *BRCA2* genes account for the majority of familial breast and ovarian cancers. In recent years, numerous studies have assessed the prevalence of germline mutations in *BRCA1* and *BRCA2* genes in various cohorts. However, both inherited and somatic mutations occur in *BRCA1* and *BRCA2*. Somatic mutations occur in non-reproductive cells and are passed on to other cells through mitosis, creating a clone of cells with the mutant gene, whereas germline mutations occur in cells that give rise to gametes. The frequency of somatic BRCA1/2 mutations and expression loss is sufficiently common in ovarian cancer to warrant assessment of tumors in addition to germline DNA for patient selection for clinical trials.[34,35]

Single-Molecule Real-Time Sequencing

High-throughput sequencing technologies have made deep transcriptome sequencing and transcript quantification, whole genome sequencing, and resequencing possible.[36] Although the cost and time have been greatly reduced, the error profiles and limitations of the new platforms differ significantly from those of previous sequencing technologies.[36] The selection of an appropriate sequencing platform for particular types of experiments is an important consideration and requires a detailed understanding of the technologies available, including sources of error, error rate, and the speed and cost of sequencing.[36] New approaches such as single-molecule, real-time (SMRT) sequencing have the potential to bypass this challenge. SMRT sequencing is done on a chip that contains many zero-mode waveguides (ZMWs). Inside each ZMW, a single active DNA polymerase with a single molecule of single-stranded DNA template is immobilized to the bottom, through which light can penetrate and create a visualization chamber that allows monitoring of the activity of the DNA polymerase at a single-molecule level.[37] The signal from a phospho-linked nucleotide incorporated by the DNA polymerase is detected as the DNA synthesis proceeds, which results in the DNA sequencing in real time.[37] Although this technology has the potential to change the face of worldwide collaborative efforts such as International Cancer Genome Consortium (ICGC) and TCGA, high costs currently restrict the technology to in-depth studies of a limited number of patients.

Whole-genome sequencing studies of breast cancer genomes have revealed additional candidate mutations and gene rearrangements.[38] Systems such as the Illumina® MiSeq® and Life Technologies Ion Torrent™ next-generation sequencers have supplied the field of cancer research with an overwhelming amount of molecular data. These data have provided a catalog of somatic alterations in more than 3500 breast tumors.[39] Banerji and colleagues[38] used the Illumina sequencing platform to sequence the exomes of 103 primary breast tumors and an additional five breast cancer specimens by whole-genome sequencing.[39] The authors identified six recurrently mutated genes within this cohort: *CBFB*, *TP53*, *PIK3CA*, *AKT1*, *GATA3*, and *MAP3K1*.[39] All of these, with the exception of *CBFB*, have been previously identified as recurrently mutated in breast cancer.[39] The CBFB/RUNX1 transcriptional complex appears to be frequently inactivated, as a hemizygous deletion of *RUNX1* at the genomic level co-occurred with *CBFB* mutations.[39] In addition, several cancers with homozygous deletions of *RUNX1* were identified. *CBFB* and *RUNX1* mutations were also identified by Ellis and colleagues[40] in a TCGA study, suggesting that disruption of *CBFB/RUNX1* function is involved in breast cancer progression.[39]

In order to significantly impact patient management it is pertinent to evaluate the frequency of mutations, determine mutations that are coordinated and mutually exclusive, establish mutational events that signal prognosis or respond to specific targeted therapies, and find out whether coordinate mutations (co-mutations) alter clinical outcomes or consequences of therapy.

MassARRAY

A mass spectroscopy-based approach (MassARRAY®, Sequenom) aimed at evaluating single-nucleotide polymorphisms (SNPs) can facilitate rapid, high-throughput, and cost-effective detection of hot-spot gene mutations in cancer cells (e.g., PIK3CA, AKT1).[41,42] However, this latter approach is not readily applicable to genes targeted by non-hot-spot mutations in tumor suppressors (e.g., TP53, PTEN). Using this technology, investigators have determined the frequency, breast cancer subtype specificity, and signaling effects of *PIK3CA* and *AKT* mutations in human breast tumors and breast cancer cell lines. MassARRAY technology (iPLEX®) constitutes a highly sensitive, high-throughput tool for the genotyping of single-nucleotide polymorphisms[43–48] and for mutation screening.[49–52] To detect nucleic acid changes, target regions are initially amplified using multiplex PCR and subsequently hybridized to custom-designed primers, then subjected to a single-base extension reaction using single mass-modified nucleotides.[52] Spotting the products onto a matrix chip and subsequent ionization then enables real-time detection by the MassARRAY mass spectrometer.[52] The high-throughput nature of the technology is due to a combination of the ability to multiplex polymerase chain reactions (PCRs) (up to 36-plex, with as little as 10 ng per multiplex) and rapid analysis.[52] Furthermore, small PCR amplicons (70 to 120 bp) are suitable for the assessment of formalin-fixed, paraffin-embedded (FFPE) tissue, facilitating the identification of recurrent fusion genes in large annotated cohorts.[52] Some special types of breast cancer have recently been shown to be characterized by the presence of recurrent fusion genes resulting from chromosomal translocations, including *ETV6–NTRK3* in secretory carcinomas[41,42,53–56] and *MYB–NFIB* in adenoid cystic carcinomas.[52,57–60] The MassARRAY-based approach can be employed as a high-throughput screening tool for known fusion genes in human cancer.

There is considerable interest in defining the population of patients who have the greatest chance of benefiting from tamoxifen. Because germline markers have the potential to be used in therapy selection, *CYP2D6* polymorphisms were investigated to predict patient responsiveness to tamoxifen. Early clinical investigation of the pharmacogenetics of tamoxifen metabolism showed promise that a pharmacogenetic testing of cytochrome P450 2D6 (CYP2D6) phenotype to identify patients with reduced tamoxifen metabolism could predict poorer responsiveness to tamoxifen in terms of disease recurrence.[61,62] However, Regan et al.[61] reported that the CYP2D6 metabolism phenotype is not the correct surrogate for predicting symptoms and outcome of tamoxifen-treated postmenopausal women, and that the relationship of tamoxifen metabolism with symptoms and disease control is not adequately understood. These results are conflicting[63] in a number of clinical investigations, and the evidence base is inconclusive.[61] With CYP2D6 pharmacogenetic testing now clinically available, there is uncertainty among patients, healthcare providers, health authorities, and insurers with regard to its utility for patient care.[61]

Epigenetic Profiling

Epigenetic changes, such as histone modifications and DNA methylation of tumor suppressor genes, are considered a hallmark of certain cancers, including breast cancer.[64,65] Unlike germline mutations, epigenetic modifications can potentially be reversed, making them very appealing for preventative care and therapeutics against cancers.[64,65] Among the genes commonly hypermethylated in breast cancer are *p16NK4A*, estrogen receptor (*ER*) alpha, progesterone receptor (*PR*), BRCA1, GSTP1, TIMP-3, and E-cadherin.[66] The steroid receptor genes, *ER* and *PR*, have long been associated with breast cancer.[66] Methylation studies of these have shown that the *ER* gene has a CpG island in its promoter and first exon areas.[66,67] The *ER* gene is unmethylated in normal cells and in *ER*-positive cell lines but shows a high degree of methylation in more than half of primary cancers.[66] The *BRCA1* gene, located at chromosome 17q21, is one of the more commonly associated genes in breast cancer, and the protein product is reduced or absent.[66] DNA methylation has been proposed as one of the causes of its inactivation.[66,68] The CpG island of *RASSF1A* is hypermethylated in 60% to 77% of breast cancers, and its transcripts are frequently inactivated in cancer cell lines and primary tissues.[65,69,70] Literature suggests that *RASSF1A* hypermethylation may be a promising biomarker to screen putative cancer patients.[65,71] Gene-specific epigenetic changes for breast cancer are likely to occur early in tumorigenesis and have the potential to be used as early detection and prevention methods.[65,72] This underscores the need to identify "epigenetic signatures" specific to breast cancer using high-throughput techniques.

Methylation has proven to be a promising predictive and prognostic biomarker,[73] but it is especially promising as a biomarker for early cancer detection in biological fluids[74] for various reasons.[75] First, methylation aberrations occur with high frequency and in early stages of tumor development.[75–77] Second, methylation changes have been demonstrated in noncancerous cells adjacent to the tumor.[75,78] This so-called field defect facilitates detection in heterogeneous biological samples.[75] Finally, methylation detection is applicable to biological fluids that contain low amounts of DNA.[75,79–81] Analysis of DNA methylation has been advanced recently by the application of high-throughput DNA sequencing technology that allows robust, quantitative, and cost-effective functional genomic strategies.[82] This has in recent years led to the development of a large variety of PCR-based methylation assays interrogating methylation of cytosine (methyl-C) in CpG dinucleotides that cluster in CpG islands in the regulatory sequences of gene promoters.[75,83]

QM-MSP

Quantitative multiplex methylation-specific polymerase chain reaction (QM-MSP) is a sensitive technique to quantitate cumulative gene promoter hypermethylation in multiple genes. With this technique it is possible to use samples that contain a limited amount of DNA, such as ductal lavage, nipple aspiration fluids, and fine-needle aspirates.[79,84] It has been reported that specific molecular alterations typifying tumor can be more sensitive than and precede the appearance of morphologic abnormalities detected by cytology.[79]

MS-MLPA

A powerful alternative approach to QM-MSP is the semiquantitative methylation-specific multiplex ligation-dependent probe amplification (MS-MLPA), which relies on methylation-sensitive endonucleases that discriminate between methylated and unmethylated DNA sequences.[75,85] Like MLPA,[86] MS-MLPA is relatively fast and inexpensive.[75] However, for biological samples with scarce DNA, QM-MSP is the method of choice.[75]

RNA Profiling

Breast cancer is clinically heterogeneous with varying response to treatment.[87] The established methods that are suited to study one gene at a time do not seem to have the power to overcome this clinical heterogeneity, which is likely to be due to a complex set of multiple somatic mutations, epigenetic changes, and genomic rearrangements.[87–89] To overcome the limitation of single-gene or protein biomarkers, the implementation of microarray technology nearly a decade ago has enabled the quantitative measurement of complex gene expression patterns (i.e., gene expression profiling) in breast and other cancers and has paved the way to new pattern-based biomarker strategies.[87] The conceptual changes resulting from gene expression profiling studies of breast cancer have led to a new paradigm in the way breast cancer is perceived,[90–93] and, importantly, have provided a rationale for a change in the way clinical trials are undertaken and patients are stratified for treatment decision making.[94,95] Furthermore, some tests that have emerged from these analyses provide an incremental increase in the reproducibility and accuracy of the assessment of variables that are crucial to determine prognosis of disease and tailor therapy.[94]

RNA Microarrays

Gene expression profiling with RNA microarrays enables investigators to semiquantitatively measure, in a single experiment, the expression of most mRNAs expressed in a small piece of cancer tissue.[96] With the help of this technology one can identify individually predictive genes and combine these into a multivariate prediction model that will be more accurate than any single gene.[96] There are several established statistical methods for combining variables into prediction models, including the commonly used logistic regression analysis and the Cox proportional hazards regression model.[96,97]

One of the first applications of microarray-based gene expression profiling analysis to the study of breast cancer was an assessment of the diversity of the disease at the molecular level. The hierarchical cluster analysis of genes that vary more between tumors than between repeated samples of the same tumor, the so-called intrinsic genes, initially revealed the existence of at least four molecular subtypes of breast cancer.[94,98] The "intrinsic" classification[98] proposes four molecular classes of breast cancer: (1) basal-like breast cancers, mostly corresponding to estrogen receptor (ER)-negative, progesterone-receptor (PR)-negative, and HER2-negative tumors, or "triple-negative" tumors; (2) luminal-A breast cancers, which are mostly ER positive and histologically low grade; (3) luminal-B cancers, which are also mostly ER positive but may express hormone receptors and proliferation markers and are often high grade; and (4) HER2-positive cancers, which show amplification and high expression of the ERBB2 gene as well as other genes of the ERBB2 amplicon.[99]

MicroRNAs (miRNAs) show differential expression across breast cancer subtypes and have both oncogenic and tumor-suppressive roles.[16,100–105] Dvinge et al.[22,100] have reported the miRNA expression profiles of 1302 breast tumors with matching detailed clinical annotation, long-term follow-up, and genomic and messenger RNA expression data. Their report has provided a comprehensive overview of the quantity, distribution, and variation of the miRNA population and information on the extent to which genomic, transcriptional, and posttranscriptional events contribute to the miRNA expression architecture, suggesting an important role for posttranscriptional regulation.[100]

RNA sequencing has revolutionized the exploration of gene expression. Advances in the RNA sequencing workflow, from sample preparation through data analysis, enable rapid profiling and deep investigation of the transcriptome. Using microarray technology limits the researcher to detecting transcripts that correspond to existing genomic sequencing information; RNA-seq experiments, on the other hand, work well for investigating both known transcripts and exploring new ones. Therefore, RNA-seq is ideal for discovery-based experiments. Using RNA-seq and Ingenuity® Pathway Analysis (IPA®), Randovich et al.[106] demonstrated how comprehensive network and pathway analysis revealed novel insights into the tumor biology of triple-negative breast cancers and has informed rational drug targeting for therapeutic development.

PAM50

The PAM50 Breast Cancer Intrinsic Classifier™ is an reverse transcription (RT)-qPCR assay that measures the expression of 50 classifier genes and five control genes to identify the intrinsic subtypes known as luminal-A, luminal-B, HER2-enriched, and basal-like.[107] PAM50 on the nCounter® platform represents the next generation in genomic testing for breast cancer, providing a powerful new tool for reliable and accurate genomic testing. The two preferred technologies for gene expression profiling from FFPE tissues are RT-qPCR[108,109] and NanoString's nCounter®.[110,111] The nCounter system uses color-coded probes that bind directly to the RNA transcript without reverse transcription and PCR amplification.[110] Although these methods have high agreement for gene quantification, other methodologies may lead to different conclusions and treatment decisions.[110] For example, in the NCIC CTG MA.12 clinical trial that randomized premenopausal women with primary breast cancer to tamoxifen versus placebo, it was found that panel 6 immunohistochemistry (IHC) antibodies for subtyping were not prognostic, but the PAM50 RT-qPCR subtypes were prognostic.[110,112] The PAM50 gene set is often used for gene expression-based subtyping; however, surrogate subtyping using panels of IHC markers are still widely used clinically.[110] Discrepancies between these methods may lead to different treatment decisions.[110]

Although up to 70% of patients with breast cancer can be cured today, a significant proportion of these patients are overtreated.[87] It remains a challenge to identify those patients who will indeed profit from current treatment strategies and also to develop innovative concepts for patients currently at high risk for relapse after treatment.[87] For this reason, the identification of reliable prognostic biomarkers and the development of clinically efficient therapies are urgently needed.[87,113] Gene-expression profiling has also been used to develop genomic tests that may provide better predictions of clinical outcome than the traditional clinical and pathological standards.[99,114]

MammaPrint

MammaPrint (Agendia), the first successfully developed prognostic signature, is a microarray-based test approved by the U.S. Food and Drug Administration (FDA) that can be used for the prognostication of patients with stage 1 or 2, node-negative, invasive breast cancer of tumor size less than 5.0 cm.[94] The assay measures the expression of 70 genes and calculates a prognostic score that categorizes patients into "good" or "poor" risk groups; it requires fresh or frozen samples containing tumor cell content greater than 30%.[94] The challenges in prospective validation of this prognostic signature stem from the requirement for fresh or frozen samples. In an early feasibility study of MammaPrint (MicroarRAy PrognoSTics in Breast CancER [RASTER] study), 158 of 585 patients were excluded because of sampling failure ($n = 128$) or incorrect procedure ($n = 30$).[94] To circumvent the challenges of tissue procurement and shipping of snap-frozen tumor specimens, a new procurement method (RNA Retain®, Asuragen) has been adopted.[94,115]

Genomic Grade Index

Histologic grading of breast carcinomas is an important prognostic factor.[116,117] High tumor grade is associated with decreased overall survival,[118] but it also predicts increased response to neoadjuvant chemotherapy.[116,119] Lack of sufficient reproducibility and objectivity limit the clinical utility of histologic grade as a prognostic or predictive factor.[116,120] Particularly, tumors of intermediate grade display a low degree of reproducibility and are of poor prognostic and predictive value.[116] These imperfections have recently been addressed by the development of a multigene index representing a genomic correlate of histologic tumor grade.[116,121] Comparison of gene expression profiles between breast cancers of low versus high histologic grade identified a panel of differentially expressed genes, 97 of which were combined into the genomic grade index (GGI).[116] It has been demonstrated that a high GGI is capable of assigning breast cancers of intermediate grade into two groups, whose prognoses resemble those of either high or low histologic grade, and is predictive of higher risk of recurrence than a low index in both untreated and tamoxifen-treated patients.[116,122]

RNA microarray technology renders it possible to assay the expression of thousands of genes simultaneously.[123] Gene-specific probes (i.e., oligonucleotides) representing thousands of genes are arrayed on an inert substrate (microarray platform).[123] Messenger RNA (mRNA) extracted from a tissue of interest is amplified, fluorescently labeled, and further hybridized with the gene-specific probes in the microarray platform.[123] Fluorescent detectors coupled with computers are used for scanning and are able to estimate the gene expression for a given sample.[123,124] When GGI was applied to previously defined breast cancer molecular subtypes, its ability to classify the subgroups in high or low risk was demonstrated.[123] In the dataset of Van De Vijver, even the population that was previously classified molecularly as "undefined" could be classified by the application of GGI.[123,125] Luminal-A and normal-like subtypes were categorized as low-GGI. HER2, basal-like, luminal-B, and the subgroup of patients previously unclassified were categorized as high-GGI.[122,123]

Oncotype DX®

In parallel with the development of microarray-based prognostic signatures, Paik and colleagues[126] developed Oncotype DX® (ODX), a qRT-PCR-based signature that measures the expression of 21 genes (16 cancer-related and five reference genes) that can be performed with RNA extracted from formalin-fixed, paraffin-embedded tissue samples.[94] The recurrence score (RS) is used to predict patient prognosis (i.e., the likelihood of recurrence at 10 years);[126] scores range from 0 to 100.[127] The assay also categorizes patients into three risk groups: (1) low-risk group (RS = 0 to 18), in which the score correlates with a risk of distant recurrence of less than 10%; (2) intermediate-risk group (18 < RS < 31), in which the risk score correlates with a risk of distant recurrence of between 10% and 20%; (3) high-risk group (RS ≥ 31), in which the score correlates with a risk of distant recurrence of greater than 20%.[127]

This test can be used in women of all ages with newly diagnosed ER-positive stage I or II breast cancer.[127] In addition to providing prognostic information, it predicts benefit from hormonal therapy (tamoxifen and/or aromatase inhibitors) as well from chemotherapy.[126–131]

Oncotype DX provides information that can be directly used to establish the outcome of patients with ER-positive disease.[94] High-risk patients have a poor outcome and derive significant benefit from adjuvant cyclophosphamide, methotrexate, and fluorouracil-based chemotherapy, whereas low-risk patients have a good outcome when treated with tamoxifen alone and the benefit these patients derive from chemotherapy is small, if any.[94,126,131,132] The management of the intermediate-risk group remains uncertain and is being addressed in the Trial Assigning IndividuaLized Options for Treatment (TAILORx).[94] The TAILORx and the RxPONDER trials will validate the clinical utility of Oncotype DX to assign ER-positive, node-negative and node-positive patients to chemotherapy plus endocrine therapy versus endocrine therapy alone.[133,134]

Proteomic Assays

Mammostrat®

The multiparameter immunohistochemical (IHC) assay Mammostrat® (Clarient) combines novel information in a five-biomarker assay measuring SLC7A5, HTF9C, p53, NDRG1, and CEACAM5.[135] Each marker assesses independent features of tumor biology distinct from HER2, proliferation, or hormone receptor status, and the combined risk measured has been evaluated in multiple cohorts.[135–138] The five markers in the Mammostrat panel (SLC7A5, HTF9C, p53, NDRG1, and CEACAM5) assess aspects of DNA damage, stress response, and nutritional and differentiation pathways that are not determined by conventional assays for ER/PR, HER2, and proliferation.[135–138] Thus, Mammostrat may provide novel information relevant to the assessment of residual risk after adjuvant endocrine therapy, at moderate costs, and by using conventional formalin-fixed pathology samples.[135] It has been reported that, for postmenopausal women with ER-positive early breast cancers, irrespective of nodal status, the Mammostrat panel provided independent information on residual risk of distant recurrence or death as a result of breast cancer after treatment with exemestane or a switch regimen (tamoxifen followed by exemestane) in a retrospective analysis of the Tamoxifen versus Exemestane Adjuvant Multicenter (TEAM) trial pathology study cohort.[135]

Reverse-Phase Protein Array

Proteins are the direct effectors of cellular function.[139] As protein levels and function depend not only on translation but also on posttranslational modifications, functional proteomic profiling may theoretically yield more direct answers to functional and pharmacological questions than transcriptional profiling alone.[139] Reverse-phase protein array (RPPA) is a useful tool to identify and validate proteins and phosphoproteins.[139,140] RPPA offers the potential to profile potentially hundreds of phosphorylation events in very small quantities of tumor materials, such as those that might be obtained from laser-capture microdissection from a biopsy.[141,142] Using RPPA, Gonzalez-Angulo et al.[139] developed a ten-protein biomarker panel that classifies breast cancer into prognostic groups that may have potential utility in the management of patients who receive anthracycline–taxane-based neoadjuvant systemic therapy (NST). Gonzalez et al.[143] have also used RPPA to determine the molecular characteristics of residual breast cancer, in general, and in hormone receptor (HR)-positive tumors after NST, and their relationship with patient outcomes, in order to identify potential therapeutic targets. Though RPPA is useful for the objective quantification of protein expression in cell lines and tumor tissues, it does not provide information on intratumoral or cellular localization of the evaluated proteins nor on the effect of different protein localization patterns on clinical outcomes.[143]

IHC4+C

The immunohistochemical (IHC) 4+C score is a prognostic tool based on quantitative values of four standard laboratory IHC assays (ER, PR, HER2, and Ki67), and the clinicopathologic parameters of tumor grade, size, nodal burden, patient age, and treatment with aromatase inhibitor or tamoxifen—hence, IHC4+clinical (IHC4+C) score.[144,145] The IHC4+C score was developed in a retrospective analysis from the TransATAC trial after recognition that these IHC assays independently hold prognostic power in endocrine-treated patients.[144,146,147] IHC4+C gives a prediction of the residual risk of distant recurrence at 9 years in postmenopausal women with node-negative, hormone-receptor-positive disease treated with 5 years of adjuvant endocrine therapy.[144,145] IHC4+C has also been shown to be at least as good as Oncotype Dx.[144,145] Not only is it cost effective compared to gene-expression profiling tools such as Oncotype Dx, but it can also be easily carried out at the majority of oncology clinical centers, as it utilizes existing laboratory assays.[144] However, there are quality assurance issues with the qualitative assessment of ER, PR, HER2, and Ki67 IHC, with the potential for interlaboratory variation in values.[144] In this regard the International Ki67 in Breast Cancer Working Group recently proposed guidelines to reduce interlaboratory variability and improve interstudy comparability of Ki67, mostly using IHC with monoclonal antibody MIB1.[148]

Significance of Prognostic Signatures

Several groups have analyzed prognostic biological pathways across breast cancer molecular subtypes;[149–151] a tacit assumption is that if a gene signature is associated with prognosis, it is likely to encode a biological signature driving carcinogenesis.[152] Recent work by Venet et al.[152,153] has questioned the validity of this assumption by showing that most random gene sets are able to separate breast cancer cases into groups exhibiting significant survival differences. This suggests that it is not valid to infer the biologic significance of a gene set in breast cancer based on its association with breast cancer prognosis and, further, that new rigorous statistical methods are needed to identify biologically informative prognostic pathways.[152] To this end, Significance Analysis of Prognostic Signatures (SAPS) has been developed.[152] It is an algorithm that helps to more accurately identify prognostic signatures associated with patient survival.[152] When Beck et al.[152] used SAPS to analyze previously identified prognostic signatures in breast and ovarian cancer, they found that only a small subset of the signatures that were considered statistically significant by standard measurements also achieved statistical significance when evaluated by SAPS. A gene set may appear to be important based on its survival association, when in reality it does not perform significantly better than random genes.[152] This can be a serious problem, as it can lead to false conclusions regarding the biological and clinical significance of a gene set.[152] The SAPS procedure ensures that a significant prognostic gene set not only is associated with patient survival but also performs significantly better than random gene sets.[152]

USING TARGETED THERAPY TO PERSONALIZE CANCER TREATMENT

The current wave of excitement about targeted cancer therapy[154–158] was initiated by the success of imatinib in the treatment of chronic myeloid leukemia (CML).[159–161] Four decades of research passed between the discovery of the Philadelphia chromosome and the first treatment to target an activated oncogene in a human cancer.[159] Targeted therapies against many different types of cancer are now being developed at a fast pace.[159] These include gefitinib and erlotinib for non-small-cell lung cancer patients with epidermal growth factor receptor (EGFR) mutations,[158] panitumumab and cetuximab for metastatic colon cancer,[162] vemurafenib for patients with melanomas harboring BRAF mutations,[154] and crizotinib for lung cancer patients with EML4-ALK translocations.[156,159] At present, dozens of other targeted cancer therapies have either been approved or are being evaluated in clinical trials.[159]

Although numerous systemic agents are available to treat metastatic breast cancer (MBC), most tumors eventually become unresponsive to systemic therapy.[163] In recent years, several targeted agents have become available that have improved the outcomes of patients with solid tumors.[163] A greater understanding of the underlying biology of breast cancer has resulted in the identification of a number of molecular targets and development of novel therapeutics.[164] Among them are tyrosine kinase inhibitors (TKIs) directed at a number of targets (HER1, HER2, HER3, IGF receptor [IGFR], C-MET, FGF receptor [FGFR]), inhibitors of intracellular signaling pathways (PI3K, AKT, mammalian target of rapamycin [mTOR], ERK), angiogenesis inhibitors, and agents that interfere with DNA repair.[164] Some of these agents have shown remarkable activity and have already become part of the standard of care in patients with breast cancer (exemplified by the anti-HER2 agents trastuzumab and lapatinib).[164] A large group of compounds are still in an early phase of development, but in some cases, indications of clinical responses have already been observed.[164] Others have shown clinical activity but are not yet approved for clinical practice.[164]

Modulation of Estrogen Receptor Signaling

Estrogen receptor-positive and progesterone receptor-positive breast cancer has, for more than three decades, been the prime example of cancer amenable to targeted drug approaches. Hormone receptor (HR)-positive breast cancers are largely driven by the estrogen/ER pathway, and endocrine therapy targeting this pathway has been most successful.[165] Endocrine therapy (ET) is a key treatment modality in the management of ER alpha-positive breast cancer.[166] ET can be given preoperatively (neoadjuvant), postoperatively (adjuvant), and in the metastatic/advanced disease setting (palliative treatment).[166] Historically, ET is the oldest systemic therapy for the treatment of breast cancer.[166] Current ET constitutes treatments that modulate or disrupt the process of estrogen production or the function or presence of the ER in breast cancer cells.[166] Selective estrogen response modulators (SERMs) structurally resemble estrogens.[167] Upon binding to estrogen receptors, they exert functionally different effects in normal tissue and cancer cells.[167] They function as ER agonists in some tissues but oppose the action of estrogen in others.[167] For many decades, the SERM tamoxifen was the gold standard for treating both pre- and postmenopausal patients with hormone receptor-positive breast cancer.[167]

The 2011 metaanalyses from the Early Breast Cancer Trialists' Collaborative Group (EBCTCG), with a median of 13 years' follow-up, have shown that 5 years of tamoxifen, compared to none, reduced recurrence rates by almost half throughout the first 10 years (rate ratio (RR), 0.53 [SE 0.03]).[166] Furthermore, yearly breast-cancer mortality was reduced by about a third throughout the first 15 years (RR, 0.70 [0.05]; $p < 0.00001$).[166]

These effects of tamoxifen were independent of a patient's sex, age, and menopausal status but were absolutely dependent on ER/PR expression, as measured by immunohistochemistry.[167,168] ER response modulation with tamoxifen or raloxifene has also demonstrated value in the prevention of breast cancer in women at moderate to high risk of developing the disease.[167,169,170] Whereas tamoxifen acts as an estrogen antagonist in breast tissue, it has partial agonist activity in other tissues.[167] Such dichotomy results in an increased risk of endometrial cancer and thromboembolic disease but an improvement in bone health and reduced cholesterol levels in postmenopausal women.[167]

For patients who become postmenopausal after five years of tamoxifen, extended therapy with an aromatase inhibitor (AI) is another option.[165] As an alternative to tamoxifen, ovarian ablation or suppression could be considered as an adjuvant therapy for premenopausal women.[165] In postmenopausal women, AIs have been shown to improve overall survival (OS), compared with tamoxifen, in the metastatic setting.[165,171] All three AIs—letrozole and anastrozole (nonsteroidal) and exemestane (steroidal)—have shown similar efficacy in the clinical setting, although non-cross-resistance exists between the nonsteroidal and the steroidal AIs.[165] Options for second or later lines of endocrine therapy include another AI, fulvestrant, tamoxifen, testosterone, megestrol acetate (Megace®, Bristol-Myers Squibb), or (paradoxically) estradiol, as well as the recently approved combination of everolimus and exemestane.[165] In postmenopausal women with early-stage disease, multiple large adjuvant trials have demonstrated that monotherapy with an AI for five years or a switching strategy (from AI to tamoxifen or from tamoxifen to AI, with a total duration of therapy of five years) is superior to tamoxifen.[165,172] AI has become a preferred approach, or at least part of the adjuvant hormonal therapy approach, in postmenopausal women with ER-positive breast cancer.[165]

Phosphorylation of the retinoblastoma protein (Rb), mediated by cyclin-dependent kinase 4 (CDK4) or CDK6 (complexed with the activating subunit cyclin D), is required for entry of a cell into the cell cycle.[173] One of the most commonly deregulated checkpoints, in hormone-positive breast cancer, involves the cyclin D–CDK4/CDK6/Rb pathway.[173] Miller et al.[174] identified an estrogen-independent role for ER and the CDK4/Rb/E2F transcriptional axis in the hormone-independent growth of breast cancer cells. Using a small interfering RNA (siRNA) screen they found that CDK4, which activates E2F transcription, is required for hormone independent cell growth.[174] They also reported that CDK4 inhibition suppressed the hormone-independent growth of both fulvestrant-sensitive and -insensitive ER-positive cell lines.[174] Their data support the development of CDK4 inhibitors for the treatment of antiestrogen-resistant breast cancers.[174] Palbociclib (PD-0332991, a CDK4/CDK6 inhibitor) is currently being evaluated to overcome this resistance mechanism. Pfizer has initiated a randomized, multi-center, double-blind Phase III study (known as Study 1008) evaluating palbociclib in combination with letrozole versus letrozole alone as a first-line treatment for postmenopausal patients with ER-positive, HER2-negative locally advanced or metastatic breast cancer.[175]

Targeting the HER Signaling Pathway

The human epidermal growth factor receptor (HER) family of proteins is comprised of four receptors (EGFR/HER1 and HER2–4) activated by numerous extracellular ligands.[164] Upon ligand binding, the receptors dimerize, become phosphorylated, and transduce intracellular signals that regulate a variety of cellular processes including proliferation and survival.[164] HER2 overexpression is associated with an aggressive clinical phenotype that includes high-grade tumors, increased growth rates, early systemic metastasis, and decreased rates of disease-free and overall survival.[176–178] Preclinical data indicate that this adverse clinical picture results from fundamental changes in the biologic features of breast-cancer cells containing the alteration, including increased proliferation, suppression of apoptosis, increased motility, greater invasive and metastatic potential, accelerated angiogenesis, and steroid hormone independence.[176,179–186]

Trastuzumab (Herceptin®, Genentech) is a recombinant humanized monoclonal antibody against the extracellular domain of HER2.[167] Trastuzumab inhibits cancer cell proliferation, induces apoptosis, and reduces tumor-induced angiogenesis in preclinical breast cancer models.[167,187] Introduction of the monoclonal antibody trastuzumab has led to significant improvement in the outcome of this disease.[165] Alone and in combination with chemotherapy, trastuzumab has been shown to have an acceptable safety record and to be active in advanced HER2-positive disease.[167,188–190]

In the Phase III study H0648g (Advanced Metastatic Breast Cancer), women who received Herceptin plus chemotherapy (either an anthracycline and cyclophosphamide or paclitaxel) lived nearly three months longer without their disease worsening compared to women who received chemotherapy alone (median time to disease progression: 7.4 months versus 4.6 months).[191,192] This study suggests that trastuzumab augments the effects of chemotherapy.[191]

The optimum duration of treatment with adjuvant trastuzumab has been, and remains, unclear.[193] In patients with metastatic disease, withholding trastuzumab in a responding patient almost always leads to disease progression.[193] This observation would support administering trastuzumab for a longer period.[193] Conversely, in women with operable breast cancer, two small studies suggested that when trastuzumab is administered concomitantly with chemotherapy between 9 weeks and 6 months the reduction in the risk of relapse is similar to longer treatment regimens.[193,194] A shorter period of trastuzumab treatment would be an attractive option for several reasons, including reduced toxicity, inconvenience to patients, and costs.[193]

The Herceptin Adjuvant (HERA) trial compared 1-year versus 2-year trastuzumab added sequentially to adjuvant chemotherapy and found no additional benefit of 2-year treatment.[193,195] The Protocol for Herceptin as Adjuvant therapy with Reduced Exposure (PHARE) trial[196] could not prove the non-inferiority of 6-month versus 12-month adjuvant trastuzumab on disease-free survival, the primary study endpoint.[193] Although the results of PHARE must not alter current clinical practice, they support the notion that the treatment of patients with HER2-positive operable breast cancer requires more individualized approaches.[193] In this respect, trastuzumab treatment duration remains a potential component of tailored strategies.[193]

Compared with ER-positive/HER2-negative disease, ER-positive/HER2-positive breast cancer is associated with a higher risk of relapse on adjuvant endocrine therapy.[165] This is explained by the finding of incomplete cell-cycle arrest under treatment with endocrine agents alone in the neoadjuvant setting.[165,197] The benefit of adding HER2-targeted agents in this patient population was demonstrated in studies of adjuvant trastuzumab in HER2-positive breast cancer; the ER-positive/HER2-positive subset derived a significant benefit from trastuzumab in reducing relapse.[165] Thus, adjuvant trastuzumab, in addition to hormonal therapy, is a standard of care for these patients.[165] In addition to trastuzumab, several HER2-targeted agents, including laptinib, pertuzumab, and trastuzumab emtansine, have been approved for treatment of advanced HER2 positive disease.[165]

Despite achieving notable success by adding trastuzumab to chemotherapy in HER2-positive early breast cancer, 70% of patients demonstrate intrinsic or secondary resistance to trastuzumab.[198,199] Understanding the mechanisms behind trastuzumab resistance is a critical step toward the development of novel anti-HER2 strategies.[199] To date, known mechanisms of resistance to anti-HER2 agents include aberrant activation of the downstream phosphoinositide 3-kinase (PI3K)[200,201] and Src[202] pathways, co-expression of the truncated p95HER2 receptor,[203] co-expression and dimerization with other RTKs,[204] and cyclin E amplification.[205,206] These mechanisms are clinically relevant;[200–203,206] therefore, specific therapeutic approaches are being investigated in patients.[205,207]

PI3K/AKT/mTOR Signaling Pathway Inhibitors

Phosphatidylinositol 3-kinase (PI3K)/Akt/mTOR (mammalian target of rapamycin) is a critical intracellular signaling pathway that is involved in numerous normal cellular processes.[166] Aberrations in this pathway are well described in multiple cancers.[166,208] The PI3K/Akt/mTOR pathway is emerging as a novel target in breast cancer.[209] Activation of the pathway has been implicated in tumorigenesis and breast cancer progression,[210] as well as in resistance to standard therapies.[200,201,209,211] Acquired resistance may occur as tumor cells adapt to the stress of treatment by using alternative cellular signaling pathways.[212–214] Potential mechanisms for resistance to targeted agents include steric inhibition imposed by other cellular elements, molecular changes in the target receptor, alterations in the regulation of downstream signaling components, compensatory cross-talk with other signaling pathways, and pharmacogenetic alterations in the host.[212,213,215] Deregulation of the PI3K/Akt/mTOR pathway is an important mechanism of endocrine resistance.[165,216] Gain-of-function mutations in the PI3 kinase α catalytic subunit gene (PIK3CA) occur at a frequency of 30 to 40% and represent the most frequent genetic abnormality in ER-positive breast cancer.[16,165] In preclinical models, ER-positive breast cancer carrying PIK3CA mutations was highly dependent on PI3Kα (alias p110α) for cell survival.[165,217] Knockdown of PIK3CA using RNAi or inhibition of PI3K or AKT with small molecule inhibitors induced apoptosis in the presence of estrogen deprivation in ER-positive breast cancer cell lines.[165,217,218] In addition, the development of acquired endocrine resistance was accompanied by activation of the PI3K pathway in studies of long-term estradiol-deprived breast cancer cell lines, and inhibition of PI3K pathway signaling reduced cancer cell growth and survival.[165,218,219]

Aberrant activation of the PI3K pathway has also been shown to correlate with diminished responses to HER2-directed therapies.[220] Hanker et al.[220] reported that mice expressing both human HER2 and mutant PIK3CA in the mammary epithelium developed tumors with shorter latencies compared with mice expressing either oncogene alone. They demonstrated that *PIK3CA*[H1047R] accelerates HER2-mediated breast epithelial transformation and metastatic progression, alters the intrinsic phenotype of HER2-overexpressing cancers, and generates resistance to approved combinations of anti-HER2 therapies.[220] Addition of a PI3K inhibitor reversed resistance in these tumors, suggesting that combining anti-HER2 therapies with PI3K inhibitors may be beneficial for the clinical treatment of HER2+/PIK3CA-mutant breast cancers.[220]

As indicated above, evidence suggests that both hormone receptor-positive tumors and HER2-overexpressing tumors use the PI3K/Akt/mTOR pathway to escape control of anti-hormone and anti-HER2 therapies.[213] The combination of mTOR inhibitors, with hormone-targeted or HER2-targeted therapies, appears to be a promising strategy for overcoming resistant disease and preventing the development of resistance.[221]

Three mTOR antagonists are being studied for breast cancer treatment:[222] everolimus, a mammalian target of rapamycin inhibitor with better oral availability than sirolimus; temsirolimus, a water-soluble ester of sirolimus; and deforolimus, a nonrapamycin analog prodrug that has been tested in Phase I and II clinical trials and shows promising results in several tumor types, including sarcoma.[163]

Growing evidence supports a close interaction between the mTOR pathway and ER signaling. A substrate of mTOR complex 1 (mTORC1), called S6 kinase 1, phosphorylates the activation function domain 1 of the ER, which is responsible for ligand-independent receptor activation.[223,224] In the Phase III BOLERO-2 (Breast cancer trials of OraLEveROlimus-2) trial, Baselga et al.[221] compared everolimus and exemestane versus exemestane and placebo (randomly assigned in a 2:1 ratio) in 724 patients with hormone-receptor-positive advanced breast cancer who had recurrence or progression while receiving previous therapy with a nonsteroidal aromatase inhibitor in the adjuvant setting or to treat advanced disease (or both). They found that everolimus combined with an aromatase inhibitor improved progression-free survival.[221] Based on this study, on July 20, 2012, the FDA approved everolimus tablets (Afinitor®, Novartis) for the treatment of postmenopausal women with advanced hormone-receptor-positive, HER2-negative breast cancer in combination with exemestane, after failure of treatment with letrozole or anastrozole.[221] In a Phase III BOLERO-3 trial, the addition of everolimus to trastuzumab and vinorelbine significantly extended progression-free survival in women with HER2-positive advanced breast cancer, compared to treatment with placebo plus trastuzumab and vinorelbine.[225] Data from this study demonstrate that everolimus also has a meaningful impact in heavily pretreated HER2-positive advanced breast cancer patients.[225]

Targeting VEGF for the Treatment of Breast Cancer

Angiogenesis is implicated in the pathogenesis of malignancy and metastasis.[226] Inhibition of angiogenesis has demonstrated clinically significant improvements in outcomes in a variety of malignancies, including breast cancer.[226] E2100 was a randomized Phase III trial to assess bevacizumab in patients with newly diagnosed metastatic breast cancer (MBC).[155] The addition of bevacizumab to weekly paclitaxel chemotherapy as first-line therapy for MBC doubled progression-free survival and significantly improved the response rate, leading to its accelerated approval by the FDA for this patient cohort.[155,227] Soon this regimen became widely adopted by clinicians who treated thousands of patients and felt comfortable with using the drug.[155] However, the two post-approval studies designed to confirm the outcomes in E2100-AVADO (docetaxel with and without bevacizumab)[228] and RIBBON1 (chemotherapy [capecitabine, a taxane, or an anthracycline] with and without bevacizumab)[229] did not demonstrate the magnitude of benefit observed in E2100, despite meeting their predefined endpoints. In addition, no trial using bevacizumab in patients with MBC has shown a significant improvement in overall survival when compared with standard chemotherapy. These observations, and the reports of "substantial adverse reactions," prompted the FDA to rescind its approval based on an unfavorable risk–benefit profile.[230] In contrast to the enthusiasm for vascular endothelial growth factor (VEGF)-targeted therapies in 2004 and 2005, views have vacillated. However, despite the negative view of VEGF-targeted therapies in 2011, we must remember that this therapeutic approach has led to significant advances and changes in the standard of care for patients with the most highly angiogenic tumors.[155] We need to consider that certain drugs could work better in combination with bevacizumab than others, impacting both safety and efficacy.[155] By combining bevacizumab with the appropriate chemotherapeutic agent (such as dose-dense paclitaxel), the risk for serious adverse events could be circumvented.[155]

The metaanalysis of 16 randomized trials in advanced-stage solid tumors led researchers to conclude that the use of bevacizumab was associated with a 1.46-fold increase in the rate of fatal adverse events compared with chemotherapy alone (95% CI, 1.09 to 1.94; $p = 0.01$; incidence, 2.5% versus 1.7%).[155,231] However, the comparisons of bevacizumab and chemotherapy combination have been carried out against single-agent chemotherapies, whereas a metaanalysis of the toxic effects of combination chemotherapy versus single-agent chemotherapy has not been carried out.[155] The serious adverse events reported with bevacizumab are rare and certainly less common than those seen with any combination chemotherapy regimens used to treat MBC.[155,231] It is our responsibility as oncologists to consider the relative risk–benefit ratio of any regimen for the individual patients in our clinics.[155] As we appear to have hit the ceiling with the use of bevacizumab, one way to break through this ceiling would be to identify predictive biomarkers.[232] Clinical studies should be undertaken with the prospective use of biomarkers for patient selection that will help target the appropriate patients for therapy, offer alternatives to those patients unlikely to benefit from bevacizumab, and avoid the toxicities and costs for patients who will not benefit.[232]

PERSONALIZED THERAPY FOR BREAST CANCER: ARE WE THERE YET?

Although personalizing the treatment of breast and other cancers is a promising goal, individualizing treatments will require a wealth of new molecular data and therapeutic options.[233] Personalized medicine for metastatic breast cancer presents hurdles due to the complexity, heterogeneity, and genomic instability of metastatic breast cancer cells which make their evaluation and therapy a challenging process.[233]

Drawbacks in Evaluating Prognostic Signatures

Not only did the advent of high-throughput gene expression profiling techniques result in the molecular classification of breast cancer into separate molecular subtypes, but it also enabled an improvement in the prognostication of the disease, beyond the prognostic information provided by the traditional clinicopathological parameters.[92,234] The clinical utility of two signatures, namely MammaPrint and Oncotype DX, is being assessed in two large international Phase III randomized trials aiming to provide level I evidence to support their clinical implementation: the MINDACT (assessing MammaPrint)[235] study and the TAILORx study (assessing Oncotype DX).[134,234] The aforementioned gene signatures exhibit two major conceptual drawbacks: They do not take into consideration the molecular heterogeneity of breast cancer, as their generation took place in parallel with the major class-discovery studies, and they are restricted to the epithelial compartment of the disease, disregarding important molecular contributors to the malignant progression, namely the stromal and immune components of the disease.[234]

It is pertinent to understand whether signatures based on characteristics other than proliferation (e.g., dormancy, stemness, metastatic colonization potential) may hold greater potential for personalizing the prevention of metastasis.[233] A starting point would be to determine what tumor cohorts with what follow-up data are needed to be collected as a centralized resource for validation of potential signatures.[233] Before ultimately striving toward cure, genomic profiling and screening for molecular aberrations serve to match patients with specific drugs.[236] Trial designs need to incorporate biomarker-driven enrollments in order to better treat the patients while saving resources and "wasted" toxicity.[236] In a recent analysis, the odds of toxic death were found to be greater for new agents as were the odds of treatment discontinuation.[236]

Challenges for Targeted Therapy

Administering anticancer drugs on the assumption of homogeneity among individuals leads to unwanted adverse side effects after treatment without attaining maximum drug efficacy. Such adverse drug reactions impose a huge burden not only on the patient but also on the health care system. Implementation of personalized medicine requires transition from a "one drug treats all" philosophy into a more tailored approach to drug development involving enrichment of treatment cohorts with patients most likely to have therapeutic benefit.[237] High-throughput technologies, for comprehensive molecular characterization of tumors as well as the individual's own genetic makeup have the potential to select appropriate therapies for each patient.[237] Thus, the time is right to implement personalized molecular medicine.[238] Despite the exciting potential of personalized medicine, there are several challenges that must be overcome before personalized cancer therapy can be widely implemented: lack of effective drugs against most genomic aberrations, limitations of molecular tests, lack of a validated predictive biomarker of efficacy for several molecularly targeted agents, tumor heterogeneity and molecular evolution, costs, quality of and potential morbidity of tumor biopsies, and reimbursement and regulatory challenges.[238,239] Additionally, challenges are also associated with tumor assessment tools, clinical trial designs, and the drug development and approval processes.[240] Overcoming these challenges is critical to improving on the early success achieved during the past two decades.[240]

Substituting oral small molecule inhibitors for traditional chemotherapy eliminates some treatment costs, including those associated with vascular access and intravenous infusions; however, targeted therapy is often used in addition to, rather than in place of, traditional chemotherapy. If targeted therapy includes monoclonal antibodies, costs can escalate exponentially.[241]

Some of the attributes of an ideal targeted compound include optimal target selectivity, validation of the biologic target, a predictable pharmacokinetic profile (oral formulation or monthly/annual parenteral/subcutaneous administration), minimal toxicity, minimal drug–drug interactions, and a low cost–efficacy ratio. Determining optimal target concentrations and intracellular drug levels is difficult and is not performed routinely.[240,241] Modifying the physical properties of anticancer agents to improve their pharmacodynamics behavior is a continuous challenge.[241]

There are a number of other challenges that still need to be addressed, such as the identification of biomarkers of response and early markers of clinical benefit.[164] The study of resistance mechanisms is also critically important.[164] A frequent mechanism of primary resistance is lack of dependency on the targeted gene or pathway, such as the lack of activity of PARP inhibitors in breast tumors with intact BRCA function.[164] This provides a strong argument for the development of early biomarkers of response and for the development of novel agents only in the subpopulation of breast tumors that may be dependent on the targeted gene.[164]

In patients with metastatic disease, the therapeutic action of trastuzumab and lapatinib tends to be short lived. Even though some patients treated in the adjuvant setting will likely be cured of their cancer, it is anticipated that a fraction will eventually recur. This suggests that tumors harbor *de novo* or acquired mechanisms of resistance to therapeutic inhibitors of HER2. Acquired resistance can be the result of acquired mutations that "overrule" the mechanism of action of the anticancer agent, such as mutations in the *PI3K* gene, downstream from HER2, which render cells insensitive to the effects of trastuzumab and lapatinib.[164,242] This would require a combined therapeutic approach against the primary activating event (HER2 in this case) and the acquired mechanism of resistance (PI3K).[164] There is an additional mechanism of resistance that relates to the activation of compensatory pathways that allow cells to "escape" the effects of therapeutic agents.[164] Inhibition of certain molecular targets and/or pathways may result in activation of compensatory signaling pathways that prevent cell death.[164] Combining agents directed against different targets is a natural option for bypassing therapeutic limitations such as tumor heterogeneity and multiple resistance mechanisms.[240] Potential combinations of targeted therapies include agents affecting one or several mechanisms of action and individual or multiple signaling pathways through modulation of different molecular targets.[240,243]

More than 800 drugs are now in clinical development for cancer indications, yet success rates in bringing drugs to market remain in the range of only 5 to 8%.[244] Many factors may contribute to these low success rates: little scientific insight into the determinants of drug sensitivity and resistance; poorly conceived and executed clinical development plans; heterogeneous patient populations and lack of biomarkers to identify patients most likely to benefit from specific treatments; unclear, conflicting, or burdensome regulatory requirements; and lack of agreement among clinicians, investigators, and regulators as to what constitutes clinical benefit in some circumstances.[244] In order to solve vexing problems in contemporary cancer drug development, an inclusive, collaborative effort is needed among clinical investigators, statisticians, regulatory scientists, laboratory researchers, patients, and drug and device manufacturers, who should be convened around a common goal: to translate insights in cancer biology into clinically useful, safer, and more effective products for patients.[244]

References

1. Chan IS, Ginsburg GS. Personalized medicine: progress and promise. Ann. Rev. Genom. Hum. Genet. 2011;12:217–44.
2. Miller FA, Hayeems RZ, Bytautas JP, et al. Testing personalized medicine: patient and physician expectations of next-generation genomic sequencing in late-stage cancer care. Eur. J. Hum. Genet. 2013;22(3):391–5.
3. Hamburg MA, Collins FS. The path to personalized medicine. New Engl. J. Med. 2010;363(4):301–4.
4. Borden EC, Raghavan D. Personalizing medicine for cancer: the next decade. Nat. Rev. Drug Discov. 2010;9(5):343–4.
5. Roychowdhury S, Iyer MK, Robinson DR, et al. Personalized oncology through integrative high-throughput sequencing: a pilot study. Science Transl. Med. 2011;3(111):111ra21.
6. Schilsky RL. Personalized medicine in oncology: the future is now. Nat. Rev. Drug Discov. 2010;9(5):363–6.
7. Leary RJ, Kinde I, Diehl F, et al. Development of personalized tumor biomarkers using massively parallel sequencing. Sci. Transl. Med. 2010;2(20):20ra14.
8. Tsimberidou AM, Iskander NG, Hong DS, et al. Personalized medicine in a phase I clinical trials program: the MD Anderson Cancer Center initiative. Clin. Cancer Res. 2012;18(22):6373–83.
9. Von Hoff DD, Stephenson JJ Jr, Rosen P, et al. Pilot study using molecular profiling of patients' tumors to find potential targets and select treatments for their refractory cancers. J. Clin. Oncol. 2010;28(33):4877–83.
10. Chang JC, Hilsenbeck SG, Fuqua SA. Pharmacogenetics of breast cancer: toward the individualization of therapy. Cancer Invest. 2009;27(7):699–703.
11. The Cancer Genome Atlas, http://cancergenome.nih.gov/.
12. Siddiq A, Couch FJ, Chen GK, et al. A meta-analysis of genome-wide association studies of breast cancer identifies two novel susceptibility loci at 6q14 and 20q11. Hum. Mol. Genet. 2012;21(24):5373–84.
13. Theodoratou E, Montazeri Z, Hawken S, et al. Systematic meta-analyses and field synopsis of genetic association studies in colorectal cancer. J. Natl. Cancer Inst. 2012;104(19):1433–57.
14. Hertz DL, McLeod HL. Use of pharmacogenetics for predicting cancer prognosis and treatment exposure, response and toxicity. J. Hum. Genet. 2013;58(6):346–52.
15. Gonzalez-Angulo AM, Hennessy BT, Mills GB. Future of personalized medicine in oncology: a systems biology approach. J. Clin. Oncol. 2010;28(16):2777–83.
16. Koboldt DC, Fulton RS, McLellan MD, et al. Comprehensive molecular portraits of human breast tumours. Nature 2012;490(7418):61–70.
17. Collins FS, Barker AD. Mapping the cancer genome: pinpointing the genes involved in cancer will help chart a new course across the complex landscape of human malignancies. Sci. Am. 2007;296(3):50–7.
18. Walter V, Nobel AB, Wright FA. DiNAMIC: a method to identify recurrent DNA copy number aberrations in tumors. Bioinformatics 2011;27(5):678–85.
19. Hennessy BT, Gonzalez-Angulo AM, Carey MS, Mills GB. A systems approach to analysis of molecular complexity in breast cancer. Clin. Cancer Res. 2009;15(2):417–9.
20. Shih IeM, Sheu JJ, Santillan A, et al. Amplification of a chromatin remodeling gene, Rsf-1/HBXAP, in ovarian carcinoma. Proc. Natl. Acad. Sci. U.S.A. 2005;102(39):14004–9.
21. Wang TL, Maierhofer C, Speicher MR, et al. Digital karyotyping. Proc. Natl. Acad. Sci. U.S.A. 2002;99(25):16156–61.
22. Curtis C, Shah SP, Chin SF, et al. The genomic and transcriptomic architecture of 2,000 breast tumours reveals novel subgroups. Nature 2012;486(7403):346–52.
23. Leyland-Jones B, editor. Pharmacogenetics of Breast Cancer: Towards the Individualization of Therapy. New York: Informa Healthcare; 2008.
24. Lucito R, Healy J, Alexander J, et al. Representational oligonucleotide microarray analysis: a high-resolution method to detect genome copy number variation. Genome Res. 2003;13(10):2291–305.
25. Iljin K, Wolf M, Edgren H, et al. TMPRSS2 fusions with oncogenic ETS factors in prostate cancer involve unbalanced genomic rearrangements and are associated with HDAC1 and epigenetic reprogramming. Cancer Res. 2006;66(21):10242–6.
26. Sharp AJ, Hansen S, Selzer RR, et al. Discovery of previously unidentified genomic disorders from the duplication architecture of the human genome. Nature Genet. 2006;38(9):1038–42.
27. Zhou X, Mok SC, Chen Z, Li Y, Wong DT. Concurrent analysis of loss of heterozygosity (LOH) and copy number abnormality (CNA) for oral premalignancy progression using the Affymetrix 10K SNP mapping array. Hum. Genet. 2004;115(4):327–30.

28. Oosting J, Lips EH, van Eijk R, et al. High-resolution copy number analysis of paraffin-embedded archival tissue using SNP BeadArrays. Genome Res. 2007;17(3):368–76.

29. Selzer RR, Richmond TA, Pofahl NJ, et al. Analysis of chromosome breakpoints in neuroblastoma at sub-kilobase resolution using fine-tiling oligonucleotide array CGH. Genes Chromosomes Cancer 2005;44(3):305–19.

30. Wang Y, Moorhead M, Karlin-Neumann G, et al. Allele quantification using molecular inversion probes (MIP). Nucleic Acids Res. 2005;33(21):e183.

31. Albertson DG. Profiling breast cancer by array CGH. Breast Cancer Res. Treat. 2003;78(3):289–98.

32. Bergamaschi A, Kim YH, Wang P, et al. Distinct patterns of DNA copy number alteration are associated with different clinicopathological features and gene-expression subtypes of breast cancer. Genes Chromosomes Cancer 2006;45(11):1033–40.

33. Hennessy BT, Gonzalez-Angulo AM, Stemke-Hale K, et al. Characterization of a naturally occurring breast cancer subset enriched in epithelial-to-mesenchymal transition and stem cell characteristics. Cancer Res. 2009;69(10):4116–24.

34. Gonzalez-Angulo AM, Timms KM, Liu S, et al. Incidence and outcome of BRCA mutations in unselected patients with triple receptor-negative breast cancer. Clin. Cancer Res. 2011;17(5):1082–9.

35. Hennessy BT, Timms KM, Carey MS, et al. Somatic mutations in BRCA1 and BRCA2 could expand the number of patients that benefit from poly (ADP ribose) polymerase inhibitors in ovarian cancer. J. Clin. Oncol. 2010;28(22):3570–6.

36. Kircher M, Kelso J. High-throughput DNA sequencing—concepts and limitations. BioEssays 2010;32(6):524–36.

37. Eid J, Fehr A, Gray J, et al. Real-time DNA sequencing from single polymerase molecules. Science 2009;323(5910):133–8.

38. Banerji S, Cibulskis K, Rangel-Escareno C, et al. Sequence analysis of mutations and translocations across breast cancer subtypes. Nature 2012;486(7403):405–9.

39. Balko JM, Stricker TP, Arteaga CL. The genomic map of breast cancer: which roads lead to better targeted therapies? Breast Cancer Res. 2013;15(4):209.

40. Ellis MJ, Ding L, Shen D, et al. Whole-genome analysis informs breast cancer response to aromatase inhibition. Nature 2012;486(7403):353–60.

41. Makretsov N, He M, Hayes M, et al. A fluorescence *in situ* hybridization study of ETV6–NTRK3 fusion gene in secretory breast carcinoma. Genes Chromosomes Cancer 2004;40(2):152–7.

42. Reis-Filho JS, Natrajan R, Vatcheva R, et al. Is acinic cell carcinoma a variant of secretory carcinoma? A FISH study using ETV6 "split apart" probes. Histopathology 2008;52(7):840–6.

43. Deininger MW, Goldman JM, Lydon N, Melo JV. The tyrosine kinase inhibitor CGP57148B selectively inhibits the growth of BCR-ABL-positive cells. Blood 1997;90(9):3691–8.

44. Falzoi M, Mossa A, Congeddu E, Saba L, Pani L. Multiplex genotyping of CYP3A4, CYP3A5, CYP2C9 and CYP2C19 SNPs using MALDI-TOF mass spectrometry. Pharmacogenomics 2010;11(4):559–71.

45. Humeny A, Rodel F, Rodel C, et al. MDR1 single nucleotide polymorphism C3435T in normal colorectal tissue and colorectal carcinomas detected by MALDI-TOF mass spectrometry. Anticancer Res. 2003;23(3B):2735–40.

46. James MR, Hayward NK, Dumenil T, Montgomery GW, Martin NG, Duffy DL. Epidermal growth factor gene (EGF) polymorphism and risk of melanocytic neoplasia. J. Invest. Dermatol. 2004;123(4):760–2.

47. Werner M, Sych M, Herbon N, Illig T, Konig IR, Wjst M. Large-scale determination of SNP allele frequencies in DNA pools using MALDI-TOF mass spectrometry. Hum. Mutat. 2002;20(1):57–64.

48. Yu JT, Mao CX, Zhang HW, et al. Genetic association of rs11610206 SNP on chromosome 12q13 with late-onset Alzheimer's disease in a Han Chinese population. Clin. Chim. Acta. 2011;412(1-2):148–51.

49. Fumagalli D, Gavin PG, Taniyama Y, et al. A rapid, sensitive, reproducible and cost-effective method for mutation profiling of colon cancer and metastatic lymph nodes. BMC Cancer 2010;10:101.

50. MacConaill LE, Campbell CD, Kehoe SM, et al. Profiling critical cancer gene mutations in clinical tumor samples. PloS ONE 2009;4(11):e7887.

51. Thomas RK, Nickerson E, Simons JF, et al. Sensitive mutation detection in heterogeneous cancer specimens by massively parallel picoliter reactor sequencing. Nature Med. 2006;12(7):852–5.

52. Lambros MB, Wilkerson PM, Natrajan R, et al. High-throughput detection of fusion genes in cancer using the Sequenom MassARRAY platform. Lab. Invest. 2011;91(10):1491–501.

53. Euhus DM, Timmons CF, Tomlinson GE. ETV6-NTRK3—Trk-ing the primary event in human secretory breast cancer. Cancer Cell. 2002;2(5):347–8.

54. Lambros MB, Tan DS, Jones RL, et al. Genomic profile of a secretory breast cancer with an ETV6-NTRK3 duplication. J. Clin. Pathol. 2009;62(7):604–12.
55. Letessier A, Ginestier C, Charafe-Jauffret E, et al. ETV6 gene rearrangements in invasive breast carcinoma. Genes Chromosomes Cancer 2005;44(1):103–8.
56. Tognon C, Knezevich SR, Huntsman D, et al. Expression of the ETV6-NTRK3 gene fusion as a primary event in human secretory breast carcinoma. Cancer Cell. 2002;2(5):367–76.
57. Marchio C, Weigelt B, Reis-Filho JS. Adenoid cystic carcinomas of the breast and salivary glands (or "The strange case of Dr Jekyll and Mr Hyde" of exocrine gland carcinomas). J. Clin. Pathol. 2010;63(3):220–8.
58. Mitani Y, Li J, Rao PH, et al. Comprehensive analysis of the MYB–NFIB gene fusion in salivary adenoid cystic carcinoma: incidence, variability, and clinicopathologic significance. Clin. Cancer Res. 2010;16(19):4722–31.
59. Persson M, Andren Y, Mark J, Horlings HM, Persson F, Stenman G. Recurrent fusion of MYB and NFIB transcription factor genes in carcinomas of the breast and head and neck. Proc. Natl. Acad. Sci. U.S.A. 2009;106(44):18740–4.
60. West RB, Kong C, Clarke N, et al. MYB expression and translocation in adenoid cystic carcinomas and other salivary gland tumors with clinicopathologic correlation. Am. J. Surg. Pathol. 2011;35(1):92–9.
61. Regan MM, Leyland-Jones B, Bouzyk M, et al. CYP2D6 genotype and tamoxifen response in postmenopausal women with endocrine-responsive breast cancer: the breast international group 1-98 trial. J. Natl. Cancer Inst. 2012;104(6):441–51.
62. Goetz MP, Rae JM, Suman VJ, et al. Pharmacogenetics of tamoxifen biotransformation is associated with clinical outcomes of efficacy and hot flashes. J. Clin. Oncol. 2005;23(36):9312–8.
63. Higgins MJ, Stearns V. Pharmacogenetics of endocrine therapy for breast cancer. Annu. Rev. Med. 2011;62:281–93.
64. Dworkin AM, Huang TH, Toland AE. Epigenetic alterations in the breast: implications for breast cancer detection, prognosis and treatment. Sem. Cancer Biol. 2009;19(3):165–71.
65. Dworkin AM, Huang TH, Toland AE. The role of epigenetics in breast cancer: implications for diagnosis, prognosis, and treatment. In: Leyland-Jones B, editor. Pharmacogenetics of Breast Cancer—Towards the Individualization of Therapy. New York: Informa Healthcare; 2008. p. 45–60.
66. Das PM, Singal R. DNA methylation and cancer. J. Clin. Oncol. 2004;22(22):4632–42.
67. Yang X, Yan L, Davidson NE. DNA methylation in breast cancer. Endocr. Relat. Cancer. 2001;8(2):115–27.
68. Catteau A, Morris JR. BRCA1 methylation: a significant role in tumour development? Sem. Cancer Biol. 2002;12(5):359–71.
69. Oka M, Rodic N, Graddy J, Chang LJ, Terada N. CpG sites preferentially methylated by Dnmt3a *in vivo*. J. Biol. Chem. 2006;281(15):9901–8.
70. Vincent-Salomon A, Ganem-Elbaz C, Manie E, et al. X inactive-specific transcript RNA coating and genetic instability of the X chromosome in BRCA1 breast tumors. Cancer Res. 2007;67(11):5134–40.
71. Pfeifer GP, Dammann R. Methylation of the tumor suppressor gene RASSF1A in human tumors. Biochemistry (Moscow) 2005;70(5):576–83.
72. Balch C, Montgomery JS, Paik HI, et al. New anti-cancer strategies: epigenetic therapies and biomarkers. Front. Biosci. 2005;10:1897–931.
73. Sharma G, Mirza S, Yang YH, et al. Prognostic relevance of promoter hypermethylation of multiple genes in breast cancer patients. Cell. Oncol. 2009;31(6):487–500.
74. Suijkerbuijk KP, van Diest PJ, van der Wall E. Improving early breast cancer detection: focus on methylation. Ann. Oncol. 2011;22(1):24–9.
75. Suijkerbuijk KP, Pan X, van der Wall E, van Diest PJ, Vooijs M. Comparison of different promoter methylation assays in breast cancer. Analyt. Cell. Pathol. 2010;33(3):133–41.
76. Lewis CM, Cler LR, Bu DW, et al. Promoter hypermethylation in benign breast epithelium in relation to predicted breast cancer risk. Clin. Cancer Res. 2005;11(1):166–72.
77. Pasquali L, Bedeir A, Ringquist S, Styche A, Bhargava R, Trucco G. Quantification of CpG island methylation in progressive breast lesions from normal to invasive carcinoma. Cancer Lett. 2007;257(1):136–44.
78. Yan PS, Venkataramu C, Ibrahim A, et al. Mapping geographic zones of cancer risk with epigenetic biomarkers in normal breast tissue. Clin. Cancer Res. 2006;12(22):6626–36.
79. Fackler MJ, Malone K, Zhang Z, et al. Quantitative multiplex methylation-specific PCR analysis doubles detection of tumor cells in breast ductal fluid. Clin. Cancer Res. 2006;12(11, Pt. 1):3306–10.
80. Hoque MO, Feng Q, Toure P, et al. Detection of aberrant methylation of four genes in plasma DNA for the detection of breast cancer. J. Clin. Oncol. 2006;24(26):4262–9.

IV. NOVEL APPROACHES FOR CANCER THERAPIES

81. Suijkerbuijk KP, van der Wall E, van Diest PJ. Oxytocin: bringing magic into nipple aspiration. Ann. Oncol. 2007;18(10):1743–4.

82. Ruike Y, Imanaka Y, Sato F, Shimizu K, Tsujimoto G. Genome-wide analysis of aberrant methylation in human breast cancer cells using methyl-DNA immunoprecipitation combined with high-throughput sequencing. BMC Genom. 2010;11:137.

83. Laird PW. The power and the promise of DNA methylation markers. Nat. Rev. Cancer. 2003;3(4):253–66.

84. Fackler MJ, McVeigh M, Mehrotra J, et al. Quantitative multiplex methylation-specific PCR assay for the detection of promoter hypermethylation in multiple genes in breast cancer. Cancer Res. 2004;64(13):4442–52.

85. Nygren AO, Ameziane N, Duarte HM, et al. Methylation-specific MLPA (MS-MLPA): simultaneous detection of CpG methylation and copy number changes of up to 40 sequences. Nucleic Acids Res. 2005; 33(14):e128.

86. Moelans CB, de Weger RA, van Blokland MT, et al. HER-2/neu amplification testing in breast cancer by multiplex ligation-dependent probe amplification in comparison with immunohistochemistry and *in situ* hybridization. Cell. Oncol. 2009;31(1):1–10.

87. Mallmann MR, Staratschek-Jox A, Rudlowski C, et al. Prediction and prognosis: impact of gene expression profiling in personalized treatment of breast cancer patients. EPMA J. 2010;1(3):421–37.

88. Stephens PJ, McBride DJ, Lin ML, et al. Complex landscapes of somatic rearrangement in human breast cancer genomes. Nature. 2009;462(7276):1005–10.

89. Zhao Q, Caballero OL, Levy S, et al. Transcriptome-guided characterization of genomic rearrangements in a breast cancer cell line. Proc. Natl. Acad. Sci. U.S.A. 2009;106(6):1886–91.

90. Iwamoto T, Pusztai L. Predicting prognosis of breast cancer with gene signatures: are we lost in a sea of data? Genome Med. 2010;2(11):81.

91. Reis-Filho JS, Weigelt B, Fumagalli D, Sotiriou C. Molecular profiling: moving away from tumor philately. Sci. Transl. Med. 2010;2(47):47ps3.

92. Sotiriou C, Pusztai L. Gene-expression signatures in breast cancer. New Engl. J. Med. 2009;360(8):790–800.

93. Weigelt B, Baehner FL, Reis-Filho JS. The contribution of gene expression profiling to breast cancer classification, prognostication and prediction: a retrospective of the last decade. J. Pathol. 2010;220(2):263–80.

94. Reis-Filho JS, Pusztai L. Gene expression profiling in breast cancer: classification, prognostication, and prediction. Lancet 2011;378(9805):1812–23.

95. Pusztai L, Broglio K, Andre F, Symmans WF, Hess KR, Hortobagyi GN. Effect of molecular disease subsets on disease-free survival in randomized adjuvant chemotherapy trials for estrogen receptor-positive breast cancer. J. Clin. Oncol. 2008;26(28):4679–83.

96. Liedtke C, Pusztai L. Gene expression profiling as an emerging diagnostic tool to personalize chemotherapy selection for early stage breast cancer. In: Leyland-Jones B, editor. Pharmacogenetics of Breast Cancer—Towards the Individualizatoin of Therapy. New York: Informa Healthcare; 2008. p. 77–96.

97. Kattan MW, Scardino PT. Prediction of progression: nomograms of clinical utility. Clin. Prostate Cancer 2002;1(2):90–6.

98. Perou CM, Sorlie T, Eisen MB, et al. Molecular portraits of human breast tumours. Nature. 2000;406(6797): 747–52.

99. Babiera GV, Skoracki RJ, Esteva FJ. Advanced Therapy of Breast Disease. 3rd ed Shelton, CT: People's Medical Publishing House; 2012.

100. Dvinge H, Git A, Graf S, et al. The shaping and functional consequences of the microRNA landscape in breast cancer. Nature. 2013;497(7449):378–82.

101. Buffa FM, Camps C, Winchester L, et al. microRNA-associated progression pathways and potential therapeutic targets identified by integrated mRNA and microRNA expression profiling in breast cancer. Cancer Res. 2011;71(17):5635–45.

102. Enerly E, Steinfeld I, Kleivi K, et al. miRNA-mRNA integrated analysis reveals roles for miRNAs in primary breast tumors. PloS ONE 2011;6(2):e16915.

103. Farazi TA, Horlings HM, Ten Hoeve JJ, et al. MicroRNA sequence and expression analysis in breast tumors by deep sequencing. Cancer Res. 2011;71(13):4443–53.

104. Le Quesne J, Caldas C. Micro-RNAs and breast cancer. Mol. Oncol. 2010;4(3):230–41.

105. Lyng MB, Laenkholm AV, Sokilde R, Gravgaard KH, Litman T, Ditzel HJ. Global microRNA expression profiling of high-risk ER+ breast cancers from patients receiving adjuvant tamoxifen mono-therapy: a DBCG study. PloS ONE 2012;7(5):e36170.

106. Radovich M, Atale R, Clare SE, Sledge GW, Schneider BP. Next-generation RNA-sequencing of triple negative breast cancer compared to donated microdissected normal epithelium and adjacent normal tissues. Cancer Res. 2012;72(24).
107. ARUP Laboratories, www.aruplab.com/PAM50.
108. Mullins M, Perreard L, Quackenbush JF, et al. Agreement in breast cancer classification between microarray and quantitative reverse transcription PCR from fresh-frozen and formalin-fixed, paraffin-embedded tissues. Clin. Chem. 2007;53(7):1273–9.
109. Perreard L, Fan C, Quackenbush JF, et al. Classification and risk stratification of invasive breast carcinomas using a real-time quantitative RT-PCR assay. Breast Cancer Res. 2006;8(2):R23.
110. Bastien RR, Rodriguez-Lescure A, Ebbert MT, et al. PAM50 breast cancer subtyping by RT-qPCR and concordance with standard clinical molecular markers. BMC Med. Genom. 2012;5:44.
111. Geiss GK, Bumgarner RE, Birditt B, et al. Direct multiplexed measurement of gene expression with color-coded probe pairs. Nat. Biotechnol. 2008;26(3):317–25.
112. Chia SK, Bramwell VH, Tu D, et al. A 50-gene intrinsic subtype classifier for prognosis and prediction of benefit from adjuvant tamoxifen. Clin. Cancer Res. 2012;18(16):4465–72.
113. Golubnitschaja O, editor. Predictive Diagnostics and Personalized Treatment: Dream or Reality. Hauppauge, NY: Nova Biomedical Books; 2009.
114. van't Veer LJ, Dai H, van de Vijver MJ, et al. Gene expression profiling predicts clinical outcome of breast cancer. Nature 2002;415(6871):530–6.
115. Bueno-de-Mesquita JM, van Harten WH, Retel VP, et al. Use of 70-gene signature to predict prognosis of patients with node-negative breast cancer: a prospective community-based feasibility study (RASTER). Lancet Oncol. 2007;8(12):1079–87.
116. Liedtke C, Hatzis C, Symmans WF, et al. Genomic grade index is associated with response to chemotherapy in patients with breast cancer. J. Clin. Oncol. 2009;27(19):3185–91.
117. Rakha EA, El-Sayed ME, Lee AH, et al. Prognostic significance of Nottingham histologic grade in invasive breast carcinoma. J. Clin. Oncol. 2008;26(19):3153–8.
118. Trudeau ME, Pritchard KI, Chapman JA, et al. Prognostic factors affecting the natural history of node-negative breast cancer. Breast Cancer Res. Treat. 2005;89(1):35–45.
119. Fisher ER, Wang J, Bryant J, Fisher B, Mamounas E, Wolmark N. Pathobiology of preoperative chemotherapy: findings from the National Surgical Adjuvant Breast and Bowel (NSABP) protocol B-18. Cancer 2002;95(4):681–95.
120. Singletary SE, Allred C, Ashley P, et al. Revision of the American Joint Committee on Cancer staging system for breast cancer. J. Clin. Oncol. 2002;20(17):3628–36.
121. Sotiriou C, Wirapati P, Loi S, et al. Gene expression profiling in breast cancer: understanding the molecular basis of histologic grade to improve prognosis. J. Natl. Cancer Inst. 2006;98(4):262–72.
122. Loi S, Haibe-Kains B, Desmedt C, et al. Definition of clinically distinct molecular subtypes in estrogen receptor-positive breast carcinomas through genomic grade. J. Clin. Oncol. 2007;25(10):1239–46.
123. Metzger Filho O, Ignatiadis M, Sotiriou C. Genomic Grade Index: an important tool for assessing breast cancer tumor grade and prognosis. Crit. Rev. Oncol. Hematol. 2011;77(1):20–9.
124. Quackenbush J. Microarray analysis and tumor classification. New Engl. J. Med. 2006;354(23):2463–72.
125. van de Vijver MJ, He YD, van't Veer LJ, et al. A gene-expression signature as a predictor of survival in breast cancer. New Engl. J. Med. 2002;347(25):1999–2009.
126. Paik S, Shak S, Tang G, et al. A multigene assay to predict recurrence of tamoxifen-treated, node-negative breast cancer. New Engl. J. Med. 2004;351(27):2817–26.
127. Gökmen-Polar Y, Badve S. Molecular profiling assays in breast cancer: are we ready for prime time? Oncology (Williston Park) 2012;26(4):350–7.
128. Albain KS, Barlow WE, Shak S, et al. Prognostic and predictive value of the 21-gene recurrence score assay in postmenopausal women with node-positive, oestrogen-receptor-positive breast cancer on chemotherapy: a retrospective analysis of a randomised trial. Lancet Oncol. 2010;11(1):55–65.
129. Dowsett M, Cuzick J, Wale C, et al. Prediction of risk of distant recurrence using the 21-gene recurrence score in node-negative and node-positive postmenopausal patients with breast cancer treated with anastrozole or tamoxifen: a TransATAC study. J. Clin. Oncol. 2010;28(11):1829–34.
130. Goldstein LJ, Gray R, Badve S, et al. Prognostic utility of the 21-gene assay in hormone receptor-positive operable breast cancer compared with classical clinicopathologic features. J. Clin. Oncol. 2008;26(25):4063–71.

IV. NOVEL APPROACHES FOR CANCER THERAPIES

131. Paik S, Tang G, Shak S, et al. Gene expression and benefit of chemotherapy in women with node-negative, estrogen receptor-positive breast cancer. J. Clin. Oncol. 2006;24(23):3726–34.

132. Kim C, Paik S. Gene-expression-based prognostic assays for breast cancer. Nat. Rev. Clin. Oncol. 2010;7(6):340–7.

133. Hormone Therapy With or Without Combination Chemotherapy in Treating Women Who Have Undergone Surgery for Node-Negative Breast Cancer (The TAILORx Trial), https://www.clinicaltrials.gov/ct2/show/NCT00310180.

134. Sparano JA, Paik S. Development of the 21-gene assay and its application in clinical practice and clinical trials. J. Clin. Oncol. 2008;26(5):721–8.

135. Bartlett JM, Bloom KJ, Piper T, et al. Mammostrat as an immunohistochemical multigene assay for prediction of early relapse risk in the tamoxifen versus exemestane adjuvant multicenter trial pathology study. J. Clin. Oncol. 2012;30(36):4477–84.

136. Bartlett JM, Thomas J, Ross DT, et al. Mammostrat as a tool to stratify breast cancer patients at risk of recurrence during endocrine therapy. Breast Cancer Res. 2010;12(4):R47.

137. Ring BZ, Seitz RS, Beck R, et al. Novel prognostic immunohistochemical biomarker panel for estrogen receptor-positive breast cancer. J. Clin. Oncol. 2006;24(19):3039–47.

138. Ross DT, Kim CY, Tang G, et al. Chemosensitivity and stratification by a five monoclonal antibody immuno-histochemistry test in the NSABP B14 and B20 trials. Clin. Cancer Res. 2008;14(20):6602–9.

139. Gonzalez-Angulo AM, Hennessy BT, Meric-Bernstam F, et al. Functional proteomics can define prognosis and predict pathologic complete response in patients with breast cancer. Clin. Proteom. 2011;8(1):11.

140. Hennessy BT, Lu Y, Poradosu E, et al. Pharmacodynamic markers of perifosine efficacy. Clin. Cancer Res. 2007;13(24):7421–31.

141. Boyd ZS, Wu QJ, O'Brien C, et al. Proteomic analysis of breast cancer molecular subtypes and biomark-ers of response to targeted kinase inhibitors using reverse-phase protein microarrays. Mol. Cancer Ther. 2008;7(12):3695–706.

142. Espina V, Wulfkuhle J, Calvert VS, Liotta LA, Petricoin EF 3rd. Reverse phase protein microarrays for theranos-tics and patient-tailored therapy. Methods Mol. Biol. 2008;441:113–28.

143. Gonzalez-Angulo AM, Liu S, Chen H, et al. Functional proteomics characterization of residual breast cancer after neoadjuvant systemic chemotherapy. Ann. Oncol. 2013;24(4):909–16.

144. Barton S, Zabaglo L, A'Hern R, et al. Assessment of the contribution of the IHC4+C score to decision making in clinical practice in early breast cancer. Br. J. Cancer 2012;106(11):1760–5.

145. Cuzick J, Dowsett M, Pineda S, et al. Prognostic value of a combined estrogen receptor, progesterone receptor, Ki-67, and human epidermal growth factor receptor 2 immunohistochemical score and comparison with the Genomic Health recurrence score in early breast cancer. J. Clin. Oncol. 2011;29(32):4273–8.

146. Dowsett M, Allred C, Knox J, et al. Relationship between quantitative estrogen and progesterone receptor expression and human epidermal growth factor receptor 2 (HER-2) status with recurrence in the Arimidex, Tamoxifen, Alone or in Combination trial. J. Clin. Oncol. 2008;26(7):1059–65.

147. Dowsett M, Salter J, Zabaglo L, et al. Predictive algorithms for adjuvant therapy: TransATAC. Steroids 2011;76(8):777–80.

148. Dowsett M, Nielsen TO, A'Hern R, et al. Assessment of Ki67 in breast cancer: recommendations from the Inter-national Ki67 in Breast Cancer working group. J. Natl. Cancer Inst. 2011;103(22):1656–64.

149. Desmedt C, Haibe-Kains B, Wirapati P, et al. Biological processes associated with breast cancer clinical outcome depend on the molecular subtypes. Clin. Cancer Res. 2008;14(16):5158–65.

150. Iwamoto T, Bianchini G, Booser D, et al. Gene pathways associated with prognosis and chemotherapy sensitiv-ity in molecular subtypes of breast cancer. J. Natl. Cancer Inst. 2011;103(3):264–72.

151. Wirapati P, Sotiriou C, Kunkel S, et al. Meta-analysis of gene expression profiles in breast cancer: toward a uni-fied understanding of breast cancer subtyping and prognosis signatures. Breast Cancer Res. 2008;10(4):R65.

152. Beck AH, Knoblauch NW, Hefti MM, et al. Significance analysis of prognostic signatures. PLoS Comput. Biol. 2013;9(1):e1002875.

153. Venet D, Dumont JE, Detours V. Most random gene expression signatures are significantly associated with breast cancer outcome. PLoS Comput. Biol. 2011;7(10):e1002240.

154. Chapman PB, Hauschild A, Robert C, et al. Improved survival with vemurafenib in melanoma with BRAF V600E mutation. New Engl. J. Med. 2011;364(26):2507–16.

155. Gonzalez-Angulo AM, Hortobagyi GN, Ellis LM. Targeted therapies: peaking beneath the surface of recent bevacizumab trials. Nat. Rev. Clin. Oncol. 2011;8(6):319–20.

156. Kwak EL, Bang YJ, Camidge DR, et al. Anaplastic lymphoma kinase inhibition in non-small-cell lung cancer. New Engl. J. Med. 2010;363(18):1693–703.

157. Sawyers C. Targeted cancer therapy. Nature 2004;432(7015):294–7.

158. Sequist LV, Martins RG, Spigel D, et al. First-line gefitinib in patients with advanced non-small-cell lung cancer harboring somatic EGFR mutations. J. Clin. Oncol. 2008;26(15):2442–9.

159. Bozic I, Reiter JG, Allen B, et al. Evolutionary dynamics of cancer in response to targeted combination therapy. eLife 2013;2:e00747.

160. Druker BJ, Guilhot F, O'Brien SG, et al. Five-year follow-up of patients receiving imatinib for chronic myeloid leukemia. New Engl. J. Med. 2006;355(23):2408–17.

161. Gambacorti-Passerini C, Antolini L, Mahon FX, et al. Multicenter independent assessment of outcomes in chronic myeloid leukemia patients treated with imatinib. J. Natl. Cancer Inst. 2011;103(7):553–61.

162. Amado RG, Wolf M, Peeters M, et al. Wild-type KRAS is required for panitumumab efficacy in patients with metastatic colorectal cancer. J. Clin. Oncol. 2008;26(10):1626–34.

163. Alvarez RH, Valero V, Hortobagyi GN. Emerging targeted therapies for breast cancer. J. Clin. Oncol. 2010;28(20):3366–79.

164. Higgins MJ, Baselga J. Targeted therapies for breast cancer. J. Clin. Invest. 2011;121(10):3797–803.

165. Mohamed A, Krajewski K, Cakar B, Ma CX. Targeted therapy for breast cancer. Am. J. Pathol. 2013;183(4): 1096–112.

166. Palmieri C, Patten DK, Januszewski A, Zucchini G, Howell SJ. Breast cancer: current and future endocrine therapies. Mol. Cell. Endocrinol. 2013;382(1):695–723.

167. Kurzrock R, Markman M, editors. Targeted Cancer Therapy. Totowa, NJ: Humana Press; 2008.

168. Hortobagyi GN. Opportunities and challenges in the development of targeted therapies. Sem. Oncol. 2004;31(1, Suppl. 3):21–7.

169. Fisher B, Costantino JP, Wickerham DL, et al. Tamoxifen for prevention of breast cancer: report of the National Surgical Adjuvant Breast and Bowel Project P-1 Study. J. Natl. Cancer Inst. 1998;90(18):1371–88.

170. Vogel VG, Costantino JP, Wickerham DL, et al. Effects of tamoxifen vs. raloxifene on the risk of developing invasive breast cancer and other disease outcomes: the NSABP Study of Tamoxifen and Raloxifene (STAR) P-2 trial. JAMA 2006;295(23):2727–41.

171. Mauri D, Pavlidis N, Polyzos NP, Ioannidis JP. Survival with aromatase inhibitors and inactivators versus standard hormonal therapy in advanced breast cancer: meta-analysis. J. Natl. Cancer Inst. 2006;98(18): 1285–91.

172. Rao RD, Cobleigh MA. Adjuvant endocrine therapy for breast cancer. Oncology (Williston Park) 2012;26(6): 541–7. 50, 52 passim.

173. Flaherty KT, Lorusso PM, Demichele A, et al. Phase I dose-escalation trial of the oral cyclin-dependent kinase 4/6 inhibitor PD 0332991, administered using a 21-day schedule in patients with advanced cancer. Clin. Cancer Res. 2012;18(2):568–76.

174. Miller TW, Balko JM, Fox EM, et al. ERα-dependent E2F transcription can mediate resistance to estrogen deprivation in human breast cancer. Cancer Discov. 2011;1(4):338–51.

175. Pfizer. Study 1008 a study of Palbociclib (PD-0332991) in combination with letrozole vs. letrozole for first line treatment of postmenopausal women with ER+ and HER-2 advanced breast cancer. Pfizer Oncol. May 1, 2013 (http://www.pfizer.com/files/news/asco/palbociclib_study_1008_backgrounder.pdf).

176. Slamon D, Eiermann W, Robert N, et al. Adjuvant trastuzumab in HER2-positive breast cancer. New Engl. J. Med. 2011;365(14):1273–83.

177. Slamon DJ, Clark GM, Wong SG, Levin WJ, Ullrich A, McGuire WL. Human breast cancer: correlation of relapse and survival with amplification of the HER-2/neu oncogene. Science 1987;235(4785):177–82.

178. Slamon DJ, Godolphin W, Jones LA, et al. Studies of the HER-2/neu proto-oncogene in human breast and ovarian cancer. Science. 1989;244(4905):707–12.

179. Arboleda MJ, Lyons JF, Kabbinavar FF, et al. Overexpression of AKT2/protein kinase Bbeta leads to up-regulation of beta1 integrins, increased invasion, and metastasis of human breast and ovarian cancer cells. Cancer Res. 2003;63(1):196–206.

180. Benz CC, Scott GK, Sarup JC, et al. Estrogen-dependent, tamoxifen-resistant tumorigenic growth of MCF-7 cells transfected with HER2/neu. Breast Cancer Res. Treat. 1992;24(2):85–95.

181. De Luca A, Carotenuto A, Rachiglio A, et al. The role of the EGFR signaling in tumor microenvironment. J. Cell. Physiol. 2008;214(3):559–67.

182. Feigin ME, Muthuswamy SK. ErbB receptors and cell polarity: new pathways and paradigms for understanding cell migration and invasion. Exp. Cell Res. 2009;315(4):707–16.

183. Izumi Y, Xu L, di Tomaso E, Fukumura D, Jain RK. Tumour biology: herceptin acts as an anti-angiogenic cocktail. Nature 2002;416(6878):279–80.

184. Marcotte R, Muller WJ. Signal transduction in transgenic mouse models of human breast cancer—implications for human breast cancer. J. Mammary Gland Biol. neoplasia. 2008;13(3):323–35.

185. Pietras RJ, Arboleda J, Reese DM, et al. HER-2 tyrosine kinase pathway targets estrogen receptor and promotes hormone-independent growth in human breast cancer cells. Oncogene. 1995;10(12):2435–46.

186. She QB, Chandarlapaty S, Ye Q, et al. Breast tumor cells with PI3K mutation or HER2 amplification are selectively addicted to Akt signaling. PloS ONE 2008;3(8):e3065.

187. Emens LA, Davidson NE. Trastuzumab in breast cancer. Oncology (Williston Park) 2004;18(9):1117–28. discussion, 31–2, 37–8.

188. Arteaga CL, Ramsey TT, Shawver LK, Guyer CA. Unliganded epidermal growth factor receptor dimerization induced by direct interaction of quinazolines with the ATP binding site. J. Biol. Chem. 1997;272(37):23247–54.

189. Moulder SL, Yakes FM, Muthuswamy SK, Bianco R, Simpson JF, Arteaga CL. Epidermal growth factor receptor (HER1) tyrosine kinase inhibitor ZD1839 (Iressa) inhibits HER2/neu (erbB2)-overexpressing breast cancer cells *in vitro* and *in vivo*. Cancer Res. 2001;61(24):8887–95.

190. Nicholson S, Sainsbury JR, Halcrow P, Chambers P, Farndon JR, Harris AL. Expression of epidermal growth factor receptors associated with lack of response to endocrine therapy in recurrent breast cancer. Lancet 1989;1(8631):182–5.

191. Genentech. *Herceptin® (Trastuzumab) in Early-Stage and Advanced Breast Cancer*, 2014, http://www.gene.com/media/product-information/herceptin-breast#5.

192. Slamon DJ, Leyland-Jones B, Shak S, et al. Use of chemotherapy plus a monoclonal antibody against HER2 for metastatic breast cancer that overexpresses HER2. New Engl. J. Med. 2001;344(11):783–92.

193. Montemurro F, Aglietta M. Duration of trastuzumab for HER2–positive breast cancer. Lancet Oncol. 2013;14(8):678–9.

194. Moja L, Tagliabue L, Balduzzi S, et al. Trastuzumab containing regimens for early breast cancer. Cochrane Database Syst. Rev. 2012;4:CD006243.

195. Goldhirsch A, Gelber RD, Piccart-Gebhart MJ, et al. 2 years versus 1 year of adjuvant trastuzumab for HER2-positive breast cancer (HERA): an open-label, randomised controlled trial. Lancet 2013;382(9897):1021–8.

196. Pivot X, Romieu G, Deble d M, et al. 6 months versus 12 months of adjuvant trastuzumab for patients with HER2-positive early breast cancer (PHARE): a randomised phase 3 trial. Lancet Oncol. 2013;14(8):741–8.

197. Ellis MJ, Tao Y, Young O, et al. Estrogen-independent proliferation is present in estrogen-receptor HER2-positive primary breast cancer after neoadjuvant letrozole. J. Clin. Oncol. 2006;24(19):3019–25.

198. Arribas J, Baselga J, Pedersen K, Parra-Palau JL. p95HER2 and breast cancer. Cancer Res. 2011;71(5):1515–9.

199. Wong AL, Lee SC. Mechanisms of resistance to trastuzumab and novel therapeutic strategies in HER2-positive breast cancer. Int. J. Breast Cancer 2012;2012:415170.

200. Berns K, Horlings HM, Hennessy BT, et al. A functional genetic approach identifies the PI3K pathway as a major determinant of trastuzumab resistance in breast cancer. Cancer Cell. 2007;12(4):395–402.

201. Nagata Y, Lan KH, Zhou X, et al. PTEN activation contributes to tumor inhibition by trastuzumab, and loss of PTEN predicts trastuzumab resistance in patients. Cancer Cell. 2004;6(2):117–27.

202. Zhang S, Huang WC, Li P, et al. Combating trastuzumab resistance by targeting SRC, a common node downstream of multiple resistance pathways. Nat. Med. 2011;17(4):461–9.

203. Scaltriti M, Rojo F, Ocana A, et al. Expression of p95HER2, a truncated form of the HER2 receptor, and response to anti-HER2 therapies in breast cancer. J. Natl. Cancer Inst. 2007;99(8):628–38.

204. Nahta R, Yuan LX, Zhang B, Kobayashi R, Esteva FJ. Insulin-like growth factor-I receptor/human epidermal growth factor receptor 2 heterodimerization contributes to trastuzumab resistance of breast cancer cells. Cancer Res. 2005;65(23):11118–28.

205. Garcia-Garcia C, Ibrahim YH, Serra V, et al. Dual mTORC1/2 and HER2 blockade results in antitumor activity in preclinical models of breast cancer resistant to anti-HER2 therapy. Clin. Cancer Res. 2012;18(9):2603–12.

206. Scaltriti M, Eichhorn PJ, Cortes J, et al. Cyclin E amplification/overexpression is a mechanism of trastuzumab resistance in HER2+ breast cancer patients. Proc. Natl. Acad. Sci. U.S.A. 2011;108(9):3761–6.

207. Bendell JC, Rodon J, Burris HA, et al. Phase I dose-escalation study of BKM120, an oral pan-Class I PI3K inhibitor, in patients with advanced solid tumors. J. Clin. Oncol. 2012;30(3):282–90.

208. Vivanco I, Sawyers CL. The phosphatidylinositol 3-kinase AKT pathway in human cancer. Nat. Rev. Cancer 2002;2(7):489–501.

209. Gonzalez-Angulo AM, Blumenschein GR Jr. Defining biomarkers to predict sensitivity to PI3K/Akt/mTOR pathway inhibitors in breast cancer. Cancer Treat. Rev. 2013;39(4):313–20.

210. Agarwal R, Carey M, Hennessy B, Mills GB. PI3K pathway-directed therapeutic strategies in cancer. Curr. Opin. Invest. Drugs 2010;11(6):615–28.

211. Miller TW, Perez-Torres M, Narasanna A, et al. Loss of phosphatase and tensin homologue deleted on chromosome 10 engages ErbB3 and insulin-like growth factor-I receptor signaling to promote antiestrogen resistance in breast cancer. Cancer Res. 2009;69(10):4192–201.

212. Hurvitz SA, Pietras RJ. Rational management of endocrine resistance in breast cancer: a comprehensive review of estrogen receptor biology, treatment options, and future directions. Cancer 2008;113(9):2385–97.

213. Mayer I. Role of mTOR inhibition in preventing resistance and restoring sensitivity to hormone-targeted and HER2–targeted therapies in breast cancer. Clin. Adv. Hematol. Oncol. 2013;11(4):217–24.

214. Nahta R, Yu D, Hung MC, Hortobagyi GN, Esteva FJ. Mechanisms of disease: understanding resistance to HER2-targeted therapy in human breast cancer. Nat. Clin. Pract. Oncol. 2006;3(5):269–80.

215. Pegram M. Can we circumvent resistance to ErbB2-targeted agents by targeting novel pathways? Clin. Breast Cancer 2008;8(Suppl. 3):S121–30.

216. Ma CX, Crowder RJ, Ellis MJ. Importance of PI3-kinase pathway in response/resistance to aromatase inhibitors. Steroids 2011;76(8):750–2.

217. Crowder RJ, Phommaly C, Tao Y, et al. PIK3CA and PIK3CB inhibition produce synthetic lethality when combined with estrogen deprivation in estrogen receptor-positive breast cancer. Cancer Res. 2009;69(9):3955–62.

218. Sanchez CG, Ma CX, Crowder RJ, et al. Preclinical modeling of combined phosphatidylinositol-3-kinase inhibition with endocrine therapy for estrogen receptor-positive breast cancer. Breast Cancer Res. 2011;13(2):R21.

219. Miller TW, Hennessy BT, Gonzalez-Angulo AM, et al. Hyperactivation of phosphatidylinositol-3 kinase promotes escape from hormone dependence in estrogen receptor-positive human breast cancer. J. Clin. Invest. 2010;120(7):2406–13.

220. Hanker AB, Pfefferle AD, Balko JM, et al. Mutant PIK3CA accelerates HER2-driven transgenic mammary tumors and induces resistance to combinations of anti-HER2 therapies. Proc. Natl. Acad. Sci. U.S.A. 2013;110(35):14372–7.

221. Baselga J, Campone M, Piccart M, et al. Everolimus in postmenopausal hormone-receptor-positive advanced breast cancer. New Engl. J. Med. 2012;366(6):520–9.

222. Meric-Bernstam F, Gonzalez-Angulo AM. Targeting the mTOR signaling network for cancer therapy. J. Clin. Oncol. 2009;27(13):2278–87.

223. Yamnik RL, Digilova A, Davis DC, Brodt ZN, Murphy CJ, Holz MK. S6 kinase 1 regulates estrogen receptor alpha in control of breast cancer cell proliferation. J. Biol. Chem. 2009;284(10):6361–9.

224. Yamnik RL, Holz MK. mTOR/S6K1 and MAPK/RSK signaling pathways coordinately regulate estrogen receptor alpha serine 167 phosphorylation. FEBS Lett. 2010;584(1):124–8.

225. O'Regan R, Ozguroglu M, Andre F, et al. Phase III, randomized, double-blind, placebo-controlled multicenter trial of daily everolimus plus weekly trastuzumab and vinorelbine in trastuzumab-resistant, advanced breast cancer (BOLERO-3). J. Clin. Oncol. 2013;31. (Suppl.; Abstract 505).

226. Schneider BP, Sledge GW Jr. Drug insight: VEGF as a therapeutic target for breast cancer. Nat. Clin. Pract. Oncol. 2007;4(3):181–9.

227. Miller K, Wang M, Gralow J, et al. Paclitaxel plus bevacizumab versus paclitaxel alone for metastatic breast cancer. New Engl. J. Med. 2007;357(26):2666–76.

228. Miles DW, Chan A, Dirix LY, et al. Phase III study of bevacizumab plus docetaxel compared with placebo plus docetaxel for the first-line treatment of human epidermal growth factor receptor 2-negative metastatic breast cancer. J. Clin. Oncol. 2010;28(20):3239–47.

229. Robert NJ, Dieras V, Glaspy J, et al. RIBBON-1: randomized, double-blind, placebo-controlled, phase III trial of chemotherapy with or without bevacizumab for first-line treatment of human epidermal growth factor receptor 2-negative, locally recurrent or metastatic breast cancer. J. Clin. Oncol. 2011;29(10):1252–60.

230. Pazdur, R. Memorandum to the file BLA 125085 Avastin (bevacizumab). FDA Center for Drug Evaluation and Research, December 15, 2010 (http://www.fda.gov/downloads/Drugs/DrugSafety/PostmarketDrugSafetyInformationforPatientsandProviders/UCM237171.pdf).

231. Ranpura V, Hapani S, Wu S. Treatment-related mortality with bevacizumab in cancer patients: a meta-analysis. JAMA 2011;305(5):487–94.

232. Maru D, Venook AP, Ellis LM. Predictive biomarkers for bevacizumab: are we there yet? Clin. Cancer Res. 2013;19(11):2824–7.

233. Marino N, Woditschka S, Reed LT, et al. Breast cancer metastasis: issues for the personalization of its prevention and treatment. Am. J. Pathol. 2013;183(4):1084–95.

234. Zardavas D, Pugliano L, Piccart M. Personalized therapy for breast cancer: a dream or a reality? Future Oncol. 2013;9(8):1105–19.

235. Cardoso F, Van't Veer L, Rutgers E, Loi S, Mook S, Piccart-Gebhart MJ. Clinical application of the 70-gene profile: the MINDACT trial. J. Clin. Oncol. 2008;26(5):729–35.

236. Awada A, Aftimos PG. Targeted therapies of solid cancers: new options, new challenges. Curr. Opin. Oncol. 2013;25(3):296–304.

237. Moulder S, Yan K, Huang F, et al. Development of candidate genomic markers to select breast cancer patients for dasatinib therapy. Mol. Cancer Therap. 2010;9(5):1120–7.

238. Meric-Bernstam F, Farhangfar C, Mendelsohn J, Mills GB. Building a personalized medicine infrastructure at a major cancer center. J. Clin. Oncol. 2013;31(15):1849–57.

239. Meric-Bernstam F, Mills GB. Overcoming implementation challenges of personalized cancer therapy. Nat. Rev. Clin. Oncol. 2012;9(9):542–8.

240. Camacho LH. Drug development in cancer medicine: challenges for targeted approaches. In: Kurzrock R, Markman M, editors. Targeted Cancer Therapy. Totowa, NJ: Humana Press; 2008. p. 383–410.

241. Gerber DE. Targeted therapies: a new generation of cancer treatments. Am. Fam. Physician 2008;77(3):311–9.

242. Dave B, Migliaccio I, Gutierrez MC, et al. Loss of phosphatase and tensin homolog or phosphoinositol-3 kinase activation and response to trastuzumab or lapatinib in human epidermal growth factor receptor 2-overexpressing locally advanced breast cancers. J. Clin. Oncol. 2011;29(2):166–73.

243. Hainsworth JD, Sosman JA, Spigel DR, Edwards DL, Baughman C, Greco A. Treatment of metastatic renal cell carcinoma with a combination of bevacizumab and erlotinib. J. Clin. Oncol. 2005;23(31):7889–96.

244. Schilsky RL, Allen J, Benner J, Sigal E, McClellan M. Commentary: tackling the challenges of developing targeted therapies for cancer. Oncologist 2010;15(5):484–7.

CHAPTER

14

Hunting Molecular Targets for Anticancer Reagents by Chemical Proteomics

Bin Sun[1,2], Qing-Yu He[2]

[1]Southern Medical University, Guangzhou, China
[2]Key Laboratory of Functional Protein Research of Guangdong Higher Education Institutes, Institute of Life and Health Engineering, College of Life Science and Technology, Jinan University, Guangzhou, China

INTRODUCTION

Cancer, the uncontrolled growth of abnormal cells, is a global public health issue that profoundly affects more than 1 million people and their families each year. According to the American Cancer Society, in 2010 there were 569,490 cancer deaths overall, and the number of deaths caused by cancer is second place only to deaths caused by cardiovascular disease.[1] Surgery, chemotherapy, and radiotherapy are the general, conventional approaches to

Novel Approaches and Strategies for Biologics, Vaccines and Cancer Therapies. DOI: 10.1016/B978-0-12-416603-5.00014-6

effectively treating most types of cancer. Among these strategies, chemotherapeutics plays a major role in the discovery and development of innovative anticancer strategies.

The dawning of cancer chemotherapy began in the first half of the 20th century with the serendipitous discovery of the nitrogen mustard family of agents.[2] In 1971, President Richard Nixon launched the so-called War on Cancer, and, after 20 years of unremitting efforts, researchers have made substantial and important progress.[3-5] More and more compounds with anticancer properties are appearing from the laboratories of leading experts in medicinal chemistry and the research and development (R&D) departments of pharmaceutical companies. However, in recent years, the efficiency–cost ratio of inventing and developing new anticancer agents within the traditional paradigms of drug discovery is an issue. When confronted with such challenges, we need new knowledge and concepts, along with technological advances, to arm us in the war against cancer.

Sun Tzu, a military general and the author of *The Art of War* (~500 B.C.), once said, "Know your enemy as completely as possible; locate your enemy as soon as possible; strike your enemy as hard as possible, you can win a hundred battles without a single loss." Such a strategy can similarly be applied by drug developers seeking to address the discovery of new targets. The better we understand the roles that various enemies play in tumors, the better we can shape a precise strategic plan for a debilitating strike against cancer. The recent growth in omics technologies has brought about a revolution in new drug target identification, giving rise to rapid changes in the paradigms of anticarcinogen discovery toward molecularly targeted therapeutics.

Chemical proteomics, combining current proteomics techniques and affinity chromatography, as well as analytical measures such as mass spectrometry (MS) and bioinformatics tools, have been successfully applied to comprehensively and unbiasedly interrogate the precise mechanism of action (MOA) of bioactive anticancer compounds, such as natural products, kinase inhibitors, and other compounds efficacious against cancer. Such an approach allows the identification of thus far undetected target proteins and provides information regarding potential side-effects, including unanticipated adverse reactions caused by off-target interactions for an established anticancer agent.[6,7] Two distinctly different strategies are widely used in the field of chemical proteomics. The first is compound-oriented protein profiling (COPP), where the target proteins for the anticarcinogen of interest can be captured and identified with the aid of solid matrix and mass spectrometry. The second is affinity-based protein profiling, also known as photoaffinity labeling (PAL), which is accomplished by characterizing drug targets (and off-targets) of small molecule compounds possessing antitumor activities by means of affinity-based probes (AfBPs) in native biological systems on a global scale.[8]

In this chapter, we briefly discuss the general principles, current developments, and strengths and weaknesses of these two approaches. We also provide several examples of how chemical proteomics can facilitate target identification and quantification of small molecule compounds possessing antitumor activities. In addition, a systems-level approach comprised of chemical proteomics and other omics technologies for mapping anticarcinogen–target networks is introduced.

CHEMICAL PROTEOMICS STRATEGIES

Compound-Oriented Protein Profiling Strategies

Most bioactive medicaments exert their pharmacologic actions via directly targeting the disease-related proteins to modulate the pathways involved in the pathological process. Knowledge about the relationship between bioactive molecules and their binding targets is not only pivotal to gaining insight into the therapeutic and adverse mechanism of medicament action at the pathway level but also useful for predicting novel targets pertinent to the bioactivity of medicaments. Two affinity chromatography-based compound-oriented protein profiling (COPP) strategies are routinely applied to aid in unraveling the medicament receptors (see Figure 14.1).

The first COPP strategy, sometimes termed a *pull-down experiment*, is a relatively easy, straightforward method to identify potential medicament-binding partners,[9–13] including off-targets.[14–17] Immobilization of selected medicaments bearing reactive functional chemical groups (typically amino, carboxyl, epoxy, hydroxyl, or sulfhydryl groups) as linkable moieties through spacer arms with optimal lengths onto stationary matrices is a key step of the pull-down experiment.[6,18–20] The entire medicament-bound matrix serves as drug target-fishing system (DTF) to capture a proteome on the basis of a specific interaction (typically, hydrogen, ionic, hydrophobic, or covalent bonding) between the target proteins and medicaments from cell or tissue extracts. By extensive washing to eliminate the unbound proteins, the target proteome can be obtained with excess free medicament or under highly denaturing conditions. Followed by subsequent digestion and MS identification, only the overlapping proteins identified after two experiments are supposed to be valid. Results from pull-down experiments should be validated as reliable and accurate by other complementary biology experiments.

In 1996, Schreiber and coworkers[21] reported an example of revealing the binding proteins targeting histone deacetylase in the case of the anticancer drug trapoxin. Fleischer et al.[22] made use of a MPI-0479883–Sepharose® matrix to capture target proteins of CB30865, a potent, selective cytotoxic compound with an unknown MOA from cell extracts. The authors reported that a 55-kDa protein nicotinamide phosphoribosyltransferase (Nampt) may be a primary target for CB30865 cytotoxicity. Based on the data from biochemical and cellular pharmacology experiments, the authors suggested that CB30865 cytotoxicity is due to subnanomolar inhibition of Nampt within the nicotinamide adenine dinucleotide (NAD) biosynthetic pathway, thus assisting cancer cells in sustaining their incremental energy metabolism.

Based on the extremely tight binding interaction of the avidin/streptavidin–biotin system, another widely employed COPP strategy was designed to facilitate targeted proteome purification of biotin labeling medicament.[23–26] Wang and coworkers[23] presented a biotinylated form of diazonamide A attached to agarose beads to unravel its molecular mechanism of perturbing spindle assembly in mammalian cell cultures. Binding profiles obtained for such strategy suggest that a mitochondrial enzyme ornithine δ-amino transferase may be a primary target of diazonamide A. Subsequent biochemical studies disclosed that ornithine δ-amino transferase was responsible for mediating the mitotic arrest caused by diazonamide A in human cancer cells. Oridonin, an active diterpene isolated from the traditional Chinese herbal medicine *Isodon rubescens*, has attracted attention for its remarkable chemopreventive and antitumor activity in cancer therapy. Several research groups have suggested that the MOA of oridonin may be related to its ability to interfere with several pathways involved in cell proliferation, cell-cycle arrest, apoptosis, and autophagy.[24] To gain a better understanding of the MOA of oridonin, a mass spectrometry-based chemical proteomics approach was applied to explore the targets of oridonin in leukemia-derived Jurkat cells. Among the identified four potential partners of oridonin, the multifunctional, stress-inducible molecular chaperone HSP701A was suggested to be the most likely anticancer drug target. Moreover, the binding site of oridonin on the chaperone was identified by a mass-based approach combined with molecular dynamics simulations.[25]

IV. NOVEL APPROACHES FOR CANCER THERAPIES

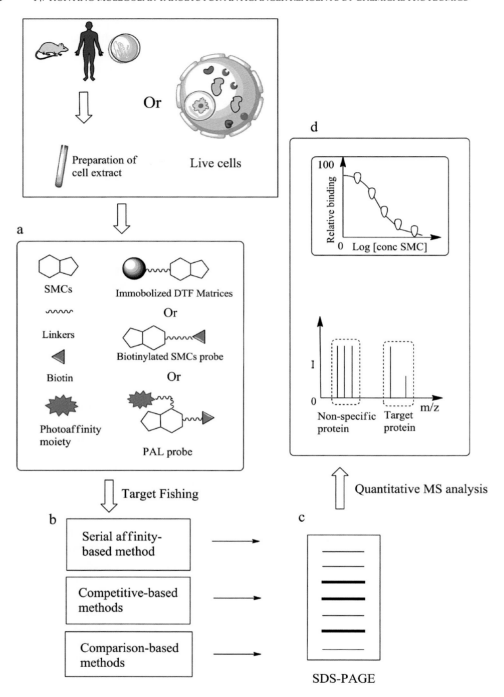

Limitations and Solutions

As illustrated by the above examples, the convenience and efficacy of the COPP strategies have provided new opportunities for proteomic analysis of novel cellular receptors. Despite the many successes achieved with this technique, there are drawbacks to its use. The primary limitation of a COPP strategy is in the chemical design of the derivatives of selected small molecule compounds which is guided through extensive structure–activity relationship (SAR) studies. A SAR study is a tedious and time-consuming method for selecting an appropriate functional group or site on a candidate that tethers to the linker without negatively affecting its molecule bioactivity, thus sometimes the end result is never guaranteed. Many small molecule compounds (SMCs) cannot be modified without influencing their inherent bioactivity, or it is difficult to obtain their derivatives or synthesize them in quantities sufficient to perform subsequent studies.[26] Seeking guidances from seasoned medicinal chemistry experts could resolve many of these problems.

Also, due to the introduction of spacer arms and a stationary matrix in the DTF synthesis procedure, relevant proteins with the mode of physical adsorption to the above affinity matrices[27] would appear in the list of identified interactors and confuse our target mining. Furthermore, the instability of the conventional stationary matrices (such as resin, agarose, polyglycidylmethacrylate, and magnetic particles[28–34]) might lead to low efficiency in affinity-based target identification. In order to overcome such drawbacks, many researchers have sought to develop innovative solutions for eliminating the unfavorable nonspecifically bound proteins, termed background proteins. Tanaka et al.[35–37] described the use of a substituted heptanoic acid spacer that is hydrophilic enough to improve selectivity and capacity (i.e., density of the effectively immobilized ligand on matrices). Reduction of natively biotinylated proteins and nonselectively bound proteins is important for the success of biotin/streptavidin-based profiling systems. Yang et al.[38] developed a powerful, highly reliable, easily synthesized, and inexpensive cleavable linker to address this issue. Honda et al.[30] have presented an overview on the development of the high-performance affinity beads that enable one-step affinity purification of drug targets. A classic example is the identification of a novel target protein of the anticancer agent methotrexate (MTX) by using magnetic nanocarriers. The authors also

◀ FIGURE 14.1 **Experimental workflows in chemical proteomics.** Figure illustrates the major affinity chromatography approaches to compound-oriented protein profiling (COPP), which is used to identify receptor proteins of anticancer SMCs *in vitro* and *in vivo*. (a) In SMC-immobilized affinity chromatography, SMCs are directly immobilized onto a solid support via a spacer arm to reduce steric hindrance. In the biotin-based affinity approach, SMCs coupled with a biotin moiety are regarded as a biotinylated probe to selectively enrich the target proteins with the aid of a streptavidin-coated matrix. In a PAL experiment, the probe is incubated with protein extracts for noncovalent interactions with target proteins. Upon irradiation, the noncovalent probe–target interactions are converted to covalent binding through photo-induced crosslinking of the reactivity function. (b) To distinguish specific target proteins from nonspecific binding components, one of the three methods (serial-based, competitive-based, or comparison-based technologies) could be applied to the target proteins isolated from the three affinity-enrichment approaches above. (c) Specific target proteins isolated from these three approaches could be visualized on sodium dodecyl sulfate polyacrylamide gel electrophoresis (SDS-PAGE) and subsequently identified with MS analysis. (d) Quantitative mass spectrometry is ideally suited to determine the identity and quantity of the captured proteins. The IC_{50} value for SMC-bound specific target proteins can be determined through the MS-based SILAC competition experiment with increasing amounts of SMCs and subsequently with the affinity-matrices containing SMCs.

discussed the advantages of their affinity products (SG and FG beads) compared to other conventional matrices.

A number of nonspecific binding proteins to several commonly used affinity matrices were presented in the work of Trinkle-Mulcahy et al.[39] Their research results serve as a valuable reference, and the authors describe methods for differentiating specific protein binding partners from background proteins in chemical proteomics experiments. By taking advantage of a 7.5-Å polyethylene glycol spacer to prevent steric hindrance between the protein targets and the deguelin-bearing matrix, Garcia et al.[40] investigated the targets of deguelin and related rotenoids. Two biotin conjugates immobilized on streptavidin resin exhibited strong cellular colocalization with mitochondria, a result consistent with binding to mitochondrial complex 1 (i.e., NADH/ubiquinone oxidoreductase). Hale and coworkers[41,42] promulgated a creative strategy—immuno-chemo-proteomics—for target selection with a peptide-coupled small molecule probe from cells or tissues. Introducing peptides with a hydrophilic nature can dramatically modify the behavior of nonspecific binding.

Two cases of immuno-chemo-proteomics have been utilized in target-fishing studies of bisindolyl maleimide III (Bis-III): a protein kinase Cα (PKCα) and a glycogen synthase kinase 3β (GSK3β) inhibitor.[41,42] The first scenario was used to compare the effects of peptide-based immuno-chemo-proteomics and traditional solid support matrix-based chemical proteomics on searching target proteins of Bis-III in high-salt HeLa cell lysates.[41] Both traditional chemical proteomics techniques and immuno-chemo-proteomics captured several identical proteins, including PKCα, GSK3α/β, CaMKII-γ, NQO2, VDAC, and prohibitin; however, the FLAG-coupled–Bis-III probes exhibited raised activity levels in enriching proteins with lower binding affinity. A strategy for target elimination was applied to reduce false positives in this work. In subsequent research, a 5-FAM-TAT-coupled–Bis-III probe with the ability of cell permeability was developed and used to pursue the viable targets of Bis-III from live cells. The introduction of fluorophore (i.e., 5-FAM) appending the probe offers the fascinating opportunity to image the probe inside the live cells, providing valuable information about target location and distribution by means of high-resolution microscope.[42]

A novel yet simple tactic for discriminating target proteins from the nonspecific binding of irrelevant proteins is a comparison-based target-fishing method that introduces blank control of affinity matrices without immobilized parent ligand or negative control of affinity matrices that contain a nonbioactive analog sharing structural similarities to the parent ligand.[28,43] Due to the vast structural diversity and complexity of biologically active small molecules, the production of such a nonbioactive analog would involve arduous work to modify or remove functional groups necessary for drug activity. Yamamota et al.[44] offered general guidelines of an alternative serial affinity chromatography strategy for distinguishing specific binding components from nonspecific ones. The cell lysates were loaded onto the same amount of affinity matrix bearing the same ligand in sequence. There is little difference in the amounts of nonspecific binders between the two affinity matrices because most nonspecific binders remained in the lysates due to their low affinity for the matrices. However, the amount of specific binders on the second matrix was expected to be drastically reduced, on the basis of the theory that the first affinity matrix should be preferentially enriched for specific target binders. It is worth noting that such a strategy could lead to confusing results when the ligand-immobilized affinity matrix has low affinity for the specific binding proteins.

Another significant source of unfavorable nonspecific proteins is from high abundance proteins, sometimes referred to as *core-proteome proteins*,[45] which are not direct targets or downstream receptors of the affected signaling cascade under the drug treatment but are often present in many cell lines involved in stress response or housekeeping functions. These undesirable high-abundance proteins may cloud the real higher affinity targets with low abundance. A competition-based target-fishing strategy is often described as a clear and effective way to deal with the problem of nonspecific binding. In the competition method, cell lysates are incubated in the presence or absence of the excess free test ligands to enrich the target proteins in parallel. The presence of free ligands competes with the target proteins so as to allow a decline in the amount of bound proteins from the immobilized-ligand affinity matrices. The capture assays of specific proteins by competition experiment sometimes include proteins that bind indirectly to test ligands through protein–protein interactions. In this situation, it is necessary, by combining the proteomic results of competition and comparison-based affinity target profiling approaches, to refine the interacting target list and to obtain more reliable information on target proteins. Furthermore, multiple confirmatory biological experiments (such as immunoblotting or coimmunoprecipitation)[15] or using databases such as IntAct or Mint[46] to recognize proteins that undergo protein–protein interactions with other proteins on the list are also promising solutions.

Most of the COPP strategies have been extensively performed on lysate samples from various cell types for comprehensive analysis of target and off-target proteome activities, so the requirement of a large amount of cell materials is key to elucidating the MOA as well as pharmacological pathways of selected drug candidates. Moreover, considering that the bioactivity of some target proteins would be reduced or would disappear due to the release of the activators and inhibitors during disruption of cellular organelles and various compartments in the cell lysis process,[47] COPP strategies performed in intact cells with membrane-permeable affinity matrices are gaining renewed interest as a widely applicable technique. Hu et al.[48] devised an affinity-permeating plan with the aid of the nanopolymer-G4 poly(amidoamine) dendrimer to identify drug targets of the antimetabolite and anticancer drug methotrexate (MTX) from cells in culture. Two proteins known to interact with MTX (DHFR and dCK) were identified by this approach.

Photoaffinity Labeling Strategies

Photoaffinity labeling (PAL) is another successful and widespread strategy that facilitates the implement of target-fishing with AfBP probes. The three components of a universal model of AfBP probes are (1) parent molecule compound derivates as the core segment, (2) photoreactive moiety (e.g., benzopheno, 3-trifluoromethyl-3-phenyl diazirine, arylazides) as a photoactivatable segment, and (3) biotin or fluorophore as a report segment. Upon activation by ultraviolet irradiation, the selected AfBP probes interacting irreversibly to the target proteins begins to stabilize by forming a new covalent bond at the binding site. Isolation of the labeled proteins can be accomplished by avidin or streptavidin affinity chromatography with a biotin affinity tag. An important advantage of such AfBP probes is that unspecific background proteins attached to the probes can be eliminated by extensive washing without dissociating the biotinylated ligand–protein complexes.

Using PAL, Taylor and coworkers[49–51] studied the effect of quercetin, a natural flavonoid possessing antioxidative, antiinflammatory, and anticancer bioactivity. The intrinsic photoactive characteristics of quercetin[52] and the weak interaction between most known enzymes and quercetin make the PAL strategy an attractive solutions. O7-biotinylated AfBP probes of quercetin (BioQ) were prepared to purify possible binding proteins from cells.[53] Several possible quercetin protein targets, including HSP70, HSP90, ubiquitin-activating enzyme E1, splicesomal protein SPA-130, RuvBL2 ATPases, and eukaryotic translation initiation factors 3, have been identified from normal and heat-shocked Jurkat cells under stringent washing conditions. Most of the binding partners collected by PAL are potent cancer therapeutic targets accounting for the apoptotic and antitumor activities of quercetin. The authors inferred that quercetin exerts its effect through simultaneous but low-level inhibition of multiple therapeutic targets, which could explain quercetin's positive therapeutic effect with low specificity and toxicity.

Gexia (herboxidiene), first obtained from a cultured broth of *Streptomyces* sp.,[54] has been found to be a potentially potent antitumor product associated with the induction of cell-cycle arrest in G_1 and G_2/M phases in normal human fibroblast cell line WI-38[55] and human cervix adenocarcinoma cell line HeLa.[56] Mizukami and coworkers[56] applied the PAL assay to search for the protein targets of gexia. A 143-kDa protein was isolated and identified as SAP155 by LC–MS/MS analysis; the protein is a component of SF3b complexes that participate in pre-mRNA splicing. These data indicated that gexia inhibited splicing of the pre-mRNA by binding with SAP155.

The delivery of small molecule probes into live cells for the identity and cellular location imaging of specific target binders continues to be a challenge in the field of PAL. The implementation of click chemistry has driven the development of new AfBP probes for this purpose. Over the past several years, these potent tools have brought revolutionary changes to many fields.[57–61] Nacamura et al.[62,63] developed two multifunctional photoaffinity probes to profile the target proteins of the HIF-1α inhibitor o-carboranylphenoxyacetanilide. Hypoxia response element (HRE) reporter gene assay with two such probes, followed by immunoblot analysis, confirmed that the modification to an efficient functional group (i.e., boronic acid) of o-carboranylphenoxyacetanilide in the probe synthesis correlated with negative reductions on HIF-1α activation to some extent. Tryptic digestion and subsequent peptide mass fingerprinting (PMF) analysis of the enriched proteins from these photoaffinity probes inserting AlexathFluor488 through click reaction were performed. A 55-kDa HSP60 as a primary target of o-carboranylphenoxyacetanilide was identified. Competition-based photoaffinity labeled assay in HeLa cell lysates with or without o-carboranylphenoxyacetanilide has also provided striking insights into specific protein targets by proportionally diminishing the extent of the fluorescent band of the labeled proteins.

Another aspect of AfBP probes possessing remarkable features of cell-permeable, clickable, photoaffinity was presented by Yao et al.[64] By comparing results obtained from different proteomic settings (live cells, cell lysates, and traditional affinity method by immobilizing ligands to matrix), one of the two AfBPs probes based on dasatinib would contribute considerably to identifying significantly more putative kinase targets. In addition to Abl and Src family tyrosine kinases, a number of previously unknown dasatinib targets have been identified, including several serine/threonine kinases (PCTK3, STK25, eIF-2A, PIM-3, PKA C-α, and PKN2). They concluded that the clickable, cell-permeable affinity probe was capable of accessing to the intended protein targets more easily and capturing more kinase targets than traditional affinity matrix methods. The choice of an alkyl diazirine was critical in shrinking the overall probe size and preventing poor cell permeability.

CHEMICAL PROTEOMIC-BASED QUANTIFICATION

Chemical proteomic-based COPP strategies have proven to be powerful for elucidating the function of potential anticarcinogens and the intricacies of multiple pharmacological signal pathways. Although the use of COPP strategies has provided a wealth of information, their inability to provide quantitative information about ligand–target complexes (K_d values and half-maximal inhibitory values) has slowed down the pace of adopting COPP strategies. Recent work has focused on a new field that uses quantitative MS strategy to deliver complementary sets of results obtained by traditional affinity-based chemical proteomics approaches. In this section, we briefly discuss several examples with a view toward target identification and quantification of anticarcinogens by employing a variety of quantitative proteomic techniques

Isotope-Coded Affinity Tags

In 1999, Gelb and coworkers[65] described a gel-free method for identifying and quantifying proteins in two cell populations. The method was based on the fact that only free cysteine thiols tend to be labeled by iodoacetamide-like reagents, known as isotope-coded affinity tags (ICATs). Mass spectroscopy can be adopted to quantify the relative labeling of free thiols. The ICAT method involves a trifunctional probe containing a reactive unit with specificity toward sulfhydryl groups, an linker unit with either eight hydrogens (the light form of the reagent, D_0) or eight deuteriums (the heavy form of the reagent, D_8), and an affinity unit for the isolation of labeled peptides. The traditional ICAT method is carried out as follows. First, two protein mixtures in different cell states are labeled with the heavy and light reagents, respectively. These two labeled protein mixtures are then combined together. After digestion with trypsin to generate peptide fragments, the labeled peptides (cysteine-containing) are enriched by avidin affinity chromatography. Finally, the enriched peptides are subjected to MS for analysis, and the relative abundances of proteins in the two samples are determined by the intensity ratio of the labeled peptide pairs (light and heavy).[66] The ease of working with cysteine residues makes them ideal for ICAT methods.

Nagasu et al.[67] developed a systematic strategy of combining the comparison-based affinity target-fishing method with the fluorescent two-dimensional differential in gel electrophoresis (2D-DIGE) method, as well as a newly developed cleavable ICAT method to identify the primary binding protein targets of indisulam. Indisulam (i.e., N-(-3-chloro-7-indolyl)-1,4-benzenedisulfonamide, or E7070) is an experimental sulfonamide anticancer agent that disrupts the G_1/S phase of the cell cycle.[68] Recent reports have indicated that Phase II studies of indisulam on some solid tumors have been completed.[69] Based on the results of MTT assays in E7070-sensitive human colon cancer cell line HCT116-C9 and E7070-resistant subclone HCT116-C9-C1, two of the synthesized indisulam derivates were chosen to play the role of positive or negative ligands, which were immobilized to the affinity matrix. Because highly abundant proteins correlate to E7070 in a nonspecific binding manner and represent a very large proportion of identified proteins, thus interfering with target analysis, 2D-DIGE and improved ICAT methods were applied to overcome the issue of nonspecific binding proteins. The quantitative proteome experiments suggested that several metabolic enzymes, including cytosolic malate dehydrogenase (MDH), cartilage oligomeric matrix protein, and G protein-α inhibiting activity polypeptide 3, were selective binders to an E7070-coupled matrix. The verification experiment with surface plasmon resonance (SPR) proved that cytosolic MDH was the most specific binding partner, in agreement with data measured by ICAT.

Stable Isotope Labeling by Amino Acids in Cell Culture

Stable isotope labeling by amino acids in cell culture (SILAC), first demonstrated by Mann's group,[70] has emerged as a new theme in quantitative proteomics with the advantage of eliminating the need to visualize the target proteins by gel staining. The rationale is that two groups of cell materials are differentially labeled by growing them in culture media containing heavy isotopes (stable isotope ^{2}H/^{13}C/^{15}N-code amino acid or ^{15}N-enriched culture media) or normal amino acids (normal ^{1}H/^{12}C/^{14}N-code amino acid or ^{14}N-minimal culture media). After a number of cell divisions, cells are encoded with the label as they grow in cell culture. When both samples are combined in the same amount and processed for MS analysis, the ratio of peak intensities in the mass spectrum reflects the relative protein abundance.[71]

A novel powerful approach combining SILAC with a competition-based target-fishing strategy was reported by Carr et al.,[72] who described full-scale identification and quantification of the proteins that bind to small molecule probes and test compounds. A unique feature of this strategy is that free test compounds compete with the binding interaction of the compound-coupled probes in the same amount of normal and heavy cell populations. By comparison of the target's pull-down in normal and heavy culture conditions, true target proteins can be more easily distinguished through relevant differential ratios in MS. Many nonspecific binders, however, due to their equivalent enrichment could be collected in both samples with ratios close to 1. Using quantitative SILAC in tandem with a target affinity measurement approach, Daub et al.[73] proposed an elegant means for providing potent quantitative information, including the target-specific dissociation constants (K_d) and IC$_{50}$ values.[73] In this method, triple encoding SILAC containing light arginine and lysine (Arg^0 and Lys^0) and two heavy isotopic variants (Arg^{10} and Lys^8 or Arg^6 and Lys^4) can be separately applied to label three groups of HeLa cell material instead of two, thus allowing the comparison of protein enrichments with control beads and different levels (one or two times) of affinity beads containing selected kinase inhibitors in a single pull-down experiment. The three elution fractions are amalgamated and analyzed by quantitative liquid chromatography-MS to identify specific binding partners at full scale with relevant quantitative information. Such results were strengthened through calculating the potency of inhibition values IC$_{50}$ by means of fitting the inhibition curves with different levels of test compounds and extrapolating the individual target binding affinities (K_d) for free kinase inhibitors according to the Cheng–Prusoff equation. To eliminate the false-positive output and verify the reproducibility of binding partners, an inverse experiment must be performed by switching the incubation frequency with affinity beads in heavy (Arg^{10}–Lys^8) and light (Arg^0–Lys^0) labeled lysates.

Isobaric Tags for Relative and Absolute Quantification and Tandem Mass Tags

Reporter ion-based quantification strategies, such as isobaric tags for relative and absolute quantification (iTRAQ)[74] and tandem mass tags (TMTs),[75] have become popular in biological studies. The two most commonly encountered isobaric labeling technologies, iTRAQ and TMTs, allow for multiplexing up to eight samples and six samples, respectively.[76] In these quantification methods, peptides are chemically labeled with isobaric tagging reagents in varying masses.[77] The labeling samples are pooled together, followed by cation exchange fractionation and reversed-phase separation, and are then subjected to MS analysis. Differentiation of the diagnostic mass reporter ions occurs upon label fragmentation in the MS detecting process and is used to obtain quantitative information.

Aberrant protein kinases have been identified as key regulators of signal transduction and are an important class of drug targets in human diseases, particularly in cancer and inflammation. Exploring how kinases interact with kinase inhibitors is thus common in drug discovery. Many small molecule inhibitors have been developed against protein kinases.[78] Immobilized nonselective kinase inhibitors (Kinobeads™) are widely used for tracking the actions of kinase inhibitor drug candidates on treated cells in culture and animals to identify their mechanisms of action and potential side-effects. Kinobeads were created by immobilizing a combination of seven broad-selective kinase inhibitors (including *bis*-(3-indolyl) maleimide, purvalanol B, staurosporine, CZC8004, and analogs of PD173955, sunitinib, and vandetanib) to Sepharose beads through covalent bonds using amino and carboxyl groups. Kinobeads could be a complementary technology for overcoming major bottlenecks in traditional chemoproteomics, such as altered potency and selectivity of the selected SMC due to the modification and immobilization procedures and the biased results toward abundant proteins of low affinity. Kinobeads are also a powerful tool for capturing all members of targeted classes of interest that can be used to measure quantitatively the binding interaction of a compound with more than 300 different kinases at the same time. Up to 200 protein kinases and 600 additional chemically tractable proteins can be identified in Kinobead pull-down assays from any given cell type, indicating that Kinobeads could cover a wide range of protein kinases located on different branches of the kinome tree.

Kinase drug selectivity screens by reporter ion-based quantification strategies have gained attention. Kinobeads in combination with iTRAQ quantification have been reported as a useful chemical proteomics approach to describe the binding of small molecule inhibitors to their targeted protein kinases. Bantscheff et al.[79] detected novel targets of three Abl family kinase inhibitors, including the recently accepted for FDA evaluation drug bosutinib (SKI-606) and the marketed drugs imatinib (Gleeved) and dasatinib (Sprycel®), and determined IC_{50} values in K562 chronic myelogenous leukemia cells. In their studies, cells or cell extracts were exposed to increasing concentrations ranging from 100 pM to 10 μM of the free kinase inhibitor drugs. After immobilization of the drugs, the beads were incubated with lysates of K562 cells to allow protein binding. Due to competition between the free kinase inhibitors and immobilized ligands attached to Kinobeads, special target proteins relevant to the selected inhibitors on the Kinobeads were reduced and quantified by iTRAQ and MS. The obtained data collected from the quantitative iTRAQ method were applied to evaluate the selective profiles and relevant drug–protein affinity parameters, as well as potential downstream effectors of the selected inhibitor drugs. Through this approach, many novel kinase and nonkinase target candidates for all the three selected drugs were proposed. Dasatinib and bosutinib exhibited broad spectrum target profiles with 39 and 53 proteins, respectively. Imatinib showed much more selectivity: 13 proteins exhibited >50% competition on Kinobeads when the drug concentration was at 1 μM in the lysate. Among these target protein candidates of imatinib, except the known primary target proteins Abl/Bcr-Abl and the Abl family kinase Arg, two novel target candidates—the receptor tyrosine kinase DDR1 and the quinone oxidoreductase NQO2—were detected by the quantitative chemical proteomic approach.

Bantscheff et al. reported another similar research strategy, which was adopted to identify potential targets and target complexes of the 16 HDAC inhibitors and their potencies by combining the histone deacetylase (HDAC) probe matrix (capable of capturing class I and class IIb HDACs and the majority of known subunits of HDAC complexes) with quantitative isobaric tandem mass tags (TMTs).[80] The parasite *Trypanosoma brucei* is invariably fatal if left untreated. Parasite protein kinases are attractive drug targets for this disease. Urbaniak and his group[81] employed a Kinobead-based chemoproteomics profiling strategy, enabling the simultaneous assessment of kinase inhibitor potencies against more than 50 endogenously expressed *T. brucei* kinases in parasite cell extracts, which by far exceeds any currently available enzyme panels. A Kinobead-based chemical proteomics approach was also applied to assess the binding capacity of clinical-stage kinase inhibitors for their target protein complexes directly in patient-derived samples. The results pointed toward a positive transcription elongation factor (P-TEFb) complex consisting of four proteins as main targets of BMS-387032 and BTF2/TFIIH complexes as additional targets in chronic lymphoid leukemia (CLL) cells.[82] The Kinobeads approach is generally applicable to chemical proteomics, providing strong support in selectivity profiling of kinase inhibitors.

SYSTEMATIC AND EFFICACIOUS TARGET IDENTIFICATION

In this postgenomic era, advances in the generation and interpretation of chemical proteomics data have spurred expectations of novel targets for anticancer drug discovery. Considering the apparent deficiencies within the chemical proteomics field resulting in high attrition rates for the identified targets in subsequent validation phases, a multitiered systems-level method guided by chemical proteomic technologies is necessary to illuminate novel candidate anticancer targets and shed light on novel therapeutic schedules.

Most cancers feature dysregulation of kinase signaling pathways.[83] Phosphorylation profiling is a promising technique complementary to chemical proteomics via identifying aberrantly activated kinases and their downstream substrates. Haura et al.[84] utilized a renewed integrated system of quantitative phosphoproteomics and targeted chemical proteomics to mine the target proteome and related downstream substrates for dasatinib. Results from such combined experiments indicate that almost 40 direct kinase targets of dasatinib have been identified through the enrichment of dasatinib-containing probe. Quantitative phosphoproteomics was considered to be a versatile tool to evaluate the effects of dasatinib on the kinase phosphorylation sites in multiple lung cancer cell lines. Src family kinases and epidermal growth factor receptor (EGFR) were found to be crucial for dasatinib action by using this combinational approach.[84] Following a similar strategy, Daub's group[85] studied the molecular determinants downstream of the affected signaling cascade underlying the antileukemic effects of erlotinib and gefitinib in acute myeloid leukemia (AML) cells.

Winter et al.[86] extended the range of a systems-level approach by integrating phosphoproteomics, transcriptomics, and chemical proteomics to analyze the underlying mechanisms of the two known kinase inhibitors (bosutinib and danusertib). This work is the first description of a comprehensive dissection of a synergistic drug interaction using three different large-scale omics datasets. Chemical proteomics was committed to profile drug-binding proteomes, and then genome-wide transcriptomics was employed in conjunction with phosphoproteomics to reveal the reduced c-Myc activity as key to the synergistic effect of these two inhibitors. Cho et al.[87] introduced a reintegrated approach encompassing multi-omics-based target identification and validation (MOTIV) and phenotypic screening for characterizing the targets and effectors of bioactive compounds at the organism level. MOTIV provided cross-validation of the myriad candidates resulting from various omics methods; in this system, chemical proteomics or genetics/genomics-based target identification methods were applied to compensate for each other's limitations.

CONCLUSIONS

Developing a new anticancer drug is a complicated, time-consuming task that continues to challenge the pharmaceutical industry. Although over the last decade advances in technology and methodology have accelerated several stages of the anticancer drug discovery process, the efficiency in the production of star molecules in the anticancer field is still unsatisfactory. The difficulty in searching for new targets, the broad capability of the new synthesized compounds beyond that originally anticipated, and the elusive mechanisms of clinical-used reagents have all contributed to the problem. The chemoproteomics approach is gradually gaining acceptance as a potent and promising strategy to circumvent such issues by directly discovering and evaluating the target proteins in an unbiased and comprehensive way. Better integration of other orthogonal omics technologies with MS-based quantitative techniques would not only expand the target proteome but also provide a systems-level understanding of precise pharmacological mechanisms of action of anticarcinogens and downstream effectors of compound-target interactions.

Several research groups are pushing forward in the development and application of chemical proteomics in three ways. The first involves introducing the COPP strategy into intact living cells with the aid of biorthogonal chemistry and cleavable linkers, thus significantly lowing the risk of disrupting signaling complexes in the cell lysis process. The second involves allowing chemical proteomics to reach its full potential as a truly systematic method by drawing on its strengths in combination with other omics technologies. Researchers believe that the integration of information from various omics technologies could provide valuable clues for identifying targets for small molecule anticarcinogens, exploring the related signaling networks, and completing a pharmacological map to obtain deep insights into the intricacies of drug action. The third improvement lies in developing the high-throughput techniques necessary to achieve large-scale target identification.

As chemical proteomics continues to evolve at a rapid pace, it promises to make a significant contribution to more efficient profiling of tumor-promoting molecules and the design of more potent and less toxic anticancer treatments.

References

1. NCI. *Cancer Trends Progress Report – 2011/2012 Update*. Rockville, MD: National Cancer Institute; 2012. (http://progressreport.cancer.gov/).
2. Goodman LS, Wintrobe MM, et al. Nitrogen mustard therapy; use of methyl-*bis* (beta-chloroethyl) amine hydrochloride and *tris* (beta-chloroethyl) amine hydrochloride for Hodgkin's disease, lymphosarcoma, leukemia and certain allied and miscellaneous disorders. JAMA 1946;132:126–32.
3. Nathan DG. The cancer treatment revolution. Trans. Am. Clin. Climatol. Assoc. 2007;118:317–23.
4. Hanahan D, Weinberg RA. Hallmarks of cancer: the next generation. Cell. 2011;144(5):646–74.
5. Cantley LC, et al. AACR cancer progress report 2012. Clin. Cancer Res. 2012;18(21, Suppl.):S1–100.
6. Bantscheff M, Scholten A, Heck AJ. Revealing promiscuous drug-target interactions by chemical proteomics. Drug Discov. Today 2009;14(21-22):1021–9.
7. Raida M. Drug target deconvolution by chemical proteomics. Curr. Opin. Chem. Biol. 2011;15(4):570–5.
8. Shi H, et al. Small molecule microarray-facilitated screening of affinity-based probes (AfBPs) for gamma-secretase. Chem. Commun. (Camb.) 2009;(33):5030–2.
9. Schirle M, Bantscheff M, Kuster B. Mass spectrometry-based proteomics in preclinical drug discovery. Chem. Biol. 2012;19(1):72–84.
10. Hsieh TC, et al. Identification of glutathione sulfotransferase-pi (GSTP1) as a new resveratrol targeting protein (RTP) and studies of resveratrol-responsive protein changes by resveratrol affinity chromatography. Anticancer Res. 2008;28(1A):29–36.
11. Xing C, et al. Identification of GAPDH as a protein target of the saframycin antiproliferative agents. Proc. Natl. Acad. Sci. U.S.A. 2004;101(16):5862–6.
12. Wang Z, et al. Identification and purification of resveratrol targeting proteins using immobilized resveratrol affinity chromatography. Biochem. Biophys. Res. Commun. 2004;323(3):743–9.
13. Uga H, et al. A new mechanism of methotrexate action revealed by target screening with affinity beads. Mol. Pharmacol. 2006;70(5):1832–9.
14. Ito T, Ando H, Handa H. Teratogenic effects of thalidomide: molecular mechanisms. Cell. Mol. Life Sci. 2011;68(9):1569–79.
15. Ito T, et al. Identification of a primary target of thalidomide teratogenicity. Science 2010;327(5971):1345–50.
16. Missner E, et al. Off-target decoding of a multitarget kinase inhibitor by chemical proteomics. Chembiochem 2009;10(7):1163–74.
17. Hoffmann BR, et al. Chemical proteomics-based analysis of off-target binding profiles for rosiglitazone and pioglitazone: clues for assessing potential for cardiotoxicity. J. Med. Chem. 2012;55(19):8260–71.
18. Rix U, Superti-Furga G. Target profiling of small molecules by chemical proteomics. Nat. Chem. Biol. 2009;5(9):616–24.
19. Mondal K, Gupta MN. The affinity concept in bioseparation: evolving paradigms and expanding range of applications. Biomol. Eng. 2006;23(2-3):59–76.
20. Guiffant D, et al. Identification of intracellular targets of small molecular weight chemical compounds using affinity chromatography. Biotechnol. J. 2007;2(1):68–75.
21. Taunton J, Hassig CA, Schreiber SL. A mammalian histone deacetylase related to the yeast transcriptional regulator Rpd3p. Science 1996;272(5260):408–11.
22. Fleischer TC, et al. Chemical proteomics identifies Nampt as the target of CB30865, an orphan cytotoxic compound. Chem. Biol. 2010;17(6):659–64.
23. Wang G, et al. Diazonamide toxins reveal an unexpected function for ornithine delta-amino transferase in mitotic cell division. Proc. Natl. Acad. Sci. U.S.A. 2007;104(7):2068–73.
24. Li CY, et al. Oridonin: an active diterpenoid targeting cell cycle arrest, apoptotic and autophagic pathways for cancer therapeutics. Int. J. Biochem. Cell. Biol. 2011;43(5):701–4.
25. Dal Piaz F, et al. Chemical proteomics reveals HSP70 1A as a target for the anticancer diterpene oridonin in Jurkat cells. J. Proteomics. 2013;82:14–26.
26. Lomenick B, Olsen RW, Huang J. Identification of direct protein targets of small molecules. ACS Chem. Biol. 2011;6(1):34–46.
27. Hofstee BH. Immobilization of enzymes through non-covalent binding to substituted agaroses. Biochem. Biophys. Res. Commun. 1973;53(4):1137–44.

28. Margarucci L, et al. Chemical proteomics discloses petrosapongiolide M, an antiinflammatory marine sesterterpene, as a proteasome inhibitor. Angew. Chem. Int. Ed. Engl. 2010;49(23):3960–3.

29. Kuramori C, et al. Capsaicin binds to prohibitin 2 and displaces it from the mitochondria to the nucleus. Biochem. Biophys. Res. Commun. 2009;379(2):519–25.

30. Sakamoto S, et al. Development and application of high-performance affinity beads: toward chemical biology and drug discovery. Chem. Rec. 2009;9(1):66–85.

31. Kuramochi K, et al. Identification of small molecule binding molecules by affinity purification using a specific ligand immobilized on PEGA resin. Bioconjug. Chem. 2008;19(12):2417–26.

32. von Rechenberg M, et al. Ampicillin/penicillin-binding protein interactions as a model drug-target system to optimize affinity pull-down and mass spectrometric strategies for target and pathway identification. Proteomics 2005;5(7):1764–73.

33. Tamura T, Terada T, Tanaka A. A quantitative analysis and chemical approach for the reduction of nonspecific binding proteins on affinity resins. Bioconjug. Chem. 2003;14(6):1222–30.

34. Shimizu N, et al. High-performance affinity beads for identifying drug receptors. Nat. Biotechnol. 2000;18(8): 877–81.

35. Takahashi T, et al. Development of chemically stable solid phases for the target isolation with reduced nonspecific binding proteins. Bioorg. Med. Chem. Lett. 2006;16(2):447–50.

36. Mori T, et al. An easy preparation of "monolithic type" hydrophilic solid phase: capability for affinity resin to isolate target proteins. Bioorg. Med. Chem. 2006;14(16):5549–54.

37. Iwaoka E, et al. Improvement of monolithic solid material by utilization of spacer for identification of the target using affinity resins. Bioorg. Med. Chem. Lett. 2009;19(5):1469–72.

38. Yang Y, et al. A simple and effective cleavable linker for chemical proteomics applications. Mol. Cell. Proteomics 2013;12(1):237–44.

39. Trinkle-Mulcahy L, et al. Identifying specific protein interaction partners using quantitative mass spectrometry and bead proteomes. J. Cell Biol. 2008;183(2):223–39.

40. Garcia J, et al. Synthesis of deguelin-biotin conjugates and investigation into deguelin's interactions. Bioorg. Med. Chem. 2012;20(2):672–80.

41. Saxena C, et al. An immuno-chemo-proteomics method for drug target deconvolution. J. Proteome Res. 2008;7(8):3490–7.

42. Saxena C, et al. Capture of drug targets from live cells using a multipurpose immuno-chemo-proteomics tool. J. Proteome Res. 2009;8(8):3951–7.

43. Wang Z, et al. Identification and purification of resveratrol targeting proteins using immobilized resveratrol affinity chromatography. Biochem. Biophys. Res. Commun. 2004;323(3):743–9.

44. Yamamoto K, et al. A versatile method of identifying specific binding proteins on affinity resins. Anal. Biochem. 2006;352(1):15–23.

45. Burkard TR, et al. Initial characterization of the human central proteome. BMC Syst. Biol. 2011;5:17.

46. Shoemaker BA, Panchenko AR. Deciphering protein-protein interactions. Part I. Experimental techniques and databases. PLoS Comput. Biol. 2007;3(3):e42.

47. Baruch A, Jeffery DA, Bogyo M. Enzyme activity—it's all about image. Trends Cell Biol. 2004;14(1):29–35.

48. Hu L, et al. Identification of drug targets *in vitro* and in living cells by soluble-nanopolymer-based proteomics. Angew. Chem. Int. Ed. Engl. 2011;50(18):4133–6.

49. Vargas AJ, Burd R. Hormesis and synergy: pathways and mechanisms of quercetin in cancer prevention and management. Nutr. Rev. 2010;68(7):418–28.

50. Murakami A, Ashida H, Terao J. Multitargeted cancer prevention by quercetin. Cancer Lett. 2008;269(2):315–25.

51. Boots AW, Haenen GR, Bast A. Health effects of quercetin: from antioxidant to nutraceutical. Eur. J. Pharmacol. 2008;585(2-3):325–37.

52. Fahlman BM, Krol ES. UVA and UVB radiation-induced oxidation products of quercetin. J. Photochem. Photobiol. B 2009;97(3):123–31.

53. Wang RE, et al. Biotinylated quercetin as an intrinsic photoaffinity proteomics probe for the identification of quercetin target proteins. Bioorg. Med. Chem. 2011;19(16):4710–20.

54. Sakai Y, et al. GEX1 compounds, novel antitumor antibiotics related to herboxidiene, produced by *Streptomyces* sp. I. Taxonomy, production, isolation, physicochemical properties and biological activities. J. Antibiot. (Tokyo) 2002;55(10):855–62.

55. Sakai Y, et al. GEX1 compounds, novel antitumor antibiotics related to herboxidiene, produced by *Streptomyces* sp. II. The effects on cell cycle progression and gene expression. J. Antibiot. (Tokyo) 2002;55(10):863–72.

56. Hasegawa M, et al. Identification of SAP155 as the target of GEX1A (Herboxidiene), an antitumor natural product. ACS Chem. Biol. 2011;6(3):229–33.

57. Rana S, Cho JW. Functionalization of carbon nanotubes via Cu(I)-catalyzed Huisgen [3+2] cycloaddition "click chemistry.". Nanoscale 2010;2(12):2550–6.

58. Hoyle CE, Lowe AB, Bowman CN. Thiol-click chemistry: a multifaceted toolbox for small molecule and polymer synthesis. Chem. Soc. Rev. 2010;39(4):1355–87.

59. El-Sagheer AH, Brown T. Click chemistry with DNA. Chem. Soc. Rev. 2010;39(4):1388–405.

60. Decreau RA, Collman JP, Hosseini A. Electrochemical applications. How click chemistry brought biomimetic models to the next level: electrocatalysis under controlled rate of electron transfer. Chem. Soc. Rev. 2010;39(4):1291–301.

61. Hein CD, Liu XM, Wang D. Click chemistry, a powerful tool for pharmaceutical sciences. Pharm. Res. 2008;25(10):2216–30.

62. Ban HS, et al. Identification of HSP60 as a primary target of *o*-carboranylphenoxyacetanilide, an HIF-1alpha inhibitor. J. Am. Chem. Soc. 2010;132(34):11870–1.

63. Shimizu K, et al. Boron-containing phenoxyacetanilide derivatives as hypoxia-inducible factor (HIF)-1alpha inhibitors. Bioorg. Med. Chem. Lett. 2010;20(4):1453–6.

64. Shi H, et al. Cell-based proteome profiling of potential dasatinib targets by use of affinity-based probes. J. Am. Chem. Soc. 2012;134(6):3001–14.

65. Gygi SP, et al. Quantitative analysis of complex protein mixtures using isotope-coded affinity tags. Nat. Biotechnol. 1999;17(10):994–9.

66. Tao WA, Aebersold R. Advances in quantitative proteomics via stable isotope tagging and mass spectrometry. Curr. Opin. Biotechnol. 2003;14(1):110–8.

67. Oda Y, et al. Quantitative chemical proteomics for identifying candidate drug targets. Anal. Chem. 2003;75(9):2159–65.

68. Tsukahara K, et al. Anticancer agent E7070 inhibits amino acid and uracil transport in fission yeast. Mol. Pharmacol. 2001;60(6):1254–9.

69. Ozawa Y, et al. Therapeutic potential and molecular mechanism of a novel sulfonamide anticancer drug, indisulam (E7070) in combination with CPT-11 for cancer treatment. Cancer Chemother. Pharmacol. 2012;69(5): 1353–62.

70. Ong SE, et al. Stable isotope labeling by amino acids in cell culture, SILAC, as a simple and accurate approach to expression proteomics. Mol. Cell. Proteomics. 2002;1(5):376–86.

71. Ong SE, Mann M. A practical recipe for stable isotope labeling by amino acids in cell culture (SILAC). Nat. Protoc. 2006;1(6):2650–60.

72. Ong SE, et al. Identifying the proteins to which small-molecule probes and drugs bind in cells. Proc. Natl. Acad. Sci. U.S.A. 2009;106(12):4617–22.

73. Sharma K, et al. Proteomics strategy for quantitative protein interaction profiling in cell extracts. Nat. Methods. 2009;6(10):741–4.

74. Ross PL, et al. Multiplexed protein quantitation in *Saccharomyces cerevisiae* using amine-reactive isobaric tagging reagents. Mol. Cell. Proteomics 2004;3(12):1154–69.

75. Thompson A, et al. Tandem mass tags: a novel quantification strategy for comparative analysis of complex protein mixtures by MS/MS. Anal. Chem. 2003;75(8):1895–904.

76. Breitwieser FP, et al. General statistical modeling of data from protein relative expression isobaric tags. J. Proteome Res. 2011;10(6):2758–66.

77. Vaudel M, et al. Integral quantification accuracy estimation for reporter ion-based quantitative proteomics (iQuARI). J. Proteome Res. 2012;11(10):5072–80.

78. Lemeer S, et al. Comparing immobilized kinase inhibitors and covalent ATP probes for proteomic profiling of kinase expression and drug selectivity. J. Proteome Res. 2013;12(4):1723–31.

79. Bantscheff M, et al. Quantitative chemical proteomics reveals mechanisms of action of clinical ABL kinase inhibitors. Nat. Biotechnol. 2007;25(9):1035–44.

80. Bantscheff M, et al. Chemoproteomics profiling of HDAC inhibitors reveals selective targeting of HDAC complexes. Nat. Biotechnol. 2011;29(3):255–65.

81. Urbaniak MD, et al. Chemical proteomic analysis reveals the drugability of the kinome of *Trypanosoma brucei*. ACS Chem. Biol. 2012;7(11):1858–65.
82. Kruse U, et al. Chemoproteomics-based kinome profiling and target deconvolution of clinical multi-kinase inhibitors in primary chronic lymphocytic leukemia cells. Leukemia. 2011;25(1):89–100.
83. Harsha HC, Pandey A. Phosphoproteomics in cancer. Mol. Oncol. 2010;4(6):482–95.
84. Li J, et al. A chemical and phosphoproteomic characterization of dasatinib action in lung cancer. Nat. Chem. Biol. 2010;6(4):291–9.
85. Weber C, Schreiber TB, Daub H. Dual phosphoproteomics and chemical proteomics analysis of erlotinib and gefitinib interference in acute myeloid leukemia cells. J. Proteomics. 2012;75(4):1343–56.
86. Winter GE, et al. Systems-pharmacology dissection of a drug synergy in imatinib-resistant CML. Nat. Chem. Biol. 2012;8(11):905–12.
87. Cho YS, Kwon HJ. Identification and validation of bioactive small molecule target through phenotypic screening. Bioorg. Med. Chem. 2012;20(6):1922–8.

Cancer Vaccines

Teresa Ramirez-Montagut

Genomics Institute of the Novartis Research Foundation, San Diego, CA, USA

INTRODUCTION

The premise for cancer immunotherapy is the notion that the immune system is able to recognize and reject cancerous tissue. Cancer immunity exists because the immune system's repertoire contains immune cells that, when properly activated, will kill malignant cells. Immune recognition of tumor cells is driven by the expression of unaltered, altered, or mutated self-antigens. Cancer antigens can be divided in four broad types: unique antigens, germ-cell antigens, differentiation antigens, and overexpressed antigens.

Unique tumor antigens are generated upon mutations in genes that create new gene products with or without altered function. Mutations that confer a selective growth advantage to the tumor cell are called *driver* mutations, and mutations that have no effect on the neoplastic process are defined as *passenger* mutations. In the context of immune recognition, the functionality of the mutations is not as relevant as the presentation of these neoantigens to the immune system. Alterations in mutated/altered self presented in the context of a human leukocyte antigen (HLA) protein will make the mutations visible to the immune system. It has

Novel Approaches and Strategies for Biologics, Vaccines and Cancer Therapies. DOI: 10.1016/B978-0-12-416603-5.00015-8

been estimated that a typical breast or colorectal cancer contains 7 to 10 mutations that can be presented in an individual patient's HLA type.[1] Recent experimental data have indicated that, indeed, many somatic mutations in tumors are recognized by the immune system.[2] Considering that common solid tumors including colon, breast, brain, and pancreas present an average of 33 to 66 somatic mutations,[3] the potential for the immune system to recognize tumor-restricted neoantigens is significant.

Germ-cell antigens, or cancer-testis (CT) antigens, are normally expressed in male germ cells and are silenced in healthy somatic cells but are re-expressed in certain cancers. CT antigens were initially identified in melanoma cells but are also expressed broadly in other cancer types. The first human cancer antigen recognized by CD8+ cytotoxic T-cell lymphocytes (CTLs) was the melanoma antigen MAGE-1.[4] The cellular strategy utilized for the identification of MAGE-1 (MAGE-A1) led to the discovery of other CT genes, including MAGE-A2, MAGE-A3, BAGE, and GAGE.[5–8] Subsequently, development of a serological analysis of tumor cDNA expression libraries (SEREX) with patient-derived sera enabled the discovery of other novel and highly immunogenic antigens members of the CT family, including New York esophageal squamous cell carcinoma 1 (NY-ESO-1).[9] Since then, different techniques have been used to identify more CT antigens, and the list has expanded to at least 70 families containing over 140 different members. The highly restricted expression of CT antigens exclusively at adult tumor tissues (excluding testis and placenta, both sites of immune privilege), together with their strong immunogenicity in human patients, identifies these antigens as ideal targets for cancer vaccine strategies.

The third category, the *differentiation antigens*, are entities expressed both in tumor cells and in their normal cellular counterparts. These antigens define a cell lineage and distinct stages of differentiation within a lineage. Differentiation antigens were initially described in melanoma where proteins in the pigmentation pathway—namely, TYRP-1/gp75 (mouse *brown* locus), tyrosinase (*albino* locus), gp100/pMEL17 (*silver* locus), TYRP-2 (*slaty* locus), and Melan-A/MART-1—that are expressed at different stages of melanocyte/melanoma differentiation, were recognized by patients' immune systems. Although differentiation antigens are the most frequent tumor antigens recognized by antibodies and T cells,[10] their expression is not restricted exclusively to the tumor tissue; therefore, immunotherapies may induce autoimmunity. Evidence in the literature indicates that development of autoimmunity in patients with malignant melanoma has been linked to tumor regression following interleukin-2 (IL-2), interferon alpha (IFNα), or blocking antibodies to cytotoxic T-lymphocyte antigen 4 (CTLA-4).[11–16] In particular, the development of vitiligo in melanoma patients is associated with better prognosis and when associated with therapy predicts objective response to the treatment.[17–19]

Overexpressed antigens, the fourth group of cancer antigens, are proteins with low levels of expression in normal tissues but which are overexpressed in tumor tissues and may be immunogenic if presented to the immune system. More than 30 genes have been found to be overexpressed in various cancers, and some have been demonstrated to be recognized by the immune system, including EPHA3, ERBB2, PRAME, BIRC5, and TERT.

As the understanding of the field develops, the definition of an "ideal" tumor antigen has evolved from only tumor-specific, to the inclusion of non-tumor-specific targets. Moreover, in an effort to understand the clinical relevance of cancer antigens, the U.S. National Cancer Institute (NCI), through a panel of members from academia, industry, and government, convened a project to prioritize a list of "ideal" cancer antigens. Utilizing an analytic hierarchy process based on pre-identified criteria and weighted by a panel of experts, Cheever and colleagues[20] constructed a priority-ranked list of 75 cancer antigens. The major criteria for formulating this ranking included the following:

1. Evidence of antitumor activity from human clinical trials
2. Evidence of immune responses *in vivo* or elicited as a results of immunization
3. Role of the antigen in the oncogenic process to assess the possibility of antigen-loss variants
4. Specificity of the antigen expression to tumor cells
5. Frequency of antigen expression in tumor cells
6. Antigen expression in cancer stem cells
7. Frequency of patients with antigen-positive tumors
8. Number of potential antigenic epitopes
9. Surface expression of the antigen.

The authors concluded that none of the 75 antigens had all of the characteristics of an "ideal" cancer antigen. Forty-six antigens had documented immunogenicity in clinical trials, and 20 had suggestive clinical efficacy in the therapeutic function category, with documented vaccine-induced clinical responses in at least a small number of patients or suggestive evidence of benefit versus controls. The pilot prioritization project focuses on known and well-studied candidate antigens and does not include recently identified cancer antigens. Moreover, the work in antigen identification is continuing; therefore, future ranking may be modified based on the results of investigations currently in progress.[21] For example, sipuleucel-T, a vaccine that targets PAP ranked 26th in the predefined and preweighted criteria, indicating that the characteristics of an ideal cancer vaccine antigen are not completely understood. However, the NCI investigators attribute the limited efficacy of cancer vaccines to immunologic tolerance and the inability of robust activation and expansion of effector cells. More active vaccine formulations and/or combinations of vaccine strategies with immunomodulator agents may circumvent tolerance, tumor-induced immune suppression, and lack of activation.

LIMITED POTENCY OF CANCER VACCINES

It is generally believed that for a cancer vaccine to be optimally efficacious it must generate antigen-specific CD8$^+$ CTLs, which require cytokines produced by antigen-specific CD4$^+$ helper cells 1 (Th1). Generation of memory CTL responses against a self-antigen is challenging, and, although CTLs may be generated efficiently and be detected in peripheral blood, these cells may encounter a local tumor immunosuppressive environment which may inhibit effective killing of the tumor cells. Many active immunosuppressive cell types have been described to be present at the tumor microenvironment, including Treg, MDSC, TAMs/M2 macrophages, and Bregs. A second mechanism of immune evasion induced directly by the tumor cells has also been described, and it includes soluble factors (e.g., IL-10, TGFβ, VEGF) and membrane-bound negative regulators such as B7 family members (i.e., PD-L1, VTCN1, and B7-H3), tumor necrosis factor receptor (TNFR) and receptor ligands (i.e., HVEM and LIGHT[22]), carbohydrate-binding proteins (i.e., galectin-1, galectin-3, and galectin-9), and various enzymes (e.g., enzymes IDO, TDO, iNOS) whose products block T-cell responses. Therefore, progress in the cancer vaccination field resides in developing novel and more potent vaccine adjuvants that generate CTLs capable of overcoming systemic and local suppressive mechanisms. Additionally, identifying rational clinical combinations with other therapies including standard-of-care chemotherapeutics, targeted therapies, and novel immunomodulators that will generate a more permissive environment for immune-mediated rejection may be of paramount importance for positive clinical outcomes.

VACCINE PLATFORMS

Current vaccine platforms include many different modalities from cellular products, viral vectors, proteins, and peptides of different sizes. Each strategy has specific advantages and disadvantages.[23] However, it is expected that platforms with a multiprong approach, where a vaccine platform activates several effector arms of the immune system and not exclusively CD8 T cells, may be more efficacious. For example, vaccination strategies that stimulate T cells (both CD4 and CD8) will generate long-lasting immunity, and vaccination strategies that also recruit B-cell activation may prove more efficacious because antigen–antibody (Ab) complexes will help in antigen cross-presentation and CTL maintenance.

Peptide Vaccines

Vaccines based on peptides that exclusively target CD8 T cells are usually administered with an adjuvant and/or with an immunomoudulator. This strategy assumes that strong adjuvanticity will bypass the requirement for CD4 help. However, clinical trials have demonstrated that repeated peptide vaccination with a strong adjuvant has failed to induce sustained antigen-specific CD8 T cells.[24] Despite the setbacks, a few trials assessing the efficacy of peptides have reported consistent rates of objective, long-term clinical responses.[25–29] These peptide vaccines with better clinical outcomes tend to incorporate either longer peptides that include epitopes for CD4 activation or pooled peptides specific for both CD4 and CD8 T cells.[28,30]

Recombinant Proteins

Vaccine platforms that include a whole antigen will present both MHC class I and class II epitopes to CD8 and CD4 cells, respectively, and will have the potential of also generating antibody responses. However, there is a significant challenge in generating CTL responses when an antigen is delivered exogenously rather than delivered to the cytoplasm of the target cells. The process of delivering an exogenous antigen with the ultimate goal of having CTL activation is called *cross-presentation*. Activation of CTLs in peripheral tissues is limited to presentation of intracellular peptides on MHC class I. This activation is typically exemplified as an antiviral response—that is, when viral proteins derived from the intracellular compartments of the infected cells are processed and presented on MHC class I molecules, CTL surveying peptides presented on class I will identify a foreign epitope and kill the infected cell. The capture of an extracellular protein and presentation of peptides derived from it onto MHC class I is a task that exclusively antigen-presenting cells (APCs) can accomplish. The role of APCs in activation of the immune system and CTL induction is to survey and capture pathogens, phagocytose infected cells and cancerous cells, and then process and present these extracellular entities onto MHC class I and class II molecules.

The challenge for cancer immunotherapies is providing a soluble recombinant protein in a manner that stimulates APCs to present the exogenous protein in the context of a class I molecule (cross-presentation). Stimulation of APCs to cross-present antigen to CTLs depends on the adjuvant utilized. There are only two adjuvants in clinical use in the United States: aluminum salts (alum), which have been employed as a human vaccine adjuvant for eight decades, and the Adjuvant System 04 (AS04),[31] which has been approved for clinical use and consists of alum with monophosphoryl lipid A (MPLA), a derivative of lipopolysaccharide that signals through the activation of toll-like receptor 4 (TLR4). Aluminum adjuvants were thought to activate the immune response by acting as an antigen depot, and only recently has it been demonstrated that regulation of immune signals triggered by alum requires the activation of intracellular innate immune responses and the Nalp3 inflammasome.[32] In human vaccines, alum adjuvants are weak in their capacity to induce cross-presentation of recombinant protein antigens, resulting in a lack of generation of CTL responses and primarily inducing CD4 help for development of strong humoral immunity (CD4 Th2 help). Incorporation of MPLA to the alum adjuvant, as in the case of AS04, has demonstrated a significant increase of humoral and memory B-cell immunity in humans vaccinated with HPV16/18 virus-like particles compared to the aluminum salt only.[33] How aluminum adjuvants initiate immune responses that favor Th2 and humoral immunity as opposed to Th1 and CTL responses remains unresolved.

The finding that the addition of TLR4 signaling mediated by MPLA enhanced immune responses has led to the search for stronger adjuvants for cancer vaccination that necessitate strong CTL responses for tumor rejection. Mixtures of MPLA with other agents including various TLR agonists have been tested in clinical trials with some success. AS02B contains MPLA and QS21, a saponin extracted from the South American tree *Quillaja saponaria Molina*, and was used to vaccinate non-small-cell lung cancer (NSCLC) patients against the CT antigen MAGE-A3. Patients with resected IB-IIIA NSCLC vaccinated with AS02B/MAGE-A3 in a multicenter, double-blind, randomized, placebo-controlled Phase II trial exhibited prolonged disease free-survival rates.[34,35] A more complex mixture, AS15, which includes MPLA, QS21, TLR9 agonist deoxycytidyl-deoxyguanosin oligodeoxynucleotides (CpG ODNs), and liposomes, has been compared to AS02B in clinical trials. A randomized Phase II trial in which patients with unresectable metastatic melanoma were vaccinated with MAGE-A3 adjuvanted with either AS02B or AS15 showed that AS15 yielded higher immunological and clinical responses compared to AS02B.[36] Based on the results of this trial, large, double-blind, Phase III clinical trials testing MAGE/AS15 in patients with stage IB–IIIA resected NSCLC (MAGRIT trial)[37] or in patients with advanced melanoma (DERMA trial) were initiated and are in progress. In Europe, the first oil-in-water adjuvant, MF59, was approved in Italy in 1997 for use in influenza vaccines and is now licensed in 30 countries.[38] Comparison of MF59 with alum-based vaccinations indicates that MF59 induces superior titers and broader Ab profiles in both mouse models[39] and human trials,[40] and its U.S. licensure is expected in the coming years.

Tumor Cell Vaccines

Whole cell cancer vaccines represent one form of active cancer immunotherapy undergoing clinical development. This approach is based on the rationale that tumor cells will contain proteins expressed in the patient's cancer lesions and will provide multiple tumor antigens for immune recognition. Vaccine platforms based on autologous tumor cells have proven difficult to produce because harvesting patient-specific tumor cells is technically challenging and can be financially costly and time consuming.[41] An alternative has been the utilization of cell lines as an allogeneic vaccination strategy where it is expected that the patient's tumor shares antigens express by the cell lines that will induce immune recognition. Whole cell vaccines are rendered more immunogenic when the tumor cells are genetically modified to express cytokines, chemokines, or costimulatory molecules for immune stimulation. Historically, one cytokine, granulocyte–macrophage colony-stimulation factor (GM-CSF), was found to be superior in the induction of immune responses when compared to other cytokines tested.[42] The GM-CSF-secreting whole tumor cell vaccine recruits dendritic cells (DCs) to the site of injection and stimulates antigen uptake, processing, and cross-presentation to CD8 CTLs.[43] A recent analysis of studies published in the last 10 to 15 years of clinical experience with gene-modified whole cell vaccines concluded that this strategy lacked sufficient evidence for efficacy in inducing both a strong immune response and a therapeutic response.[44]

Dendritic Cells and Antigen-Presenting Cells

Vaccination strategies targeting APCs have been mostly limited to utilizing DCs as a vaccination platform. The special properties of these cells in coordinating innate and adaptive immunity are used to initiating antitumor immune responses. The earliest studies began in 1993 and utilized whole blood leukapheresis products with enrichment procedures to isolate rare immature DC precursors before antigen loading and maturation.[45] Due to low yield in DC procurement, clinical development was initially limited. Subsequently, few clinical studies assessed the generation of DCs from $CD34^+$ hematopoietic progenitors in the presence of GM-CSF and tumor necrosis factor alpha (TNFα).[46–49] Currently, the preferred and generally accepted method of generating DCs is from $CD14^+$ peripheral blood monocytes, as large numbers are obtained without the necessity for pretreatment of donors with cytokines to mobilize precursors. The combination of GM-CSF with IL-4 is a well-established combination to most efficiently induce immature DCs (imDCs) from monocytes. Adequate activation and maturation of DCs is required because imDCs are no longer considered competent candidates for vaccination trials due to low potential for Th1 polarized responses and CTL induction.[50–52] The "gold standard" cocktail of cytokines to induce DC maturation was first proposed by Jonuleit et al.[53] and included IL-1β, IL-6, TNFα, and PGE$_2$. Maturation induced with this combination has consistently induced superior T-cell priming compared to imDCs; however, the use of PGE$_2$ remains controversial. Although PGE$_2$ increases expression of CCR7 necessary for migration of DC into the lymph nodes to prime T-cell responses, it also inhibits IL-12p70 secretion necessary for adequate CTL induction. Since then, several cytokine cocktails have been proposed indicating that the "ideal" maturation mix is yet to be defined.

Although an impressive amount of information has been obtained from clinical trials completed thus far, the outcome has not delivered results aligned with the initial expectations. It has gradually become clear that DCs are a heterogeneous population, with the first distinction being whether the origin is either plasmocytoid and myeloid or conventional. Plasmocytoid DCs (pDCs) are capable of secreting large amounts of type I interferons (IFNs) in response to viral and autologous nucleic acids. Conversely, conventional DCs (cDCs) recognize bacterial components and produce proinflammatory cytokines, Th1/Th17 CD4 T cells, and induction of CTL responses. Recently, several groups have identified a unique myeloid human DC subset that produces high levels of bioactive IL-12p70 and has a superior capacity for antigen cross-presentation. CD11c+ BDCA-3+ DCs are homologous to mouse CD8a+ DCs and are well accepted as a unique DC subset that effectively activates CTL responses.[54–56] The potential key role for the myeloid BDCA-3+ DC subset in immunity to viruses and robust CTL generation may have important implications in the design of human DC vaccines. The first cancer vaccine approved by the Food and Drug Administration (FDA) in the United States is Dendreon's Provenge® (also known as sipuleucel-T). The strategy is based on an enriched cellular product manufactured from autologous APC-containing peripheral blood mononuclear cells (PBMCs) obtained from leukapheresis that are co-cultured with a recombinant fusion protein of human prostatic acid phosphatase (PAP)–GM-CSF prior to reinfusion into the patient. Phase III clinical trials demonstrated approximately 4.1 months in median overall survival (OS) in castration-resistant prostate cancer patients treated with the vaccine.[57] Of note, Provenge is comprised of multiple types of mononuclear cells, including APCs, CD4, CD8, natural killer (NK), and B cells, and was introduced in the U.S. market with a regimen of three infusions given over one month. However, the company has faced several hurdles, including significant investment required to overcome considerable development costs and launching numerous FDA-certified centers across the U.S. for production.

Recombinant Vectors

Genetic engineering has led to the exploitation of viruses, which are intrinsically immunogenic pathogens, as vectors for delivering non-immunogenic antigens. These vaccine platforms have been modified to express cancer antigens and are aimed at intramuscular or subcutaneous delivery. Most modifications have focused on members of the Adenoviridae, Poxviridae, and Herpesviridae families. Early attempts at vaccination with adenovirus used replication-incompetent variants of the serotypes Ad2 and Ad5. However, most humans have preexisting immunity against these viruses, which explains the small therapeutic benefit observed clinically.[58–60] Poxviruses have broad cell tropism and are highly immunogenic, and preexisting immunity is present only in patients who received the smallpox vaccine. Initial studies that tested the clinical activity of vaccinia virus, fowlpox virus, and canarypox virus demonstrated weak induction of T-cell and B-cell responses,[61,62] including the preferred vaccine strategy, the modified vaccinia Ankara (MVA), which demonstrated limited clinical activity when encoding the 5T4 antigen in a Phase III trial.[63] It has been speculated that its low efficacy may be due to its limited replication in primary human cells.

These vectors have been further modified to increase their potency by coexpressing costimulatory molecules necessary for T-cell activation. Thus far, the most promising strategy is the TRIACOM platform, which encodes a triad of costimulatory molecules (B7.1, ICAM-1, and LFA3) in poxviruses. PROSTVAC-VF includes vaccinia and fowlpox viruses encoding TRIACOM and prostate-specific antigen (PSA) and is administered in a prime-boost approach (i.e., vaccinia-prime and fowlpox-boost). This vaccine demonstrated an increase in median OS in a Phase II clinical trial but failed to improve progression-free survival (PFS); however, an ongoing Phase III trial will provide more insight into current levels of efficacy. A similar approach is being tested in pancreatic cancer, where the virus vectors encode one antigen, either carcinoembryonic antigen (CEA) or MUC1, alongside TRIACOM costimulatory genes. Although this platform was unable to demonstrate increased survival in Phase III trials, recent studies provide evidence of survival benefit in a particular patient subgroup.[64] A different strategy to increase efficacy has been the incorporation of IL-2 alongside the cancer antigen. The TG4010 vaccine is a MVA vector encoding MUC1 and IL-2 that was tested in a Phase IIB study as an adjunct to conventional chemotherapy and demonstrated some increase in PFS.[65] Given the lack of robust efficacy but promising results with these viral vectors, it has been postulated that the use of recombinant vectors delivered directly to the tumor site may enhance antitumor immunity. In pilot experiments, injection of recombinant vaccinia virus (rVV) encoding TRIACOM at the tumor site induced clinical responses in ~30% of patients.[66] This strategy is now expanded to include intratumoral delivery of rVV encoding PSA and TRIACOM.

Other vectors currently under development include platforms that deliver antigen encoded in *Listeria*,[67] *Salmonella*,[68] and alpha viruses such as the Venezuelan equine encephalitis (VEE) virus,[69] which are attractive vectors for cancer vaccination because once the cells are infected the virus replicates its RNA in the cytoplasm and expresses high levels of transgenes.

LIMITED CLINICAL EFFICACY OF CANCER VACCINES

One of the hurdles of cancer vaccination is the notion that preclinical model systems are poor at translating or predicting clinical efficacy. Careful consideration of the literature makes evident that preclinical models lack rigor in (1) modeling self-tolerance, (2) assessing the efficacy of immunotherapies as therapeutic agents rather than prophylactic settings, and (3) determining the compatibility of standard-of-care with immunomodulation. Even when cancer vaccines have progressed into Phase I and Phase II clinical trials, essentially all but one have failed to achieve FDA approval. In 2007, Finke et al.[70] performed a thorough analysis of cancer vaccines that demonstrated promising Phase II trials but eventually failed the Phase III trials. Relevant to clinical trial design, the authors indicated that (1) patients were not stratified appropriately and the heterogeneity of the studied cancers may have masked efficacy in certain subgroups, (2) utilization of historical data instead of randomized controls may underestimate the actual survival outcomes of prospective studies due to baseline shift, (3) time to establish an effective immune response may exceed the observation period, and (4) studies may have been underpowered due to late separation of the curves (late separation of time-to-event curves) and the assumption that the hazard ratio applies immediately after randomization. Similarly, Wolchock et al.[71] assessed the kinetics of clinical responses in cancer immunotherapies and determined that the clinical effects may be present past 12 weeks from therapy initiation. It was noted that patients with an early increase in tumor burden may not necessarily signify tumor progression, and the authors hypothesized that it may signify lymphocytic infiltration. Additionally, it was observed that clinical benefit was possible even under the appearance of new lesions. Based on these observations and in an attempt to capture all observed response patterns, a new "immune-related" RECIST criteria (irRC) has been proposed.[72] The novelty of the irRC lies in the measurement of new lesions, which are included in the overall tumor burden, allowing for the levels of tumor burden to be described as a continuous variable (before and after conventional progression).

Given that patients with heavy tumor burden may be immunocompromised as a result of their underlying disease, it has been postulated that patients with lower tumor burden, fewer metastasis, and superior overall health may be better candidates for mounting an effective and durable immune response to active cancer immunotherapy. Recognizing that cancer vaccines may be more effective if administered to patients with minimal residual disease, several investigators are conducting trials in the adjuvant setting. Moreover, increasing data support the concept of vaccination patients with biologically less aggressive disease or at earlier stages of disease.[73] For example, prostate cancer is indolent; therefore, a vaccine such as Provenge may be successful in a metastatic setting. Conversely, a similar approach may not be successful in metastatic pancreatic cancer, which is biologically more aggressive. For patients with aggressive malignancies, it may be more critical to vaccinate in the adjuvant setting or to investigate strategies of immunotherapy in combination with other therapies. Of importance, these clinical experiences have culminated in new recommendations and a new paradigm in clinical trial design,[74] as well as new immune-related response criteria.[71] Recently, the FDA issued its Guidance for Industry–Clinical Considerations for Therapeutic Cancer Vaccines.

Several fundamental challenges remain in the clinical development of cancer vaccines. Phase I and II studies have stumbled on two crucial issues: inadequate monitoring of immune responses and lack of reliable biomarkers to define correlates. An effort to harmonize several immunological methods has been applied to ELISPOT analysis,[75] tetramer analysis,[76] and intracellular cytokine analysis by flow cytometry-based assays.[77] Furthermore, it has been proposed that guidelines for minimal information about T-cell assays (MIATA) be followed to improve data reporting and adequate interpretation of immune monitoring.[78–80] Oncology drug developers are increasingly required to consider the use of different biomarkers in development of targeted therapies. The FDA Critical Path initiative, which was launched in 2004, has proposed this paradigm, but according to data obtained recently only 3% of clinical trials had incorporated a novel biomarker of efficacy into their clinical trial design, and there continues to be significant delays with development of diagnostic companion tests.

In 2009, the U.S.–Japan Workshop on Immunological Biomarkers in Oncology was held.[81] The objective was to identify strategies for biomarker discovery and validation in the field of biotherapy of cancer. The primary goal of the workshop was to define the status of the science in biomarker discovery by identifying emerging concepts in human tumor immune biology that could predict responsiveness to immunotherapy and/or explain its mechanisms. Examples of predictive biomarkers (those that will predict immunotherapy efficacy), prognostic biomarkers (those that will assess disease progression independent of therapy and are used in patient stratification according to likelihood of survival), and mechanistic biomarkers (those that will provide a mechanistic explanation of drug function) were provided.

Although the analysis was relatively unrefined, there was some concordance in biomarkers that represented conceptually similar pathways involved in tissue rejection or tolerance. The first attempt to identify classifiers of immune responsiveness was an analysis of melanoma metastasis biopsied before and after vaccination with cancer antigens and concomitant systemic administration of IL-2.[82] Analysis of pretreatment biopsies compared to posttreatment identified a set of genes differentially expressed by the tumors that subsequently responded to treatment. Therefore, some metastatic nodules were predetermined to respond to immunotherapy by a preexisting inflammatory process conducive to immune stimulation. A subsequent small prospective mechanistic study confirmed these findings.[83] Surprisingly, several transcripts identified during tumor rejection were simultaneously described as markers of acute kidney allograft rejection in patient samples.[84]

Marincola and his colleagues[85] have proposed an immunologic constant of rejection (ICR) as a set of genes identifying a convergent pathway required for tissue-specific destruction (TSD) to occur. This constant dictates *how* immune-mediated rejection occurs but it is not predictive of *why* it may or may not occur in different tumors. However, during deconvolution of tumor rejection through a specific group of genes necessary for TSD, a polymorphism in interferon regulatory factor 5 (IRF5) was determined to be a key identifier for non-responders to adoptive T-cell therapy.[86] Consistent with the fine line that separates autoimmunity from tumor immunity, the same polymorphism has been reported to be protective against the development of systemic lupus erythematosus (SLE). The identification of a single predictor gene is not common, and, more likely, highly predictive signatures will be the outcome of combined over- or underexpression of different immune-related genes. The combination of a host's genetic background, the somatic mutations present in the heterogeneous tumor mass, and the influence of environmental factors may determine immune responsiveness.[87] An algorithm has been proposed where initial study of the tumor in the context of peripheral circulation is followed by analysis of the host's genetic background together with the genetics of the tumor lesion. Finally, integrative bioinformatics approaches are applied in search of complex relationships rather than univariate class comparisons.

Similar to challenges faced in cancer vaccine strategies and critical for infectious vaccine development is the related field of system immunogenetics which explores the interplay of immune systems and genetics and is focused on the immunological compartment.[88] Rather than analyzing individual components within a larger process, systems-level approaches attempt to model the entire set of interactions among individual components of a system. These models are then used to predict the behavior (i.e., host response) that results from these interactions. Systems-level research is dependent on having a complete inventory of the components of the system. The large amount of genomic and proteomic generated through high-throughput technologies has improved the ability to construct models of the host's immune system and its interaction with pathogens. In addition to the high-throughput omics readouts, there is also the development of high-throughput, high-dimensional immune phenotypes. A new technology derived from flow or mass cytometry (CyTOF®) has the capacity for analysis of as many as 100 protein biomarkers in parameters in individual cells.[89] Because the major objective of systems immunogenetics is the identification of molecular signatures associated with immune responses after vaccination, these approaches were used to analyze a yellow fever vaccine and two influenza vaccines.[90–92] Simple correlations and sophisticated machine learning algorithms were applied to the datasets to produce a high prediction accuracy even with small training sets. The results from these studies are of seminal importance because markers of vaccine protection could be predicted soon after vaccination. This approach could potentially allow, during the clinical development of cancer vaccinations, for the refinement and validation of immune markers for protection, which could guide vaccine optimization and increase the success rate of therapeutic vaccines in human subjects.

NEW TRENDS IN VACCINE STRATEGIES

An analysis and data mining of cancer vaccine trials performed in 2008[93] has shown that since the first tumor vaccine using autologous tumor cells in a lung cancer trial in 1971 the field re-emerged in the 1990s and grew rapidly until 2000, with more than 30 vaccine trials starting that year. Since then, new cancer vaccine trials have shown a steady increase in number, reaching more than 60 vaccine trials each year. Moreover, the number of Phase III clinical vaccine trials has increased steadily since then. The top five cancers targeted by cancer vaccination are melanoma, cervical, prostate, breast, and leukemia. Melanoma is the main indication for vaccine trials, accounting for 25% of all vaccine trials; it is followed in number of trials by cervical cancer. The study also indicated that most clinical vaccine trials target cancers with high incidence rates and also those associated with high rates of 5-year survival. Analysis of the technology platforms used in vaccine strategies indicated that the majority of the trials use antigens to directly stimulate the immune system, with the format most commonly being full-length proteins or peptides, and the second most common platform being cellular-based vaccines.

An example of a successful Phase III clinical trial using recombinant protein as a vaccine platform is the antiidiotype vaccine in patients with follicular lymphoma (FL).[25] This platform includes three components in the formulation: the patient- and tumor-specific idiotype protein conjugated to the highly immunogenic carrier keyhole limpet hemocyanin (KLH) adjuvanted with GM-CSF. The trial required untreated advance-stage FL patients who were treated with uniform PACE chemotherapy to induce remission.[94] Those achieving a complete remission were randomized at a ratio of 2:1 to receive Id-KLH plus GM-CSF or KLH plus GM-CSF as controls. The median time to relapse after randomization for the Id-KLH/GM-CSF arm was 44.2 months versus 30.6 months for the control arm, suggesting a benefit associated with use of the vaccine ($p = .045$; hazard ratio [HR] = 1.6). Of interest, although there were no statistically significant differences in the baseline patient characteristics between individuals who received the IgM Id-vaccine versus the IgG Id-vaccine, the latter group demonstrated a significantly longer time to relapse after randomization: 52.9 months versus 28.7 months in the IgM tumor isotype control-treated patients ($p = 0.001$; HR = 0.34, $p = .002$). Among patients receiving the IgG Id-vaccine, the median time to relapse after randomization was not significant: 35.1 versus 32.4 months in the IgG tumor isotype control-treated patients ($p = 0.807$; HR = 1.1).

The results in the successful clinical trial are in contrast to two other Phase III studies that have used recombinant idiotype vaccine for FL.[95,96] One of several key differences in the positive study compared to the two negative ones was the low tumor burden required for all vaccinated patients in the successful trial, although other issues may have contributed to survival outcomes. Nonetheless, Biovest is currently seeking formal regulatory approval for BiovaxID™ in Europe.[97]

A second example of a successful Phase III clinical trial utilizing protein or peptides as a platform is based on peptide vaccination for melanoma.[27] The study compared locally advanced stage III or IV melanoma patients treated with a modified gp100 peptide delivered in Montanide™ ISA-15 and adjuvanted with high-dose of IL-2 to patients treated with high dose IL-2 alone. The group vaccinated with peptide and IL-2 had superior objective clinical response rate (16% versus 6%; $p = 0.03$) and slightly improved progression-free survival

(2.2 versus 1.6 months; $p = 0.008$) when compared to the patients treated exclusively with high-dose IL-2. These findings were not observed in three previous independent Phase II clinical trials where there was no detected benefit in the combination treatment; however, these trials were not powered to assess a progression-free endpoint.[98] In the successful trial, serious adverse events in both groups were consistent with high-dose IL-2 therapy. The results underscore the need for novel potent and safe vaccine adjuvant systems in the field of cancer vaccination.

New Adjuvant Systems

Given that the majority of vaccine trials are based on protein/peptide vaccination, there is a paramount need for stronger adjuvants that can break tolerance to self-antigens and also overcome tumor-induced local immune suppression. An adjuvant is any component added to a vaccine that enhances immune responses, and are divided in two groups: immune potentiators and delivery systems. It is well established that the innate immune response regulates the initiation, quality, and magnitude of the adaptive immune response. Activation of innate immune responses is mediated by pattern recognition receptors (PRRs), which recognize and bind ligands associated with pathogens. The essential role of PRRs on the modulation of adaptive immune responses has steered the development of immune poteintiators that agonize PRR as novel adjuvants. There are many different classes of PRRs, including Toll-like receptors (TLRs), NOD-like receptors (NLRs), RIG-I-like receptors (RIRs), and C-type lectin receptors (CLRs). The canonical PRRs critical for the activation of adaptive immunity are the TLRs, which can be classified into extracellular (TLR 1, 2, 4, 5, 6), which recognize bacterial components, and intracellular (TLR 3, 7, 8, and 9), which serve as nucleic acid sensors. Specific TLR agonists or different combinations of agonists can direct the type of immune response that will be induced. For example, the TLR agonist flagellin can promote cellular immunity without inducing a Th1 or Th2 bias; conversely, TLR4, 4, 7, 8, and 9 agonists induce a Th1 bias and CTL responses. Approximately 13 TLRs have been identified, 10 of which are expressed by human cells. Experiments assessing downstream signaling of TLRs have demonstrated that all TLRs, except for TLR3 and some TLR4 ligands, signal through MyD88 to activate NF-κB and mitogen-activated protein kinase (MAPK). TLR7, 8, and 9 also utilize MyD88 to activate interferon (IFN) regulatory factors. TRIF is the adaptor molecule through which TLR3 and some TLR4 ligands activate the production of type I IFNs. As mentioned previously, some of these TLR agonists have been tested clinically as vaccine adjuvants. MPLA, a TLR4 agonist, is included in the AS04 utilized in Cervarix® and Fendrix®, which are approved for vaccination against human papillomavirus (HPV) and hepatitis B virus (HBV).

Several groups have demonstrated that vaccines comprised of more than one TLR agonist stimulate broader and stronger immune responses (reviewed in Mount et al.[99] and Mutwiri et al.[100]). For example, recent studies by Zhu et al.[101] described novel T-cell activation mechanisms by which the quality of immune response is enhanced by a combination of the three different TLRs (ligands MALP2, poly(I:C), and CpG), as opposed to double combinations that increase the quantity but not quality of T-cell responses. The triple combination induced higher functional avidity CD8+ T cells against antigens as well as higher IL-15 production, known for inducing high-avidity T cells during the priming phase.[102] Of note, negative cross-regulation of TLR pathways has also been reported. A clear example of negative cross-regulation was demonstrated by Simmons et al.,[103] where TLR2 signaling inhibited production of type I IFNs and antigen cross-presentation induced by TLR9 agonism. Similarly, other PRRs have also been described to inhibit TLR signaling; for example, NOD2 is a negative regulator of TLR2-induced Th2 cellular responses.[104] Therefore, the limited understanding of TLR agonism and lack of insight into synergistc and negative cross-regulation of different combinations have limited the rational design and development of multi-adjuvanted vaccines. However, findings supporting enhanced immune responses with multi-adjuvanted vaccines have substantiated clinical testing of TLR agonist combinations for the treatment of chronic infections and cancer.[105] In the cancer vaccine field, the most advanced multi-adjuvanted vaccine is MAGE-A3/AS15, which, as previously noted, combines TLR4 and TLR9 agonism to enhance immunity against MAGE-A3 protein. Resiquimod, a small molecule imidazoquinoline that activates TLR7 signaling, is being utilized alone or in combination with poly-ICLC (TLR3 agonist) as adjuvants for the DEC205–NY-ESO-1 fusion protein (NCT00948961). Nonetheless, the larger part of cancer vaccine trials are adjuvanted with a single TLR agonist. For example, NY-ESO-1 protein delivered in Montanide™ ISA-51 is being adjuvanted with topical resiquimod (NCT00821652) or poly-ICLC (NCT01079741). Peptide vaccines are also most commonly formulated with Montanide adjuvants and a TLR agonist. Several examples include melanoma peptides delivered in Montanide ISA-51 in combination with either LPS (TLR4 agonist) or poly-ICLC (NCT01585350), and with CpG7909 (NCT00085189). As the field develops, a deeper understanding of the mechanism of action of novel immune potentiators will lead the way toward novel vaccine adjuvants and the development of efficacious multi-adjuvanted vaccines. However, careful consideration will have to be given to ensure the safety of multi-adjuvanted vaccines, especially in early-stage cancer patients where the potential for adverse events and impact on patient safety may outweigh the potential for clinical benefit.

Oncolytic Viruses

The traditional approach of viral vectors for cancer vaccination utilizes viruses as a means of antigen delivery and leverages the proinflammatory signals of the virus itself for immune stimulation. Based on the latter characteristic of viral infections, new approaches are exploring intratumor delivery of viral vectors and oncolytic virotherapy. Oncolytic viruses demonstrate significant replication and destruction preferentially of cancer cells with little pathology to normal tissues.[106] Replicating viruses often induce better immune responses than non-replicating vectors. The antineoplasic potential of oncolytic virotherapy is not exclusively a consequence of the cytopathic activity but rather involves the induction of antitumor immunity.[107] Their potency relies in spreading to infect adjacent cells and repeating the process. Oncolytic viral vaccines show particular promise in addressing local immune suppression by inducing inflammatory cytokine expression that can enhance innate and adaptive antitumor immune responses and reduce tumor-mediated immune suppression. In murine models, oncolytic vaccinia virus has demonstrated a reduction of immunosuppressive cells, including myeloid-derived suppressor cells (MDSCs), Tregs, and tumor-associated macrophages (TAMs).[108]

In recent years, new and enhanced oncolytic viruses have been developed through genetic modification by deletion of viral genes involved in pathogenesis and insertion of novel transgenes that enhance antitumor activity. The most frequent modification approach for immunomodulation is the insertion of GM-CSF to stimulate an inflammatory response that facilitates DC recruitment.[109–112] Several viruses have progressed into clinical trials and have demonstrated varying degrees of success. Adenoviruses and herpes simplex viruses (HSVs) are the most commonly and extensively investigated platforms in nonclinical models and in clinical trials.[113–115] Clinical testing of adenoviruses included conditionally replicating viruses engineered to replicate in p53 null cancers with marked attenuation for normal cells (ONYX-015). Some tumor responses were observed in patients with accessible head and neck cancer that triggered a combination of the virus with chemotherapy in a Phase II study. The trial suggested improved outcomes compared with what was expected from chemotherapy alone, and tumor biopsies demonstrated tumor-specific viral replication.[116,117] However, further successes have been elusive and further development of ONYX-15 waned.

An identical vaccine platform (H101) demonstrated positive outcomes in a Phase III clinical trial and achieved licensure in China. The trial included patients with nasopharyngeal carcinoma in combination with platinum and 5-florouracil and demonstrated more than doubling of the response rate in the vaccinated group.[118] The furthest developed oncolytic virus tested in Western countries is an oncolytic HSV engineered to express GM-CSF, named talimogene laherparevec (T-VEC). This platform constitutes the first oncolytic immunotherapy to demonstrate therapeutic benefit against melanoma in a Phase III clinical trial. The interim results from the study indicate that patients treated with T-VEC significantly improved in durable response rate compared with GM-CSF-treated patients with metastatic disease (16.3% versus 2.1%; $p > 0.0001$), thus meeting the study's primary endpoint. A durable response was defined as a complete or partial response that began within 12 months of treatment initiation and lasted 6 months or more. Encouragingly, there is a hint of a survival benefit, as the interim data based on more than 85% of the required events revealed that median overall survival reached 23.3 months with the viral treatment compared to 19.0 months with GM-CSF (HR = 0.79; 95% CI, 0.61 to 1.02). However, the final assessment requires reporting of overall survival information, and there is a concern that the comparator arm of the study, GM-CSF alone, is not the standard treatment option for melanoma patients. It has been suggested that comparing T-VEC with Yervoy® or in combination with Yervoy may be the required next steps.

Currently, official sources list more than 50 recent and ongoing clinical trials assessing the safety and antineoplastic potential of several oncolytic viruses, although mostly in early development. The approaches include modified vaccinia virus, modified adenovirus, modified HSV, modified retrovirus, modified vesicular stomatitis virus (VSV), naturally occurring coxsackievirus A, wild-type reovirus, the Seneca Valley virus (a replication-competent oncolytic picornavirus), nonpathogenic recombinant poliovirus, attenuated lentogenic isolate of the Newcastle virus, and variants of naturally occurring parvovirus (H1) (reviewed in Vacchelli et al.[119]). The safety of oncolytic viruses will be the determining factor in progression into clinical development. The requirement to protect the host from overwhelming viral infection is of the outmost importance and may preclude clinical development of novel platforms in preclinical and early clinical stages. Remarkably, both H101 and T-VEC were delivered into the tumor, and data from these and other several oncolytic viruses delivered locally to the tumor have shown that clinical responses are possible even in distant, non-injected tumor lesions. These data seem to indicate that the local route, as opposed to systemic route of administration, may be a safe and efficient alternative in some clinical settings.

Prophylactic Vaccines

When assessing the origins of cancer it is clear that a significant proportion of human tumors worldwide are caused by infection of pathogens. It is estimated that HBV, HCV, human T-lymphotropic virus (HTLV), HPV, Kaposi's sarcoma-associated herpesvirus (KSHV), Merkel cell polyomavirus (MCV), and Epstein–Barr virus (EBV) are responsible for more than 11% of all diagnosed cancers worldwide.[120] Therefore, developing vaccines against infectious agents can be considered as the development of prophylactic vaccines for neoplasms caused by viral infections. Within this line of thought, one can recognize the recent FDA approval of two prophylactic vaccines against human papillomavirus (HPV) (Gardasil® and Cervarix®) as successful prophylactic cancer vaccines. These vaccines protect against infection by the two types of HPV (type 16 and 18) that cause approximately 70% of all cases of cervical cancer worldwide. Over the last 20 years, HPV has been identified as a cause of oropharyngeal cancer (OPC); HPV types 16 and 18 are responsible for almost all HPV-positive OPCs.[121] Primary prevention of OPC is feasible given that the parenterally administered vaccine prevents mucosal HPV infection at all genital sites, making it likely that a direct effect can be observed against oral/oropharyngeal HPV.

A proof-of-principle clinical study was performed in the Costa Rica Vaccine Trial, as a value-added component was introduced at the final randomized blinded study visit four year following initial vaccination.[122,123] Among the women who attended the study and accepted oral specimen collection, vaccine efficacy against oral HPV16/18 infection was 93%. The data are encouraging but not definitive because no pre-vaccination oral specimens were obtained and the trial included only one-time detection of oral HPV evaluated at the endpoint. Moreover, current vaccine schedules are based on the epidemiology of cervical HPV infection being highest in the mid- to late teens; however, the prevalence of HPV does not peak in early ages but instead remains stable or increases with increasing age.[124,125]

The FDA has also approved a cancer prophylactic vaccine against HBV infection. Chronic HBV infection causes 80% of all liver cancers worldwide, making it the ninth leading cause of death. The original anti-HBV vaccine was approved in 1981, is based on the recombinant HBV surface antigen (HBsAg), is highly immunogenic, and has been shown to convey lifelong immunity. Some of the obstacles hindering the development of effective vaccines against hepatitis C virus (HCV) and Epstein-Barr virus are an incomplete understanding of protective immune responses and genomic instability. For example, an attempt to develop a vaccine that generates neutralizing antibody responses against the viral envelope glycoprotein gp340 was unsuccessful;[126] however, although protection from primary infection was not observed, there was some protection and reduction in the risk of developing infectious mononucleosis. It has been suggested that a successful vaccine will require a robust CTL component able to recognize and destroy the *de novo* B-cell infections and avoidance of carrier state. Nonetheless, the successful development of anti-HBV and anti-HPV vaccines has demonstrated that effective prophylactic vaccines targeting cancer-associated infectious agents can be produced.

Among the general population, certain individuals carry a hereditary propensity to develop specific tumor types,[127] and because these individuals are at risk there may be significant benefits of prophylactic vaccination. Animal studies have shown that cancer vaccines are most effective in a prophylactic setting with immunization occurring before tumor implantation or, in the case of genetically predisposed animals, prior to spontaneous tumor development. Consistent throughout the literature, therapeutic vaccination in animal models has seldom been efficacious; however, genetically engineered mouse models (GEMMs) that express or overexpress mutated or oncogenic factors have provided sound evidence on the efficacy of the prophylactic approach. Females transgenic for the oncogenic or protoncogenic gene encoding ratHer-2/*neu* develop mammary tumors with 50 to 100% penetrance at ~5 months of age, depending on the model. Different vaccination strategies, including peptides, proteins, and DNA immunization, have demonstrated a block in tumor development.

Similar to the previous example, several MUC1 transgenic models have demonstrated protection from tumor development upon prophylactic vaccination. Mice transgenic for human MUC1 driven by the human promoter, express the endogenous protein similar to the human tissue distribution demonstrate both cellular and humoral responses against the self-antigen when immunized with strong vaccine platforms and CTL induction that resulted in tumor rejection and long-term protection. In a different murine model, the p48^{Cre}/LSL-*Kras*/MUC1 mouse, immunotherapy with MUC1 vaccination in combination with a cyclooxygenase-2 inhibitor and low-dose gemcitabine was reported to be effective in preventing progression from pancreatic intraepithelial neoplasia (PanIN) to invasive pancreatic ductal adenocarcinoma (PDAC).[128,129] In a mouse model of inflammatory bowel disease, a prophylactic MUC1 vaccine protected from progression to dysplasia and cancer development.[130,131]

Another GEMM model that resembles human disease is the TRAMP model. Males transgenic for SV40 driven under the probasin promoter, which restricts expression to prostate epithelial cells, are protected from primary tumors upon vaccination. Finally, mice engineered to express the human carcinoembryonic antigen (CEA) under its human promoter when immunized with optimal vaccine strategies are able to mount an immune response against the self-antigen sufficient to protect from a tumor challenge.

Of importance, autoimmunity is rarely observed in any of the experimental models described above. The translatability of these findings resides in the fact that these are expressed early in the process of transformation and even at the premalignant stage of the disease.[132-134] Necessary for the development of prophylactic cancer vaccines is the early detection of at-risk target populations. Patients with familial history where the progression of genetic alterations and cancer antigen expression is well defined may be ideal candidates for this approach. Hereditary propensity has been described in colon, breast, prostate, and pancreatic cancers, among others. As noted above, HER2/*neu*, MUC1, and CEA have been proposed as potential candidates for preventive vaccines. HER2/*neu* overexpression has been detected in ovarian, breast, non-small cell lung cancer, and pancreatic cancer.

With respect to breast cancer, a point of clinical insertion may be the ductal intraepithelial neoplasia (DIN) stage. DIN lesions represent an early stage of the disease where invasion and malignancy are not fully established. These are intermediary lesions without significant tumor burden. A window clinical trial tested the role of HER-2/*neu* DC-pulsed vaccination prior to surgery in patients immunized once a week for four weeks.[135] Results showed that vaccination was safe and well tolerated and induced a decline and/or eradication of HER2/*neu* expression. MUC1 is overexpressed in 90% of all adenocarcinomas, including breast, lung pancreas, prostate, stomach, colon, and ovary. A hypoglycosylated form of MUC1 is expressed in epithelial cancers and preneoplastic lesions in colon and pancreas. Expression of CEA is one of the key features of aberrant crypt foci, the precursors of colon cancer. Increased CEA expression is not associated with the degree of dysplasia but is associated with the size of the foci. It has been postulated that the altered location of CEA may disrupt colonic epithelial cell–cell interactions. Other antigens postulated for prophylactic vaccination in breast cancer include the CT antigens and alpha-lactalbumin.[136–139] Of importance, a high prevalence of expression of the CT antigens NY-ESO-1 and MAGE-A3 has been demonstrated in triple-negative (TN) breast cancers.[140,141] TN tumors are more commonly associated with BRCA1 mutations, and mutations in BRCA1 and BRCA2 confer a high lifetime risk for developing breast and ovarian cancer. Therefore, women with BRCA germline mutations may represent a target population for prophylactic vaccine based on CT antigens.

The efficacy of prophylactic vaccination with alpha-lactalbumin was demonstrated in two mouse models of spontaneous breast cancer, the MMTV-ratHER2/*neu* and the MMTV-PyVT transgenic mice.[138] In the first model, vaccination of 2-month-old females completely prevented the appearance of spontaneous tumors at 10 months of age. Of note, the authors indicated that no detectable inflammation of the normal breast and other tissues was detected. However, whether normal healthy cancer-free women will demonstrate no signs of autoimmunity remains to be elucidated.

In prostate cancer, differentiation antigens have been proposed for prophylactic vaccination. Utilizing the TRAMP mouse model it has been demonstrated that immunization against the prostate stem-cell antigen (PSCA) protected 90% of the mice for up to 340 days compared to 10% of control animals.[142] As with the previous models, male mice were immunized at a young age (eight weeks) prior to development of prostate tumors but in the presence of prostate intraepithelial neoplasia. If vaccination was initiated at 16 weeks of age, when the lesions had progressed to full adenocarcinomas, protection was significantly reduced.[143] Similar results in the prophylactic setting have been observed in mice immunized with yet another differentiation antigen, the six-transmembrane epithelial antigen of the prostate (STEAP).[144]

In the search for novel cancer antigens expressed at early stages of colorectal cancer (CRC) genes upregulated in adenoma relative to normal tissue that maintained increased expression in CRC have been postulated as possible targets for prevention of the disease.[145] Microarray analysis identified 160 genes with this profile that were greater than twofold upregulated. Of these, 23 genes with confirmed protein overexpression in CRC and the most highly upregulated ones were progressed into validation. Silencing of CDH3, CLDN1, KRT23, and MMP7 resulted in a significant decrease in viability. To determine whether these proteins could be utilized as antigens, immunogenicity was assessed by elevated serum detection in early-stage CRC patients compared to control individuals. This study is encouraging in that a high-throughput approach was utilized to identify biologically relevant antigens suitable for prophylactic vaccination strategies.

Although most experiments conducted in mice are promising, there is some evidence in the literature indicating the possibility of vaccination inducing inflammatory reactions that may enhance tumor growth.[146–148] Given that a low threshold for adverse events is inherent in prophylactic treatments, further definition and understanding of the inflammation that enhances carcinogenesis are necessary. Overall, the future of prophylactic cancer vaccines will depend on stringent and reliable methods to identify patients eligible to receive a specific vaccine intervention. Investment in infrastructure necessary to develop standard screening assays and tools to define the propensity of developing cancerous lesions may be significant. Such workflow may only be applicable to patients with defined inherited oncogenic drivers or patients with early nonmalignant lesions, whereas a workflow to identify individuals at risk as a consequence of their occupation and behavior patterns may be an insurmountable hurdle.

SUMMARY

Given that our understanding of the mechanism of action of superior vaccine adjuvants and tumor-mediated immune suppression is increasing and given the exciting developments in vaccine delivery systems, the potential for harnessing immune responses as a therapeutic force against cancer is ever improving. Of note, in virtually all of the therapeutic cancer vaccines trials reported to date, there have been extremely low levels of toxicity (grade I and II levels), and virtually no evidence of autoimmunity has been observed, with the exception of the vitiligo resulting from administration of some melanoma vaccines.

References

1. Segal NH, Parsons DW, Peggs KS, et al. Epitope landscape in breast and colorectal cancer. Cancer Res. 2008;68(3):889–92.
2. Castle JC, Kreiter S, Diekmann J, et al. Exploiting the mutanome for tumor vaccination. Cancer Res. 2012;72(5):1081–91.
3. Vogelstein B, Papadopoulos N, Velculescu VE, Zhou S, Diaz LA Jr, Kinzler KW. Cancer genome landscapes. Science. 2013;339(6127):1546–58.
4. Traversari C, van der Bruggen P, Luescher I, et al. A nonapeptide encoded by human gene MAGE-1 is recognized on HLA-A1 by cytolytic T lymphocytes directed against tumor antigen MZ2-E. J. Exp. Med. 1992;176:1453–7.
5. Boel P, Wildmann C, Sensi ML, et al. BAGE: a new gene encoding an antigen recognized on human melanomas by cytolytic T lymphocytes. Immunity 1995;2(2):167–75.
6. De Backer O, Arden KC, Boretti M, et al. Characterization of the GAGE genes that are expressed in various human cancers and in normal testis. Cancer Res. 1999;59(13):3157–65.
7. Chomez P, De Backer O, Bertrand M, De Plaen E, Boon T, Lucas S. An overview of the MAGE gene family with the identification of all human members of the family. Cancer Res. 2001;61(14):5544–51.
8. Gaugler B, van den Eynde B, van der Bruggen P, et al. Human gene MAGE-3 codes for an antigen recognized on a melanoma by autologous cytolytic T lymphocytes. J. Exp. Med. 1994;179:921–30.
9. Chen YT, Scanlan MJ, Sahin U, et al. A testicular antigen aberrantly expressed in human cancers detected by autologous antibody screening. Proc. Natl. Acad. Sci. U.S.A. 1997;94(5):1914–8.
10. Houghton AN, Gold JS, Blachere NE. Immunity against cancer: lessons learned from melanoma. Curr. Opin. Immunol. 2001;13(2):134–40.
11. Gogas H, Ioannovich J, Dafni U, et al. Prognostic significance of autoimmunity during treatment of melanoma with interferon. N. Engl. J. Med. 2006;354(7):709–18.
12. Atkins MB, Mier JW, Parkinson DR, Gould JA, Berkman EM, Kaplan MM. Hypothyroidism after treatment with interleukin-2 and lymphokine-activated killer cells. N. Engl. J. Med. 1988;318(24):1557–63.
13. Phan GQ, Attia P, Steinberg SM, White DE, Rosenberg SA. Factors associated with response to high-dose interleukin-2 in patients with metastatic melanoma. J. Clin. Oncol. 2001;19(15):3477–82.
14. Naldi L, Locati F, Finazzi G, Barbui T, Cainelli T. Antiphospholipid syndrome associated with immunotherapy for patients with melanoma. Cancer 1995;75(11):2784–5.
15. Chan C, O'Day J. Melanoma-associated retinopathy: does autoimmunity prolong survival? Clin. Exp. Ophthalmol. 2001;29(4):235–8.
16. Rosenberg SA, White DE. Vitiligo in patients with melanoma: normal tissue antigens can be targets for cancer immunotherapy. J. Immunother. Emphasis Tumor Immunol. 1996;19(1):81–4.
17. Nordlund JJ, Kirkwood JM, Forget BM, Milton G, Albert DM, Lerner AB. Vitiligo in patients with metastatic melanoma: a good prognostic sign. J. Am. Acad. Dermatol. 1983;9(5):689–96.
18. Bystryn JC, Rigel D, Friedman RJ, Kopf A. Prognostic significance of hypopigmentation in malignant melanoma. Arch. Dermatol. 1987;123(8):1053–5.
19. Richards JM, Mehta N, Ramming K, Skosey P. Sequential chemoimmunotherapy in the treatment of metastatic melanoma. J. Clin. Oncol. 1992;10(8):1338–43.
20. Cheever MA, Allison JP, Ferris AS, et al. The prioritization of cancer antigens: a national cancer institute pilot project for the acceleration of translational research. Clin. Cancer Res. 2009;15(17):5323–37.

21. Lang JM, Andrei AC, McNeel DG. Prioritization of cancer antigens: keeping the target in sight. Expert Rev. Vaccines. 2009;8(12):1657–61.

22. Pasero C, Olive D. Interfering with coinhibitory molecules: BTLA/HVEM as new targets to enhance anti-tumor immunity. Immunol. Lett. 2013;151(1-2):71–5.

23. Vergati M, Intrivici C, Huen NY, Schlom J, Tsang KY. Strategies for cancer vaccine development. J. Biomed. Biotechnol. 2010;1–13.

24. Rezvani K, Yong AS, Mielke S, et al. Repeated PR1 and WT1 peptide vaccination in Montanide-adjuvant fails to induce sustained high-avidity, epitope-specific CD8+ T cells in myeloid malignancies. Haematologica. 2011;96(3):432–40.

25. Schuster SJ, Neelapu SS, Gause BL, et al. Vaccination with patient-specific tumor-derived antigen in first remission improves disease-free survival in follicular lymphoma. J. Clin. Oncol. 2011;29(20):2787–94.

26. Mittendorf EA, Clifton GT, Holmes JP, et al. Clinical trial results of the HER-2/neu (E75) vaccine to prevent breast cancer recurrence in high-risk patients: from U.S. Military Cancer Institute Clinical Trials Group Study I-01 and I-02. Cancer 2012;118(10):2594–602.

27. Schwartzentruber DJ, Lawson DH, Richards JM, et al. gp100 peptide vaccine and interleukin-2 in patients with advanced melanoma. N. Engl. J. Med. 2011;364(22):2119–27.

28. Walter S, Weinschenk T, Stenzl A, et al. Multipeptide immune response to cancer vaccine IMA901 after single-dose cyclophosphamide associates with longer patient survival. Nat. Med. 2012;18(8):1254–61.

29. Kenter GG, Welters MJ, Valentijn AR, et al. Phase I immunotherapeutic trial with long peptides spanning the E6 and E7 sequences of high-risk human papillomavirus 16 in end-stage cervical cancer patients shows low toxicity and robust immunogenicity. Clin. Cancer Res. 2008;14(1):169–77.

30. Melief CJ, van der Burg SH. Immunotherapy of established (pre)malignant disease by synthetic long peptide vaccines. Nat. Rev. Cancer. 2008;8(5):351–60.

31. Garcon N, Morel S, Didierlaurent A, Descamps D, Wettendorff M, Van Mechelen M. Development of an AS04-adjuvanted HPV vaccine with the adjuvant system approach. BioDrugs 2011;25(4):217–26.

32. Eisenbarth SC, Colegio OR, O'Connor W, Sutterwala FS, Flavell RA. Crucial role for the Nalp3 inflammasome in the immunostimulatory properties of aluminium adjuvants. Nature 2008;453(7198):1122–6.

33. Giannini SL, Hanon E, Moris P, et al. Enhanced humoral and memory B cellular immunity using HPV16/18 L1 VLP vaccine formulated with the MPL/aluminium salt combination (AS04) compared to aluminium salt only. Vaccine 2006;24(33-34):5937–49.

34. Vansteenkiste J, Zielinski M, Linder A, et al. Adjuvant MAGE-A3 immunotherapy in resected non-small-cell lung cancer: phase II randomized study results. J. Clin. Oncol. 2013;31(19):2396–403.

35. Ulloa-Montoya F, Louahed J, Dizier B, et al. Predictive gene signature in MAGE-A3 antigen-specific cancer immunotherapy. J. Clin. Oncol. 2013;31(19):2388–95.

36. Kruit WH, Suciu S, Dreno B, et al. Selection of immunostimulant AS15 for active immunization with MAGE-A3 protein: results of a randomized phase II study of the European Organisation for Research and Treatment of Cancer Melanoma Group in Metastatic Melanoma. J. Clin. Oncol. 2013;31(19):2413–20.

37. Tyagi P, Mirakhur B. MAGRIT: the largest-ever phase III lung cancer trial aims to establish a novel tumor-specific approach to therapy. Clin. Lung Cancer 2009;10(5):371–4.

38. O'Hagan DT, Ott GS, Nest GV, Rappuoli R, Giudice GD. The history of MF59(®) adjuvant: a phoenix that arose from the ashes. Expert Rev. Vaccines. 2013;12(1):13–30.

39. Wack A, Baudner BC, Hilbert AK, et al. Combination adjuvants for the induction of potent, long-lasting antibody and T-cell responses to influenza vaccine in mice. Vaccine 2008;26(4):552–61.

40. Khurana S, Chearwae W, Castellino F, et al. Vaccines with MF59 adjuvant expand the antibody repertoire to target protective sites of pandemic avian H5N1 influenza virus. Sci. Transl. Med. 2010;2(15):15ra5.

41. Simons JW, Jaffee EM, Weber CE, et al. Bioactivity of autologous irradiated renal cell carcinoma vaccines generated by *ex vivo* granulocyte-macrophage colony-stimulating factor gene transfer. Cancer Res. 1997;57(8):1537–46.

42. Dranoff G, Jaffee E, Lazenby A, et al. Vaccination with irradiated tumor cells engineered to secrete murine granulocyte-macrophage colony-stimulating factor stimulates potent, specific, and long-lasting anti-tumor immunity. Proc. Natl. Acad. Sci. U.S.A. 1993;90(8):3539–43.

43. Thomas AM, Santarsiero LM, Lutz ER, et al. Mesothelin-specific CD8[+] T cell responses provide evidence of *in vivo* cross-priming by antigen-presenting cells in vaccinated pancreatic cancer patients. J. Exp. Med. 2004;200(3):297–306.

44. Parmiani G, Pilla L, Maccalli C, Russo V. Autologous versus allogeneic cell-based vaccines? Cancer J. 2011;17(5):331–6.

45. Reichardt VL, Brossart P, Kanz L. Dendritic cells in vaccination therapies of human malignant disease. Blood Rev. 2004;18(4):235–43.

46. Caux C, Dezutter-Dambuyant C, Schmitt D, Banchereau J. GM-CSF and TNF-alpha cooperate in the generation of dendritic Langerhans cells. Nature 1992;360(6401):258–61.

47. Lardon F, Snoeck HW, Berneman ZN, et al. Generation of dendritic cells from bone marrow progenitors using GM-CSF, TNF-alpha, and additional cytokines: antagonistic effects of IL-4 and IFN-gamma and selective involvement of TNF-alpha receptor-1. Immunology 1997;91(4):553–9.

48. Banchereau J, Palucka AK, Dhodapkar M, et al. Immune and clinical responses in patients with metastatic melanoma to CD34$^+$ progenitor-derived dendritic cell vaccine. Cancer Res. 2001;61(17):6451–8.

49. Titzer S, Christensen O, Manzke O, et al. Vaccination of multiple myeloma patients with idiotype-pulsed dendritic cells: immunological and clinical aspects. Br. J. Haematol. 2000;108(4):805–16.

50. McIlroy D, Gregoire M. Optimizing dendritic cell-based anticancer immunotherapy: maturation state does have clinical impact. Cancer Immunol. Immunother. 2003;52(10):583–91.

51. Giermasz AS, Urban JA, Nakamura Y, et al. Type-1 polarized dendritic cells primed for high IL-12 production show enhanced activity as cancer vaccines. Cancer Immunol. Immunother. 2009;58(8):1329–36.

52. Lee JJ, Foon KA, Mailliard RB, Muthuswamy R, Kalinski P. Type 1-polarized dendritic cells loaded with autologous tumor are a potent immunogen against chronic lymphocytic leukemia. J. Leukoc. Biol. 2008;84(1):319–25.

53. Jonuleit H, Kuhn U, Muller G, et al. Pro-inflammatory cytokines and prostaglandins induce maturation of potent immunostimulatory dendritic cells under fetal calf serum-free conditions. Eur. J. Immunol. 1997;27(12): 3135–42.

54. Jongbloed SL, Kassianos AJ, McDonald KJ, et al. Human CD141$^+$ (BDCA-3)+ dendritic cells (DCs) represent a unique myeloid DC subset that cross-presents necrotic cell antigens. J. Exp. Med. 2010;207(6):1247–60.

55. Poulin LF, Salio M, Griessinger E, et al. Characterization of human DNGR-1+ BDCA3+ leukocytes as putative equivalents of mouse CD8alpha+ dendritic cells. J. Exp. Med. 2010;207(6):1261–71.

56. Crozat K, Guiton R, Contreras V, et al. The XC chemokine receptor 1 is a conserved selective marker of mammalian cells homologous to mouse CD8α$^+$ dendritic cells. J. Exp. Med. 2010;207(6):1283–92.

57. Higano CS, Schellhammer PF, Small EJ, et al. Integrated data from 2 randomized, double-blind, placebo-controlled, phase 3 trials of active cellular immunotherapy with sipuleucel-T in advanced prostate cancer. Cancer 2009;115(16):3670–9.

58. Zhai Y, Yang JC, Kawakami Y, et al. Antigen-specific tumor vaccines. Development and characterization of recombinant adenoviruses encoding MART1 or gp100 for cancer therapy. J. Immunol. 1996;156(2):700–10.

59. Rosenberg SA, Zhai Y, Yang JC, et al. Immunizing patients with metastatic melanoma using recombinant adenoviruses encoding MART-1 or gp100 melanoma antigens. J. Natl. Cancer Inst. 1998;90(24):1894–900.

60. Lubaroff DM, Konety BR, Link B, et al. Phase I clinical trial of an adenovirus/prostate-specific antigen vaccine for prostate cancer: safety and immunologic results. Clin. Cancer Res. 2009;15(23):7375–80.

61. Tsang KY, Zaremba S, Nieroda CA, Zhu MZ, Hamilton JM, Schlom J. Generation of human cytotoxic T cells specific for human carcinoembryonic antigen epitopes from patients immunized with recombinant vaccinia-CEA vaccine. J. Natl. Cancer Inst. 1995;87(13):982–90.

62. Conry RM, Allen KO, Lee S, Moore SE, Shaw DR, LoBuglio AF. Human autoantibodies to carcinoembryonic antigen (CEA) induced by a vaccinia-CEA vaccine. Clin. Cancer Res. 2000;6(1):34–41.

63. Amato RJ, Hawkins RE, Kaufman HL, et al. Vaccination of metastatic renal cancer patients with MVA-5T4: a randomized, double-blind, placebo-controlled phase III study. Clin. Cancer Res. 2010;16(22):5539–47.

64. Gulley JL, Arlen PM, Tsang KY, et al. Pilot study of vaccination with recombinant CEA-MUC-1-TRICOM poxviral-based vaccines in patients with metastatic carcinoma. Clin. Cancer Res. 2008;14(10):3060–9.

65. Quoix E, Ramlau R, Westeel V, et al. Therapeutic vaccination with TG4010 and first-line chemotherapy in advanced non-small-cell lung cancer: a controlled phase 2B trial. Lancet Oncol. 2011;12(12):1125–33.

66. Kaufman HL, Cohen S, Cheung K, et al. Local delivery of vaccinia virus expressing multiple costimulatory molecules for the treatment of established tumors. Hum. Gene Ther. 2006;17(2):239–44.

67. Dubensky TW Jr, Skoble J, Lauer P, Brockstedt DG. Killed but metabolically active vaccines. Curr. Opin. Biotechnol. 2012;23(6):917–23.

68. Shahabi V, Maciag PC, Rivera S, Wallecha A. Live, attenuated strains of Listeria and Salmonella as vaccine vectors in cancer treatment. Bioeng. Bugs. 2010;1(4):235–43.

69. MacDonald GH, Johnston RE. Role of dendritic cell targeting in Venezuelan equine encephalitis virus pathogenesis. J. Virol. 2000;74(2):914–22.

70. Finke LH, Wentworth K, Blumenstein B, Rudolph NS, Levitsky H, Hoos A. Lessons from randomized phase III studies with active cancer immunotherapies—outcomes from the 2006 meeting of the Cancer Vaccine Consortium (CVC). Vaccine 2007;25(Suppl. 2):B97–109.

71. Wolchok JD, Hoos A, O'Day S, et al. Guidelines for the evaluation of immune therapy activity in solid tumors: immune-related response criteria. Clin. Cancer Res. 2009;15(23):7412–20.

72. Tuma RS. New response criteria proposed for immunotherapies. J. Natl. Cancer Inst. 2008;100(18):1280–1.

73. Hale DF, Clifton GT, Sears AK, et al. Cancer vaccines: should we be targeting patients with less aggressive disease? Expert Rev. Vaccines 2012;11(6):721–31.

74. Hoos A, Parmiani G, Hege K, et al. A clinical development paradigm for cancer vaccines and related biologics. J. Immunother. 2007;30(1):1–15.

75. Janetzki S, Panageas KS, Ben-Porat L, et al. Results and harmonization guidelines from two large-scale international Elispot proficiency panels conducted by the Cancer Vaccine Consortium (CVC/SVI). Cancer Immunol. Immunother. 2008;57(3):303–15.

76. Britten CM, Janetzki S, van der Burg SH, Gouttefangeas C, Hoos A. Toward the harmonization of immune monitoring in clinical trials: *quo vadis?* Cancer Immunol. Immunother. 2008;57(3):285–8.

77. McNeil LK, Price L, Britten CM, et al. A harmonized approach to intracellular cytokine staining gating: results from an international multiconsortia proficiency panel conducted by the Cancer Immunotherapy Consortium (CIC/CRI). Cytometry A 2013;83(8):728–38.

78. Britten CM, Janetzki S, Butterfield LH, et al. T cell assays and MIATA: the essential minimum for maximum impact. Immunity 2012;37(1):1–2.

79. Hoos A, Janetzki S, Britten CM. Advancing the field of cancer immunotherapy: MIATA consensus guidelines become available to improve data reporting and interpretation for T-cell immune monitoring. Oncoimmunology 2012;1(9):1457–9.

80. Janetzki S, Hoos A, Melief CJ, Odunsi K, Romero P, Britten CM. Structured reporting of T cell assay results. Cancer Immun. 2013;13:13.

81. Tahara H, Sato M, Thurin M, et al. Emerging concepts in biomarker discovery; the U.S.–Japan Workshop on Immunological Molecular Markers in Oncology. J. Transl. Med. 2009;7:45.

82. Wang E, Miller LD, Ohnmacht GA, et al. Prospective molecular profiling of melanoma metastases suggests classifiers of immune responsiveness. Cancer Res. 2002;62(13):3581–6.

83. Weiss GR, Grosh WW, Chianese-Bullock KA, et al. Molecular insights on the peripheral and intratumoral effects of systemic high-dose rIL-2 (aldesleukin) administration for the treatment of metastatic melanoma. Clin. Cancer Res. 2011;17(23):7440–50.

84. Sarwal M, Chua MS, Kambham N, et al. Molecular heterogeneity in acute renal allograft rejection identified by DNA microarray profiling. N. Engl. J. Med. 2003;349(2):125–38.

85. Wang E, Worschech A, Marincola FM. The immunologic constant of rejection. Trends Immunol. 2008;29(6):256–62.

86. Uccellini L, De Giorgi V, Zhao Y, et al. IRF5 gene polymorphisms in melanoma. J. Transl. Med. 2012;10:170.

87. Wang E, Uccellini L, Marincola FM. A genetic inference on cancer immune responsiveness. Oncoimmunology. 2012;1(4):520–5.

88. Mooney M, McWeeney S, Sekaly RP. Systems immunogenetics of vaccines. Semin. Immunol. 2013;25(2):124–9.

89. Bandura DR, Baranov VI, Ornatsky OI, et al. Mass cytometry: technique for real time single cell multitarget immunoassay based on inductively coupled plasma time-of-flight mass spectrometry. Anal. Chem. 2009;81(16):6813–22.

90. Querec TD, Akondy RS, Lee EK, et al. Systems biology approach predicts immunogenicity of the yellow fever vaccine in humans. Nat. Immunol. 2009;10(1):116–25.

91. Nakaya HI, Wrammert J, Lee EK, et al. Systems biology of vaccination for seasonal influenza in humans. Nat. Immunol. 2011;12(8):786–95.

92. Gaucher D, Therrien R, Kettaf N, et al. Yellow fever vaccine induces integrated multilineage and polyfunctional immune responses. J. Exp. Med. 2008;205(13):3119–31.

93. Cao X, Maloney KB, Brusic V. Data mining of cancer vaccine trials: a bird's-eye view. Immunome Res. 2008;4:7.

94. Bendandi M. Idiotype vaccines for lymphoma: proof-of-principles and clinical trial failures. Nat. Rev. Cancer 2009;9(9):675–81.

IV. NOVEL APPROACHES FOR CANCER THERAPIES

95. Freedman A, Neelapu SS, Nichols C, et al. Placebo-controlled phase III trial of patient-specific immunotherapy with mitumprotimut-T and granulocyte-macrophage colony-stimulating factor after rituximab in patients with follicular lymphoma. J. Clin. Oncol. 2009;27(18):3036–43.

96. Inoges S, Rodriguez-Calvillo M, Zabalegui N, et al. Clinical benefit associated with idiotypic vaccination in patients with follicular lymphoma. J. Natl. Cancer Inst. 2006;98(18):1292–301.

97. Anon. Biovest initiates formal regulatory approval process for BiovaxID in Europe. Hum. Vaccin. Immunother. 2012;8(8):1017.

98. Sosman JA, Carrillo C, Urba WJ, et al. Three phase II cytokine working group trials of gp100 (210M) peptide plus high-dose interleukin-2 in patients with HLA-A2-positive advanced melanoma. J. Clin. Oncol. 2008;26(14):2292–8.

99. Mount A, Koernig S, Silva A, Drane D, Maraskovsky E, Morelli AB. Combination of adjuvants: the future of vaccine design. Expert Rev Vaccines 2013;12(7):733–46.

100. Mutwiri G, Gerdts V, van Drunen Littel-van den Hurk S, et al. Combination adjuvants: the next generation of adjuvants? Expert. Rev. Vaccines 2011;10(1):95–107.

101. Zhu Q, Egelston C, Gagnon S, et al. Using 3 TLR ligands as a combination adjuvant induces qualitative changes in T cell responses needed for antiviral protection in mice. J. Clin. Invest. 2010;120(2):607–16.

102. Oh S, Perera LP, Burke DS, Waldmann TA, Berzofsky JA. IL-15/IL-15Ralpha-mediated avidity maturation of memory CD8$^+$ T cells. Proc. Natl. Acad. Sci. U.S.A. 2004;101(42):15154–9.

103. Simmons DP, Canaday DH, Liu Y, et al. Mycobacterium tuberculosis and TLR2 agonists inhibit induction of type I IFN and class I MHC antigen cross processing by TLR9. J. Immunol. 2010;185(4):2405–15.

104. Watanabe T, Kitani A, Murray PJ, Strober W. NOD2 is a negative regulator of Toll-like receptor 2-mediated T helper type 1 responses. Nat. Immunol. 2004;5(8):800–8.

105. Galluzzi L, Vacchelli E, Eggermont A, et al. Trial watch: experimental Toll-like receptor agonists for cancer therapy. Oncoimmunology 2012;1(5):699–716.

106. Vaha-Koskela MJ, Heikkila JE, Hinkkanen AE. Oncolytic viruses in cancer therapy. Cancer Lett. 2007;254(2):178–216.

107. Russell SJ, Peng KW, Bell JC. Oncolytic virotherapy. Nat. Biotechnol. 2012;30(7):658–70.

108. Thorne SH, Liang W, Sampath P, et al. Targeting localized immune suppression within the tumor through repeat cycles of immune cell-oncolytic virus combination therapy. Mol Ther. 2010;18(9):1698–705.

109. Malhotra S, Kim T, Zager J, et al. Use of an oncolytic virus secreting GM-CSF as combined oncolytic and immunotherapy for treatment of colorectal and hepatic adenocarcinomas. Surgery 2007;141(4):520–9.

110. Simpson GR, Han Z, Liu B, Wang Y, Campbell G, Coffin RS. Combination of a fusogenic glycoprotein, prodrug activation, and oncolytic herpes simplex virus for enhanced local tumor control. Cancer Res. 2006;66(9):4835–42.

111. Kasuya H, Takeda S, Nomoto S, Nakao A. The potential of oncolytic virus therapy for pancreatic cancer. Cancer Gene Ther. 2005;12(9):725–36.

112. Kim JH, Oh JY, Park BH, et al. Systemic armed oncolytic and immunologic therapy for cancer with JX-594, a targeted poxvirus expressing GM-CSF. Mol. Ther. 2006;14(3):361–70.

113. Cerullo V, Diaconu I, Romano V, et al. An oncolytic adenovirus enhanced for toll-like receptor 9 stimulation increases antitumor immune responses and tumor clearance. Mol. Ther. 2012;20(11):2076–86.

114. Kaur B, Chiocca EA, Cripe TP. Oncolytic HSV-1 virotherapy: clinical experience and opportunities for progress. Curr. Pharm. Biotechnol. 2012;13(9):1842–51.

115. Li H, Zhang X. Oncolytic HSV as a vector in cancer immunotherapy. Methods Mol. Biol. 2010;651:279–90.

116. Nemunaitis J, Khuri F, Ganly I, et al. Phase II trial of intratumoral administration of ONYX-015, a replication-selective adenovirus, in patients with refractory head and neck cancer. J. Clin. Oncol. 2001;19(2):289–98.

117. Khuri FR, Nemunaitis J, Ganly I, et al. A controlled trial of intratumoral ONYX-015, a selectively-replicating adenovirus, in combination with cisplatin and 5-fluorouracil in patients with recurrent head and neck cancer. Nat. Med. 2000;6(8):879–85.

118. Xia ZJ, Chang JH, Zhang L, et al. Phase III randomized clinical trial of intratumoral injection of E1B gene-deleted adenovirus (H101) combined with cisplatin-based chemotherapy in treating squamous cell cancer of head and neck or esophagus [in Chinese]. Ai Zheng. 2004;23(12):1666–70.

119. Vacchelli E, Eggermont A, Sautes-Fridman C, et al. Trial watch: oncolytic viruses for cancer therapy. Oncoimmunology 2013;2(6):e24612.

120. Parkin DM. The global health burden of infection-associated cancers in the year. 2002. Int. J. Cancer 2006;118(12):3030–44.

121. Chaturvedi AK, Engels EA, Pfeiffer RM, et al. Human papillomavirus and rising oropharyngeal cancer incidence in the United States. J. Clin. Oncol. 2011;29(32):4294–301.

122. Herrero R, Hildesheim A, Rodriguez AC, et al. Rationale and design of a community-based double-blind randomized clinical trial of an HPV 16 and 18 vaccine in Guanacaste, Costa Rica. Vaccine 2008;26(37): 4795–808.

123. Herrero R, Quint W, Hildesheim A, et al. Reduced prevalence of oral human papillomavirus (HPV) 4 years after bivalent HPV vaccination in a randomized clinical trial in Costa Rica. PLoS ONE 2013;8(7):e68329.

124. Kreimer AR, Villa A, Nyitray AG, et al. The epidemiology of oral HPV infection among a multinational sample of healthy men. Cancer Epidemiol Biomarkers Prev. 2011;20(1):172–82.

125. Gillison ML, Broutian T, Pickard RK, et al. Prevalence of oral HPV infection in the United States, 2009-2010. JAMA 2012;307(7):693–703.

126. Moutschen M, Leonard P, Sokal EM, et al. Phase I/II studies to evaluate safety and immunogenicity of a recombinant gp350 Epstein–Barr virus vaccine in healthy adults. Vaccine 2007;25(24):4697–705.

127. American Society of Clinical, Oncology. American Society of Clinical Oncology policy statement update: genetic testing for cancer susceptibility. J. Clin. Oncol. 2003;21(12):2397–406.

128. Finn OJ, Jerome KR, Henderson RA, et al. MUC-1 epithelial tumor mucin-based immunity and cancer vaccines. Immunol. Rev. 1995;145:61–89.

129. Kadayakkara DK, Beatty PL, Turner MS, Janjic JM, Ahrens ET, Finn OJ. Inflammation driven by overexpression of the hypoglycosylated abnormal mucin 1 (MUC1) links inflammatory bowel disease and pancreatitis. Pancreas. 2010;39(4):510–5.

130. Beatty PL, Narayanan S, Gariepy J, Ranganathan S, Finn OJ. Vaccine against MUC1 antigen expressed in inflammatory bowel disease and cancer lessens colonic inflammation and prevents progression to colitis-associated colon cancer. Cancer Prev. Res. (Phila.) 2010;3(4):438–46.

131. Beatty P, Ranganathan S, Finn OJ. Prevention of colitis-associated colon cancer using a vaccine to target abnormal expression of the MUC1 tumor antigen. Oncoimmunology 2012;1(3):263–70.

132. Reis CA, David L, Correa P, et al. Intestinal metaplasia of human stomach displays distinct patterns of mucin (MUC1, MUC2, MUC5AC, and MUC6) expression. Cancer Res. 1999;59(5):1003–7.

133. Salem RR, Wolf BC, Sears HF, et al. Expression of colorectal carcinoma-associated antigens in colonic polyps. J. Surg. Res. 1993;55(3):249–55.

134. Schmitt FC, Andrade L. Spectrum of carcinoembryonic antigen immunoreactivity from isolated ductal hyperplasias to atypical hyperplasias associated with infiltrating ductal breast cancer. J. Clin. Pathol. 1995;48(1):53–6.

135. Sharma A, Koldovsky U, Xu S, et al. HER-2 pulsed dendritic cell vaccine can eliminate HER-2 expression and impact ductal carcinoma *in situ*. Cancer 2012;118(17):4354–62.

136. Theurillat JP, Ingold F, Frei C, et al. NY-ESO-1 protein expression in primary breast carcinoma and metastases: correlation with CD8$^+$ T-cell and CD79a$^+$ plasmacytic/B-cell infiltration. Int. J. Cancer 2007;120(11):2411–7.

137. Mischo A, Kubuschok B, Ertan K, et al. Prospective study on the expression of cancer testis genes and antibody responses in 100 consecutive patients with primary breast cancer. Int. J. Cancer 2006;118(3):696–703.

138. Jaini R, Kesaraju P, Johnson JM, Altuntas CZ, Jane-Wit D, Tuohy VK. An autoimmune-mediated strategy for prophylactic breast cancer vaccination. Nat. Med. 2010;16(7):799–803.

139. Sugita Y, Wada H, Fujita S, et al. NY-ESO-1 expression and immunogenicity in malignant and benign breast tumors. Cancer Res. 2004;64(6):2199–204.

140. Grigoriadis A, Caballero OL, Hoek KS, et al. CT-X antigen expression in human breast cancer. Proc. Natl. Acad. Sci. U.S.A. 2009;106(32):13493–8.

141. Curigliano G, Viale G, Ghioni M, et al. Cancer-testis antigen expression in triple-negative breast cancer. Ann. Oncol. 2011;22(1):98–103.

142. Garcia-Hernandez Mde L, Gray A, Hubby B, Klinger OJ, Kast WM. Prostate stem cell antigen vaccination induces a long-term protective immune response against prostate cancer in the absence of autoimmunity. Cancer Res. 2008;68(3):861–9.

143. Gray A, de la Luz Garcia-Hernandez M, van West M, Kanodia S, Hubby B, Kast WM. Prostate cancer immunotherapy yields superior long-term survival in TRAMP mice when administered at an early stage of carcinogenesis prior to the establishment of tumor-associated immunosuppression at later stages. Vaccine 2009;27(Suppl. 6):G52–9.

IV. NOVEL APPROACHES FOR CANCER THERAPIES

144. Garcia-Hernandez Mde L, Gray A, Hubby B, Kast WM. *In vivo* effects of vaccination with six-transmembrane epithelial antigen of the prostate: a candidate antigen for treating prostate cancer. Cancer Res. 2007;67(3): 1344–51.
145. Broussard EK, Kim R, Wiley JC, et al. Identification of putative immunologic targets for colon cancer prevention based on conserved gene upregulation from preinvasive to malignant lesions. Cancer Prev. Res. 2013;6(7):666–74.
146. Siegel CT, Schreiber K, Meredith SC, et al. Enhanced growth of primary tumors in cancer-prone mice after immunization against the mutant region of an inherited oncoprotein. J. Exp. Med. 2000;191(11):1945–56.
147. Lin EY, Nguyen AV, Russell RG, Pollard JW. Colony-stimulating factor 1 promotes progression of mammary tumors to malignancy. J. Exp. Med. 2001;193(6):727–40.
148. Moore RJ, Owens DM, Stamp G, et al. Mice deficient in tumor necrosis factor-alpha are resistant to skin carcinogenesis. Nat. Med. 1999;5(7):828–31.

T-Cell Immunotherapy for Cancer

Conrad Russell Y. Cruz, Catherine M. Bollard

Children's National Health System, Washington DC, USA

BRIEF HISTORY OF T-CELL THERAPY

Like most immune-based therapies, William Coley's work using streptococcal cultures ("Coley's toxins") to mediate regression in patients with inoperable sarcomas[3] was instrumental in ushering the use of T cells to the clinic. However, the proof-of-principle studies suggesting that adoptive T-cell transfer can eradicate tumors was first observed in murine transplant models and validated clinically in patients receiving allogeneic hematopoietic stem cell transplants (allo-HSCTs).

A study by Barnes et al.[4] first showed evidence for a graft-versus-tumor effect using transplanted allogeneic T cells to eradicate malignancy. Mice injected with leukemic cells and subsequently transplanted with allogeneic splenocytes following total body irradiation exhibited the characteristic symptoms (i.e., a diarrhea syndrome) of what is now known as graft-versus-host disease (GVHD). The development of this syndrome, however, also correlated with an eradication of the malignant cells in mice who received the allogeneic cells in contrast to mice who received autologous splenocytes.[4] Subsequently, Fefer et al.[5] demonstrated that donor splenocytes from mice immunized against leukemia by subcutaneous injection were capable

Novel Approaches and Strategies for Biologics, Vaccines and Cancer Therapies. DOI: 10.1016/B978-0-12-416603-5.00016-X

of protecting recipient mice from an otherwise aggressive intraperitoneal tumor challenge. Because these studies suggested that allogeneic bone marrow transplantation could exert an antileukemic effect, Weiden et al.[6] reviewed the results from 242 bone marrow transplant patients and observed that relapse rates were significantly less in patients who developed GVHD after allo-HSCT.

Efforts to exploit this graft-versus-leukemia (GVL) effect accelerated upon recognition of the central role of lymphocytes in mediating antitumor activity. A series of studies by Southam et al.,[7] for example, on autotransplantation of cancer in incurable patients, identified the cell-mediated immune response by lymphocytes as the crucial mechanism involved in tumor autograft rejection. Various institutions then used donor lymphocyte infusions (DLIs) in an attempt to induce post-transplant antileukemia activity and treat relapsed disease.[8–10] Although early attempts failed to separate GVL from GVHD,[10] subsequent studies in chronic myelogenous leukemia (CML) showed more promising results.[8] For example, Kolb et al.[8] successfully infused cells from buffy coats into three CML patients with hematologic relapse following bone marrow transplantation. Following infusion, patients showed complete clinical and cytological remission lasting from 32 to 91 weeks.

Hence, allogeneic transplantation and DLI are the most potent demonstrations of the potential for adoptive cell therapies,[11] and this is most evident in the setting of CML patients relapsing after transplant.[12,13] Poorer response to DLI in other hematologic malignancies (particularly acute leukemia and myeloma) may be attributed to poor antigen presentation by the tumor cells and complications of GVHD,[11] an important limiting factor in the use of this therapy. Several strategies have been proposed to eliminate unwanted cells and enrich tumor-specific T cells, including: (1) depletion of alloreactive cells by initial depletion with anti-CD25 immunotoxin,[14] (2) photodynamic purging,[15] or (3) *ex vivo* irradiation/psoralen treatment.[16] But, the most successful strategies arguably involve the generation of antigen-specific T cells, where prolonged expansion to selectively increase tumor specific cells eliminates residual alloreactive T cells from the final infusion product. Efforts to balance potent graft-versus-tumor effects and graft-versus-host disease thus led to the development of various T-cell therapies as described below.[17]

TUMOR-INFILTRATING LYMPHOCYTES

The original tumor-specific cells were derived from tumor-infiltrating lymphocytes, which, presumably, recognize the various antigens present but are merely incapable of eradicating the cancer because of chronic activation and active immunosuppression within the tumor microenvironment.[18] Removing T cells from this environment for *ex vivo* expansion therefore (theoretically) allowed for their reactivation and formed the basis for the pioneering work by Rosenberg et al.[19] against metastatic melanoma.

Discoveries in the late 1980s documenting infiltrating lymphocytes in melanoma[20] encouraged the use of tumor-infiltrating T cells in adoptive immunotherapy. Autologous tumor-infiltrating lymphocytes (TILs) were harvested and expanded *in vitro* from resected tumor nodules of metastatic melanoma patients in the presence of IL-2. Of 86 patients with metastatic melanoma treated at the Surgery Branch at the National Institutes of Health, 29 showed objective clinical responses with TIL therapies (34%).[19,21,22] Although TILs were infused regardless of their ability to lyse autologous fresh tumor, subsequent *in vitro* analysis showed a positive correlation between clinical response and *in vitro* antitumor activity. Additionally, TILs from younger cultures and shorter doubling times were found to correlate with favorable responses.[19,21,22]

To maximize T-cell persistence and function *in vivo*, a subsequent cohort of metastatic melanoma patients received a conditioning lymphodepleting regimen prior to infusion of TILs. Following non-myeloablative treatment with cyclophosphamide and fludarabine, patients were given TILs along with high-dose IL-2. Improvements in response rate in this cohort were immediately evident: 21 of 42 patients with no total body irradiation, 13 of 25 patients with 2 Gy of irradiation, and 18 of 25 with 12 Gy of irradiation showed objective clinical responses by Response Evaluation Criteria In Solid Tumors (RECIST) criteria. Ten of these patients had complete responses. Survival in the study was positively correlated to the degree of lymphodepletion.[23] Persistence of T cells after infusion correlated with disappearance of the malignancy, and tumor-specific T cells persisted in the peripheral blood for up to 6 to 12 months following infusion.[22] However, patients in this melanoma study experienced significant toxicities, likely as a result of the high doses of IL-2 necessary for maintaining T-cell function *in vivo*.[22]

Efforts to extend these approaches to other solid tumors with infiltrating lymphocytes have not been as successful. In the case of ovarian cancers, where the presence of intratumoral T cells has correlated with survival,[24] attempts have been made to improve outcomes by infusing *ex vivo* expanded tumor-infiltrating lymphocytes but to no avail.[25] However, subsequent studies in patients with no clinically detectable tumors showed higher 3-year disease-free survival rates in patients treated with TIL (82.1%) versus control (54.5%) to prevent relapse following chemotherapy and surgery.[26] In contrast, tumor-infiltrating T cells given to patients with metastatic colorectal cancer following radical hepatic resection did not show improved survival compared to non-T-cell-treated patients.[27]

Although the utility of TIL therapy appears to be limited to metastatic melanoma, it encouraged the development of T-cell immune therapies by providing direct evidence that these cells are capable of curing patients with metastatic disease. However, because most solid tumors and hematologic malignancies do not harbor TILs, attention has shifted to the identification of tumor-associated targets for T cells.

ANTIGEN-SPECIFIC T CELLS

Virus-Specific T Cells

The association of certain tumors with viruses presents an ideal opportunity to target tumor-associated viral antigens with T-cell therapeutic approaches because they present an immunogenic protein on the surface and they have generally limited expression that is specific to the malignant cells.

Epstein–Barr virus (EBV) is a ubiquitous virus present as a latent infection in approximately 90% of the population. EBV encodes several tumorigenic proteins and is associated with several malignancies, including Hodgkin's lymphoma, non-Hodgkin's lymphoma, Burkitt's lymphoma, and nasopharyngeal carcinoma in the immune-competent host[28] and post-transplant lymphoproliferative disease in the immune-deficient host.[29]

Investigators used B cells infected with the B95-8 laboratory strain of EBV to generate EBV-infected B cells (lymphoblastoid cell lines) to use as antigen-presenting cells in order to expand EBV-specific T cells in sufficient numbers for adoptive T-cell transfer. Because these lymphoblastoid cell lines express lytic and latent antigens that can also be seen in EBV-associated post-transplant lymphoproliferative disease (PTLD), it serves as an excellent antigen presenting cell for expanding EBV-specific T cells to administer to patients.

Epstein–Barr virus-specific T cells have been given to more than 120 patients either at high risk for PTLD or with active disease after allogeneic HSCT. Analysis of the outcomes demonstrated that these cells expanded a thousand-fold or more *in vivo*,[30–33] persisted as long as ten years,[31] prevented EBV lymphoma in the immunocompromised host by destroying EBV-infected target cells,[34] and eradicated established EBV-associated lymphomas.[31,34]

The success of EBV-specific T cells spurred efforts to make them available as off-the-shelf therapies using third-party, allogeneic EBV cytotoxic T lymphocytes (CTLs) matched through at least one HLA type. In a clinical trial, overall response rates of 52% were obtained after infusing third-party CTLs to post-transplant recipients who failed conventional therapies for lymphoproliferative disease.[35] Similarly in another trial, human leukocyte antigen (HLA)-disparate EBV-specific T cells resulted in complete and partial remissions in 68% of treated patients.[36] Finally, CTL recognizing EBV, as well as cytomegalovirus (CMV) and adenovirus, were able to treat rituximab-resistant EBV-associated PTLD, resulting in four complete remissions and two partial remissions in eight treated patients.[37]

Having thus demonstrated activity against immunogenic EBV lymphomas occurring after transplant, attempts were made to extend use of EBV CTLs to EBV-associated cancers arising in immune-competent individuals that expressed a more restricted array of EBV antigens. The use of EBV-specific cytotoxic T cells (EBV-CTLs) in patients after allo-HSCT is an ideal model for this therapeutic approach because these patients lack competing endogenous T cells and are already lymphopenic (which facilitates expansion and persistence of adoptively transferred cells). Moreover, the viral tumor antigens have not undergone immune editing, thus rendering these tumor cells highly immunogenic and easily recognized by the infused EBV-CTLs.[38,39]

Although such favorable conditions are not present in immune-competent patients with EBV-associated malignancies, several modifications allow for the application of the viral antigen-specific CTL platform to this population. In follow-up studies, EBV-specific CTL therapies were extended to patients with EBV-associated Hodgkin's lymphomas (HL). In this setting, the Hodgkin/Reed–Sternberg cell expresses EBV antigens associated with type II latency proteins: LMP1, LMP2, BARF1, and EBNA1. After infusion of EBV-CTLs, small numbers of latent membrane protein (LMP)-specific T cells present in the bulk EBV-CTL cultures were sufficient to produce long-term disease control, but only in patients with minimal residual disease.[40] Improved methods then utilized highly enriched CTLs specific for the EBV LMP antigens expressed by the tumors. In two trials administering CTLs recognizing the LMP2 antigen or both LMP1 and LMP2 antigens, impressive response rates in patients with advanced/relapsed EBV-positive lymphomas (Hodgkin's lymphoma, natural killer T-cell lymphoma, and B-cell lymphoma) were observed, with approximately 50% of patients with relapsed/refractory disease attaining a complete or partial remission with CTL therapy alone.[41] Further, when used in the adjuvant setting, 28 of 29 high-risk or multiply-relapsed HL and non-HL patients remained in durable remissions (>80% 3-year progression-free survival) following infusion of LMP-specific CTLs.[42]

Epstein–Barr virus-specific CTLs have also been used in nasopharyngeal cancer, where more than 95% of tumors express the EBV proteins associated with type II viral latency. Among patients with active disease, 48% had a complete response and 15% had a partial response, with a two-year disease-free survival of more than 60% versus the expected 5 to 20% in published series.[43,44] Moreover, this approach was successfully exported to other institutions abroad through a collaborative study in Singapore showing the same 60% two-year survival in the CTL treatment group.[45] Several clinical trials using EBV-specific T cells for malignancies are currently ongoing (Table 16.1).

TABLE 16.1   Clinical Trials with EBV Specific T Cells

Clinical Trial	Indication	Group
NCT00078546	Nasopharyngeal cancer (following CD45 antibody)	Baylor College of Medicine
NCT00058773	Relapsed Hodgkin's disease	Baylor College of Medicine
NCT01430390	Residual/relapsed ALL	Memorial Sloan-Kettering Cancer Center
NCT00953420	Nasopharyngeal carcinoma (following carboplatin and docetaxel)	Baylor College of Medicine
NCT00058617	Relapsed lymphoma	Baylor College of Medicine
NCT01195480	Childhood acute lymphoblastic leukemia	University College, London I European Union Framework 6 Specific Targeted Research Project Initiative I The Leukemia and Lymphoma Society I Children with Leukaemia I Department of Health, United Kingdom I JP Moulton Charitable Foundation I Deutsche Krebshilfe
NCT00609219	Nasopharyngeal cancer	Baylor College of Medicine
NCT00006100	Progressive, relapsed, or refractory Hodgkin's lymphoma	National Cancer Institute (NCI) I Milton S. Hershey Medical Center
NCT00690872	Metastatic/locally recurrent nasopharyngeal cancer	National Cancer Institute (NCI) I National Cancer Centre, Singapore
NCT00002663	Lymphoma, lymphoproliferative disease	Memorial Sloan-Kettering Cancer Center
NCT01823718	Lymphoma	Nantes University Hospital
NCT00779337	Relapsed/refractory lymphoma	Queensland Institute of Medical Research I The Atlantic Philanthropies I Australian Department of Industry, Tourism and Resources I British Society for Haematology I National Health and Medical Research Council, Australia
NCT00005606	Lymphoproliferative disease	Northwestern University I National Cancer Institute (NCI)
NCT00058604	Lymphoma following solid organ transplant	Baylor College of Medicine
NCT00706316	Nasopharyngeal cancer	University Health Network, Toronto
NCT00063648	Lymphoproliferative disorder after liver transplant	National Institute of Diabetes and Digestive and Kidney Diseases (NIDDK)

(Continued)

TABLE 16.1   Clinical Trials with EBV Specific T Cells (*cont.*)

Clinical Trial	Indication	Group
NCT00709033	Advanced B cell NHL/CLL	Baylor College of Medicine
NCT01636388	Recurrent/refractory Hodgkins lymphoma	New York Medical College ∣ Children's Research Institute ∣ Baylor College of Medicine ∣ M.D. Anderson Cancer Center ∣ Beckman Research Institute ∣ Johns Hopkins University ∣ Ohio State University ∣ University of Utah ∣ University of Michigan
NCT01460901	Neuroblastoma	Children's Mercy Hospital Kansas City/NHLBI
NCT01447056	Hodgkin's/non Hodgkin's lymphoma, lymphoproliferative disease, nasopharyngeal carcinoma, leiomyosarcoma (third party)	Baylor College of Medicine

Efforts to extend results from the EBV setting into other virus-associated malignancies are now underway. Preclinical development of T cells recognizing cytomegalovirus (CMV) for CMV-expressing glioblastoma (GBM)[46] and human papilloma virus type 16 (HPV16) for HPV-associated tumors such as cervical carcinoma[47] have been encouraging. CMV-specific T cells were expanded to clinically sufficient numbers from GBM patients using monocytes that have been transduced with an adenoviral vector expressing the immunogenic CMV proteins IE1 and pp65, and these cells showed CMV-specific cytokine secretion and cytotoxicity against HLA-matched GBM cells infected with CMV VR1814 *in vitro*.[46] HPV-specific T cells, on the other hand, were expanded using monocyte-derived dendritic cells loaded with an overlapping peptide library spanning the E6/E7 protein of HPV, and released cytokines in response to E6/E7-expressing autologous targets and lysed partially matched HPV16+ cervical cancer cell lines.[47]

Although these results are promising, the majority of tumors are not associated with viral antigens or caused by a viral etiology.[48] The challenge, therefore, is to extend T-cell therapy toward the treatment of tumors expressing weaker, tumor-associated self-antigens.

Tumor Antigen-Specific T Cells

In contrast to highly immunogenic viral antigens, tumor antigens are often self-proteins that are mostly weakly immunogenic. A majority of T cells do not have the receptors capable of avidly binding to self antigens.[49] Selection processes mediated early in life and through central and peripheral tolerance ensure that only a small percentage of cells are able to recognize self proteins, reflecting the body's efforts to curtail possible autoimmune reactions.[1]

Four groups of non-viral tumor antigens are frequently recognized: (1) antigens associated with mutations, where the mutated peptide is able to bind to HLA (or the wild-type does not) or the modified HLA–peptide configuration creates a new epitope for T cells; (2) cancer–testis antigens, germline proteins expressed by different tumors and immune-privileged germ cells; (3) differentiation antigens, with tissue-specific expression; and (4) overexpressed antigens, which are seen at much higher levels in tumors as a result of the genomic imbalance.[50] For these antigens, investigators generally use one of three methods of expanding tumor-specific T cells *ex vivo*: (1) antigen-presenting cells (APCs) loaded with whole tumor lysates,[51] (2) electroporation/transfection of mRNA[52] or plasmid DNA[53] containing the antigen as a transgene into APCs, and (3) APCs pulsed with immunogenic peptides, either as specific epitopes or as overlapping libraries spanning the protein of interest.[54]

Upon closer examination, however, the list of known tumor antigens is very limited and hardly representative of the various malignancies oncologists wish to target.[55] Roughly 55% of tumor antigens with point mutations are specific to melanoma, 34% of shared tumor specific antigens are from melanoma, and 58% of melanoma differentiation antigens found in tumors are from melanoma. Besides the fact that melanoma is more than adequately represented in the field of T-cell immunotherapy as highlighted by TIL therapies, this disease only accounts for approximately 2% of all malignancies.[56]

Still, clinical trials using tumor antigen-specific T cells directed against metastatic melanoma are extremely important proof-of-principle studies. Meidenbauer et al.[57] infused eight patients with T cells specific for a Melan-A epitope recognized through HLA-A2 (ELAGIGILTV) and showed increased frequencies of tumor-specific T cells up to two weeks following transfer and preferential localization at tumor sites. Mackensen et al.,[58] using similar methods, treated 11 melanoma patients and also observed increased frequency of Melan-A-specific T cells up to two weeks. Three of the 11 patients also had documented antitumor responses. Khammari et al.[59] infused 14 patients with autologous T-cell clones specific for Melan A and also observed *in vivo* expansion of T-cell populations coupled with observed objective clinical responses (both complete and partial remissions) in six patients (two of which had long-term complete remissions).

In contrast, the use of tumor-specific antigens against non-melanoma tumors has seen more modest results. Wright et al.[60] infused seven patients with recurrent ovarian cancer with T cells specific for the MUC1 peptide GSTAPPAHGVTSAPDTRPAP, and reported that one patient was disease free for more than a year. Similarly, Dobrzanski et al.[61] adoptively transferred MUC1-specific T cells for treatment of ovarian cancer and saw at best an association between monthly treatment and enhanced survival (with 1/4 disease free and 1/4 with prolonged survival).

Several studies are seeking to improve upon tumor antigen-specific T-cell therapies and have shown promising results. WT1-specific T cells from healthy donors generated by overlapping peptide mixes spanning the protein were able to lyse WT1-expressing leukemia cells.[62] Tumor-specific T cells targeting WT1, survivin, MAGE-A3, and PRAME were expanded from patients with acute lymphoblastic leukemia despite low lymphocyte counts, with cells showing specificity for their targets and cytotoxic ability against autologous bone marrow blast sample.[63] Analogously, tumor-specific T cells targeting survivin, PRAME, NY-ESO1, SSX2, and MAGE-A4 can be expanded from lymphoma patients and this approach is currently being evaluated clinically (NCT01333046; see Table 16.3).[54,64]

GENETICALLY MODIFIED T CELLS

For all the advantages of antigen-specific T cells, their applications are inevitably limited against cancers because of the low-affinity self-antigens seen in tumors, the HLA-match dependence of tumors, and the downregulation of major histocompatibility complex (MHC) by some malignancies. To provide alternative options, genetic modification of T cells has been used to redirect specificities of T cells from their native T-cell receptors (TCRs) into the relevant antigen of choice. Two successful technologies employed are the generation of (1) known $\alpha\beta$ TCRs from high-affinity tumor antigen T-cell clones, and (2) chimeric antigen receptors recognizing proteins (or other antigens) in tumors through single-chain fragments of monoclonal antibodies.[49]

TCR Gene Transfer

T cells from both cancer patients and healthy donors seldom contain clones with high affinity directed against self-proteins and tumor antigens because of central and peripheral tolerance mechanisms. In the rare patient where such cell populations arise, a high-affinity TCR clone can provide immune protection against tumors expressing the corresponding antigen. Earlier discoveries that showed T-cell antigen specificity derived from a heterodimeric complex of two immunoglobulin-like proteins (α and β) that form part of the TCR complex,[1] coupled with advances in gene transfer technology, allowed for the genetic modification of T cells. The process described is the basis for the production of tumor-specific T cells via TCR gene transfer.[49]

Several investigators have applied TCR gene transfer with varying degrees of success.[65–71] One example of this approach was the study by Morgan et al.[72] where 31 patients with metastatic melanoma received T cells that had been modified to express TCRs recognizing the MART-1 antigen. The gene-modified T cells persisted for up to 12 months. Although objective clinical responses were only seen in 13% of the patients, this was a highly important proof-of-principle study. A follow-up study used a TCR with an even higher avidity for an HLA-A2 restricted epitope of MART-1. Better responses (30%) were noted in this study,[73] but they did not approach many of the response rates observed in the studies using lymphodepletion, unmanipulated TILs, and IL-2.[23]

One concern with this technology is that, although redirecting the T cell's specificity using TCR gene transfer may provide higher avidity receptors, the modified T cells remain limited to the HLA-restriction of the donor TCR. Further, because transgenic alpha and beta chains can theoretically pair with a T cell's own endogenous TCR chains, mispairings can potentially result in a nonfunctional TCR, thereby decreasing the effectiveness of the immune therapy. In addition, a TCR recognizing a self protein may potentially cause harmful graft-versus-host effects. Investigators have therefore used a variety of methods to address these problems: adding murine components to the TCR, adding cysteine to initiate dimers, and silencing the endogenous TCR using small interfering RNA (siRNA).[74]

Chimeric Antigen Receptors

Given the limitations of the TCR gene transfer technology, the use of chimeric antigen receptor appears an attractive alternative that allows a broader, non-HLA-restricted targeting of tumor antigens *in vivo*.[49] Chimeric antigen receptors (CARs) are composed of an extracellular region that mediates antigen recognition. This region consists of a single-chain variable fragment of a monoclonal antibody recognizing a particular antigen and an intracellular region that mediates T-cell activation and signaling upon ligand binding. The basic design for CARs was derived from studies by Eshhar et al.,[76] who investigated ways of conferring antibody specificity onto any lymphocyte.

Chimeric antigen receptor-modified T cells have several distinct advantages over virus-specific, tumor-specific, and TCR-transgenic T cells: (1) they are HLA independent; (2) they can target a wide variety of antigens, not just proteins; (3) they can redirect specificity of different T cell subsets; and (4) they can be engineered to deliver or express any protein that can enhance their antitumor activity.[77]

Early CAR-modified T cells, which incorporated so-called first-generation CAR technology, used the zeta chain of the T-cell receptor complex as the intracellular signaling moiety. These

CARs showed great promise in murine studies by mediating complete regression of tumor cells overexpressing the target antigen of CARs directed against ErbB2, for example.[78] However, the absence of additional costimulatory signals from actual tumors meant that the CAR-modified T cells did not proliferate and hence did not persist *in vivo*. Because only "signal 1" was delivered to the T cells, the often downregulated costimulatory molecules in tumors meant that "signal 2" was frequently absent.[79] This was highlighted in the initial clinical trials targeting CD19+ and CD20+ hematologic malignancies where T cells modified to express first-generation anti-CD19 and anti-CD20 CARs failed to persist in patients and had limited efficacy.[80]

Efforts to improve persistence focused on adding costimulatory molecules such as CD28 (so-called second-generation CARs). These second-generation CARs included the intracellular signaling domain from CD28 coupled to the zeta chain of the TCR complex. In the only study comparing first- and second-generation CARs, Savoldo et al.[81] administered T cells that were genetically modified to recognize CD19. Two T-cell lines were generated: one expressing a first-generation CD19 CAR and the other expressing a second-generation CD19 CAR that included the CD28 costimulatory signaling domain. By infusing both T-cell products into the same patient, comparisons were made of their persistence and *in vivo* activities. CAR T cells coexpressing the CD28 endodomain persisted longer than their first-generation counterparts, demonstrating the ability of CD28 signaling to mediate T-cell proliferation and persistence *in vivo*. However, the therapeutic efficacy even of the T cells expressing the second-generation CARs was modest in this study.

Another strategy to improve persistence utilized native TCR signaling from latent viral antigens. T cells continually receive activating signals from latent antigens expressed *in vivo*. Pule et al.[82] investigated whether or not these virus-specific TCRs provide survival signals to CAR-modified T cells. In this study, enhanced survival of EBV-specific T cells modified with a first-generation CAR recognizing GD2 in neuroblastoma patients was observed compared to non-specifically activated T cells modified with the same CARs,[82,83] with evidence of clinical efficacy.

An alternative approach evaluated the homeostatic environment of adoptively transferred T cells and utilized lymphodepleting chemotherapy regimens to enhance persistence similar to the early TIL studies. Endogenous cells from lymphoreplete hosts are believed to compete for cytokines and regulate or suppress infused T cells, causing decreased expansion and persistence of the gene-modified T cells *in vivo*. By lymphodepleting the host, cytokine sinks and regulatory cells are eliminated.[84] Using a chemotherapy regimen comprised of cyclophosphamide and fludarabine followed by infusion of CD19 CAR T cells, Kochenderfer et al.[85] observed remissions from progressive B-cell malignancies in six of eight. Following allogeneic transplant, CD19 CAR T cells mediated tumor eradication and reversion to MRD-negative status in five patients with B-cell acute lymphoblastic leukemia.[86] Finally, the group at the University of Pennsylvania utilized a second-generation CARs that used 41BBL instead of CD28 as the costimulatory moiety. They transduced CD3/28 stimulated T cells with a lentivirus expressing the CAR CD19 41BBL and following "dealers' choice" chemotherapy showed highly impressive rapid and sustained responses in two out of three patients with chronic lymphocytic leukemia.[87,88] Estimates that each infused CAR-expressing T cell eradicated more than 1000 chronic lymphoid leukemia (CLL) cells serve as a powerful illustration of the potency of CAR-modified T cells.[88] The same success was demonstrated in two patients with acute lymphoblastic leukemia, with one patient having a durable response almost a year following infusion.[89]

A large number of studies have focused on T cells expressing CARs directed against CD19 (Table 16.2). Although inevitably targeting healthy B cells along with malignant ones,

TABLE 16.2   Clinical Trials with CD19 CAR T Cells

Clinical Trial	T Cell	Groups
NCT01865617	Anti-CD19 chimeric antigen receptor (CAR) lentiviral vector-transduced autologous T lymphocytes	Fred Hutchinson Cancer Research Center, National Cancer Institute
NCT01087294	Anti-CD19 CAR-transduced T cells	National Institutes of Health Clinical Center, National Cancer Institute
NCT00586391	CD19 CAR-28-zeta T cells	Baylor College of Medicine
NCT00924326	Anti-CD19 CAR transduced peripheral blood lymphocytes	National Institutes of Health Clinical Center, National Cancer Institute
NCT01593696	Anti-CD19 CAR autologous peripheral blood lymphocytes	National Institutes of Health Clinical Center, National Cancer Institute
NCT00840853	CD19 CAR virus-specific T cells	Baylor College of Medicine
NCT01683279	Autologous CD19 CAR+ EGFTt+ T cells	Seattle Children's Hospital
NCT01815749	CD19 CAR-specific/truncated epidermal growth factor receptor (EGFR) lentiviral vector-transduced autologous T cells	City of Hope Medical Center, National Cancer Institute
NCT01864889	Anti-CD19 CAR vector-transduced T cells	Chinese PLA General Hospital
NCT01475058	Anti-CD19 CAR cytomegalovirus-specific cytotoxic T lymphocytes (CTLs)	Fred Hutchinson Cancer Research Center, University of Washington Cancer Consortium, National Cancer Institute
NCT01195480	Donor-derived Epstein–Barr virus (EBV)-specific cytotoxic T cells (EBV-CTLs) transduced with the retroviral vector SFGalpha-CD19-CD3zeta	University College, London; European Union Framework 6 Specific Targeted Research Project Initiative; Leukemia and Lymphoma Society; Children with Leukemia; Department of Health, United Kingdom; J.P. Moulton Charitable Foundation; Deutsche Krebshilfe
NCT01029366	Anti-CD19 CAR retroviral vector-transduced autologous T cells	Abramson Cancer Center of the University of Pennsylvania
NCT01430390	Anti-CD19 CAR EBV-specific CTLs	Memorial Sloan–Kettering Cancer Center
NCT01853631	CD19-specific CAR T cells 2nd versus 3rd generation	Baylor College of Medicine
NCT01840566	Anti-CD19-28z CAR T cells	Memorial Sloan–Kettering Cancer Center
NCT01860937	Anti-CD19-28z CAR T cells	Memorial Sloan–Kettering Cancer Center
NCT01626495	Anti-CD19 CAR 41BBz autologous T cells	Children's Hospital of Philadelphia, University of Pennsylvania
NCT01318317	Anti-CD19 CAR T cells	City of Hope Medical Center, National Cancer Institute
NCT00466531	Anti-CD19 CAR T cells	Memorial Sloan–Kettering Cancer Center, National Cancer Institute

previous experience with monoclonal antibodies (rituximab) directed against B-cell antigens suggest that the accompanying B-cell ablation is tolerable and B-cell counts can be expected to recover.[90] However as shown in Table 16.2, the treatment of patients with B-cell malignancies using autologous[81,85,88,91] and allogeneic[92,93] CD19 CAR-modified T cells has yielded mixed results. It is difficult to dissect the precise reasons for these differences, as each protocol varies in terms of CAR design, T-cell production, prior conditioning chemotherapy, and tumor burden.[94]

The future of this field is focused not only on proving the efficacy of the CD19 CAR strategy in Phase II/III studies but also on evaluating this approach utilizing other targets. For example, CARs targeting CD138 are being investigated in a clinical trial targeting chemotherapy-refractory multiple myeloma (NCT01886976), while T cells recognizing Her2 have been developed for the treatment of glioblastoma and lung cancer.[95] Ongoing trials with other chimeric antigen receptors are listed in Table 16.3. Finally, in an attempt to further improve the efficacy of the CAR-modified T cells, third-generation CARs incorporating two or more costimulatory molecules have been developed,[77,79] and comparisons with second-generation CARs are currently underway in clinical trials.

TABLE 16.3   Other Ongoing Clinical Trials with T Cell Immunotherapies for Cancer

	NCT Number	Phase	Indication	Product	Groups
Activated T cells, donor lymphocyte infusion (DLI)	NCT01802138		Refractory, relapsed neuroblastoma	Activated T cells	Seoul National University Hospital
	NCT01897610	Phase II	Advanced hepatocellular carcinoma	Activated T cells	Green Cross Cell Corporation
	NCT01144247	Phase I	Glioma, anaplastic astrocytoma, anaplastic oligodendroglioma, anaplastic mixed glioma, glioblastoma multiforme, malignant meningioma	Alloreactive cytotoxic T lymphocytes	Jonsson Comprehensive Cancer Center; National Institutes of Health Clinical Center; National Cancer Institute
	NCT01943188	Phase I	Clear-cell carcinoma, renal-cell cancer	Autologous T cells	Stanford University; National Cancer Institute
	NCT01426828	Phase II	Multiple myeloma	CD3/CD28 activated T cells	Abramson Cancer Center
	NCT00242515	Phase I/II	Acute myeloid leukemia, myelodysplastic syndrome	Donor lymphocyte infusion	National University Hospital Singapore; Singapore General Hospital

(Continued)

TABLE 16.3   Other Ongoing Clinical Trials with T Cell Immunotherapies for Cancer *(cont.)*

NCT Number	Phase	Indication	Product	Groups
NCT01627275	Phase I	Hematologic malignancies	Donor lymphocyte infusion	Duke University
NCT01518153	Phase II	Leukemia, lymphoma, myeloma, myeloproliferative disease	Donor lymphocyte infusion	MD Anderson Cancer Center
NCT01131169	Phase II	Multiple myeloma	Donor lymphocyte infusion	Memorial Sloan–Kettering Cancer Center; Otsuka America Pharmaceutical; Ludwig Institute of Cancer Research
NCT00534118		Hematologic malignancies	Donor lymphocyte infusion	Roswell Park Cancer Institute
NCT01240525	Phase II	Hematologic malignancies	Donor lymphocyte infusion	University College London
NCT00167180	Phase II	Chronic myeloid leukemia (CML), lymphomas, multiple myeloma, myelodysplastic syndrome, acute lymphoblastic leukemia, chronic lymphocytic leukemia, acute myeloid leukemia	Donor lymphocyte infusion	Masonic Cancer Center
NCT00376480	Phase I	Leukemia, myelodysplastic syndrome	Donor lymphocyte infusion	National Cancer Institute; Dana Farber Cancer Institute
NCT01794299	Phase II	Acute myeloid leukemia, acute lymphoblastic leukemia, myelodysplastic syndrome	Donor lymphocyte infusion	Kiadis Pharma
NCT01875237	Phase I/II	Leukemia, myeloma, myeloproliferative disease	iCasp9 donor lymphocyte infusion	MD Anderson Cancer Center; Bellicum Pharmaceuticals
NCT01839916	Phase II	Hematologic malignancies	Donor T cells	University of Chicago; National Cancer Institute

TABLE 16.3 Other Ongoing Clinical Trials with T Cell Immunotherapies for Cancer (*cont.*)

	NCT Number	Phase	Indication	Product	Groups
	NCT01630564	Phase I	Leukemia, lymphoma, myeloprooliferative disease	Expanded cord blood T cells	MD Anderson Cancer Center
	NCT01140373	Phase I	Castrate metastatic prostate cancer	Engineered autologous T cells	Memorial Sloan–Kettering Cancer Center; Department of Defense
	NCT00914628	Phase III	High-risk acute leukemia	HSVTk donor lymphocyte infusion	MolMed SPA
	NCT00602693	Phase I	Hematologic malignancies	Regulatory T cells	Masonic Cancer Center
	NCT01946373	Phase I	Melanoma	T cells	Karolinska University Hospital
	NCT01685606	Phase II	Leukemia, lymphoma	T cells	Brown University
	NCT00937625	Phase I	Melanoma	T cells	Herlev Hospital
	NCT00986518	Phase I/II	Colorectal cancer	Treg-depleted T cells	Assistance Publique–Hopitaux de Paris
	NCT01513109	Phase I/II	Acute myeloid leukemia	Treg-depleted T cells	Jules Bordet Institute
Tumor-infiltrating lymphocytes	NCT01814046	Phase II	Metastatic ocular melanoma	Tumor-infiltrating lymphocytes	National Institutes of Health Clinical Center; National Cancer Institute
	NCT01462903	Phase I	Nasopharyngeal carcinoma, hepatocellular carcinoma, breast carcinoma	Tumor-infiltrating lymphocytes	Sun Yat-sen University
	NCT01659151	Phase II	Melanoma	Tumor-infiltrating lymphocytes	H. Lee Moffitt Cancer Center and Research Institute
	NCT01460901	Phase I	Neuroblastoma	Trivirus-specific cytotoxic T lymphocytes	Children's Mercy Hospital Kansas City; National Heart, Lung, and Blood Institute
Tumor Ag cytotoxic T lymphocytes	NCT01333046	Phase I	Hodgkin's lymphoma, non-Hodgkin's lymphoma	Tumor-associated antigen-specific cytotoxic T lymphocytes	Baylor College of Medicine

(Continued)

TABLE 16.3   Other Ongoing Clinical Trials with T Cell Immunotherapies for Cancer (*cont.*)

	NCT Number	Phase	Indication	Product	Groups
T-cell receptor (TCR) transgenic T cells	NCT01343043	Phase I	Synovial sarcoma	NY-ESO-1 HLA-A2 T-cell receptor transgenic cytotoxic T lymphocytes	Adaptimmune; National Cancer Institute
	NCT01273181	Phase I/II	Metastatic cancer	MAGE A3/12 HLA-A2 T-cell receptor transgenic cytotoxic T lymphocytes	National Cancer Institute
	NCT01967823	Phase II	Metastatic cancer	NY-ESO-1 mouse T-cell receptor transgenic cytotoxic T lymphocytes	National Cancer Institute
	NCT01621724	Phase I/II	Acute myeloid leukemia, chronic myeloid leukemia	WT1 HLA-A2 T-cell receptor transgenic cytotoxic T lymphocytes	University College, London
	NCT00670748	Phase II	Metastatic melanoma and renal cancer	NY-ESO-1 HLA-A2 T-cell receptor transgenic cytotoxic T lymphocytes	National Cancer Institute
	NCT01350401	Phase I/II	Melanoma	NY-ESO-1 HLA-A2 T-cell receptor transgenic cytotoxic T lymphocytes	Adaptimmune
Other chimeric antigen receptor (CAR) T cells	NCT01886976	Phase I/II	Multiple myeloma	Anti-CD138 chimeric antigen receptor T cells	Chinese PLA General Hospital
	NCT01735604		Hematologic malignancies	Anti-CD20 chimeric antigen receptor T cells	Chinese PLA General Hospital
	NCT01316146	Phase I	Hodgkin's lymphoma, non-Hodgin's lymphoma	Anti-CD30 chimeric antigen receptor T cells	Baylor College of Medicine

TABLE 16.3   Other Ongoing Clinical Trials with T Cell Immunotherapies for Cancer *(cont.)*

NCT Number	Phase	Indication	Product	Groups
NCT01864902	Phase I/II	CD33+ acute myeloid leukemia	Anti-CD33 chimeric antigen receptor T cells	Chinese PLA General Hospital
NCT01822652	Phase I	Neuroblastoma	Anti-GD2 chimeric antigen receptor T cells with iCasp9	Baylor College of Medicine
NCT01109095	Phase I	Glioblastoma multiforme	Anti-Her2 chimeric anti-gen receptor cytomegalo-virus-specific cytotoxic T lymphocytes	Baylor College of Medicine
NCT00881920	Phase I	Lymphoma, myeloma, leukemia	Anti-kappa chimeric antigen receptor T cells	Baylor College of Medicine
NCT01318317	Phase I/II	B-cell non-Hodgkin's lymphoma	Engineered T cells	City of Hope medical Center; National Cancer Institute
NCT01586403	Phase I	Melanoma	Engineered T cells	Loyola University; National Cancer Institute
NCT01740557	Phase I/II	Melanoma	CXCR2 or nerve growth factor receptor-transduced T cells	MD Anderson Cancer Center; National Institutes of Health Clinical Center; National Cancer Institute
NCT01081808	Phase I	Advanced solid tumors	EGFRBi-armed activated T cells	Roger Williams Medical Center
NCT00569296	Phase I	Non-small cell lung cancer	EGFRBi-armed activated T cells	Roger Williams Medical Center
NCT01022138	Phase II	Metastatic breast cancer	Her2Bi-armed activated T cells	Barbar Ann Karmanos Cancer Institute; National Cancer Institute
NCT00889954	Phase I	Her2+ malignancies	TGF-β DNRII-transduced Her2/ Epstein–Barr virus cytotoxic T lymphocytes	Baylor College of Medicine

(Continued)

IV. NOVEL APPROACHES FOR CANCER THERAPIES

TABLE 16.3   Other Ongoing Clinical Trials with T Cell Immunotherapies for Cancer *(cont.)*

NCT Number	Phase	Indication	Product	Groups
NCT00368082	Phase I	Lymphoma	TGF-β DNRII-transduced latent membrane protein-specific cytotoxic T lymphocytes	Baylor College of Medicine
NCT01723306	Phase II	Adenocarcinoma	Anti-CEA chimeric antigen receptor T cells	Roger Williams Medical Center
NCT01955460	Phase I	Melanoma	TGF-β DNRII-transduced tumor-infiltrating lymphocytes	MD Anderson Cancer Center

CHALLENGES IN T-CELL IMMUNOTHERAPIES

Despite its successes, several obstacles still must be overcome to enable the successful translation of T-cell immunotherapies into mainstream clinical practice.

Persistence of T Cells

Chief among the limitations is the issue of persistence. Although virus-specific T cells in the lymphodepleted setting seem to have maximal persistence, the same cannot be said of other T cells (tumor-specific T cells, CAR T cells, etc.). The ideal scenario involves the long-term persistence of T cells in the memory compartment, providing life-long protection against infections and cancer. However, outside of latent viruses that continually express the antigens *in vivo*, infused T cells do not get the required antigenic stimulation to maintain their populations. Tumors, for example, downregulate antigens on their surface, inactivate professional antigen-presenting cells, or release antiinflammatory molecules that prevent T cells from receiving proliferative signals.[21,38,49] Most human cancers secrete transforming growth factor β (TGF-β), a cytokine that prevents proliferation of both CD4+ Th1 cells and cytotoxic T cells, effectively inducing tolerance.[96] Inherent limitations in the cell culture process may also limit the activities of T cells *in vivo*, as *in vitro* expansion requires multiple stimulations, a process that may decrease the telomere lengths of T cells and thereby hasten their early senescence *in vivo*.[97]

A number of approaches have been employed that seek to mitigate poor T-cell persistence *in vivo*. Genetic modification of T cells to express antiapoptotic genes such as Bcl-2[98] or to overexpress human telomerase to lengthen their telomeres[99] have been reported in the literature. T cells rendered resistant to the negative effects of TGF-β through expression of a dominant negative TGF-β receptor on their surface have been developed and are currently being evaluated clinically.[100] Similarly, T cells rendered resistant to the apoptotic signals of FasL have shown enhanced persistence in murine models.[101] Finally, the depletion of regulatory T cells that have homeostatic negative effects on antigen-specific T cells is another strategy to overcome the immune suppressive tumor microenvironment to improve the efficacy of adoptively transferred tumor-specific T cells.[102]

Safety of T Cells

The occurrence of severe adverse events[103,104] in the last few years highlights the fact that the potency of the T-cell-mediated effects can be a concern when there is effective tumor killing. Although a review of T-cell infusions at a single institution noted no immediate adverse events greater than grade 2 that were attributable to adoptively transferred T cells,[105] tumor-specific T cells have been shown to mediate a panoply of unintended later effects, including fever and non-specific constitutional symptoms, as a consequence of an inflammatory mediator release or cytokine secretion.[106] Hence, adoptively transferred T cells have the potential to release significant amounts of cytokines like tumor necrosis factor α (TNF-α), IL-1β, and IL-6 which may damage the host's environment.[107] Upon infusion, T cells can potentially recognize normal host cells, secrete interferon gamma, and, consequently, increase expression of HLA in other host cells. Rapid proliferation and activation of T cells ensue, resulting in more cytokines being released and more immune cells activated—the cascade known as the *systemic inflammatory response syndrome*.[89,108] Further, a highly rapid elimination of tumors by antigen-specific T cells can lead to tumor lysis syndrome.[87,109,110]

For these reasons, approaches to eliminate T cells using suicide genes have been developed. The most common suicide gene system utilized clinically employs the herpes simplex thymidine kinase (HSVtk) gene. The expression of this gene presents a substrate for ganciclovir or acyclovir which, upon administration, converts the gene product into its toxic di- and triphosphate metabolites, thus leading to death of the cell.[111] In a study using donor lymphocytes transduced with the HSVtk genes, antitumor activity remained intact, while concomitant GVHD resolved upon administration of ganciclovir.[112] In another study, a safety switch comprised of an inducible caspase 9 gene, which activates upon contact with an inert small molecule and subsequently initiates the apoptosis cascade, was cloned into a retrovirus vector and used to transduce T cells administered to high-risk leukemia patients after haploidentical stem-cell transplantation. GVHD in four (of five) patients who developed the reaction promptly resolved after infusion of a single dose of dimerizing drug. Further, more than 90% of modified T cells were eliminated within 30 minutes of drug administration.[113]

SUMMARY

Cell-based therapies have been called the "next pillar of medicine,"[114] and the promising results observed with T-cell immunotherapeutics mean that these therapies will be an important part of the treatment options for patients with cancer. Their specificity, ability to home in to tumor sites, and amenability to genetic modification make them versatile biologics. Importantly, T-cell immunotherapies can potentially be administered to prevent malignancies because T cells can persist for prolonged periods as memory cells. Hence, the improved understanding of T-cell biology should yield exciting new options for cancer treatment and, conceivably, other chronic immune-related disorders.

References

1. Janeway CA, et al. Immunobiology: The Immune System in Health and Disease. 6th ed. New York: Garland Science; 2005.
2. Rosenberg SA. Raising the bar: the curative potential of human cancer immunotherapy. Sci. Transl. Med. 2012;4(127):127ps8.
3. Coley WB. The treatment of malignant tumors by repeated inoculations of erysipelas. With a report of ten original cases. 1893. Clin. Orthop. Relat. Res. 1991;(262):3–11.
4. Barnes DW, Corp MJ, Loutit JF, Neal FE. Treatment of murine leukaemia with X rays and homologous bone marrow; preliminary communication. Br. Med. J. 1956;2:626–7.
5. Fefer A, Einstein AB, Cheever MA. Adoptive chemoimmunotherapy of cancer in animals: a review of results, principles, and problems. Ann. N.Y. Acad. Sci. 1976;277:492–504.
6. Weiden PL, Sullivan KM, Flournoy N, Storb R, Thomas ED. Antileukemic effect of chronic graft-versus-host disease: contribution to improved survival after allogeneic marrow transplantation. New Engl. J. Med. 1981;304:1529–33.
7. Brunschwig A, Southam CM, Levin AG. Host resistance to cancer. Clinical experiments by homotransplants, autotransplants and admixture of autologous leucocytes. Ann. Surg. 1965;162:416–25.
8. Kolb HJ, et al. Donor leukocyte transfusions for treatment of recurrent chronic myelogenous leukemia in marrow transplant patients. Blood 1990;76:2462–5.
9. Slavin S, Eckerstein A, Weiss L. Adoptive immunotherapy in conjunction with bone marrow transplantation—amplification of natural host defence mechanisms against cancer by recombinant IL-2. Nat. Immun. Cell Growth Reg. 1988;7:180–4.
10. Sullivan KM, et al. Graft-versus-host disease as adoptive immunotherapy in patients with advanced hematologic neoplasms. New Engl. J. Med. 1989;320:828–34.
11. Yee C. Adoptive T-cell therapy of cancer. Hematol. Oncol. Clin. North Am. 2006;20:711–33.
12. Dazzi F, et al. Durability of responses following donor lymphocyte infusions for patients who relapse after allogeneic stem cell transplantation for chronic myeloid leukemia. Blood 2000;96:2712–6.
13. Kolb HJ, et al. Graft-versus-leukemia effect of donor lymphocyte transfusions in marrow grafted patients. Blood 1995;86:2041–50.
14. Amrolia PJ, et al. Adoptive immunotherapy with allodepleted donor T-cells improves immune reconstitution after haploidentical stem cell transplantation. Blood 2006;108:1797–808.
15. Perruccio K, et al. Photodynamic purging of alloreactive T cells for adoptive immunotherapy after haploidentical stem cell transplantation. Blood Cells Mol. Dis. 2008;40:76–83.
16. Hossain MS, Roback JD, Lezhava L, Hillyer CD, Waller EK. Amotosalen-treated donor T cells have polyclonal antigen-specific long-term function without graft-versus-host disease after allogeneic bone marrow transplantation. Biol. Blood Marrow Transplant. 2005;11:169–80.
17. Kennedy-Nasser AA, Bollard CM. T cell therapies following hematopoietic stem cell transplantation: surely there must be a better way than DLI? Bone Marrow Transplant. 2007;40:93–104.
18. Restifo NP, Dudley ME, Rosenberg SA. Adoptive immunotherapy for cancer: harnessing the T cell response. Nat. Rev. Immunol. 2012;12:269–81.
19. Rosenberg SA, et al. Use of tumor-infiltrating lymphocytes and interleukin-2 in the immunotherapy of patients with metastatic melanoma. A preliminary report. N. Engl. J. Med. 1988;319:1676–80.
20. Muul LM, Spiess PJ, Director EP, Rosenberg SA. Identification of specific cytolytic immune responses against autologous tumor in humans bearing malignant melanoma. J. Immunol. 1987;138:989–95.
21. Rosenberg SA, Yang JC, Restifo NP. Cancer immunotherapy: moving beyond current vaccines. Nat. Med. 2004;10:909–15.
22. Rosenberg SA, Restifo NP, Yang JC, Morgan RA, Dudley ME. Adoptive cell transfer: a clinical path to effective cancer immunotherapy. Nat. Rev. Cancer. 2008;8:299–308.

23. Dudley ME, et al. Adoptive cell therapy for patients with metastatic melanoma: evaluation of intensive myeloablative chemoradiation preparative regimens. J. Clin. Oncol. 2008;26:5233–9.

24. Zhang L, et al. Intratumoral T cells, recurrence, and survival in epithelial ovarian cancer. New Engl. J. Med. 2003;348:203–13.

25. Freedman RS, et al. Intraperitoneal adoptive immunotherapy of ovarian carcinoma with tumor-infiltrating lymphocytes and low-dose recombinant interleukin-2: a pilot trial. J. Immunother. Emphasis Tumor Immunol. 1994;16:198–210.

26. Fujita K, et al. Prolonged disease-free period in patients with advanced epithelial ovarian cancer after adoptive transfer of tumor-infiltrating lymphocytes. Clin. Cancer Res. 1995;1:501–7.

27. Gardini A, et al. Adjuvant, adoptive immunotherapy with tumor infiltrating lymphocytes plus interleukin-2 after radical hepatic resection for colorectal liver metastases: 5-year analysis. J. Surg. Oncol. 2004;87:46–52.

28. Young LS, Rickinson AB. Epstein–Barr virus: 40 years on. Nat. Rev. Cancer 2004;4:757–68.

29. Shapiro RS, et al. Epstein–Barr virus associated B cell lymphoproliferative disorders following bone marrow transplantation. Blood 1988;71:1234–43.

30. Rooney CM, et al. Use of gene-modified virus-specific T lymphocytes to control Epstein–Barr-virus-related lymphoproliferation. Lancet 1995;345:9–13.

31. Heslop HE, et al. Long-term outcome of EBV-specific T-cell infusions to prevent or treat EBV-related lymphoproliferative disease in transplant recipients. Blood 2010;115:925–35.

32. Leen AM, et al. Monoculture-derived T lymphocytes specific for multiple viruses expand and produce clinically relevant effects in immunocompromised individuals. Nat. Med. 2006;12:1160–6.

33. Heslop HE, et al. Long-term restoration of immunity against Epstein–Barr virus infection by adoptive transfer of gene-modified virus-specific T lymphocytes. Nat. Med. 1996;2:551–5.

34. Rooney CM, et al. Infusion of cytotoxic T cells for the prevention and treatment of Epstein–Barr virus-induced lymphoma in allogeneic transplant recipients. Blood 1998;92:1549–55.

35. Haque T, et al. Allogeneic cytotoxic T-cell therapy for EBV-positive posttransplantation lymphoproliferative disease: results of a phase 2 multicenter clinical trial. Blood 2007;110:1123–31.

36. Doubrovina E, et al. Adoptive immunotherapy with unselected or EBV-specific T cells for biopsy-proven EBV+ lymphomas after allogeneic hematopoietic cell transplantation. Blood 2012;119:2644–56.

37. Leen AM, et al. Multicenter study of banked third-party virus-specific T cells to treat severe viral infections after hematopoietic stem cell transplantation. Blood 2013;121:5113–23.

38. Gattinoni L, Powell DJ Jr, Rosenberg SA, Restifo NP. Adoptive immunotherapy for cancer: building on success. Nat. Rev. Immunol. 2006;6:383–93.

39. Schreiber RD, Old LJ, Smyth MJ. Cancer immunoediting: integrating immunity's roles in cancer suppression and promotion. Science 2011;331:1565–70.

40. Bollard CM, et al. Cytotoxic T lymphocyte therapy for Epstein–Barr virus+ Hodgkin's disease. J. Exp. Med. 2004;200:1623–33.

41. Bollard CM, et al. Complete responses of relapsed lymphoma following genetic modification of tumor-antigen presenting cells and T-lymphocyte transfer. Blood 2007;110:2838–45.

42. Bollard CM, et al. Sustained complete responses in lymphoma patients receiving autologous cytotoxic T lymphocytes targeting Epstein–Barr virus latent membrane proteins. J. Clin. Oncol. 2013;32(8):798–808.

43. Louis CU, et al. Enhancing the *in vivo* expansion of adoptively transferred EBV-specific CTL with lymphodepleting CD45 monoclonal antibodies in NPC patients. Blood 2009;113:2442–50.

44. Straathof KC, et al. Treatment of nasopharyngeal carcinoma with Epstein–Barr virus-specific T lymphocytes. Blood 2005;105:1898–904.

45. Teo M, et al. Chemotherapy in combination with T-cell therapy results in significant antitumor activity and improved clinical outcomes for EBV-associated nasopharyngeal carcinoma. Mol. Ther. 2011;19:S85–6.

46. Ghazi A, et al. Generation of polyclonal CMV-specific T cells for the adoptive immunotherapy of glioblastoma. J. Immunother. 2012;35:159–68.

47. Ramos CA, et al. Human papillomavirus type 16 E6/E7-specific cytotoxic T lymphocytes for adoptive immunotherapy of HPV-associated malignancies. J. Immunother. 2013;36:66–76.

48. Weinberg RA. The Biology of Cancer. Garland Science: New York; 2007.

49. Leen AM, Rooney CM, Foster AE. Improving T cell therapy for cancer. Ann. Rev. Immunol. 2007;25:243–65.

50. Seremet T, Brasseur F, Coulie PG. Tumor-specific antigens and immunologic adjuvants in cancer immunotherapy. Cancer J. 2011;17:325–30.

51. Kandalaft LE, et al. Autologous lysate-pulsed dendritic cell vaccination followed by adoptive transfer of vaccine-primed *ex vivo* co-stimulated T cells in recurrent ovarian cancer. Oncoimmunology 2013;2:e22664.

52. Van Driessche A, Ponsaerts P, Van Bockstaele DR, Van Tendeloo VF, Berneman ZN. Messenger RNA electroporation: an efficient tool in immunotherapy and stem cell research. Folia Histochem. Cytobiol. 2005;43(4):213–6.

53. Gerdemann U, et al. Nucleofection of DCs to generate multivirus-specific T cells for prevention or treatment of viral infections in the immunocompromised host. Mol. Ther. 2009;17:1616–25.

54. Gerdemann U, et al. Cytotoxic T lymphocytes simultaneously targeting multiple tumor-associated antigens to treat EBV negative lymphoma. Mol. Ther. 2011;19:2258–68.

55. Jager D, Jager E, Knuth A. Immune responses to tumour antigens: implications for antigen specific immunotherapy of cancer. J. Clin. Pathol. 2001;54:669–74.

56. Schreiber TH, Raez L, Rosenblatt JD, Podack ER. Tumor immunogenicity and responsiveness to cancer vaccine therapy: the state of the art. Sem. Immunol. 2010;22:105–12.

57. Meidenbauer N, et al. Survival and tumor localization of adoptively transferred Melan-A-specific T cells in melanoma patients. J. Immunol. 2003;170:2161–9.

58. Mackensen A, et al. Phase I study of adoptive T-cell therapy using antigen-specific CD8+ T cells for the treatment of patients with metastatic melanoma. J. Clin. Oncol. 2006;24:5060–9.

59. Khammari A, et al. Treatment of metastatic melanoma with autologous Melan-A/MART-1-specific cytotoxic T lymphocyte clones. J. Invest. Dermatol. 2009;129:2835–42.

60. Wright SE, et al. Cytotoxic T-lymphocyte immunotherapy for ovarian cancer: a pilot study. J. Immunother. 2012;35:196–204.

61. Dobrzanski MJ, et al. Immunotherapy with IL-10- and IFN-γ-producing CD4 effector cells modulate "natural" and "inducible" CD4 TReg cell subpopulation levels: observations in four cases of patients with ovarian cancer. Cancer Immunol. Immunother. 2012;61:839–54.

62. Doubrovina E, et al. Mapping of novel peptides of WT-1 and presenting HLA alleles that induce epitope-specific HLA-restricted T cells with cytotoxic activity against WT-1+ leukemias. Blood 2012;120:1633–46.

63. Weber G, et al. Generation of tumor antigen-specific T cell lines from pediatric patients with acute lymphoblastic leukemia—implications for immunotherapy. Clin. Cancer Res. 2013;19:5079–91.

64. Cruz CR, et al. Improving T-cell therapy for relapsed EBV-negative Hodgkin lymphoma by targeting upregulated MAGE-A4. Clin. Cancer Res. 2011;17:7058–66.

65. Clay TM, et al. Efficient transfer of a tumor antigen-reactive TCR to human peripheral blood lymphocytes confers anti-tumor reactivity. J. Immunol. 1999;163:507–13.

66. Morgan RA, et al. High efficiency TCR gene transfer into primary human lymphocytes affords avid recognition of melanoma tumor antigen glycoprotein 100 and does not alter the recognition of autologous melanoma antigens. J. Immunol. 2003;171:3287–95.

67. Schaft N, et al. Peptide fine specificity of anti-glycoprotein 100 CTL is preserved following transfer of engineered TCR alpha beta genes into primary human T lymphocytes. J. Immunol. 2003;170:2186–94.

68. Mutis T, Blokland E, Kester M, Schrama E, Goulmy E. Generation of minor histocompatibility antigen HA-1-specific cytotoxic T cells restricted by nonself HLA molecules: a potential strategy to treat relapsed leukemia after HLA-mismatched stem cell transplantation. Blood 2002;100:547–52.

69. Heemskerk MH, et al. Redirection of antileukemic reactivity of peripheral T lymphocytes using gene transfer of minor histocompatibility antigen HA-2-specific T-cell receptor complexes expressing a conserved alpha joining region. Blood 2003;102:3530–40.

70. Stanislawski T, et al. Circumventing tolerance to a human MDM2-derived tumor antigen by TCR gene transfer. Nat. Immunol. 2001;2:962–70.

71. Xue SA, et al. Elimination of human leukemia cells in NOD/SCID mice by WT1-TCR gene-transduced human T cells. Blood 2005;106:3062–7.

72. Morgan RA, et al. Cancer regression in patients after transfer of genetically engineered lymphocytes. Science 2006;314:126–9.

73. Johnson LA, et al. Gene therapy with human and mouse T-cell receptors mediates cancer regression and targets normal tissues expressing cognate antigen. Blood 2009;114:535–46.

74. Govers C, Sebestyen Z, Coccoris M, Willemsen RA, Debets R. T cell receptor gene therapy: strategies for optimizing transgenic TCR pairing. Trends Mol. Med. 2010;16:77–87.

75. Eshhar Z. Tumor-specific T-bodies: towards clinical application. Cancer Immunol. Immunother. 1997;45:131–6.

76. Eshhar Z, Waks T, Gross G, Schindler DG. Specific activation and targeting of cytotoxic lymphocytes through chimeric single chains consisting of antibody-binding domains and the gamma or zeta subunits of the immunoglobulin and T-cell receptors. Proc. Natl. Acad. Sci. U.S.A. 1993;90:720–4.

77. Curran KJ, Pegram HJ, Brentjens RJ. Chimeric antigen receptors for T cell immunotherapy: current understanding and future directions. J. Gene Med. 2012;14:405–15.

78. Altenschmidt U, Klundt E, Groner B. Adoptive transfer of *in vitro*-targeted, activated T lymphocytes results in total tumor regression. J. Immunol. 1997;159:5509–11.

79. Jena B, Dotti G, Cooper LJ. Redirecting T-cell specificity by introducing a tumor-specific chimeric antigen receptor. Blood 2010;116:1035–44.

80. Jensen MC, et al. Antitransgene rejection responses contribute to attenuated persistence of adoptively transferred CD20/CD19-specific chimeric antigen receptor redirected T cells in humans. Biol. Blood Marrow Transplant. 2010;16(9):1245–56.

81. Savoldo B, et al. CD28 costimulation improves expansion and persistence of chimeric antigen receptor-modified T cells in lymphoma patients. J. Clin. Invest. 2011;121:1822–6.

82. Pule MA, et al. Virus-specific T cells engineered to coexpress tumor-specific receptors: persistence and antitumor activity in individuals with neuroblastoma. Nat. Med. 2008;14:1264–70.

83. Louis CU, et al. Antitumor activity and long-term fate of chimeric antigen receptor-positive T cells in patients with neuroblastoma. Blood 2011;118:6050–6.

84. Rosenberg SA. Cell transfer immunotherapy for metastatic solid cancer—what clinicians need to know. Nat. Rev. Clin. Oncol. 2011;8:577–85.

85. Kochenderfer JN, et al. B-cell depletion and remissions of malignancy along with cytokine-associated toxicity in a clinical trial of anti-CD19 chimeric-antigen-receptor-transduced T cells. Blood 2012;119:2709–20.

86. Brentjens RJ, et al. CD19-targeted T cells rapidly induce molecular remissions in adults with chemotherapy-refractory acute lymphoblastic leukemia. Sci. Transl. Med. 2013;5. 177ra138.

87. Porter DL, Levine BL, Kalos M, Bagg A, June CH. Chimeric antigen receptor-modified T cells in chronic lymphoid leukemia. New Engl. J. Med. 2011;365:725–33.

88. Kalos M, et al. T cells with chimeric antigen receptors have potent antitumor effects and can establish memory in patients with advanced leukemia. Sci. Transl. Med. 2011;3. 95ra73.

89. Grupp SA, et al. Chimeric antigen receptor-modified T cells for acute lymphoid leukemia. New Engl. J. Med. 2013;368:1509–18.

90. Grillo-Lopez AJ, et al. Rituximab: the first monoclonal antibody approved for the treatment of lymphoma. Curr. Pharm. Biotechnol. 2000;1:1–9.

91. Brentjens RJ, et al. Safety and persistence of adoptively transferred autologous CD19-targeted T cells in patients with relapsed or chemotherapy refractory B-cell leukemias. Blood 2011;118:4817–28.

92. Cruz CR, et al. Infusion of donor-derived CD19-redirected-virus-specific T cells for B-cell malignancies relapsed after allogeneic stem cell transplant: a phase I study. Blood 2013;122(17):2965–73.

93. Kochenderfer JN, et al. Donor-derived CD19-targeted T cells cause regression of malignancy persisting after allogeneic hematopoietic stem cell transplantation. Blood 2013;122(25):4129–39.

94. Brentjens RJ, Curran KJ. Novel cellular therapies for leukemia: CAR-modified T cells targeted to the CD19 antigen. Hematology Am Soc Hematol Educ Program 2012;2012:143–51.

95. Chow KK, et al. T cells redirected to EphA2 for the immunotherapy of glioblastoma. Mol. Ther. 2013;21:629–37.

96. Akhurst RJ, Derynck R. TGF-beta signaling in cancer—a double-edged sword. Trends Cell Biol. 2001;11:S44–51.

97. Barsov EV. Telomerase and primary T cells: biology and immortalization for adoptive immunotherapy. Immunotherapy 2011;3:407–21.

98. Charo J, et al. Bcl-2 overexpression enhances tumor-specific T-cell survival. Cancer Res. 2005;65:2001–8.

99. Eaton D, Gilham DE, O'Neill A, Hawkins RE. Retroviral transduction of human peripheral blood lymphocytes with Bcl-X(L) promotes *in vitro* lymphocyte survival in pro-apoptotic conditions. Gene Ther. 2002;9:527–35.

100. Bollard CM, et al. Adapting a transforming growth factor beta-related tumor protection strategy to enhance antitumor immunity. Blood 2002;99:3179–87.

101. Dotti G, et al. Human cytotoxic T lymphocytes with reduced sensitivity to Fas-induced apoptosis. Blood 2005;105:4677–84.

102. Attia P, Maker AV, Haworth LR, Rogers-Freezer L, Rosenberg SA. Inability of a fusion protein of IL-2 and diphtheria toxin (Denileukin Diftitox, DAB389IL-2, ONTAK) to eliminate regulatory T lymphocytes in patients with melanoma. J. Immunother. 2005;28:582–92.

103. Brentjens R, Yeh R, Bernal Y, Riviere I, Sadelain M. Treatment of chronic lymphocytic leukemia with genetically targeted autologous T cells: case report of an unforeseen adverse event in a phase I clinical trial. Mol. Ther. 2010;18:666–8.

104. Morgan RA, et al. Case report of a serious adverse event following the administration of T cells transduced with a chimeric antigen receptor recognizing ERBB2. Mol. Ther. 2010;18:843–51.

105. Cruz CR, et al. Adverse events following infusion of T cells for adoptive immunotherapy: a 10-year experience. Cytotherapy 2010;12:743–9.

106. FDA. Proposed Approach to Regulation of Cellular and Tissue-Based Products. Washington, DC: U.S. Food and Drug Administration; 1997.

107. Ferrara JL. Cytokine dysregulation as a mechanism of graft versus host disease. Curr. Opin. Immunol. 1993;5:794–9.

108. Cohen SB, Wang XN, Dickinson A. Can cord blood cells support the cytokine storm in GvHD? Cytokine Growth Factor Rev. 2000;11:185–97.

109. Porter DL, Kalos M, Zheng Z, Levine B, June C. Chimeric antigen receptor therapy for B-cell malignancies. J. Cancer. 2011;2:331–2.

110. Howard SC, Jones DP, Pui CH. The tumor lysis syndrome. New Engl. J. Med. 2011;364:1844–54.

111. Dilber MS, Gahrton G. Suicide gene therapy: possible applications in haematopoietic disorders. J. Intern. Med. 2001;249:359–67.

112. Burt RK, et al. Herpes simplex thymidine kinase gene-transduced donor lymphocyte infusions. Exp. Hematol. 2003;31:903–10.

113. Di Stasi A, et al. Inducible apoptosis as a safety switch for adoptive cell therapy. New Engl. J. Med. 2011;365:1673–83.

114. Fischbach MA, Bluestone JA, Lim WA. Cell-based therapeutics: the next pillar of medicine. Sci. Transl. Med. 2013;5. 179ps177.

Immunostimulators and Immunomodulators in Cancer Treatment

Brianna Oliver[1], Erica Jackson[1], Hatem Soliman[2]

[1]College of Medicine, University of South Florida, Tampa, FL, USA
[2]Moffitt Cancer Center and Research Institute, Women's Oncology and Experimental
Therapeutics, Tampa, FL, USA

The complexity and elegance of both the innate and adaptive immune system in multicellular organisms is staggering. The interplay among various subspecialized immune cells, host tissues, and foreign pathogens is one that has evolved over millions of years to allow organisms to survive a constant onslaught of invading pathogenic microorganisms. Recently, data about the importance of the microbiome in our overall health highlights that our immune system must also interact positively with normal flora. Now immune surveillance of transformed cells and subsequent immune evasion by cancers is a recognized hallmark in

Novel Approaches and Strategies for Biologics, Vaccines and Cancer Therapies. DOI: 10.1016/B978-0-12-416603-5.00017-1

the natural history of malignancy. Decoding the complex regulatory and signaling pathways that govern immune activation has resulted in the development of novel immunotherapeutic agents designed to awaken the host immune system against established tumors. Also, the efficacy of traditional therapies such as radiation and chemotherapy is in part due to how they modulate an antitumor immune response. Combining these traditional therapies with immune modulators is another active area of investigation. In this chapter, we delve into the role of cytokines, checkpoint inhibitors, oncolytic viruses, and the nature of the adoptive immune response against tumors to understand how these all play a role in cancer immunotherapy.

CYTOKINES AND CANCER THERAPY

Cells throughout the body communicate through release of signals that can act in an autocrine, paracrine, or endocrine manner. One of these signals used by the immune system is known as cytokines. These cytokines can recruit different types of cells to the site of infection, change the permeability of blood vessels, regulate differentiation, and stimulate proliferation.

Cytokines include molecules that have a variety of different structural characteristics and are secreted from many different types of cells that may or may not themselves have receptors for the specific cytokine. The cytokines are broadly divided into different families such as chemokines, tumor necrosis factors (TNFs), interleukins, and other hematopoetic factors. Although the individual cytokines have different characteristics, many share certain properties. One of those properties is pleiotropism, which is the ability of one molecule to have effects on multiple different cell types. Due to their effect on different cells, cytokines are intricately involved in many different related and unrelated pathways and functions. The other important property that cytokines share is redundancy. This refers to the fact that different cytokines can have the same effect on a specific target cell.[1]

The main class of cytokines that are focused on in this chapter are the interleukins. Discovered initially in the 1970s, they were initially believed to be only involved in communication between white cells, hence the name interleukin. Through subsequent research it is known that interleukins affect the behavior of other non-immune cell types as well. Most of the interleukins signal through type I cytokine receptors that share a common amino acid motif (WSWXWS) in the extracellular domain adjacent to the cell membrane. The IL-10 group, IL-1, and IL-17 interleukins belong to the type II cytokine receptor family, Ig superfamily, and IL-17 family, respectively. The interleukins can cause both immune activation and immune suppression depending on the specific interleukin and the cells that are exposed to them. The classification and function of the interleukins are outlined in Table 17.1. Because cancer causes immunosuppression, immunotherapy approaches have focused on those interleukins that broadly activate effector cells in order to overcome this problem. Examples of the types of interleukins that have been used in the clinical setting include IL-2, IL-12, IL-15, and IL-21.

Interleukin-2

Interleukin-2 (IL-2) is primarily secreted by Th1 helper T cells which primarily drive a cytotoxic T-cell response as opposed to a humoral immune response. IL-2 interacts with

TABLE 17.1 The Interleukin Family and Their Various Functions

Interleukin	Source	Target Receptors	Target Cells	Function
IL-1	Macrophages, B cells, monocytes, dendritic cells	IL1R1, IL1R2	CD4+ T cells	Costimulation
			B cells	Maturation and proliferation
			Natural killer cells	Activation
			Macrophages	Acute inflammation
IL-2	CD4+ Th1 cells	IL2RA, IL2RB, IL2RG	T cells and B cells, natural killer cells, macrophages	Stimulate growth and differentiation of T-cell response in addition to other cells
IL-3	CD4+ T cells, mast cells, natural killer cells, eosinophils	IL3RA, IL3RB	Hematopoietic stem cells	Production of erythrocytes and granulocytes
			Mast cells	Histamine release
IL-4	Th2 cells, naïve T cells, memory CD4+ cells, mast cells, macrophages	IL4R, IL2RG	Activated B cells	Proliferation and differentiation, IgG_1 and IgE synthesis
			T cells	Proliferation
IL-5	Th2 cells, mast cells, eosinophils	IL5RA, IL3RB	Eosinophils	Proliferation
			B cells	Differentiation and IgA production
IL-6	Macrophages, Th2 cells, B cells	IL6RA, IR6RB	B cells	Plasma cell differentiation
			Plasma cells	Antibody secretion
			Hematopoietic stem cells	Differentiation
			T cells	Induce inflammation
IL-7	Bone marrow and thymus stromal cells	IL7RA, IL2RG	Pre/pro-B cells, pre/pro-T cells, natural killer cells	Differentiation and proliferation of lymphoid progenitor cells
IL-8	Macrophages, lymphocytes	IL8RA, IL8RB	Neutrophils, basophils, lymphocytes	Neutrophil chemotaxis
IL-9	CD4+ helper Th2 cells	IL9R	B cells	Potentiate IgM, IgG, IgE, and mast cells
IL-10	Monocytes, Th2 cells, CD8+ T cells, mast cells, macrophages, B cells	IL10RA, IL10RB	Macrophages	Activation
			B cells	Activation
			mast cells	Inhibition
			Th1 cells	Inhibition
			Th2 cells	Stimulation
IL-11	Bone marrow stroma	IL11RA	Bone marrow stroma	Acute-phase reactions and osteoclast formation
IL-12	Dendritic cells, B cells, T cells, macrophages	IL12RB1, IR12RB2	T cells	Differentiation into CD8+ cells
			Natural killer cells	Activation

(Continued)

IV. NOVEL APPROACHES FOR CANCER THERAPIES

TABLE 17.1   The Interleukin Family and Their Various Functions *(cont.)*

Interleukin	Source	Target Receptors	Target Cells	Function
IL-13	Activated Th2 cells, mast cells, natural killer cells	IL13R	Th2-cells, B cells, macrophages	Stimulate B cells (IgE), inhibit Th1-cells, and activate macrophages
IL-14	T cells and certain malignant B cells	—	Activated B cells	Regulate B-cell growth
IL-15	Mononuclear phagocytes	IL15RA	T cells, activated B cells	Natural killer cell production
IL-16	Lymphocytes, epithelial cells, eosinophils, CD8+ T cells	CD4	CD4+ T cells	CD4+ chemoattractant
IL-17	CD4+ T helper cells (Th17)	IL17RA, IL17RB	Epithelium, endothelium	Osteoclastogenesis, angiogenesis, increased inflammation
IL-18	Macrophages	IL18R1	Th1 cells, natural killer cells	Stimulate IFN-γ and natural killer cell activity
IL-19	Monocytes	IL20R	—	inflammatory response
IL-20	Keratinocytes, monocytes	IL20R	Keratinocytes	Proliferation of keratinocytes
IL-21	Activated CD4+ T cells, natural killer cells, T cells	IL21R	All lymphocytes, dendritic cells	Activate CD8+ T cells and natural killer cells, promote Th17 cells
IL-22	Dendritic and T cells	IL22R	Multiple tissues	Acute-phase protein production
IL-23	Dendritic cells and macrophages	IL23R	T cells	Promote angiogenesis and Th17 differentiation
IL-24	Monocytes and Th2 cells	IL20R	Multiple tissues	Wound healing and tumor growth regulation
IL-25	Th2 and mast cells	LY6E	Multiple tissues	Stimulate eosinophils
IL-26	T cells	IL20R1	Epithelial cells	Promote IL-8 secretion
IL-27	Antigen-presenting cells	IL27RA	B cells and T cells	B- and T-cell regulation
IL-28	Dendritic cells and macrophages	IL28R	T cells	Antiviral immune response
IL-29	Dendritic cells and macrophages	IL29R	Multiple tissues	Innate immune response against microbial pathogens
IL-30	—	—	—	Subunit of IL-27
IL-31	Th2 cells	IL31RA	Monocytes, epithelial cells	Inflammation
IL-32	Activated T and natural killer cells	—	monocytes	Activate macrophages
IL-33	Endothelial cells	IL1RL1	Th2 and mast cells	Th2 response
IL-35	Regulatory T cells	—	T cells, Th17 cells	Suppress T-cell activation
IL-36	Keratinocytes, epithelial cells	IL1RL2	CD4+ T cells	Regulation of dendritic and activated Th1 cell response in skin inflammation

receptors on T cells, B cells, natural killer (NK) cells, and T regulatory cells.[1] IL-2 is essential for the maturation and complete activation of T cells, B cells, and NK cells. IL-2 works in collaboration with IL-12 to preferentially promote Th1 development. These cells help eradicate intracellular pathogens and promote the inflammatory processes through secretion of interferon gamma (IFN-γ).[2] The activation of B cells leads to an increase in secretion of antibodies. A change in the microenvironmental concentration of IL-2 or interaction with antigens can lead to lymphocyte death as well.[3] IL-2 promotes proliferation and differentiation of CD8+ T cells and NK cells. This leads to an increase in cytolytic activity against infected, stressed, and transformed cells.[4]

The immunosuppressive impact of IL-2 is achieved through its interaction with T regulatory cells. IL-2 is essential to the growth and differentiation of naïve CD4+ cells to become regulatory T cells. T regulatory cells downregulate the immune response of other T cells as well to protect against autoimmunity and maintain a homeostatic balance.[5]

Due to its unique characteristics, IL-2 was one of the first interleukins to be studied as a cancer immunotherapeutic and became the first therapy of its kind to be approved by the U.S. Food and Drug Association (FDA). Beginning in 1992, IL-2 was approved to be used to treat renal cell carcinoma. In 1998, IL-2 immunotherapy began to be used as a treatment modality for metastatic melanoma. In patients with renal cell carcinoma and metastatic melanoma IL-2 can induce remission in 5 to 10% of patients.[6] As a result, treatments with IL-2 in combination with other cytokines and vaccines have been evaluated.[7-9] Adoptive cell transfer with tumor-infiltrating lymphocytes is another promising strategy pioneered by Dr. Steve Rosenberg at the National Cancer Institute (NCI). Selection of tumor-reactive lymphocytes from resected tumor specimens is performed followed by rapid expansion of the T cells in a lab using IL-2. Patients also require conditioning with myeloablative chemotherapy and total body irradiation to allow for effective persistence of the infused T cells *in vivo*. This approach has resulted in durable remissions in about 20 to 40% of patients with metastatic melanoma.[6] Now other techniques of adoptive T-cell therapy such as chimeric antigen receptor (CAR) have been developed to expand the successful use of these therapies, especially in the area of hematologic malignancies.[10]

Treatment with IL-2 requires expertise and has the potential to be highly toxic. The treatment must be closely monitored due to serious side-effects such as hypotension secondary to capillary leak syndrome, cytopenias, tachycardias, pulmonary edema, renal insufficiency, transaminitis, and arrhthmias.[11] So, while IL-2 remains an important tool in cancer immunotherapy, its toxicity and modest efficacy as a single agent have driven the search for better tolerated and more potent immunotherapy agents.

Interleukin-12

Interleukin-12 (IL-12) plays an integral role in the ability of the innate and adaptive immune systems to communicate and work together. Specifically, it plays a role in the production of Th1 CD4+ helper T cells.[12] The effector T cells then assist in the promotion of the cell-mediated cytotoxic activity of CD8+ and NK cells. The Th1 response also increases IFN-γ, which leads to an increased expression of both classes of MHC proteins in antigen-presenting cells.[13] IFN-γ is involved in the inhibition of angiogenesis, which results in anti-tumor activity.[14]

When IL-12 binds its receptor, conformational changes lead to phosphorylation of sites that activate a signaling cascade via the Jak-STAT pathway. This is a key regulatory pathway in NK cells and T cells for activation, proliferation, and differentiation. IL-12 may also directly inhibit the growth of tumor cells through unknown mechanisms. Downregulation of IL-12 receptor expression by tumor cells via epigenetic silencing was shown to confer a worse prognosis in advanced-stage lung carcinoma.[15]

Lower IL-12 levels have a negative effect on the immune system's ability to attack damaged or transformed cells. With decreased levels, NK cells and macrophages are not being properly activated, resulting in an increased state of immune tolerance. Many cancers have been found to have a decrease in circulating IL-12 levels, including glioblastoma, colorectal cancer, hepatocellular carcinoma, and malignant melanoma.[4]

IL-12 therapy demonstrated promising antitumor activity in animal models using SCK carcinoma cells engineered to secrete IL-12. It appeared that secretion of IFN-γ was required for the observed antitumor effect of IL-12.[16] Over the last two decades, IL-12 has been clinically tested for its efficacy as an anticancer therapy. Unfortunately, the efficacy in clinical trials has been modest. The exact mechanism for this is unknown, but it has been proposed that the immune activation *in vivo* following IL-12 administration is not prolonged enough to mediate an effective regression of tumors.[1] Although there have been setbacks, investigators have continued evaluating IL-12 in combination with other agents. One study involved the combination of lower-dose IL-12 and trastuzumab in Her2/neu-positive patients. This Phase I trial showed antitumor activity as well as an acceptable toxicity profile.[17]

The toxicity associated with IL-12 treatment can be significant at higher doses (500 ng/kg/day) due to excessive IFN-γ release. Adverse events have included splenomegaly, leucopenia, general gastrointestinal events, and hepatic dysfunction and/or hepatomegaly.[18] To decrease the potential for treatment toxicity seen with bolus intravenous IL-12 treatment, other administration methods are being evaluated; for example, intratumoral injection of IL-12 has been studied with the goal of reducing systemic toxicity. Although the toxicity was decreased, efficacy was lost due to the rapid turnover of cytokines in the tumor microenvironment. Another strategy utilized biodegradable nanoparticle vehicles to deliver IL-12 to the tumor with less toxicity. In murine models, the encapsulated biodegradable design showed better results than the regular soluble cytokine injections.[19]

Interleukin-15

Interleukin-15 (IL-15) is in the same family as IL-2 and IL-21 and is secreted from antigen-presenting cells such as macrophages and dendritic cells.[20] Although IL-15 promotes T-cell proliferation, it does not promote the expansion of T regulatory cells to the same degree as IL-2.[21] Studies also have found that IL-15 plays an inhibitory role in activation-induced cell necrosis.[22] Therefore, IL-15 can help protect effector T cells from the activation-induced cell death and augment a cytotoxic CD8+ T cell response.

IL-15 also enhances the development and antitumor activity of NK cells.[23] The enhanced antitumor activity of NK cells is due to the increase in NKG2D receptors that IL-15 potentiates. An increase in NKG2D receptors in tumor-infiltrating NK cells may be therapeutically significant. Tumor cells have the ability to modify the expression of surface ligands, such as MICA and ULBP ligands for the NKG2D receptor. An increase in these receptors may allow for a more robust antitumor reaction from the NK cells.[24] In addition, IL-15 works through the humoral immune system by stimulation of B cells to produce antitumor antibodies.[25]

IL-15 has demonstrated a wide range of efficacy for various types of cancer in experimental murine tumor models. Meth-A fibrosarcoma cell lines transfected with IL-15 were rejected when implanted in BALB/c mice, and the surrounding tissue demonstrated a significant lymphocytic infiltrate.[26] Interestingly, N592 small cell lung cancer xenografts genetically engineered to express both IL-15 and IL-12 were completely rejected in nude mice. The infiltrates in these tumors consisted of macrophages, NK cells, and neutrophils independent of an adoptive T-cell response.[27] Combining IL-15 with chemotherapy agents such as 5-fluorouracil led to an enhanced antitumor effect in a transplantable colon cancer murine model with less toxicity.[28]

Although treatment with IL-15 has shown promise as an antitumor therapy, its use may promote the growth of neoplastic lymphocytes as well. This has been observed in a patient with chronic lymphocytic leukemia.[29] It has also been observed that overexpression of both IL-15 and the IL-15 receptor can occur in T cells in acute T-cell leukemia.[30]

IL-15 may have some functional similarities to IL-2, but IL-15 possesses a lower toxicity. Therapy with IL-15 may result in adverse events such as neutropenia, weight loss, and anemia. Generally, these side-effects are manageable and reversible. There are continuing studies to evaluate the toxicity of IV administration of IL-15.[31]

Interleukin-21

Interleukin-21 (IL-21) is primarily secreted by CD4+ helper T cells, particularly follicular helper T cells. The IL-21 secreted by these cells is important in the differentiation and function of plasma and memory B cells.[32] In addition, IL-21 is involved in the CD4+ differentiation to subtype T helper 17 cells.[33] In murine models, IL-21 has been shown to escalate cytotoxic activity of NK cells and increase other effector cells through increased IFN-γ secretions.[34] Syngeneic mice with thymoma were used to compare the antitumor activity of IL-2, IL-15, and IL-21 as monotherapies. Treatment with IL-21 resulted in the greatest survival followed by IL-15 and then IL-2.[35] Combining IL-21 and IL-15 may provide even greater antitumor efficacy, as was seen in a murine lymphoma model.[36]

IL-21 treatment is in stage I and II clinical trials for non-Hodgkin's lymphoma, metastatic melanoma, and metastatic renal cell carcinoma. Combination therapy of IL-21 with anti-CD20 monoclonal antibody rituximab was evaluated in a Phase I trial for non-Hodgkin's lymphoma and had an objective response rate of 33% and stable disease in 47%.[37]

ONCOLYTIC VIRUSES

Oncolytic viruses are viruses that preferentially infect tumor cells over non-transformed cells and replicate within them, causing cell lysis. The benefits of this approach are that it causes direct cytotoxicity in tumor cells and the subsequent viral-mediated lysis triggers a more potent immune activation within the tumor. Examples of oncolytic viruses include vesicular stomatitis virus, Newcastle disease virus, measles vaccine virus, myxoma virus, H101, poliovirus, reovirus, and talimogene laherparevec.[38] Viruses such as Newcastle disease virus and reovirus have a natural affinity for cancer cells that further aids the selectivity of these agents.[39]

When an oncolytic virus enters the cell it commandeers cell control mechanisms and dictates the use of cell resources. Once the virus has consumed all of the available resources and assembled the maximum amount of new viruses, cell lysis will result.[40] This is considered direct viral killing of the tumor cells. Viral mechanisms such as destruction of tumor blood vessels or an increase in expression of anticancer cell signals can lead to indirect viral tumor cell killing. The antiangiogenesis effects would decrease growth and metastases.[41]

Viruses used as oncolytic therapy are attenuated versions of the wild-type virus. For this reason, normal tissues cells can mount an appropriate response and destroy the virus. On the other hand, tumor cells are not able to mount this same response. The specific destruction of tumor cells can be due to activating mutations, increased expression of viral receptors, decreased antiviral interferon response, or a weakened ability to inhibit viral replication.[42]

Tumor cell destruction by viral oncolysis results in release of tumor associated antigens (TAAs). These antigens are taken up by local dendritic cells and lead to a promotion of the immune response against the tumor cells. Direct incorporation of the TAAs into viral genomes in order to prime the immune system against the tumor cells has been researched.[43] The incorporation of TAAs would lead to a greater concentration of TAAs in the tumor microenvironment and therefore opportunity for a more significant immune system response. With the greater response, combined with the lysis from the oncolytic virus, more cells will be destroyed, resulting in a positive feedback system for tumor destruction. This possible system was evaluated with vesicular stomatitis virus (VSV) that had TAAs incorporated. In this study, general tumor regression was observed. This therapeutic approach was taken one step further by combining the use of adoptive T cells selected to react against the same TAAs. In this study, it was found that CD8+ and NK cells play an essential role in the immune response. The combination of these two therapies resulted in a more effective systemic antitumor immunity than was observed with either of these as individual therapies.[44]

During the initial research into oncolytic therapies the focus was primarily focused on the antitumor activity of the virus. As the field has grown it has become apparent that the host's immune response is an integral factor in the efficacy of oncolytic viral therapy. Cytotoxic T cells are essential in this immune response.[45] Viruses inherently activate the host's immune response, which can help promote antitumor activity. This immune activation results in the production of proinflammatory cytokines such as IL-1, Il-6, IL-12, and tumor necrosis factor alpha (TNFα).[46] While using an oncolytic therapy the goal is to have a balance between an effective antitumor immune response while limiting clearance of the virus as it replicates in the tumor.[47]

Oncolytic therapy has the advantage of specifically targeting transformed tissues while leaving normal tissues relatively unaffected. The mechanisms of this specificity differ between different strains (e.g., reovirus preferentially infects Ras-activated cells; talimogene laherparevec targets rapidly proliferating cells in general). Proteomics can be used to genetically engineer viruses to be more tumor cell specific or express proteins that enhance the tumor cell lysis. Modulation of the immunogenicity of these viruses is also achieved by inserting coding sequences for cytokines such as granulocyte–macrophage colony–stimulating factor (GM-CSF) in the case of talimogene laherparevec. It is the specificity of these agents for transformed tissues that increases the therapeutic index of these agents and makes them ideal therapies to combine with other standard of care agents including cytotoxic chemotherapy and radiation.[38,39]

Talimogene laherparevec is an oncolytic HSV that is engineered to encode GM-CSF. This virus also has genetic modifications that lead to increased viral replication, increased antitumor cytotoxic effects, decreased viral ability to infect normal cells, and a decrease in antigen presentation in cells once infected. The selectivity for viral replication in tumor cells is due to a deletion in a virulence factor ICP34.5. The deletion of ICP47 is responsible for enhanced antigen presentation via MHC class I and II receptors. The ICP47 deletion also facilitates replication of the virus in cancer cells by increasing the expression of the US11 gene. The HSV in talimogene laherparevec retains the gene for thymidine kinase. The presence of thymidine kinase keeps the virus sensitive to antiviral agents (e.g., acyclovir) as a safety feature in the event that viral replication needs to be stopped. After intratumoral injection, objective responses were seen in 13 out of 50 patients in a Phase II melanoma trial. Out of the 13 patients, 10 had complete response. Again, these patients had shrinkage not only in the injected tumors but also in non-injected ones.[48] This provides proof of systemic antitumor immune activation leading to disease control outside of the injected lesions. Recently, the Phase III OP-TiM trial using talimogene laherparevec in stage III/IV melanoma reported positive results with durable response rates of 16% in the experimental arm compared to 2% in the control arm using GM-CSF alone. The therapy was very well tolerated, with the majority of adverse events at grade one or two (fevers, chills, constitutional symptoms). The most common serious adverse event was cellulitis occurring in 2.1% of the study population. This represents the first Phase III trial with proof-of-concept data for oncolytic therapy in melanoma.

Incorporation of other cytokine genes into oncolytic viruses has also been investigated. These include IL-2, IL-12, IL-24, and interferon-γ (IFN-γ) among others.[49] Like interleukins, interferons are involved in many different cell processes, including elimination of viral infections. Therapeutic interest in the use of IFN-γ is due to its antitumor effect via antiangiogenesis while also protecting adjacent normal tissues from viral infection.[50] This concept was evaluated using a VSV oncolytic virus engineered to secrete IFN-γ in a murine model with mesothelioma. It was found that the IFN-γ-secreting virus had increased antitumor activity compared to the wild-type variant.[51]

Reolysin® is a type III reovirus that is specifically cytotoxic to tumor cells with activating mutations in the Ras signaling pathway. These Ras mutations lead to the inability of the cell to phosphorylate factors that inhibit reovirus replication.[42] A mutation in Ras is seen in approximately 30% of human tumors.[52] In a Phase II trial for head and neck cancers, Reolysin was combined with carboplatin and paclitaxel. The treatment was well tolerated and demonstrated an objective response rate of 27%.[53]

Most of the success with oncolytic viruses has been seen with intratumoral injection, as this delivers the viral particles directly to the tumors and avoids the issues regarding viral clearance by the host immune system. However, in situations with diffuse metastatic disease, direct injection of all sites of disease is not feasible. The systemic immune response may also vary depending on the level of immune competence in each patient. Therefore, there is continued research into possible methods to improve systemic intravenous administration of oncolytic viruses to tumors. There are several barriers the virus faces in migrating from the bloodstream to reach the tumor cells. First, the viruses need to undergo extravasation in order to leave the blood vessels. The initiation of this process is dependent on the viral concentration reaching a threshold in the patient's blood. The levels of virus that reach the tumor microenvironment are also dependent on binding of viral surface proteins to endothelial cell receptors. It has been found that intratumoral endothelial cells have overexpression of different receptors compared to systemic blood vessels. This can be exploited to make the oncolytic virus a more "targeted" systemic therapy. Viruses can be genetically engineered to express ligands that have high affinity for these receptors in hopes of a large viral infiltration.[47]

With systemic therapy there is also an issue with the neutralization of the virus through the body's innate immune system. To protect the virus, the use of carrier cells to deliver the oncolytic viruses to the tumor cells has been studied in small clinical trials with tumor or normal primary cell lines. For example, mesenchymal stem cells have been used to protect the oncolytic virus and deliver it to the tumor cells. These cells effectively evaded neutralizing antiviral antibodies and delivered oncolytic measles viruses to intraperitoneal ovarian cancer deposits.[54] Another carrier cell transport system that has been studied is the use of immune cells that are recruited to the tumor microenvironment. To date, T cells and natural killer cells have been used with promising results. In studies using natural killer cells and the vaccinia virus, tumor regression was observed in murine models.[55]

Another barrier the viruses faces involves the body's physiological reaction to try to eradicate the virus. This includes viral sequestration in the liver and spleen. A variety of methods have been studied to deal with this issue. Changing the proteins on the viral coat can help evade the body's detection, but changes could lead to a decreased ability of the virus to infect cells. Another option that has been used with herpes simplex virus (HSV) is to deplete components of the innate immune system such as IgM and complement proteins. This can be done by administration of immunosuppresants such as cyclophosphamide. When cyclophosphamide was added to a HSV oncolytic virus therapy, an increase in viral activity within infected tumors was seen.[56]

As with any therapy potential toxicities are of concern. In order to decrease the potential toxicity, tumor-specific targeting is a large part of the development of oncolytic viruses. Another mechanism to accomplish this is to exploit the genetic differences of specific microRNA (miRNA) found in the tumor cells. When miR-122 (expressed primarily in hepatocellular carcinoma cells) binding sites were added to the 3'-UTR end of an adenoviral vector's genome, this prevented hepatotoxicity in normal murine liver tissue while preserving its oncolytic activity.[57] Sporadic mutations in either the viral genome's binding sequence or miRNAs produced in tumors may negate this form of viral replication control, so other targeting mechanisms are under investigation.[47]

The host's response to the virus may be a limiting factor in the efficacy of oncolytic viral therapy. One of the main mechanisms that cells use to eradicate the infecting viral particles is to mount an interferon response. The exact mechanism of these signals and the resulting cytokines released can significantly vary between different cells types. Different drugs have been evaluated to help improve viral resistance to this process. One of these drugs is histone deacetylase (HDAC) inhibitors. HDAC inhibitors function by epigenetically decreasing interferon signaling in transformed cells while leaving normal cells unaltered. Studies using combined therapy of HDAC inhibitors with oncolytic viruses resulted in increased propagation of oncolytic viruses. Genetically modified IFN-inhibiting viruses are being investigated as a possible therapy.[58]

Rather than using an immunosuppressant with the oncolytic therapy, genetically engineered immunosuppressing viruses are being investigated. An example of these are viruses selected for the production and secretion of viral chemokine-binding proteins (vCKBPs). These proteins downregulate the ability of chemokines to modulate the host's immune response in reaction to a viral infection. Different classes of CKBP can interact with different subsets of cytokines. This interaction can lead to a decreased presence of inflammatory cells and therefore the antiviral immune response.[59] Murine hepatocellular carcinoma models were used to evaluate VSV with engineered vectors for expression of vCKBPs. A decrease in the host's antiviral immune response in the microenvironment was seen, specifically with a reduction of NK cells. The study also showed more persistent viral activity as well as a meaningful increase in survival. The use of viruses with immune-suppressing activities raises concerns about their potential pathogenicity and toxicity. When the vCKBP-secreting VSV therapy was evaluated for host safety, it was found that there was no difference in safety between the genetically engineered virus and the wild-type form.[49]

In order to help evaluate the concentration and location of the virus once it has entered the body reporter genes are being used. These genes are engineered directly into the virus genome. So far, a large portion of studies with these genes have been focused around the use of radioactive tracers. For example, various viruses such as the measles virus have been engineered to express thyroidal sodium iodide symporter (NIS). When expressed, these channels trap radioactive iodide in the infected cell. These channels can then be detected to determine the distribution of the virus.[60] Although this approach has shown promise, it is hopeful that in the future reporter genes can be used with other detection modalities that do not include introduction of radioactive material.

There has been some concern that the viruses could mutate their genome or recombine with endogenous viral sequences to regain pathogenic abilities. Although these are rare events, this is something that must be monitored for any of these therapies. Studies have been conducted looking at viral shedding in treated patients' bodily fluids and secretions. Viral shedding in patient samples has been seen with reovirus, Newcastle virus, and HSV. Although there have been positive viral shedding samples, there is no documentation involving transmission from patients to caregivers.[61]

CHECKPOINT INHIBITORS

The immune system is constantly scanning for unwanted pathogens, infected cells, and tumor cells. Antigen-presenting cells (APCs) will process these entities and present a piece of them, an antigen, to immune cells through the major histocompatibility complex (MHC). There are two types of MHC molecules. MHC I molecules are found on all nucleated cells in the body, and recognized by the T-cell receptor (TCR) on CD8+ cells. MHC II molecules are found on APC and recognized by TCR on CD4+ cells. Due to the very specific binding, a mutation in either the MHC or TCR could lead to aberrant T-cell activation.[62] Once an MCH complex is formed, other modulating factors and costimulatory molecules come in to make it a complete immune synapse.

For complete activation of T cells, the CD28 molecule on the T cell must interact with the B7 molecule on the APC. A completed immune synapse leads to activation of T cells. The specific composition of factors and costimulatory molecules results in differentiation into the T helper cell subtypes Th1, Th2, Th17, and regulatory. Th1 and Th2 secrete cytokines that further promote cellular and humoral immunity, respectively.[63] In CD4+ cells, reciprocal activation of the APCs, such B cells, is needed. This is achieved through the expression of the CD40 ligand on the activated T cell. The receptor for the CD40 ligand is found on the APC cell.[64]

When T cells are activated by APCs there is an upregulation of cytotoxic T-lymphocyte-associated antigen 4 (CTLA-4) and programmed death 1 receptor (PD-1). These signals are important in the regulation of activated T cells. When these receptors are activated, T cell activity is decreased, thus suppressing the immune response. CTLA-4 directly competes with CD28 for the B7 molecule on the APC.[65] Blocking of CD28 results in decreased glucose uptake and downregualtion of genes that activate T-cell function. Both of these changes reduce the T cell's ability to continue with the immune response.[66] PD-1 is found on B cells and NK cells in addition to activated T cells. Regulation of T-cell activation in the periphery involves PD-1. This receptor also binds to a different subset of the B7 molecules. When PD-1 interacts with its ligand, programmed death ligand 1 (PD-L1), T cells are again downregulated.[67] CTLA-4 and PD-1 are active under normal physiological conditions and are an integral part of protection against autoimmunity.[65]

Transformed cells are under constant pressure to evade immune surveillance in the host, and immune evasion is now recognized as a hallmark of cancer. Tumor cells of different lineages have been found to express B7 molecules on their cell surface. The presence of B7 molecules was associated with a poor prognosis in these patients.[68] Researchers evaluated the presence of PD-L1 in melanoma, colon, ovarian, and lung cancers. It was found that PD-L1 was upregulated in response to IFN-γ. *In vitro* there was an increase in tumor specific T-cell apoptosis in response to the presence of PD-L1. It appears that tumor cell production of PD-L1 serves as a reactive mechanism to block the activity of tumor-infiltrating lymphocytes once they get into the tumor microenvironment.[69]

Ipilimumab (Yervoy®)

Ipilimumab was the first of these checkpoint inhibitor therapies approved by the FDA for the treatment of metastatic melanoma. It is a monocolonal antibody specifically targeted to block CTLA-4. Blockade of CTLA-4 allows T cells to activate more robustly in response to tumor-associated antigens. Although it has been used in trials with ovarian, renal, lung, breast, hematological, and castration-resistance prostate cancers, the majority of clinical significance was seen in metastatic melanoma.[70] The pivotal Phase III trial in metastatic melanoma used the following treatment regimens: ipilimumab + gp100 vaccine, ipilimumab alone, and gp100 vaccine alone. Both ipilimumab-containing arms had a significant survival benefit compared to the gp100 vaccine arm. With longer follow up of several years it appears there is a durable remission of disease in about 20% of patients. In a different Phase III trial, ipilimumab was used as a first-line therapy in previously untreated metastatic melanoma. Patients were randomly assigned to receive dacarbazine + placebo or dacarbazine + ipilimumab. Again, the treatment with ipilimumab had an increased survival when compared to the dacarbazine alone, 47% versus 36%. The ipilimumab- containing arm appeared to have an increase in autoimmune events such as colitis and hepatitis.[71]

PD-1/PD-L1 inhibitors

Expression of PD-1 on activated T cells acts as a negative feedback loop that prevents tissue damage and autoimmunity from an overactive immune response. When PD-1 binds its ligand, PD-L1, this inhibits activation of the T-cell receptor complex via decreases in ZAP70 and PKC-γ levels. Blockade of either PD-1 or PD-L1 with a monoclonal antibody prevents this inhibitory signal from activating in tumor-infiltrating lymphocytes. Multiple clinical trials have evaluated the activity of PD-1-blocking antibodies and have shown promising activity (durable response rates of 18 to 28%) in melanoma, lung, renal, and colorectal carcinoma.[72,73] The toxicity profile of these agents was similar to ipilimumab, with autoimmune events such as pneumonitis emerging as the main issue. It appears tumor expression of PD-L1 enriches for responders to PD-1 blockade, but the absence of staining does not totally preclude a response to therapy. Researchers also evaluated the use of a monoclonal antibody against PD-L1 in patients with metastatic non-small-cell lung cancer, ovarian cancer, melanoma, and renal-cell cancer. In these patients, a stability of disease was seen as well as tumor regression. In 9% of patients, adverse clinical events of grade 3 or higher was observed.[74] An additional study evaluated the PD-L1 in squamous cell carcinomas of the head and neck (SCCHN). PD-L1 was detected in 66% of SCCHN patient samples. In addition, another study assessed adoptive transfer with blocking of PD-L1 in a murine model of squamous cell carcinoma. The efficacy of CD8+ adoptive transfer therapy was enhanced when combined with monoclonal antibody against PD-L1.[75] These data are leading to some preliminary efforts to use checkpoint blockade to enhance the ability to successfully carry out adoptive immunotherapy treatments in patients.

In contrast to PD-1 and CTLA-4, CD40 promotes the activation of immune cells. Expression of CD40 has been documented in malignancies of epithelial origin and B-cell malignancies. This has led to investigation into the therapeutic use of a monoclonal anti-CD40 antibody.[64] Dacetuzumab is a monoclonal anti-CD40 IgG antibody. A Phase I trial assessed the use of dacetuzumab in patients with chronic lymphocytic leukemia. The best response seen was a stable disease in 5 out of 12 participants. Researchers suggested the use of dacetuzumab as a combination therapy in future studies.[76]

Once CD4+ activation is complete, these cells secrete cytokines that modulate the immune response. One of these cytokines is IFN-γ, which can both promote and inhibit the immune response. As previously stated, IFN-γ antitumor activity promotes expression of MHC molecules and inhibits tumor angiogenesis.[13,14] It has also been found to interrupt mechanisms for tumor cell proliferation.[77] Conversely, IFN-γ also has mechanisms that result in downregulation of the immune response. One of the ways in which it does this is to induce the production of indoleamine 2,3-dioxygenase (IDO) in dendritic cells and tumor cells. IDO is a rate-limiting step in the breakdown of tryptophan to various catabolites that exert immunosuppressive properties. Local tryptophan depletion within the tumor microenvironment also causes anergy in tumor-infiltrating lymphocytes. IDO also promotes the development of naïve T cells into immunosuppressive T regulatory cells.[78] Using HeLa cells, researchers evaluated the use of IDO inhibitor INCB024360. When this inhibitor was used an increase in T and NK cells was observed. Specifically, an increase in CD8+ proliferation was seen. In addition, there was an increase in IFNγ secretion from both CD4+ and CD8+ T cells.[79] Conventional chemotherapies in combination with IDO pathway inhibitor 1-methyl-D-tryptophan (1MT) have been evaluated in murine models transplanted with human melanoma and breast cancer. The combination treatment of 1MT with paclitaxel, doxorubicin, and cyclophosphamide resulted in increased antitumor activity when compared to the chemotherapies alone.[80] Both of these IDO inhibitor agents are undergoing clinical investigation in multiple Phase I and II trials. One of these trials is a randomized Phase II trial combining 1MT with docetaxel to test this synergistic effect with chemotherapy in the treatment of metastatic breast cancer.

The landscape of immunotherapy has changed dramatically with the advent of targeted agents that can modulate the immune system's response against established tumors. Other agents in early development include LAG-3, TIM, and PD-L2 targeting therapies, which may provide additional benefits for patients with cancer. Also, combination therapies are being explored, as it is likely that monotherapies will be inadequate in overcoming the multiple immunosuppressive pathways used by cancers to propagate. The tantalizing hint of durable, long-term survivors of metastatic cancers provides fresh hope that we can cure patients who were previously doomed to die of their disease in the near future.

IMPORTANCE OF THE Th1/Th2 RESPONSE IN CANCER IMMUNOTHERAPY

Antigen-presenting cells (APCs) recognize foreign microbes and following peptide ingestion migrate to draining lymph nodes and spleen. Naïve CD4 T cells in lymphoid organs are presented with antigens by these APCs. This activates the T cells to then proliferate and differentiate into effecter T cells. These activated T cells then enter circulation and migrate to the site of infection for further destruction of microbes. CD4 helper T cells activate phagocytes to destroy the microbes, whereas CD8 T cells can directly kill infected cells. CD4 helper T cells can differentiate into Th1 or Th2 cells depending on types of cytokines produced by the APCs. These two types of helper T cells produce different subsets of cytokines and have different effecter functions. Predominance of the Th1 or Th2 response can push the immune response toward a cell-mediated or humoral-based immunity, respectively. These differences are summarized in Table 17.2. The determination of a Th1 versus a Th2 response has a clinical impact on not only the development of cancer but also on the patient's outcome and response to cancer treatment. In this section, we will discuss the differences between the Th1 and Th2 response and the impact these responses have on the development of cancer.

TABLE 17.2   Properties of a Th1 and Th2 Immune Response

Property	Th1	Th2
Immune response activated	Cell-mediated immunity	Humoral immunity
Principle antigen cleared	Intracellular pathogens	Extracellular parasites
Clinical involvement	Autoimmunity and cancer	Asthma and allergies
Cytokines produced	IL-2, IFN-γ, TNFα	IL-4, IL-5, IL-13
Macrophage activation	Classical (microbial killing)	Alternative (tissue repair)
Dominant leukocytes recruited	Monocytes, CD8+ T cells	Eosinophils, B cells

Properties of the Th1 and Th2 Response

Helper T (CD4+) cells may differentiate into subsets of cells that are characterized by the patterns of cytokines they produce. These subsets are classified as Th1 and Th2 cells.[81] Th1 cells stimulate phagocyte-mediated killing of viruses and bacteria. This represents the host defense against intracellular microbes. Th1 produces interferon-γ (IFN-γ), a cytokine first discovered as an inhibitor of viral infection.[82] When secreted, IFN-γ activates macrophages, enhancing microbial killing. It also stimulates B cells to make opsonizing and complement-fixing antibodies. These antibodies bind directly to phagocyte Fc receptors and activate complement, promoting the phagocytosis of microbes. IFN-γ can also stimulate the expression of MHC II and the costimulatory signal, B7, on macrophages, thereby amplifying antigen presentation and T-cell activation.[83] Th1 CD4+ cells also play a role in the activation of CD8+ T cells through secretion of the cytokine IL-2. Overall, the Th1 response is considered a key player in cell-mediated immunity.

Conversely, Th2 cells mediate phagocyte-independent killing of extracellular microbes and parasites such as helminthes. Th2 cells release cytokines IL-4, IL-5, and IL-13, making them an integral part of the humoral immune response.[84] IL-4 stimulates class switching to IgE antibodies. These IgE antibodies then bind mast cells and stimulate degranulation when bound by protein antigens. IgE also coats helminthes which allows IL-5 activated eosinophils to destroy the helminthes. In addition, Th2 cytokines may play a role in barrier protection, blocking the entry of microbes at mucosal barriers by stimulating mucus secretion. They can also stimulate B cells to produce neutralizing IgG antibodies. IL-4 and IL-13 also activate macrophages; however, these cytokines do not activate macrophage killing as in the Th1 response. They participate in alternative macrophage activation, enhancing other functions such as synthesis of extracellular matrix proteins involved in tissue repair. Th2 cytokines can actually inhibit the antimicrobial properties of macrophages, causing suppression of the Th1 response. This leads us to the concept of a balance that exists between the activation of Th1 and Th2 responses that can determine the efficacy of cell-mediated immunity and the ability of the immune system to clear a microbe.

Th17 cells are a third subset of CD4 T cells. They secrete the cytokines IL-17 and IL-22.[85] These cytokines induce production of chemokines that recruit neutrophils and monocytes to sites of inflammation. These cells contribute to destruction of extracellular microbes, activation of inflammation, and the development of autoimmunity.

Differentiation into Th1 and Th2

The development of Th1 and Th2 responses is not random but driven by a combination of cytokines released when naïve CD4 T cells encounter antigens.[85] After interaction with a microbe, dendritic cells and macrophages produce the cytokine IL-12, while NK cells produce IFN-γ. These two cytokines activate transcription factors that cause naïve CD4 T cells to differentiate into Th1 T cells. In turn, Th1 cells produce IFN-γ, which activates the macrophages to kill the intracellular pathogens while also encouraging further Th1 differentiation. If a microbe does not cause IL-12 production by dendritic cells and macrophages, the T cells will produce IL-4. The cytokine IL-4 then activates transcription factors that induce Th2 differentiation. Th2 cells can also produce IL-10 which inhibits the action of Th1 while further activating Th2.[86]

Importance of Immune Response in the Tumor Microenvironment

Tumors can be distinguished by different factors such as cell type, grade, and molecular classifications. However, in order to fully understand the biology of a tumor, it is necessary to study the surrounding tumor microenvironment as well.[87] This tumor microenvironment includes cancer-associated fibroblasts, endothelial cells, and pericytes. In addition, infiltrating immune cells are now considered an integral part of the microenvironment. These cells can function as promoters of tumor growth or as growth inhibitors.

The adaptive immune response functions to destroy transformed cells before they multiply and form tumors. In order for a tumor to develop, cells must evade this immune surveillance and multiply without being detected.[88] The primary mechanism of tumor detection and destruction is by CTLs, but it can be carried out by other cells such as natural killer cells. Tumor cells express different molecules that may be recognized by the immune system as foreign antigens. These antigens are displayed as MHC I-associated peptides and are recognized by CD8 T cells. Antigen-presenting cells also present tumor antigens to CD4 T cells, which then provide signals for CTL development. CTLs can then kill tumor cells expressing the antigen. However, immune responses may be ineffective at clearing tumor cells, possibly because many tumor antigens are weakly immunogenic.[89] The tumor can also evolve ways to evade recognition by the immune response through antigen shedding. Tumors may also stop expressing MHC I molecules, prohibiting antigen presentation to T cells.[90] Other tumors overexpress inhibitory cytokines such as transforming growth factor beta (TGF-β).[91] Tumors can also activate inhibitory pathways such as CTLA-4, IDO, or PD-1, which suppress T cell activation.[92,93]

Over the past decade researchers have studied ways to manipulate genes involved in the function of immune cells to understand the role they play in tumorigenesis. Understanding the function of these cells could lead to therapies that activate immune cells that will promote tumor destruction, while downregulating cells that promote tumor growth.

Balance between Th1 and Th2

Alteration in the balance between Th1 and Th2 responses may be responsible for the occurrence or progression of cancer. A shift from Th1 to Th2 can impair cell-mediated immunity and is often seen in patients with advanced cancer. This theory has been supported by multiple studies that have looked at the cytokine profile of tumor-infiltrating lymphocytes.[94] Studies have shown that a low Th1/Th2 ratio can be found in patients with more aggressive tumors that have a lower survival rate. Those patients with a Th1-dominant response often have a lower recurrence rate and a longer disease-free survival.[95] Finding ways to push the Th1/Th2 balance toward a Th1-dominant response is key in the development of effective immunotherapeutic strategies.

Clinical Significance of Th1 and Th2 Response

Immune response has been thought to play a role in cancer risk and prognosis. Mounting an adequate immune response against tumor-associated antigens allows the host to clear foreign tumor cells. A Th1-dominant response is important for mounting this effective antitumor immune response. In one study that evaluated the ratios of Th1 to Th2 cytokines, a connection was found between a low Th1/Th2 ratio and the more aggressive estrogen receptor (ER)-type breast cancer.[96] These data can be used to generate new immunotherapy strategies. Many cancer vaccines have been designed to elicit a Th1 response in the hope of mounting a stronger immune response against tumor antigens.[97] In one study, dendritic cells were pulsed with autologous tumor lysates and matured with factors that induced cytokine production.[98] This vaccine elicited Th1 cytokine secretion and increased CD8+ IFN-γ+ cells in ER/progesterone receptor (PR)-negative breast cancer patients. The three-year progression-free survival rate was found to be 77% in the vaccinated group versus 31% in the control group.

In melanoma patients, studies have shown similar results. One group found that the majority of melanoma patients had significantly lower values of IL-2 and IFN-γ and elevated levels of IL-4, IL-6, and IL-10 as compared to healthy subjects. This would indicate an immune response skewed toward Th2. In addition, many patients who relapsed early during immunotherapy had significantly lower pretreatment levels of IL-2 and IL-12.[99] Data on malignant melanoma have generally indicated a disturbance in the balance between Th1 and Th2 responses. When this balance is tipped in the Th2 direction it may indicate more aggressive disease. A dominance of Th2 cytokines may also predict a poorer response to immunotherapy, making it possible to select patients who would benefit most from immune modulating therapies.

One group studying colorectal carcinoma analyzed the balance between cytotoxic T cells and different subsets of helper T cells and the possible effect they had on disease free survival.[95] Patients with high expression of Th17 had a poor prognosis, whereas patients with high expression of Th1 genes had longer disease-free survival. Combined analysis of cytotoxic/Th1 and Th17 clusters improved the ability to determine relapse. The correlation between tumor-infiltrating lymphocytes (TILs) and response to chemotherapy was also studied in colorectal patients with liver metastasis.[100] The density of TILs in the invasive margin of the liver metastasis predicted patient's response to chemotherapy.[101]

Immunoscore®

The significance of these data has led to a push to incorporate immunological biomarkers into the classification of cancer. Classically, risk prediction has been determined based on histopathological characteristics of the primary tumor including size, cell atypia, aberrant protein expression, and genetic markers. The TNM staging system looks at tumor burden (T), lymph node involvement (N), and evidence of distant metastasis (M) to determine prognosis.[102] This conventional system has been used to determine patient prognosis; however, outcomes can vary among patients within the same stage. This is in part due to differences in the tumor cells' biology, but this provides only part of the answer. Recent articles have determined that cancer development is influenced by the host immune system and should therefore be accounted for when staging a tumor.[103] Studies have demonstrated that the number, type, and location of infiltrating immune cells are important prognostic indicators.[104]

A large infiltration of lymphocytes has been reported to predict a better clinical outcome in multiple tumor types.[103] In particular, three cell types have been shown to improve disease free survival and/or overall survival. These include CD3+ T cells, CD8+ T cells, and

CD45RO+ memory T cells. The Immunoscore quantifies two lymphocyte subtypes within the center of the tumor (CT) and invasive margin (IM), CD3/CD45RO, or CD3/CD8, or CD8/CD45RO. The Immunoscore® ranges from I0 to I4. A score of I0 has low densities of both lymphocyte populations in both the core of the tumor (CT) and invasive margin (IM) regions. An Immunoscore of I4 has high densities of both populations in both regions. The Immunoscore was used in stage 1 and 2 colorectal patients to determine correlation with disease-free survival (DFS) and overall survival (OS). The five-year survival rate in patients with high densities of CD8 and CD45RO T cells was 86.2%. Only 4.8% of these patients had tumor recurrence. Conversely, only 27.5% of patients with low densities of these lymphocytes survived, while 75% recurred.[105] Adding immunological factors to routine tumor assessment may provide the essential data needed to provide an accurate prognosis and guide treatment decision making. Because of the improved response to chemotherapy that is noted when TILs are present at the tumor site, the Immunoscore would provide a way for oncologists to better predict a patient's response to treatment. The Immunoscore must be validated in a multicenter trial to result in its implementation as a classification of cancer called TNM-Immune (TNM-I). There is hope that this would allow for a more effective staging of cancer and a better way to predict patient outcomes. Finally, identifying which tumors require immune modulators to achieve a favorable antitumor immune response can allow for a more targeted, effective paradigm for cancer immunotherapy.

References

1. Chiba Y, et al. Interleukins and cancer immunotherapy. Immunotherapy 2009;1:825.
2. Bird JJ, et al. Helper T cell differentiation is controlled by the cell cycle. Immunity 1998;9(2):229–37.
3. Lenardo M, et al. Mature T lymphocyte apoptosis—immune regulation in a dynamic and unpredictable antigenic environment. Annu. Rev. Immunol. 1999;17:221–53.
4. Lippitz BE. Cytokine patterns in patients with cancer: a systematic review. Lancet Oncol. 2013;14(6):e218–28.
5. Littman DR, Rudensky AY. Th17 and regulatory T cells in mediating and restraining inflammation. Cell 2010;140(6):845–58.
6. Rosenberg SA. Raising the bar: the curative potential of human cancer immunotherapy. Sci. Transl. Med. 2012;4(127):127ps8.
7. Atkins MB, et al. Kidney cancer: the Cytokine Working Group experience (1986-2001). Part I. IL-2-based clinical trials. Med. Oncol. 2001;18(3):197–207.
8. Du G, et al. Human IL18–IL2 fusion protein as a potential antitumor reagent by enhancing NK cell cytotoxicity and IFN-gamma production. J. Cancer Res. Clin. Oncol. 2012;138(10):1727–36.
9. Ramlau R, et al. A phase II study of Tg4010 (Mva-Muc1-IL2) in association with chemotherapy in patients with stage III/IV non-small cell lung cancer. J. Thorac. Oncol. 2008;3(7):735–44.
10. Kebriaei P, et al. Chimeric antibody receptors (CARs): driving T-cell specificity to enhance anti-tumor immunity. Front. Biosci. 2012;4:520–31.
11. Hashmi MH, Van Veldhuizen PJ. Interleukin-21: updated review of Phase I and II clinical trials in metastatic renal cell carcinoma, metastatic melanoma and relapsed/refractory indolent non-Hodgkin's lymphoma. Expert Opin. Biol. Ther. 2010;10(5):807–17.
12. Jacobson NG, et al. Interleukin 12 signaling in T helper type 1 (Th1) cells involves tyrosine phosphorylation of signal transducer and activator of transcription (Stat)3 and Stat4. J. Exp. Med. 1995;181(5):1755–62.
13. Wigginton JM, et al. IFN-gamma and Fas/FasL are required for the antitumor and antiangiogenic effects of IL-12/pulse IL-2 therapy. J. Clin. Invest. 2001;108(1):51–62.
14. Levy EM, Roberti MP, Mordoh J. Natural killer cells in human cancer: from biological functions to clinical applications. J. Biomed. Biotechnol. 2011;2011:676198.
15. Suzuki M, et al. Aberrant methylation of IL-12Rbeta2 gene in lung adenocarcinoma cells is associated with unfavorable prognosis. Ann. Surg. Oncol. 2007;14(9):2636–42.

16. Coughlin CM, et al. Interleukin-12 and interleukin-18 synergistically induce murine tumor regression which involves inhibition of angiogenesis. J. Clin. Invest. 1998;101(6):1441–52.

17. Bekaii-Saab TS, et al. A phase I trial of paclitaxel and trastuzumab in combination with interleukin-12 in patients with HER2/neu-expressing malignancies. Mol. Cancer Ther. 2009;8(11):2983–91.

18. Car BD, et al. The toxicology of interleukin-12: a review. Toxicol. Pathol. 1999;27(1):58–63.

19. Egilmez NK, Kilinc MO. Tumor-resident CD8+ T-cell: the critical catalyst in IL-12-mediated reversal of tumor immune suppression. Arch. Immunol. Ther. Exp. (Warsz.) 2010;58(6):399–405.

20. Jakobisiak M, Golab J, Lasek W. Interleukin 15 as a promising candidate for tumor immunotherapy. Cytokine Growth Factor Rev. 2011;22(2):99–108.

21. Vang KB, et al. IL-2, -7, and -15, but not thymic stromal lymphopoeitin, redundantly govern CD4+Foxp3+ regulatory T cell development. J. Immunol. 2008;181(5):3285–90.

22. Marks-Konczalik J, et al. IL-2-induced activation-induced cell death is inhibited in IL-15 transgenic mice. Proc. Natl. Acad. Sci. U.S.A. 2000;97(21):11445–50.

23. Fehniger TA, Cooper MA, Caligiuri MA. Interleukin-2 and interleukin-15: immunotherapy for cancer. Cytokine Growth Factor Rev. 2002;13(2):169–83.

24. Cerwenka A, Lanier LL. NKG2D ligands: unconventional MHC class I-like molecules exploited by viruses and cancer. Tissue Antigens. 2003;61(5):335–43.

25. Armitage RJ, et al. IL-15 has stimulatory activity for the induction of B cell proliferation and differentiation. J. Immunol. 1995;154(2):483–90.

26. Hazama S, et al. Tumour cells engineered to secrete interleukin-15 augment anti-tumour immune responses *in vivo*. Br. J. Cancer 1999;80(9):1420–6.

27. Di Carlo E, et al. The combined action of IL-15 and IL-12 gene transfer can induce tumor cell rejection without T and NK cell involvement. J. Immunol. 2000;165(6):3111–8.

28. Cao S, Troutt AB, Rustum YM. Interleukin 15 protects against toxicity and potentiates antitumor activity of 5-fluorouracil alone and in combination with leucovorin in rats bearing colorectal cancer. Cancer Res. 1998;58(8):1695–9.

29. de Totero D, et al. The opposite effects of IL-15 and IL-21 on CLL B cells correlate with differential activation of the JAK/STAT and ERK1/2 pathways. Blood 2008;111(2):517–24.

30. Mariner JM, et al. Human T cell lymphotropic virus type I Tax activates IL-15R alpha gene expression through an NF-kappa B site. J. Immunol. 2001;166(4):2602–9.

31. Croce M, et al. Immunotherapeutic applications of IL-15. Immunotherapy 2012;4(9):957–69.

32. King C, Tangye SG, Mackay CR. T follicular helper (TFH) cells in normal and dysregulated immune responses. Annu. Rev. Immunol. 2008;26:741–66.

33. Yang L, et al. IL-21 and TGF-beta are required for differentiation of human T(H)17 cells. Nature 2008;454(7202):350–2.

34. Kasaian MT, et al. IL-21 limits NK cell responses and promotes antigen-specific T cell activation: a mediator of the transition from innate to adaptive immunity. Immunity 2002;16(4):559–69.

35. Moroz A, et al. IL-21 enhances and sustains CD8+ T cell responses to achieve durable tumor immunity: comparative evaluation of IL-2, IL-15, and IL-21. J. Immunol. 2004;173(2):900–9.

36. Kishida T, et al. Interleukin (IL)-21 and IL-15 genetic transfer synergistically augments therapeutic antitumor immunity and promotes regression of metastatic lymphoma. Mol. Ther. 2003;8(4):552–8.

37. Timmerman JM, et al. A phase I dose-finding trial of recombinant interleukin-21 and rituximab in relapsed and refractory low grade B-cell lymphoproliferative disorders. Clin. Cancer Res. 2012;18(20):5752–60.

38. Butt AQ, Miggin SM. Cancer and viruses: a double-edged sword. Proteomics. 2012;12(13):2127–38.

39. Sinkovics JG, Horvath JC. Newcastle disease virus (NDV): brief history of its oncolytic strains. J. Clin. Virol. 2000;16(1):1–15.

40. Parato KA, et al. Recent progress in the battle between oncolytic viruses and tumours. Nat. Rev. Cancer 2005;5(12):965–76.

41. Wojton J, Kaur B. Impact of tumor microenvironment on oncolytic viral therapy. Cytokine Growth Factor Rev. 2010;21(2-3):127–34.

42. Stojdl DF, et al. Exploiting tumor-specific defects in the interferon pathway with a previously unknown oncolytic virus. Nat. Med. 2000;6(7):821–5.

43. Schulz O, et al. Toll-like receptor 3 promotes cross-priming to virus-infected cells. Nature. 2005;433(7028):887–92.

44. Diaz RM, et al. Oncolytic immunovirotherapy for melanoma using vesicular stomatitis virus. Cancer Res. 2007;67(6):2840–8.
45. Prestwich RJ, et al. Immunotherapeutic potential of oncolytic virotherapy. Lancet Oncol. 2008;9(7):610–2.
46. Candido J, Hagemann T. Cancer-related inflammation. J. Clin. Immunol. 2013;33(Suppl. 1):S79–84.
47. Russell SJ, Peng KW, Bell JC. Oncolytic virotherapy. Nat. Biotechnol. 2012;30(7):658–70.
48. Senzer NN, et al. Phase II clinical trial of a granulocyte-macrophage colony-stimulating factor-encoding, second-generation oncolytic herpesvirus in patients with unresectable metastatic melanoma. J. Clin. Oncol. 2009;27(34):5763–71.
49. Altomonte J, Ebert O. Replicating viral vectors for cancer therapy: strategies to synergize with host immune responses. Microb. Biotechnol. 2012;5(2):251–9.
50. Dong Z, et al. Suppression of angiogenesis, tumorigenicity, and metastasis by human prostate cancer cells engineered to produce interferon-beta. Cancer Res. 1999;59(4):872–9.
51. Saloura V, et al. Evaluation of an attenuated vesicular stomatitis virus vector expressing interferon-beta for use in malignant pleural mesothelioma: heterogeneity in interferon responsiveness defines potential efficacy. Hum. Gene Ther. 2010;21(1):51–64.
52. Fernandez-Medarde A, Santos E. Ras in cancer and developmental diseases. Genes Cancer 2011;2(3):344–58.
53. Karapanagiotou EM, et al. Phase I/II trial of carboplatin and paclitaxel chemotherapy in combination with intravenous oncolytic reovirus in patients with advanced malignancies. Clin. Cancer Res. 2012;18(7):2080–9.
54. Mader EK, et al. Mesenchymal stem cell carriers protect oncolytic measles viruses from antibody neutralization in an orthotopic ovarian cancer therapy model. Clin. Cancer Res. 2009;15(23):7246–55.
55. Thorne SH, Negrin RS, Contag CH. Synergistic antitumor effects of immune cell-viral biotherapy. Science 2006;311(5768):1780–4.
56. Ikeda K, et al. Complement depletion facilitates the infection of multiple brain tumors by an intravascular, replication-conditional herpes simplex virus mutant. J. Virol. 2000;74(10):4765–75.
57. Cawood R, et al. Use of tissue-specific microRNA to control pathology of wild-type adenovirus without attenuation of its ability to kill cancer cells. PLoS Pathog. 2009;5(5):e1000440.
58. Diallo JS, et al. A high-throughput pharmacoviral approach identifies novel oncolytic virus sensitizers. Mol. Ther. 2010;18(6):1123–9.
59. Seet BT, McFadden G. Viral chemokine-binding proteins. J. Leukoc. Biol. 2002;72(1):24–34.
60. Dingli D, Russell SJ, Morris JC 3rd. *In vivo* imaging and tumor therapy with the sodium iodide symporter. J. Cell. Biochem. 2003;90(6):1079–86.
61. Liu TC, Galanis E, Kirn D. Clinical trial results with oncolytic virotherapy: a century of promise, a decade of progress. Nat. Clin. Pract. Oncol. 2007;4(2):101–17.
62. Kalergis AM, et al. Efficient T cell activation requires an optimal dwell-time of interaction between the TCR and the pMHC complex. Nat. Immunol. 2001;2(3):229–34.
63. Wan YY, Flavell RA. How diverse—CD4 effector T cells and their functions. J. Mol. Cell. Biol. 2009;1(1):20–36.
64. Geldart T, Illidge T. Anti-CD 40 monoclonal antibody. Leuk. Lymphoma. 2005;46(8):1105–13.
65. Pardoll DM. The blockade of immune checkpoints in cancer immunotherapy. Nat. Rev. Cancer 2012;12(4):252–64.
66. Parry RV, et al. CTLA-4 and PD-1 receptors inhibit T-cell activation by distinct mechanisms. Mol. Cell. Biol. 2005;25(21):9543–53.
67. Keir ME, et al. PD-1 and its ligands in tolerance and immunity. Annu. Rev. Immunol. 2008;26:677–704.
68. Zou W, Chen L. Inhibitory B7-family molecules in the tumour microenvironment. Nat. Rev. Immunol. 2008;8(6):467–77.
69. Dong H, et al. Tumor-associated B7-H1 promotes T-cell apoptosis: a potential mechanism of immune evasion. Nat. Med. 2002;8(8):793–800.
70. Franks HA, Wang Q, Patel PM. New anticancer immunotherapies. Anticancer Res. 2012;32(7):2439–53.
71. Lipson EJ, Drake CG. Ipilimumab: an anti-CTLA-4 antibody for metastatic melanoma. Clin. Cancer Res. 2011;17(22):6958–62.
72. Lipson EJ, et al. Durable cancer regression off-treatment and effective reinduction therapy with an anti-PD-1 antibody. Clin. Cancer Res. 2013;19(2):462–8.
73. Topalian SL, et al. Safety, activity, and immune correlates of anti-PD-1 antibody in cancer. N. Engl. J. Med. 2012;366(26):2443–54.
74. Brahmer JR, et al. Safety and activity of anti-PD-L1 antibody in patients with advanced cancer. New Engl. J. Med. 2012;366(26):2455–65.

75. Strome SE, et al. B7-H1 blockade augments adoptive T-cell immunotherapy for squamous cell carcinoma. Cancer Res. 2003;63(19):6501–5.
76. Furman RR, et al. A phase I study of dacetuzumab (SGN-40, a humanized anti-CD40 monoclonal antibody) in patients with chronic lymphocytic leukemia. Leuk. Lymphoma. 2010;51(2):228–35.
77. Kane A, Yang I. Interferon-gamma in brain tumor immunotherapy. Neurosurg. Clin. N. Am. 2010;21(1):77–86.
78. Fallarino F, Grohmann U, Puccetti P. Indoleamine 2,3-dioxygenase: from catalyst to signaling function. Eur. J. Immunol. 2012;42(8):1932–7.
79. Liu X, et al. Selective inhibition of IDO1 effectively regulates mediators of antitumor immunity. Blood 2010;115(17):3520–30.
80. Hou DY, et al. Inhibition of indoleamine 2,3-dioxygenase in dendritic cells by stereoisomers of 1-methyl-tryptophan correlates with antitumor responses. Cancer Res. 2007;67(2):792–801.
81. Mosmann TR, et al. Two types of murine helper T cell clone. I. Definition according to profiles of lymphokine activities and secreted proteins. 1986. J. Immunol. 2005;175(1):5–14.
82. Romagnani S. The Th1/Th2 paradigm. Immunol. Today 1997;18(6):263–6.
83. Greenwald RJ, Freeman GJ, Sharpe AH. The B7 family revisited. Annu. Rev. Immunol. 2005;23:515–48.
84. Reiner SL. Development in motion: helper T cells at work. Cell 2007;129(1):33–6.
85. Murphy KM, Stockinger B. Effector T cell plasticity: flexibility in the face of changing circumstances. Nat. Immunol. 2010;11(8):674–80.
86. Murphy KM, Reiner SL. The lineage decisions of helper T cells. Nat. Rev. Immunol. 2002;2(12):933–44.
87. Hanahan D, Weinberg RA. Hallmarks of cancer: the next generation. Cell 2011;144(5):646–74.
88. Teng MW, et al. Immune-mediated dormancy: an equilibrium with cancer. J. Leukoc Biol. 2008;84(4):988–93.
89. Kim R, Emi M, Tanabe K. Cancer immunoediting from immune surveillance to immune escape. Immunology 2007;121(1):1–14.
90. Harimoto H, et al. Inactivation of tumor-specific CD8(+) CTLs by tumor-infiltrating tolerogenic dendritic cells. Immunol. Cell Biol. 2013;91(10):665.
91. Sheen YY, et al. Targeting the transforming growth factor-beta signaling in cancer therapy. Biomol. Ther. (Seoul) 2013;21(5):323–31.
92. Topalian SL, Drake CG, Pardoll DM. Targeting the PD-1/B7-H1(PD-L1) pathway to activate anti-tumor immunity. Curr. Opin. Immunol. 2012;24(2):207–12.
93. Munn DH. Blocking IDO activity to enhance anti-tumor immunity. Front. Biosci. (Elite Ed.) 2012;4:734–45.
94. Shurin MR, et al. Th1/Th2 balance in cancer, transplantation and pregnancy. Springer Semin. Immunopathol. 1999;21(3):339–59.
95. Tosolini M, et al. Clinical impact of different classes of infiltrating T cytotoxic and helper cells (Th1, Th2, Treg, Th17) in patients with colorectal cancer. Cancer Res. 2011;71(4):1263–71.
96. Gu-Trantien C, et al. CD4(+) follicular helper T cell infiltration predicts breast cancer survival. J. Clin. Invest. 2013;123(7):2873–92.
97. Kaech SM, Wherry EJ, Ahmed R. Effector and memory T-cell differentiation: implications for vaccine development. Nat. Rev. Immunol. 2002;2(4):251–62.
98. Qi CJ, et al. Autologous dendritic cell vaccine for estrogen receptor (ER)/progestin receptor (PR) double-negative breast cancer. Cancer Immunol. Immunother. 2012;61(9):1415–24.
99. Miranda-Hernandez DF, et al. Expression of Foxp3, CD25 and IL-2 in the B16F10 cancer cell line and melanoma is correlated with tumor growth in mice. Oncol. Lett. 2013;6(5):1195–200.
100. Wagner P, et al. Detection and functional analysis of tumor infiltrating T-lymphocytes (TIL) in liver metastases from colorectal cancer. Ann. Surg. Oncol. 2008;15(8):2310–7.
101. Halama N, et al. Localization and density of immune cells in the invasive margin of human colorectal cancer liver metastases are prognostic for response to chemotherapy. Cancer Res. 2011;71(17):5670–7.
102. Printz C. New AJCC cancer staging manual reflects changes in cancer knowledge. Cancer 2010;116(1):2–3.
103. Angell H, Galon J. From the immune contexture to the Immunoscore: the role of prognostic and predictive immune markers in cancer. Curr. Opin. Immunol. 2013;25(2):261–7.
104. Galon J, et al. The immune score as a new possible approach for the classification of cancer. J. Transl. Med. 2012;10:1.
105. Pages F, et al. *In situ* cytotoxic and memory T cells predict outcome in patients with early-stage colorectal cancer. J. Clin. Oncol. 2009;27(35):5944–51.

IV. NOVEL APPROACHES FOR CANCER THERAPIES

Long-Circulating Therapies for Cancer Treatment

Sara Movassaghian, Vladimir P. Torchilin

Center for Pharmaceutical Biotechnology and Nanomedicine,
Northeastern University, Boston, MA, USA

OUTLINE

INTRODUCTION: CONSIDERATION OF NANOTECHNOLOGY FOR CANCER THERAPY

Rapid advances in nanotechnology, with its significant impact on therapeutic delivery systems, afford an opportunity to address some of the most complex features of human diseases at a molecular level.[1,2] A great deal of research in the nanoparticle field has been devoted to

Novel Approaches and Strategies for Biologics, Vaccines and Cancer Therapies. DOI: 10.1016/B978-0-12-416603-5.00018-3

investigation of new delivery platforms for cancer diagnosis, to imaging and treatment by providing adequate tools for early detection of the disease, and to overcoming the common bottlenecks encountered with the use of routine anticancer compounds.[3–6]

The low efficacy of many current chemotherapy regimes can be attributed to their poor physiochemical properties (poor solubility, low stability, and inadequate biocompatibility) and/or a poor pharmacokinetics and biodistribution profile (e.g., short circulating half-life, poor oral bioavailability, poor specificity, high volume of distribution, systemic toxicity, off-target uptake, high incidence of multidrug resistance).[7]

Due to their size-dependent physicochemical properties, nanoscale drug delivery carriers (liposomes, micelles, solid lipid particles, nanocapsules, polymer–drug conjugates, polymeric and protein drug delivery systems) offer the potentiality for an improved therapeutic effectiveness and safety profile of conventional forms of cancer chemotherapy and also show great promise in reconsideration of the use of existing drugs by altering their poor physicochemical and pharmacokinetic properties (Table 18.1).[8]

Nanoscopic systems encapsulate or incorporate a variety of therapeutic or imaging agents from low to high molecular weight, enhance their solubility properties, and protect the drug from inactivation, degradation, and metabolization phenomena.[9,10]

Intrinsic characteristics and extended blood circulation half-life of nanocarriers allow achievement of cellular uptake in malignant cells by passive targeting of malignant tissues due to the enhanced permeability and retention (EPR) effect.[11]

Differentials in endothelial pore size,[12] abnormal tumor vasculature and permeability, and structural changes in the interstitial matrix provide the opportunity for nano-based formulations to selectively extravasate to the tumor area relative to normal tissues, while poor lymphatic drainage helps to retain formulations at tumor sites.[13,14]

To further increase the selectivity of pharmaceutical nanocarriers, to control their biological properties in a desirable fashion, and to make them simultaneously perform various therapeutic or diagnostic functions, different surface engineering approaches have been extensively investigated to construct multifunctional nanocarriers.[15–22] These strategies are well developed to allow nanocarriers system to overcome various biological barriers from a

TABLE 18.1 Approved Long-Circulating Nanoparticles for Cancer Therapy

Composition	Trade Name	Indication
LIPOSOMAL PLATFORMS		
Liposome-PEG doxorubicin	Doxil/Caelyx	HIV-related Kaposi's sarcoma, metastatic, breast cancer, metastatic ovarian cancer
POLYMERIC PLATFORMS		
Methoxy-PEG-poly(D,L-lactide) Taxol	Genexol-PM	Metastatic breast cancer
Pegfilgrastim (PEG–GCSF)	Neulasta	Neutropenia associated with cancer chemotherapy
PEG–L-asparaginase	Oncaspar	Acute lymphoblastic leukemia

systemic level to organ and cellular levels. Detailed descriptions of the biological barriers are reviewed elsewhere.[8,23,24] These properties lead to altered biodistribution profiles and enhance the accumulation of drug-loaded nanocarriers in target sites by active targeting (e.g. receptor-mediated targeting). The net result of these altered nanocarrier properties is to reduce the amount of drug needed to reach a favorable therapeutic index and thus reduce drug-induced systemic adverse effects. Also, combining tumor targeting, tumor therapy, and tumor imaging all-in-one can provide a useful multimodal approach to conquer cancer.[25]

CHALLENGES IN RATIONAL DESIGN OF NANOCARRIERS: LONGEVITY IN THE BLOOD AS AN IMPORTANT BASIC PROPERTY OF COLLOIDAL DRUG DELIVERY SYSTEMS

An important requirement for any drug delivery system to achieve its outlined goals is to be present in the bloodstream long enough to reach or recognize the therapeutic site of action and be able to pass different level of barriers to effectiveness.[26] It is clear that maintaining therapeutic levels of nanocarriers in the blood for an acceptable interval of time will ultimately provide a higher chance of EPR-mediated drug delivery and increase the possibility of enhancing ligand-mediated targeting of nanocarriers into the areas with a limited blood supply and/or low concentration of a target antigen, when an extended time is required to allow for accumulation of a sufficient quantity of drug in the target zone.[27] However, one of the major challenges faced by colloidal drug carriers immediately after their administration is their rapid clearance by the array of defense mechanisms of the body (see Figure 18.1).[28]

Pharmaceutical nanocarriers can be detected as exogenous molecules by the immune system and quickly removed from blood circulation long before completion of their intended function.[29] Therefore, keeping track of the whole biological portrait and the nanoparticle interactions with the immune system is a rational step for the design of a long-circulating drug delivery platform. In the next section, the mechanism of particulate clearance from systemic circulation is discussed along with different factors (e.g., physicochemical properties of nanocarriers) that determine the circulation kinetics of nanoparticles.

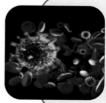

- Reduction of glomerular filtration
- Reduction of reticuloendothelial system uptake (complement activation, opsonization)
- Enhance accumulation of nanocarriers in tumor sites (take advantages of EPR effect)
- Acceleration of delivery of drugs to organs and tissues

FIGURE 18.1   Challenges in designing long-circulating nanoparticles.

Factors Affecting Clearance of Nanoparticles

The biological performance of nanotherapeutic agents used in cancer treatment, which are generally administered via the systemic circulation, is controlled by a complex array of inter-related physicochemical and biological factors. To obtain a successful clinical result with a de-signed drug delivery system, we need to understand the pharmacodynamics of nanoparticles in the body environment (absorption, distribution, metabolism, and excretion, or ADME; see Markovsky et al.[30] and Moghimi et al.[31] for a detailed review of this concept).

After intravenous administration of conventional nanoparticles, they circulate in the bloodstream and are distributed to various organs according to their properties. Interaction with blood components and opsonization are two important phenomena likely to take place. Interactions with blood protein, mainly albumin, affect particle size which could change the surface function of administrated nanoparticles. Also deposition of proteins on the surface of the nanoparticles induces aggregation, which will change the total stability of the na-nocarriers and lead to changes in the biodistribution, uptake, and clearance profile of the nanoparticles.[32]

Opsonization is an important process that typically occurs rapidly in the bloodstream af-ter introduction of the particles. It tags the foreign nanoparticles with blood serum proteins called opsonins, making them visible to macrophages. Major opsonins include complement proteins such as C3, C4, and C5; laminin; fibronectin; C-reactive protein; type I collagen, and immunoglobulins. They interact with specific receptors on monocytes and macrophages. Thus, opsonization facilitates nanoparticle recognition by the immune system by capture from the blood.[33] The mononuclear phagocytic system (MPS) (also known as the reticuloen-dothelial system, or RES) plays a key role as part of immune system that eliminates par-ticulate materials. The circulating RES and tissue macrophages in lung, spleen (sinusoidal lining cells), bone marrow, and liver (Küpffer cells)[34] are major clearance pathways for most conventional colloidal drug delivery systems. They are responsible for the very short blood circulation half-life of nanoparticles (less than 5 min) and the efficient accumulation of drug for treatment of MPS localized tumors.[35]

It has been well documented that the physicochemical properties of nanoparticles (size, shape, surface charge, hydrophobicity, and extent of rigidity/deformability) are what largely influence their biological fate and complement activation.[33,36–40]

Particle Size

Particle size is a key factor in the biological outcomes of a drug delivery system as it gov-erns the biodistribution profile and extravasation out of the circulation into the target tissue and their retention within a tumor site.[41] Upper and lower size limits should be considered when optimizing a drug delivery system for specific target zones. Particles must be small enough to avoid uptake by the RES (those >200 nm are prone to rapid clearance from the bloodstream).[42] Apart from the reticuloendothelial system, nanoparticles less than 5 nm in diameter (molecular weight of 5000 or less) are also eliminated from the circulation through renal clearance.[43] Therefore, loss associated with glomerular filtration and hepatic uptake of drug carriers should be avoided, as long as neither the kidney nor liver is a drug target. The gap size of the tumor vasculature endothelium varies from 200 to 800 nm, depending on the type of tumor and space between vessels in the same tumor.[12,44] As a rough estimation, the design of rigid and spherical nanoparticles ranging in size from 10 to 200 nm improves the blood circulation half-life of nanoparticles,[43–45] but they are small enough to efficiently accumulate in tumors through the EPR effect.[46]

Studies by Moghimi and his team[47] showed a clear-cut relationship between liposome size and liver uptake. The smaller the size of the liposomes (usually less than 100 nm), the greater the uptake by hepatocytes. It may be related to fenestration size (transcellular pores in liver sinusoidal endothelial cells), which varies from approximately 100 to 150 nm in diameter.[48,49] Ideally, long-circulating liposomes with a rigid structure should be in the range of 120 to 200 nm to avoid particle trapping in liver. If larger, then the particle must be deformable enough to bypass filtration.[47]

Particle Shape

In addition to particle size, shape is another property of a nanoparticle that can dictate the behavior of nanoparticles in various processes including blood circulation, biodistribution, targeting, cellular uptake/internalization, intracellular trafficking, and toxicity.[50–54] Recognition by macrophages is a key process in generating an immune response. Shape, geometry, and orientation of the nanoparticle play an important role in initiation of phagocytosis.[55] Remarkably, worm-shaped polymeric particles show negligible phagocytosis compared with spheres of the same volume.[56]

The effect of local geometry and shape of nanoparticles on phagocytosis was further highlighted in work by Doshi and Mitragotri.[57] They reported that worm-like particles with very high aspect ratios (>20) exhibited negligible phagocytosis compared to spherical particles of equal volume.[56] They concluded that shape-induced inhibition of phagocytosis of drug delivery particles is possible by minimizing the size-normalized curvature of the particles. Worm-like flexible micelles have also been shown to exhibit prolonged circulation in the blood.[58] The attachment propensity for opsonized particles to macrophages has also been reported to depend significantly on particle shape.[57] Devarajan et al.[59] reported the first proof of a particle shape's role with regard to *in vivo* performance of the nanocarrier systems. They proposed that control of particle shape as a parameter could lead to the development of exciting and novel approaches in passive targeting for creating macrophage-evading characteristics. Compared to spherical particles, irregular-shaped polymer lipid nanoparticles (LIPOMER) evade Küpffer cells and localize in the spleen, implying that non-spherical particles are likely to evade liver macrophages.[59] For a detailed review, see Mitragotri and Lahann,[54] Champion et al.,[60] and Venkataraman et al.[61]

Surface Characteristics (Charge, Chemistry, and Hydrophobicity)

Surface characterization of particles plays three key roles that affect the function of nanoparticles. First, there is a correlation between surface charge and chemistry and the opsonization process that dictates the RES response. Second, to obtain effective cellular targeting, target-specific ligands should be incorporated in the structure of engineered nanoparticles. Third, if organelle targeting is also required, those ligands must be included in the surface design of nanoparticles.

Studies have shown that neutrally charged particles are less prone to phagocytosis by RES compared with charged particles.[62] However, in determining clearance rates, nanoparticle size has a greater impact. Clearance of neutral particles increased considerably with an increase in size, indicating that smaller sized particles are not efficiently coated with opsonins and that surface curvature changes may affect the extent and type of the opsonin adsorption.[63]

As a general rule, the opsonization of hydrophobic particles has been shown to occur more quickly than for hydrophilic particles.[64] Serum proteins (e.g., IgG) also have a high affinity for hydrophobic particles.[65] In addition, activation of the complement system and rapid uptake of negatively charged liposomes containing certain anionic lipids (phosphatidylserine, phosphatidylglycerol, and phosphatidic acid) have been reported.[66–68]

Devine et al.[63] investigated the effect of lipid composition, membrane fluidity, and geometric characteristics of nanoparticles on the initial assembly of opsonins involved in complement activation. They suggested that, at a fixed lipid concentration, larger liposomes (400 nm) are more efficient at activating complement than smaller vesicles (50 nm). They showed that liposomal cholesterol concentration activates complement in a dose-dependent manner, and inclusion of phospholipids bearing a net charge is required to detect complement activation. They also demonstrated that the phospholipid fatty acyl chain length did not influence complement activation, while the introduction of unsaturated acyl chains markedly decreased levels of complement activation.[63]

Keeping in mind all of the above factors, the most usual way to circumvent the activation of the immune system and keep drug carriers in the blood long enough is to mask them from recognition by the immune system.[69–71] Because the initial opsonization of particles is so critical to the process of phagocytic recognition and clearance of nanoparticles, extensive efforts in the stealth drug delivery field have focused on trying to stop this process. One widely used method to change the opsonization rate is the use of surface adsorbed or grafted shielding groups that can block the interactions that opsonins use to bind to particle surfaces. These approaches are discussed in the next section.

APPROACHES TO DESIGNING LONG-CIRCULATING NANOPARTICLES

Several methods of camouflaging or masking nanoparticles have been developed which allow a drug delivery system to temporarily bypass recognition by the RES, thus prolonging their blood circulation half-life and increasing the effectiveness of stealth devices. Some of these approaches were motivated by the strategies adopted by mammalian pathogens (e.g., *Hemobartonella* and *Eperythrozoonosis*) that have several methods to escape recognition by the immune system and remain in the circulation for several hours to weeks (see next section).

As discussed, modifications on particle size, surface, shape, and flexibility of particles have been explored for this purpose.[44,58,72] The most promising method among the various strategies followed until now is sterically stabilizing the nanoparticles with a layer of hydrophilic polymer chains or non-ionic surfactants. These polymers share the common basic features—high flexiblity and hydrophilicity—that confer stealth properties to nanoparticle by repelling the opsonins, resulting in prolonged circulation half-life and selective extravasation into tumors located outside the RES. The current gold standard for stealth coating properties is polyethylene glycol (PEG).[73,74] PEGylation simply refers to the decoration of a particle surface by covalently grafting, entrapping, or adsorbing PEG chains.[75]

As a protective polymer, PEG provides a very attractive combination of properties. They are biocompatible, nontoxic, non-imunogenic, relatively inert, flexible and highly soluble and are available in various molecular weights and functionalized architectures that have led to successful clinical outcomes.[76] After the first successful report on PEG in the 1970s by Davis et al.[77] for drug delivery, a majority studies on drug delivery outcomes seem to have benefited from PEGylation.[78–80]

A wide variety of therapeutic proteins/peptides, antibody fragments, oligonucleotides, and small molecule drugs have been PEGylated.[81] The basis for these modifications is the favorable changes in size, polarity, structure, and surface properties of the drug molecule or the drug-bearing particles, as well as the capability to change the physicochemical properties of the drug molecule or drug-bearing particles themselves. Together, these effects produce significant bioavailability and pharmacokinetic/pharmacodynamics improvements (circulation life span, distribution pattern, and elimination pathway) when compared with non-PEGylated counterparts. To learn about PEGylated drugs on the market or currently under development see Pasut and Veronese,[80] Kang et al.,[82] and Jokerst et al.[83]

Different theories have been used to describe the mechanism of surface camouflaging of nanoparticles by polymers.[45] PEG was used as the most representative of the materials investigated to produce stealth nanocarriers. It is believed that PEGylation circumvents the body's defense at the opsonization step.[84] The mechanism of preventing opsonization by PEG has been thoroughly investigated and includes the shielding of the surface charge, increased surface hydrophilicity,[85] enhanced repulsive interaction between polymer-coated nanocarriers and blood components,[86] difficulties in modeling antibodies by the immune system around a flexible polymer molecule, and formation of a molecular cloud or a hydrated shell that shields the surface from attaching opsonins.[84,85,87–89] The hydrophilic and flexible chains of the PEG acquire an extended conformation and form dense conformational "clouds" over the surface of the nanoparticle and prevent the adsorption of opsonins by steric repulsion, making them "invisible" to phagocytic cells.[89]

It has been well documented that polymer composition, molecular weight, density of the polymer on the nanoparticle surface, thickness of the coating layer, conformation, flexibility, and architecture of the chains play an essential role in determining the extent of polymer–blood component interaction in biological fluids and the final *in vitro* and *in vivo* behavior of nanoparticles.[90–92] In this regard, polymer chain flexibility plays a noticeably greater role as explained by Allen.[93] Liposome coated with dextran (a highly soluble and hydrophilic but rigid structure), used in comparable quantities, does not cause an analogous decrease in liposome-protein interactions.[89,94]

Depending on the PEG density and configuration on the liposome structure, a "mushroom," "pancake," or "brush" model is expected (Figure 18.2). A mushroom-like structure is formed with full surface coverage at a low density of PEG in liposome preparation.[95]

As the PEG density increases, the PEG chains extend and avoid overlap with other PEG molecules, resulting in a brush formation.[95,96] More detailed analysis within the frame of this model is provided in a review by Torchilin and Papisov.[97] Experiments have confirmed that increasing the concentration of grafted PEG, as well as its molecular weight, improves the repulsive properties of the lipid bilayer surfaces, creating a denser, larger brush.[86,98] With further increases in PEG, however, PEG–PEG interaction will perturb the surface and cause a transition from liposomes to micelles.[95]

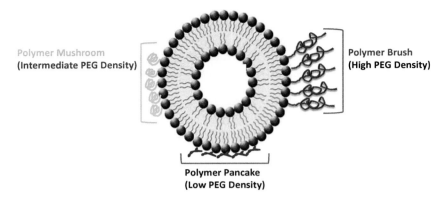

Polymer Mushroom
(Intermediate PEG Density)

Polymer Brush
(High PEG Density)

Polymer Pancake
(Low PEG Density)

FIGURE 18.2   Schematic figure of poly-(ethylene glycol) (PEG) configurations (mushroom, brush, and pancake) for polymer grafted to the surface of the liposome bilayer.

As the polymer molecular weight increases, the blood circulation half-life of the PEGylated particles increases. The optimum reported PEG content varies for different drug delivery systems. Stable stealth liposomes can be obtained with a low ratio of 3 to 5 kDa PEG-2000–DPPE.[99,100]

To ensure efficient coverage of the surface, the brush model presents an ideal model, but with this configuration integrity of the liposome membrane cannot be maintained.[95] This is related to the detergent-like effect of the PEG covering the surface of the liposome. Theoretically, for a liposome (100 nm) the ideal configuration (brush model) is obtained with >8 mol% of PEGylation.[101] PEG (2 KDa) is arranged in a mushroom conformation with <4 mol% PEG.[101]

In another study, 5 to 8 mol% PEG-2000, which is at the borderline between a mushroom and brush formation, is reported as optimal for obtaining thermodynamically stable liposomes.[95] However, Doxil®, as a stealth liposomal formulation often contains a ~5 mol% graft of PEG and is still susceptible to opsonization as liver and spleen uptake is remarkably high.[101]

In one investigation, a 10 wt% PEG density was considered optimal for poly(lactic acid) (PLA)[102] or poly(lactide-co-glycolide) (PLGA);[103,104] in another similar study, a 5 wt% of PEG was found to provide optimal surface coverage for PLA, PLGA, and PCL (polycaprolotone), and a higher amount of PEG did not further affect protein adsorption.[90,95,105] Studies have shown that a minimum effective hydrodynamic layer thickness is about 5% of the particle diameter.[106] Moghimi et al.[88] demonstrated that a 4-kDa PEG is needed to form a coating layer of 5 nm to efficiently reduce the protein adsorption of 60 to 200 nm polystyrene particles for complement activation.

Advantages and Disadvantages of PEGylation

Of all the polymers tested to date, PEG appears to be the most effective and commonly used material to provide stealth properties in drug delivery systems. PEGylated liposomes have shown extended circulation times in all mammalian species, including mice, rats, dogs, and humans.[26,107–109] However, a number of issues have been raised as a so-called "PEG dilemma," which limits the methods employed for this purpose.[110] Two important concerns about PEGylation that should be addressed are (1) interference with cellular uptake and intracellular trafficking,[111] and (2) immune system activation and the accelerated blood clearance (ABC) phenomenon, which can occur after repeated administration.[112]

After the prolonged journey through the circulation and extravasation with the help of PEGylation, there remain barriers for nanoparticles before reaching the target destination, particularly when the drug does not freely enter the cell or encounters constant removal from the cells (e.g., multidrug resistance).[113] PEGylated nanoparticles are less effective at entering cells and escaping intracellular vesicles, as it seems the PEG layers interfere with efficient nanoparticle–cell interaction at different steps (e.g., passing through the extracellular matrix, attaching to cell membrane receptors, internalization and escape from the endosome).[114] Less tumor accumulation of doxorubicin was found with PEGylated liposomes than with non-PEGylated liposomes.[115]

Furthermore, significant alterations in the pharmacokinetic behavior of a second injected PEGylated liposome appears to be a result of complement activation which may lead to rapid clearance of the liposome. Studies have demonstrated activation of the rat and human complement system with liposomes bearing PEG or poloxamer and that PEG is not an inert drug-carrying vehicle *in vivo*.[116]

In a study by Laverman et al.,[117,118] three unexpected effects were reported after *in vivo* administration of PEG-liposomes. Apart from some clinical side-effects, dose-dependent clearance of the PEG liposome was observed at lipid doses lower than 1 μmol/kg. Rapid clearance of the PEG-liposome from blood circulation was observed after repeated injection.

Accelerated blood clearance after the first injected PEGylated liposomes has been attributed to splenic synthesis of anti-PEG IgM, opsonization of the second dose of PEGylated liposomes, and then uptake by the liver.[112,119–121] Antibody against PEG–conjugate decreased the effectiveness of treatment due to rapid clearance of PEG–asparaginase in patients who were treated for acute lymphoblastic leukemia.[122]

To overcome the "PEG dilemma" and develop PEGylated nanoparticles several strategies have been designed with alternative materials to bestow immune-evasive properties on nanoparticles but inducing less ABC effects (see next section). Modifying the nanoparticles with tumor-specific ligand to enhance intracellular uptake is another approach that will be discussed later.

Alternative Polymers for Steric Protection of Nanoparticle Surfaces

Several alternatives to PEG-based coatings have been designed, in addition to poloxamers,[123] poloxamines,[124] polysorbates,[125] and polysaccharides (chitosan,[126] dextran,[127,128] hyaluronic acid,[129] and heparin[130]). These include the following:

- Single-end lipid-modified polymers, such as palmitoyl- or phosphatidylethanolamine (PE)-terminated derivatives of poly(acryl amide) (PAA), poly(vinyl pyrrolidone) (PVP), and poly(acryloyl morpholine) (PAcM), which have been found to exert comparable stealth effects on liposomes *in vivo*[66,84,131,132]
- Poly(acryloylmorpholine) (PAcM)[133]
- Zwitterionic polymers (betaines, such as sulfobetaine and carboxybetaine) that belong to zwitterionic molecules

Zwitterionic phospholipid derivatives have been shown to efficiently decrease the rate of adsorption of proteins, cells, and bacteria on the surfaces of molecules.[134] Compared to PEG, these materials bind water molecules more strongly through electrostatic interactions. Also, in contrast to PEG, which can partially insert itself in the lipid bilayer of liposomes,[135,136] zwitterionic polymers do not perturb the lipidic bilayer stability.[137,138] Moreover, poly(carboxybetaine) has multiple functional groups amenable to multivalent conjugations.[139] Liposomal formulation of a hydrophilic drug, coated with the same polymer, possessed good retention and long blood circulation and exhibited better stability in the presence of protein and better resistance to protein adsorption compared to the PEGylated counterparts.[138,140]

- Additionally, polyoxazolines have been explored as a hydrophilic segment in amphiphilic block copolymers. Poly(2-ethyl-2-oxazoline) was coupled with various polymers, including poly(caprolactone) and poly(aspartic acid), to form nanoparticles for drug delivery of paclitaxel and amphotericin B.[141,142] Poly(2-methyl-2-oxazoline) in liposome formulation also exhibited a long plasma lifetime and low hepatosplenic uptake and presented a stealth effect comparable to PEG.[143]
- Poly(amino acids) have shown prolonged blood circulation times. Poly(hydroxyethyl L-glutamine) (PHEG) and poly(hydroxyethyl L-asparagine) (PHEA) have been developed as promising enzymatically degradable stealth polymer coatings comparable to PEG. They provide some advantages over PEG, as they are biodegradable and reduce the toxicity related to PEG accumulation. Furthermore, liposomes coated with PHEA show a better pharmacokinetic pattern on repeated injection and maintain the stealth effect.[144,145]
- Polyglycerols are flexible hydrophilic aliphatic polyether polyols, with an antifouling effect comparable to that of PEG; they have been extensively studied as an alternative to PEG.[146,147] Linear poly(methyl glycerol) and polyglycerol are promising candidates to modify nanoparticles for long-circulating properties.[148,149] Less protein adsorption and higher stability have been reported for dendritic polyglycerols.[150,151] Liposomes decorated with phosphatidyl polyglycerols exhibit extended blood circulation time and decreased uptake by the phagocyte system.[146]

Bio-Inspired, Bioengineered, and Biomimetic Methods to Prepare Long Circulating Nanoparticles-A RBC Membrane-Cloaked Nanoparticles and RBC-Hitchhiking Method

One of these bio-inspired strategies was motivated by the existence of mammalian pathogens of different size (0.2 to 2 μm) that bind to the erythrocyte surface and remain in the circulation for days or weeks. Hemotrophic mycoplasmas pathogens (*Haemobartonella* and *Eperythrozoonosis*) use red blood cells (RBCs) as carriers by simply attaching to the surface of the RBC, while other types reside in the RBC (*Plasmodium falciparum*) and evade clearance by the RES.[152]

The same strategy has been used by researchers to exploit natural particulates for multiple applications in the delivery of proteins, peptides, therapeutic enzymes, and nucleic acids by nature's long circulating delivery vehicles.[153,154] Advances in molecular biology inspired modeling of nanocarriers after RBCs by taking RBC or other mammalian cell structural properties as design cues to construct effective long-circulating delivery platforms.

A team led by Mitragotri et al.[155] has successfully developed a way to harness the flexibility and mobility of RBCs to overcome the short circulation times and poor targeting associated with nanoparticles. Such RBC hitchhiking is a potentially new method for addressing rapid clearance of the nanoparticles from blood circulation.

Erythrocytes are the autologous cells of the host body and have a unique structure: (1) a non-nuclear biconcave disc, (2) a diameter of ~7 μm, (3) a thickness ~2 μm, (4) plasma membrane surface area of ~160 μm^2, (5) half-life of 120 days, and (6) widespread circulation throughout the body. These characteristics make them a potentially attractive carrier for intravascular drug delivery.[156–158] Attachment of certain drugs to erythrocytes has been used previously to prolong half-lives through covalent attachment of the drug to the erythrocyte surface.[159] This method can be used for the types of drugs that remain effective while anchored to the cell surface. However, attachment of nanoparticles to RBCs by various methods (electrostatic or hydrophobic interactions, covalent or high-affinity ligands) can combine the advantages of both systems (RBC and nanoparticle) in one platform.[160] Extended circulation half-lives of nanoparticles were dramatically achieved with little effect on erythrocyte life span and structure. The strength of binding between the particles and the RBCs was the determinant factor for the circulation lifetime of particles.[161] Eventually, detachment of the particles occurs due to shear forces, cell–cell interactions, and cell–vessel wall interactions. Once detached, the particles are cleared primarily in the liver and to some extent in the spleen.[161] The half-lives of nanoparticles attached to RBCs are comparable to those previously reported for surface-modified nanoparticles.[162] RBC–particle complex modification with PEG further increased the circulation half-life of bound particles to over 24 hours.[161]

The advantages of using RBCs to extend drug half-lives compared to common surface modification strategies are applicable for small particles (below 200 nm) with limited loading capacity. Larger particles end up in spleen. Also, this method resulted in only a few hours of extension of nanocarriers in circulation, although studies support the possibility of enhancing the circulation times of larger nanoparticles (200 to 450 nm) by orders of magnitude with non-covalent adhesion on erythrocyte membranes. This avoids the need to modify the surface chemistry of the entire particle, thus leaving opportunities for attachment of chemicals to the exposed surface for targeting applications.[32] Furthermore, a larger drug payload would be achieved with increased size of the nanoparticles and allow a sustained release profile.[161] As discussed earlier, the protective function of surface coating with PEG is reduced with repeated injections.[161] The circulation times of 220-nm particles attached to erythrocytes are comparable to those reported with surface modification strategies using poloxamine-908.[32,116,120]

Hu et al.[163] presented a new class of long-circulating nanocarriers to bridge the surface chemistry of RBCs with the versatile cargo-carrying capacity of polymeric nanoparticles. They used red blood cell membranes for stealth coating of polymeric PLGA that revealed a superior circulation time compared to particles covered with PEG–lipid. A RBC-membrane-camouflaged PLGA formed after co-extrusion of prepared PLGA nanoparticles with RBC-membrane-derived vesicles through a porous membrane.[163] Detailed explanations of RBCs utilized in drug delivery system can be found elsewhere.[154,164–166]

Almost all eukaryotic cells have a glycocalyx surface, often terminating in sialic acid residues that play a key role in non-recognition of self-tissue by low level of complement activation through the alternative pathway.[167,168] Sialic acid and its derivatives ganglioside (e.g., GM1, monosialoganglioside) and glycophorin were used in early attempts to confer stealth properties on nanoparticles, specifically liposome and micelles, for drug delivery applications.[93,116,169–173]

Allen and her coworkers[93] were the first to show this activity of GM1, and the term "stealth liposome" was applied to this class of liposomes. Liu et al.[174] showed that GM1-grafted liposomes within a specific size range (90 to 200 nm) presented longer blood retention, with consequent accumulation in tumor tissues, than those outside of this size range (>300 nm or <40 nm). GM1 concentrations in liposome will determine the degree of macrophage uptake. About a 90% decrease in uptake of liposomes by macrophage has been reported at a 10 mol% GM1 concentration in the liposome structure, while a low level of GM1 (4 mol%) failed to provide longer liposome circulation times.[175]

The use of glycolipids in drug delivery system to evade RES is apparently declining. This can be attributed to the development of better compounds such as PEG derivatives which solve the important problems associated with the use of compounds such as GM1, including their expense, and the difficulties associated with their purification to drug standards.[93] Also, *in vivo* results show that the GM1 decoration on liposome was effective in mice but failed to prove its long circulating efficacy in rats.[171]

Another approach to disguising the nanoparticle as "self" so it remains unrecognizable to the immune system is to introduce the integrin-associated protein CD47 as a coating agent for the nanoparticle. CD47 acts as a key marker of self on red blood cells (RBCs) and prevents RBC phagocytosis via interaction with a specific receptor (SIRPα) on macrophages.[176] Red blood cells that lacked CD47 were rapidly cleared from the bloodstream by macrophages.[177] This marker is also expressed by certain viruses to evade the immune system.[178,179] Hsu and his coworkers[180] showed the feasibility of reducing the phagocytosis of colloidal carriers using soluble CD47.

ENHANCING EFFICACY OF PEGYLATED NANOPARTICLES: SHEDDABLE COATINGS

As discussed earlier, steric stabilization is not desirable for all steps in the drug targeting process. After reaching a tumor site, the nanoparticle should deliver its cargo to achieve a sufficient therapeutic response. The polymer coating of nanoparticles hinders the interaction of the nanoparticle within the target zone (uptake and cytosolic delivery) and impedes release of the drug at the pathological site. Thus, attempts have been made to address this issue and enhance the therapeutic efficacy of sterically stabilized nanoparticle by various methods (see Figure 18.3).

- Selective and active targeting of PEG-coated nanoparticles involves targeting ligands, including proteins (mainly antibodies and their fragments), peptides, nucleic acids (aptamers),[181] small molecules, and others (vitamins, carbohydrates) that recognize tumor-associated antigen.[182] The proposed method minimizes the stealth nanoparticle's uptake by normal cells and enhances the influx and retention of the drug in cancer cells. In cases where the internalization of the drug (e.g., protein, gene) is required to reach the appropriate intracellular destination, other specific ligand targeting moiety-penetration enhancers (e.g., cell-penetrating peptides, or CPPs) are necessary. Recently, "smart multifunctional" nanocarriers that gather various functionalities, including stealth, ligand-targeting, cell-penetrating, and stimulus-sensitive functions, all in one platform have received much attention.[18,21,183–185]

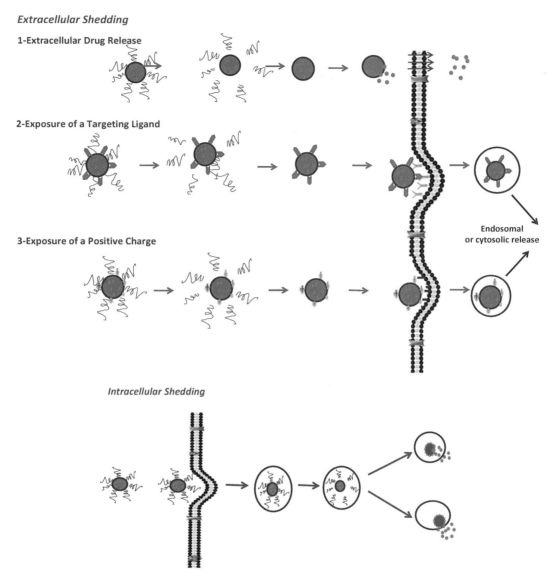

Extracellular Shedding

1-Extracellular Drug Release

2-Exposure of a Targeting Ligand

Endosomal
or cytosolic release

3-Exposure of a Positive Charge

Intracellular Shedding

FIGURE 18.3 Schematic representation of the efficacy of different shedding approaches upon the localization of sterically stabilized nanoparticles at the target site. *Adapted from Romberg, B., et al., Sheddable coatings for long-circulating nanoparticles. Pharm. Res. 2008;25(1):55–71.*[110]

- Strategies to remove the coating layer of nanoparticle upon arrival at the target zone have been developed.[186] This conditional removal of a coating layer of nanoparticles may facilitate drug release and enhance target cell interaction. The following text discusses the application and limitation of each group.

The identity of the targeting moiety and the incorporation method in the nanoparticle are important factors in determining the circulation time, affinity in the target zone, and desired cellular uptake.[187] Attempts have been made to combine longevity and targetability in one preparation step by simple incorporation of both an antibody and PEG into the membrane of the liposome (immunoliposome). By careful selection of a protective polymer/targeting moiety ratio, such an approach can be effective. The coating polymer, however, may create steric hindrances for targeting moiety recognition by cells.[188–191] In order to exclude shielding effects of the PEG chain in PEGylated nanoparticles, target ligand is designed to attach to the distal end of the PEG tips.[191,192] However, there are two important issues with regard to this type of formulation design. The presence of a high density of ligand at the terminal end of the coating particle chain will reduce the stealth properties of the nanoparticle and lead to rapid clearance from circulation.[193] Moreover, the targeting moiety will provoke an immune system reaction and restrict repeated administration of the nanoparticles.[194]

Torchilin and his team[195] reported successful enhancement of the anticancer efficacy of drug loaded in targeted long-circulating nanocarriers. The specific toxicity of doxorubicin in tumor cells (*in vitro* and *in vivo*) was increased markedly by decorating Doxil® (doxorubicin in long-circulating PEGylated liposomes) with nucleosome-specific monoclonal antibody.

Strong *in vitro* and *in vivo* antineuroblastoma activity was reported with GD2-targeted immunoliposomes, which delivered the antitumoral drug fenretinide to the target.[196] To improve intracellular trafficking of the nanoparticle, the targeted immunoliposome was combined with a pH-dependent endosome-disruptive peptide.[197] Diphtheria toxin A (DTA) chain, when used as a cargo drug, inhibits the production of protein when it reaches the cytosol of the cells and shows specific toxicity. Cytotoxicity was observed only with a liposomal formulation in which a pH-dependent fusogenic peptide helped destabilization of endosomal membranes after cellular uptake to enhance endosomal escape.[197] An anionic pH-sensitive liposome with appropriate blood stability was used for antisense oligonucleotide delivery after undergoing a phase transition at the lower pH of the endosomal environment to release a cargo to the cytoplasm.[198,199] It is clear that after internalization of therapeutic macromolecules translocation from the endosome to the cytosol is critical. Both the degradation in a harsh enzymatic environment (for DNA or protein) as well as restricted membrane transport (for hydrophilic and/or large sized cargos) can be a problem. The endosomal escape can be mediated by fusogenic liposomes (e.g., dioleoyl phosphatidylethanolamine, or DOPE). If PEG as a stealth coat is used in fusogenic liposomes, a remarkable reduction in cytosolic delivery of cargo occurs.[200] Shedding of the coating would restore the fusogenicity of the liposomes and allow for endosomal escape. Therefore, a shedding process seems to be a reasonable way to elude this limitation (discussed later).

A similar combination of longevity and targetability can also be achieved by targeting specific receptors overexpressed on the surface of cancerous cells (e.g., transferrin, folate, luteinizing hormone-releasing hormone (LHRH),[201] and human epidermal growth factor receptor 2 (HER2).[202–204]

Long-circulating liposomal daunorubicin[205,206] and doxorubicin[207] were delivered into various tumor cells via folate receptor-mediated uptake and demonstrated increased cytotoxicity. Similarly, PEG–PLGA-based particles were surface modified with trastuzumab, a monoclonal antibody against HER2. Results indicated a significantly higher cytotoxicity in HER2-positive cell lines than in nontargeted PLGA nanoparticles or with free docetaxel.[208] A sterically stabilized, mitoxantrone-loaded liposome tailored to target LHRH receptor overexpressing cells was developed to promote the efficiency of intracellular delivery of the mitoxantrone through receptor-mediated endocytosis.[209]

- To improve uptake and internalization of nanoparticles by cells, different approaches should be considered. It has been shown that a positively charged nanoparticle can efficiently interact and bind to the cell membrane of negatively charged target cells. However, using an appropriate polymer to give stealth characteristics to the delivery system will shield surface charge. At the same time, this effect helps nanoparticles to remain longer in blood circulation and prevents unfavorable interactions but also reduces cell uptake. Shedding the protective coat at the site of target cell is one possible tactic to restore the interaction characteristic of nanoparticles. Here, we focus on the conditional removal of PEG as protective and stealth components of nanocarriers at tumor sites used to achieve a better therapeutic effect.

Long-Circulating, Stimuli-Sensitive Nanoparticles

One method for preparation of long-circulating nanoparticles by surface modification with PEG is to couple the polymer to a lipid anchor and graft to the nanocarrier's structure. The presence of a cleavable linker between the polymer chain and anchoring moiety can introduce new properties to a system that already has longevity and targetability characteristics. Local environmental features unique to tumors and their extracellular matrices have been exploited to remove the protective effect of PEG in a tumor-specific manner. This smart multifunctional nanocarrier responds to intrinsic or externally applied stimuli to maximize the antitumor efficacy and minimize the drug side-effects.[210,211] These multifunctionalities can unmask the coating polymer by taking advantage of certain intrinsic local stimuli such as decreased pH, hyperthermia, and altered enzyme levels[212] or redox conditions characteristic of these zones (Table 18.2). Apart from these intrinsic local conditions, stimuli can also be applied externally to these areas, including temperature,[213] magnetic fields,[214] and ultrasound (see Figure 18.4).[215]

TABLE 18.2   Shedding Approach: Cleavage of a Linker between the Stabilizing Polymer and Its Anchor

Stimulus	Linker	Site of Shedding Action	Advantages
Low pH	Acid sensitive linkage • diorthoester • orthoester • vinyl ether • phosphoramidate • hydrazone • beta- thiopropionate	**Extracellular:** drug release, reemerging of target moiety, charge reversal **Endosome:** enhanced drug release and endosomal disrupting cell membrane	• Prolonged circulation time • Higher accumulation/exposure in tumor site via EPR effect • Higher local drug concentrations at tumor sites • upon arrival at slightly acidic tumor sites, the stealth nanocarrier is activated by pH to release its cargos[216] or to become more interactive with the targeted cells (targeted moiety re-emergence[222] or surface charge reversal to a positive charge[223])
Reducing agent	Disulfide bond	**Extracellular Intracellular (Endo/ lysosome & cytosol)**	• Extracellular stability and intracellular activity.[240–242]

(Continued)

TABLE 18.2   Shedding Approach: Cleavage of a Linker between the Stabilizing Polymer and Its Anchor (*cont.*)

Stimulus	Linker	Site of Shedding Action	Advantages
Proteolysis	Peptide	Endo/lysosome, extracellular	• Systemic stability of the carriers • Improved accumulation in tumor tissue • Increase cellular association and uptake after the accumulation of the carrier in tumor tissue[252–254]
Temperature	Thermo-sensitive block copolymer (-poly(N-isopropylacrylamide)	Extra/Intercellular	• Longer plasma half-life • Increased tumor accumulation • Controlled local drug release kinetic[255,256] • Hyperthermia also increase vascular permeability in solid tumors and may increase levels of nanoparticle accumulation[257,258]

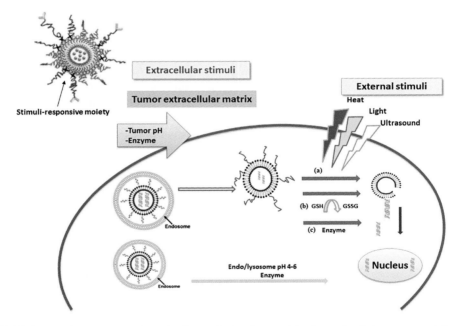

FIGURE 18.4   Schematic presentation of a "smart" stimulus-sensitive long-circulating nanoparticle and its response to internal and external stimulus.

pH-Triggered Shedding

pH-cleavable bonds can be designed to stabilize nanocarriers in circulation and in normal tissue but disintegrate and release the drug load in areas with lowered pH. The low-level pH in pathological sites such as tumors, ischemic and inflamed tissues (pH 6 to 6.5), or endosomal compartments (endosomes display a pH of 5.5 to 6 and lysosomes have a pH of around 4.5) can be applied to hydrolysis of the sensitive bond with detachment of a polymer coating chain from its anchor.[212] For nanoparticulate systems, the diorthoester, orthoester, vinyl ether, phosphoramidate, hydrazone, and beta-thiopropionate linker have been used as acid-sensitive linkers.[216–223] Among the acid-releasable coatings investigated so far, the diorthoester and the hydrazone-linked coatings are probably the most advanced. For an overview of shedding approaches using cleavable linkers see Romberg et al.[110]

The synthesis of a hydrazine-functionalized PEG–phosphatidyl–ethanolamine-based amphiphilic polymer capable of conjugating several ligands (e.g., antinucleosome 2C5 mAb, antimyosin 2G4 mAb, proteins such as concanavalin A (Con-A) and avidin) via a reversible pH-labile bond has been reported by Torchilin et al.[224,225] The PE portion of the polymer helps to integrate the polymer–ligand complex into the liposomes with targeting functionalities attached to the distal end of the PEG block, which allows targeting of the liposomes to a desired site. The pH-sensitive PEG conjugate was then detached in cancer cells due to lowered pH, resulting in improved drug delivery to the tumor.[224] The system can be modified with a cell-penetrating protein to enhance intracellular delivery. For this purpose, TAT was attached to the liposome surface via a TAT-short PEG–PE derivative. At normal pH, the TAT function was hidden by the long PEG chains; however, at lowered pH (5 to 6), after shedding of PEG due to acidic hydrolysis of PEG–HZ–PE, increased internalization of the liposome via the TAT binding was observed.[225]

pH-sensitive micelles have been developed with poly(ethylene glycol)–poly(L-histidine)–poly(L-lactide) (PEG–PH–PLLA) triblock copolymers to deliver doxorubicin. The pH-sensitive poly(L-histidine) segments swelled or shrank with the variation of pH to control the release of doxorubicin.[211,226]

A fusogenic DOPE liposome was designed with a pH-sensitive poly(ethylene glycol 2000)–diortho ester–distearoyl glycerol conjugate. The sheddable coating, which stabilizes the fusogenic DOPE in liposomes at neutral pH, hydrolyzed at low endosomal pH, promoted a phase transition, and mediated fusion of the liposome and release of the cargo in the cytoplasm.[227] Although most of the conjugate remained intact over the 3 hours of incubation at pH 7.4, complete degradation occurred within 1 hour at pH 4 and 5.[228]

Chen et al.[226]designed pH-sensitive polymersomes and micelles based on a diblock copolymer of PEG and an acid-labile polycarbonate (trimethoxybenzylidenepentaerythritol carbonate, PTMBPEC). The pH-dependent release profiles of both hydrophobic (paclitaxel) and hydrophilic drugs (doxorubicin) from the diblock polymersomes/micelle were investigated.

Significant tumor growth inhibition was evaluated in multidrug-resistant (MDR) ovarian tumor xenograft mouse models with pH-sensitive micelles composed of poly(L-histidine-co-L-phenlyalanine)–PEG-2000 and poly(L-lactic acid)–PEG-2000–folate.[229] Polyhistidine has transitions between hydrophobic properties at high pH (>7) to hydrophilic properties at low pH (<7) due to the ionization of the imidazole group at lower pH.[230]

The polyplex micelle was composed of an ABC triblock copolymer (ligand-PEG–pH-responsive segment–DNA-condensing segment) designed to be a novel targetable and endosome disruptive nonviral gene vector with pH-responsive properties.[231] The copolymer—lactosylated poly(ethyleneglycol)-block–poly(silamine)-block–poly[2–(N,N-dimethylamino) ethyl ethacrylate] (Lac–PEG–PSAO–PAMA)—consists of lactosylated poly(ethylene glycol) (A-segment), a pH-responsive polyamine segment (B-segment), and a DNA-condensing polyamine segment (C-segment). The Lac–PEG–PSAO–PAMA spontaneously associated with plasmid DNA to form three-layered polyplex micelles with a PAMA/DNA polyion complex (PIC) core, an uncomplexed PSAO inner shell, and a lactosylated PEG outer shell. The micelle underwent pH-induced conformational changes in the PSAO section, leading to swelling of the free PSAO inner shell at lowered pH while retaining the condensed pDNA in the PAMA/pDNA PIC core. The micelles exhibited a specific cellular uptake through asialoglycoprotein (ASGP) receptor-mediated endocytosis in hepatocytes and achieved a more efficient transfection ability of a reporter gene compared to the Lac–PEG–PSAO/pDNA and Lac–PEG–PAMA/pDNA polyplex micelles composed of the diblock copolymers and pDNA.[231]

An acylhydrazone-based, acid-labile PEG–lipid (HPEG2K–lipid, PEG-2000) that is stable at physiological pH but designed to lose its PEG chains at the pH of late endosomes was used to enhance transfection efficacy and endosomal escape of the cationic liposome–DNA complexes.[232] Higher transfection efficacy was observed compared with the similar but acid-stable bond formulation. This was attributed to the efficient endosomal escape, enabled by the acid-labile HPEG2K-lipid which sheds its PEG chains in the low pH environment of late endosomes, effectively switching on the electrostatic interactions that promote fusion of the membranes of complex and endosome.[232]

Enzymatic Stimuli

Another unique property common to many solid tumors is the overexpression of proteinases, such as matrix metalloproteinases (MMPs), which play a critical role in invasion of tumor cells and angiogenesis.[233] Several studies have employed MMPs to trigger PEG cleavage. Zhu et al.[234] recently designed a novel MMP-responsive multifunctional immunoliposomal nanocarrier that utilizes the upregulated levels of extracellular matrix metalloprotease 2 (MMP2) in tumors for removal of the PEG chain. The system was comprised of a TAT function shielded sterically by a long-chain PEG, a mAb 2C5 for active tumor targeting attached to the liposomal surface, and a MMP2 cleavable octapeptide (Gly–Pro–Leu–Gly–Ile–Ala–Gly–Gln) to provide a labile bond between long-chain PEG and the lipid. It was shown that the octapeptide linker was degraded by the extracellular MMP2 which exposes the TAT moiety and results in greater cellular uptake.[234]

In a series of experiments by the Hashida team,[235] galactosylated liposomes (Gal-liposome) showed delivery of incorporated antitumor drugs not only to hepatocellular carcinoma cells but also to normal liver cells. To further improve the selectivity of the delivery system, the amino group of dioleoylphosphatidylethanolamine (DOPE) was conjugated with PEGylated MMP2 substrate peptide (Gly–Pro–Leu–Gly–Ile–Ala–Gly–Gln) and MMP2–cleavable PEG–peptide–DOPE (PEG–PD).[236] Selective hepatocellular carcinoma targeting was achieved by protease activity of MMP2 and activated the liposomes in the target site. The PEG–PD in Gal–PEG–PD–liposomes can be cleaved by MMP2, exposing the galactose moieties on the liposomal surface. Consequently, they can be selectively recognized by asialoglycoprotein receptors on tumor cells.[236] By a shielding effect of PEG over the galactose ligands on the surface of the liposomes, the uptake by normal hepatocytes of Gal–liposomes containing PEG–PD (Gal–PEG–PD–liposomes) was somehow inhibited by steric hindrance.[237]

A matrix metalloproteinase-cleavable peptide-linked block copolymer was fabricated and utilized to construct PEG-sheddable polyplex micelles as smart gene delivery vectors, which were demonstrated to exhibit higher cellular uptake, improved endosomal escape, and high-efficiency gene transfection in the presence of MMP2.[238]

Redox Potential-Sensitive Systems

Based on the huge difference in redox potential between the extracellular space and the intracellular space (extracellular space is oxidative while the intracellular is reductive because of the presence of glutathione), redox-sensitive nanocarriers represent another approach for intracellular delivery.[239–242] Due to overexpression of reductase enzymes or the release of glutathione following cell death in tumor cells, the redox potential is altered largely by intracellular glutathione levels that are 4- to 100-fold greater than the normal extracellular glutathione levels.[243]

Reduction-responsive micelles were developed from a PEG–polyleucine diblock copolymer with disulfide bond-linked PEG and polyleucine and applied for trigger release of the doxorubicin.[244] The same group designed shell-sheddable micelles based on a disulfide-linked star-shaped copolymer of poly(ε-caprolactone) and poly(ethyl glycol) which shows high blood stability but rapid destabilization under a reduction environment in tumor cells.[245] Based on the same principle, shell-sheddable micelles based on a dextran-SS-poly(ε-caprolactone) diblock copolymer were also developed for efficient intracellular release of doxorubicin.[246]

Other stimulus-responsive systems can have important applications.[185] It has been proven that pathological areas show distinct hyperthermia and a thermosensitive nanocarrier can be used to selectively target the tumor area.[247,248] Liposomes can be designed to release an entrapped drug preferentially at temperatures attainable with mild local hyperthermia. Dipalmitoylphosphatidylcholine (DPPC) in liposome structures can give them temperature-sensitive functionalities.[249] Liposomes become leaky at a gel-to-liquid crystalline phase transition, and this transition for DPPC takes place at 41 °C.[250] Liposomes can also be made temperature sensitive via the incorporation of certain grafted polymers (e.g., poly-(N-isopropylacrylamide), or NIPAM) that display a lower critical solution temperature (LCST) that is slightly above the typical physiological body temperature.[249] Such polymers precipitate at temperatures above a LCST and solubilize below an LCST because they exhibit an LCST above the normal tissue. Thus, the liposome membrane breaks down during the thermal-induced precipitation and leads to the release of its cargo.[251]

CONCLUSION

Developing innovative delivery strategies for optimizing cancer therapeutics is an ongoing story. Although nanoparticle drug delivery systems have been in development for many years, many applications remain to be exploited. In this chapter, the various strategies used to improve the blood circulation half-lives of nanoparticles (mainly liposomes) are discussed, with a focus on PEG surface modification. These strategies could turn what was an impediment into a significant advantage for cancer therapy.

Despite the well-developed chemistry of PEG for use in drug delivery systems, the search for alternative polymers is ongoing. This may be explained both by current limitations of PEG and its derivatives and by hopes for achieving better control over the properties of modified drugs and drug carriers. Prolonged blood circulation and longer tissue retention are essential parts of drug delivery systems that can be used to improve the therapeutic effect, but careful consideration of the toxicity of the modified nanoparticles is required. Optimal clearance for reducing the duration of body exposure to these agents will minimize nonspecific toxicity but allow sufficient blood circulation for good tumor targeting. The transition from passive targeting via the EPR effect to selective targeting with a targeting moiety requires PEG or similar materials to promote circulation time and inhibit removal by the liver and spleen. Strategies to combine specific targeting with the long-circulation-based EPR effect for better clinical outcome remain a primary challenge in nanomedicine that is likely to be a future direction for current smart multifunctional nanocarrier systems with highly efficient and specialized delivery mechanisms for drugs, gene, and other diagnostic agents and therapeutics.

Acknowledgments

The authors would like to thank Dr. William Hartner (Center for Pharmaceutical Biotechnology and Nanomedicine, Northeastern University) for helpful advice on manuscript preparation.

References

1. Farokhzad OC, Langer R. Impact of nanotechnology on drug delivery. ACS Nano 2009;3(1):16–20.
2. Sinha R, Kim GJ, Nie S, Shin DM. Nanotechnology in cancer therapeutics: bioconjugated nanoparticles for drug delivery. Mol. Cancer Ther. 2006;5(8):1909–17.
3. Kirui DK, Khalidov I, Wang Y, Batt CA. Targeted near-IR hybrid magnetic nanoparticles for *in vivo* cancer therapy and imaging. Nanomedicine 2013;9(5):702–11.
4. Prados J, Melguizo C, Ortiz R, Perazzoli G, Cabeza L, Alvarez PJ, et al. Colon cancer therapy: recent developments in nanomedicine to improve the efficacy of conventional chemotherapeutic drugs. Anticancer Agents Med Chem. 2013;13(8):1204–16.
5. Kim TH, Lee S, Chen X. Nanotheranostics for personalized medicine. Expert Rev Mol Diagn. 2013;13(3):257–69.
6. Brigger I, Dubernet C, Couvreur P. Nanoparticles in cancer therapy and diagnosis. Adv. Drug Deliv. Rev. 2002;54(5):631–51.
7. Brown R, Links M. Clinical relevance of the molecular mechanisms of resistance to anti-cancer drugs. Expert Rev. Mol. Med. 1999;1(15):1–21.
8. Petros RA, DeSimone JM. Strategies in the design of nanoparticles for therapeutic applications. Nat. Rev. Drug Discov. 2010;9(8):615–27.
9. Sahoo SK, Labhasetwar V. Nanotech approaches to drug delivery and imaging. Drug Discov. Today 2003;8(24):1112–20.
10. Solaro R, Chiellini F, Battisti A. Targeted delivery of protein drugs by nanocarriers. Materials 2010;3(3):1928–80.
11. Torchilin V. Tumor delivery of macromolecular drugs based on the EPR effect. Adv. Drug Deliv. Rev. 2011;63(3):131–5.
12. Yuan F, Dellian M, Fukumura D, Leunig M, Berk DA, Torchilin VP, et al. Vascular permeability in a human tumor xenograft: molecular size dependence and cutoff size. Cancer Res. 1995;55(17):3752–6.
13. Hobbs SK, Monsky WL, Yuan F, Roberts WG, Griffith L, Torchilin VP, et al. Regulation of transport pathways in tumor vessels: role of tumor type and microenvironment. Proc. Natl. Acad. Sci. U.S.A. 1998;95(8):4607–12.
14. Maeda H, Wu J, Sawa T, Matsumura Y, Hori K. Tumor vascular permeability and the EPR effect in macromolecular therapeutics: a review. J. Control. Release. 2000;65(1–2):271–84.
15. Bhaskar S, Tian F, Stoeger T, Kreyling W, de la Fuente JM, Grazu V, et al. Multifunctional Nanocarriers for diagnostics, drug delivery and targeted treatment across blood–brain barrier: perspectives on tracking and neuroimaging. Particle Fibre Toxicol. 2010;7:3.
16. Liu C, Liu F, Feng L, Li M, Zhang J, Zhang N. The targeted co-delivery of DNA and doxorubicin to tumor cells via multifunctional PEI-PEG based nanoparticles. Biomaterials 2013;34(10):2547–64.
17. Wang T, Upponi JR, Torchilin VP. Design of multifunctional non-viral gene vectors to overcome physiological barriers: dilemmas and strategies. Int. J. Pharm. 2012;427(1):3–20.
18. Sawant RR, Torchilin VP. Multifunctional nanocarriers and intracellular drug delivery. Curr. Opin. Solid State Mater. Sci. 2012;16(6):269–75.

19. Koren E, Apte A, Jani A, Torchilin VP. Multifunctional PEGylated 2C5-immunoliposomes containing pH-sensitive bonds and TAT peptide for enhanced tumor cell internalization and cytotoxicity. J. Control. Release 2012;160(2):264–73.

20. Milane L, Ganesh S, Shah S, Duan Z-F, Amiji M. Multi-modal strategies for overcoming tumor drug resistance: hypoxia, the Warburg effect, stem cells, and multifunctional nanotechnology. J. Control. Release. 2011;155(2):237–47.

21. Guo M, Que C, Wang C, Liu X, Yan H, Liu K. Multifunctional superparamagnetic nanocarriers with folate-mediated and pH-responsive targeting properties for anticancer drug delivery. Biomaterials 2011;32(1):185–94.

22. Taratula O, Kuzmov A, Shah M, Garbuzenko OB, Minko T. Nanostructured lipid carriers as multifunctional nanomedicine platform for pulmonary co-delivery of anticancer drugs and siRNA. J. Control. Release. 2013;171(3):349–57.

23. Zhu L, Movassaghian S, Torchilin VP. Overcoming biological barriers with parenteral nanomedicines: physiological and mechanistic issues. In: Alonso MJ, Csaba NS, editors. Nanostructured Biomaterials for Overcoming Biological Barriers. London: Royal Society of Chemistry; 2012. p. 435–55.

24. Rabanel JM, Aoun V, Elkin I, Mokhtar M, Hildgen P. Drug-loaded nanocarriers: passive targeting and crossing of biological barriers. Curr. Med. Chem. 2012;19(19):3070–102.

25. van Vlerken LE, Amiji MM. Multi-functional polymeric nanoparticles for tumour-targeted drug delivery. Expert Opin. Drug Deliv. 2006;3(2):205–16.

26. Woodle MC. Sterically stabilized liposome therapeutics. Adv. Drug Deliv. Rev. 1995;16(2–3):249–65.

27. Torchilin VP, Trubetskoy VS. Which polymers can make nanoparticulate drug carriers long-circulating? Adv. Drug Deliv. Rev. 1995;16(2–3):141–55.

28. Ilium L, Davis SS, Wilson CG, Thomas NW, Frier M, Hardy JG. Blood clearance and organ deposition of intravenously administered colloidal particles. The effects of particle size, nature and shape. Int. J. Pharm. 1982;12(2–3):135–46.

29. Zolnik BS, González-Fernández Á, Sadrieh N, Dobrovolskaia MA. Minireview: nanoparticles and the immune system. Endocrinology 2010;151(2):458–65.

30. Markovsky E, Baabur-Cohen H, Eldar-Boock A, Omer L, Tiram G, Ferber S, et al. Administration, distribution, metabolism and elimination of polymer therapeutics. J. Control. Release 2012;161(2):446–60.

31. Moghimi SM, Hunter AC, Andresen TL. Factors controlling nanoparticle pharmacokinetics: an integrated analysis and perspective. Annu. Rev. Pharmacol. Toxicol. 2012;52:481–503.

32. Moghimi SM, Hunter AC, Murray JC. Long-circulating and target-specific nanoparticles: theory to practice. Pharmacol. Rev. 2001;53(2):283–318.

33. Vonarbourg A, Passirani C, Saulnier P, Benoit J-P. Parameters influencing the stealthiness of colloidal drug delivery systems. Biomaterials 2006;27(24):4356–73.

34. Aderem A, Underhill DM. Mechanisms of phagocytosis in macrophages. Annu. Rev. Immunol. 1999;17:593–623.

35. Moghimi SM, Hunter AC. Recognition by macrophages and liver cells of opsonized phospholipid vesicles and phospholipid headgroups. Pharm. Res. 2001;18(1):1–8.

36. Rao J. Shedding light on tumors using nanoparticles. ACS Nano. 2008;2(10):1984–6.

37. Albanese A, Tang PS, Chan WCW. The effect of nanoparticle size, shape, and surface chemistry on biological systems. Annu. Rev. Biomed. Eng. 2012;14(1):1–16.

38. Arvizo RR, Miranda OR, Thompson MA, Pabelick CM, Bhattacharya R, Robertson JD, et al. Effect of Nanoparticle Surface Charge at the Plasma Membrane and Beyond. Nano Lett. 2010;10(7):2543–8.

39. Lee H, Fonge H, Hoang B, Reilly RM, Allen C. The Effects of Particle Size and Molecular Targeting on the Intratumoral and Subcellular Distribution of Polymeric Nanoparticles. Mol. Pharm. 2010;7(4):1195–8.

40. Alexis F, Pridgen E, Molnar LK, Farokhzad OC. Factors affecting the clearance and biodistribution of polymeric nanoparticles. Mol. Pharm. 2008;5(4):505–15.

41. Yadav KS, Chuttani K, Mishra AK, Sawant KK. Effect of size on the biodistribution and blood clearance of etoposide-loaded PLGA nanoparticles. PDA J. Pharm. Sci. Technol. 2011;65(2):131–9.

42. Soo Choi H, Liu W, Misra P, Tanaka E, Zimmer JP, Itty Ipe B, et al. Renal clearance of quantum dots. Nat. Biotech. 2007;25(10):1165–70.

43. Yhee J, Koo H, Lee D, Choi K, Kwon I, Kim K. Multifunctional chitosan nanoparticles for tumor imaging and therapy. In: Jayakumar R, Prabaharan M, Muzzarelli RAA, editors. Chitosan for Biomaterials I. Berlin: Springer; 2011. p. 139–61.

44. Yoo JW, Chambers E, Mitragotri S. Factors that control the circulation time of nanoparticles in blood: challenges, solutions and future prospects. Curr. Pharm. Des. 2010;16(21):2298–307.

45. Owens DE III, Peppas NA. Opsonization, biodistribution, and pharmacokinetics of polymeric nanoparticles. Int. J. Pharm. 2006;307(1):93–102.

46. Swami A, Shi J, Gadde S, Votruba A, Kolishetti N, Farokhzad O. Nanoparticles for targeted and temporally controlled drug delivery. In: Svenson S, Prud'homme RK, editors. Multifunctional Nanoparticles for Drug Delivery Applications. New York: Springer; 2012. p. 2–29.

47. Moghimi SM, Porter CJH, Muir IS, Illum L, Davis SS. Non-phagocytic uptake of intravenously injected microspheres in rat spleen: influence of particle size and hydrophilic coating. Biochem. Biophys. Res. Commun. 1991;177(2):861–6.

48. Cogger VC, Le Couteur DG. Fenestrations in the liver sinusoidal endothelial cell. In: Arias I, Wolkoff A, Boyer J, Shafritz D, Fausto N, editors. The Liver: Biology and Pathology. 5th ed. New York: John Wiley & Sons; 2009. p. 387–404.

49. Bohrer MP, Baylis C, Humes HD, Glassock RJ, Robertson CR, Brenner BM. Permselectivity of the glomerular capillary wall. Facilitated filtration of circulating polycations. J. Clin. Invest. 1978;61(1):72–8.

50. Decuzzi P, Pasqualini R, Arap W, Ferrari M. Intravascular delivery of particulate systems: does geometry really matter? Pharm. Res. 2009;26(1):235–43.

51. Decuzzi P, Godin B, Tanaka T, Lee SY, Chiappini C, Liu X, et al. Size and shape effects in the biodistribution of intravascularly injected particles. J. Control. Release 2010;141(3):320–7.

52. Harris BJ, Dalhaimer P. Particle shape effects *in vitro* and *in vivo*. Front. Biosci. 2012;4:1344–53.

53. Tan J, Shah S, Thomas A, Ou-Yang HD, Liu Y. The influence of size, shape and vessel geometry on nanoparticle distribution. Microfluid. Nanofluidics. 2013;14(1–2):77–87.

54. Mitragotri S, Lahann J. Physical approaches to biomaterial design. Nat Mater. 2009;8(1):15–23.

55. Champion JA, Mitragotri S. Role of target geometry in phagocytosis. Proc. Natl. Acad. Sci. U.S.A. 2006;103(13):4930–4.

56. Champion JA, Mitragotri S. Shape induced inhibition of phagocytosis of polymer particles. Pharm. Res. 2009;26(1):244–9.

57. Doshi N, Mitragotri S. Macrophages recognize size and shape of their targets. PLoS ONE 2010;5(4):e10051.

58. Yan G, Paul D, Shenshen C, Richard T, Manorama T, Tamara M, et al. Shape effects of filaments versus spherical particles in flow and drug delivery. Nat. Nanotechnol. 2007;2(4):249–55.

59. Devarajan PV, Jindal AB, Patil RR, Mulla F, Gaikwad RV, Samad A. Particle shape: a new design parameter for passive targeting in splenotropic drug delivery. J. Pharm. Sci. 2010;99(6):2576–81.

60. Champion JA, Katare YK, Mitragotri S. Particle shape: a new design parameter for micro- and nanoscale drug delivery carriers. J. Control. Release. 2007;121(1–2):3–9.

61. Venkataraman S, Hedrick JL, Ong ZY, Yang C, Ee PLR, Hammond PT, et al. The effects of polymeric nanostructure shape on drug delivery. Adv. Drug Deliv. Rev. 2011;63(14–15):1228–46.

62. Roser M, Fischer D, Kissel T. Surface-modified biodegradable albumin nano- and microspheres. II. Effect of surface charges on in vitro phagocytosis and biodistribution in rats. Eur. J. Pharm. Biopharm. 1998;46(3):255–63.

63. Devine DV, Wong K, Serrano K, Chonn A, Cullis PR. Liposome—complement interactions in rat serum: implications for liposome survival studies. Biochim. Biophys. Acta. 1994;1191(1):43–51.

64. Carrstensen H, Muller RH, Muller BW. Particle size, surface hydrophobicity and interaction with serum of parenteral fat emulsions and model drug carriers as parameters related to RES uptake. Clin. Nutr. 1992;11(5):289–97.

65. Chen H, Langer R, Edwards DA. A film tension theory of phagocytosis. J. Colloid. Interface Sci. 1997;190(1):118–33.

66. Chonn A, Semple SC, Cullis PR. Association of blood proteins with large unilamellar liposomes *in vivo*. Relation to circulation lifetimes. J. Biol. Chem. 1992;267(26):18759–65.

67. Juliano RL, Stamp D. The effect of particle size and charge on the clearance rates of liposomes and liposome encapsulated drugs. Biochem. Biophys. Res. Commun. 1975;63(3):651–8.

68. Bradley AJ, Brooks DE, Norris-Jones R, Devine DV. C1q binding to liposomes is surface charge dependent and is inhibited by peptides consisting of residues 14-26 of the human C1qA chain in a sequence independent manner. Biochim. Biophys. Acta. 1999;1418(1):19–30.

69. Moghimi SM, Hunter C. Capture of stealth nanoparticles by the body's defences. Crit. Rev. Ther. Drug Carrier Syst. 2001;18(6):527–50.

70. Schneider GF, Subr V, Ulbrich K, Decher G. Multifunctional cytotoxic stealth nanoparticles. a model approach with potential for cancer therapy. Nano Lett. 2009;9(2):636–42.

71. Duan X, Li Y. Physicochemical characteristics of nanoparticles affect circulation, biodistribution, cellular internalization, and trafficking. Small 2013;9(9–10):1521–32.

72. Alexis F, Pridgen E, Molnar LK, Farokhzad OC. Factors affecting the clearance and biodistribution of polymeric nanoparticles. Mol. Pharm. 2008;5(4):505–15.

73. Peer D, Karp JM, Hong S, Farokhzad OC, Margalit R, Langer R. Nanocarriers as an emerging platform for cancer therapy. Nat. Nano. 2007;2(12):751–60.

74. Davis ME, Chen ZG, Shin DM. Nanoparticle therapeutics: an emerging treatment modality for cancer. Nat. Rev. Drug Discov. 2008;7(9):771–82.

75. Immordino ML, Dosio F, Cattel L. Stealth liposomes: review of the basic science, rationale, and clinical applications, existing and potential. Int. J. Nanomed. 2006;1(3):297–315.

76. Zhang L, Gu FX, Chan JM, Wang AZ, Langer RS, Farokhzad OC. Nanoparticles in medicine: therapeutic applications and developments. Clin. Pharmacol. Ther. 2008;83(5):761–9.

77. Davis FF, Abuchowski A, Van Es T. Enzyme–polyethylene glycol adducts: modified enzymes with unique properties. Enzyme Eng. 1978;4:169–73.

78. Greenwald RB. PEG drugs: an overview. J. Control. Release. 2001;74(1–3):159–71.

79. Pasut G, Veronese FM. Polymer–drug conjugation, recent achievements and general strategies. Prog. Polym. Sci. 2007;32(8–9):933–61.

80. Pasut G, Veronese FM. PEG conjugates in clinical development or use as anticancer agents: an overview. Adv. Drug Deliv. Rev. 2009;61(13):1177–88.

81. Ryan SM, Mantovani G, Wang X, Haddleton DM, Brayden DJ. Advances in PEGylation of important biotech molecules: delivery aspects. Expert Opin. Drug Deliv. 2008;5(4):371–83.

82. Kang JS, Deluca PP, Lee KC. Emerging PEGylated drugs. Expert Opin. Emerg. Drugs. 2009;14(2):363–80.

83. Jokerst JV, Lobovkina T, Zare RN, Gambhir SS. Nanoparticle PEGylation for imaging and therapy. Nanomedicine (Lond). 2011;6(4):715–28.

84. Lasic DD, Martin FJ, Gabizon A, Huang SK, Papahadjopoulos D. Sterically stabilized liposomes: a hypothesis on the molecular origin of the extended circulation times. Biochim. Biophys. Acta. 1991;1070(1):187–92.

85. Gabizon A, Papahadjopoulos D. The role of surface charge and hydrophilic groups on liposome clearance *in vivo*. Biochim. Biophys. Acta. 1992;10(1):94–100.

86. Needham D, McIntosh TJ, Lasic DD. Repulsive interactions and mechanical stability of polymer-grafted lipid membranes. Biochim. Biophys. Acta. 1992;8(1):40–8.

87. Gabizon A, Papahadjopoulos D. Liposome formulations with prolonged circulation time in blood and enhanced uptake by tumors. Proc. Natl. Acad. Sci. U.S.A. 1988;85(18):6949–53.

88. Moghimi SM, Muir IS, Illum L, Davis SS, Kolb-Bachofen V. Coating particles with a block co-polymer (poloxamine-908) suppresses opsonization but permits the activity of dysopsonins in the serum. Biochim. Biophys. Acta. 1993;1179(2):157–65.

89. Torchilin VP, Omelyanenko VG, Papisov MI, Bogdanov AA Jr, Trubetskoy VS, Herron JN, et al. Poly(ethylene glycol) on the liposome surface: on the mechanism of polymer-coated liposome longevity. Biochim. Biophys. Acta. 1994;12(1):11–20.

90. Gref R, Luck M, Quellec P, Marchand M, Dellacherie E, Harnisch S, et al. "Stealth" corona-core nanoparticles surface modified by polyethylene glycol (PEG): influences of the corona (PEG chain length and surface density) and of the core composition on phagocytic uptake and plasma protein adsorption. Colloids Surf. B Biointerfaces 2000;18(3–4):301–13.

91. Mosqueira VC, Legrand P, Morgat JL, Vert M, Mysiakine E, Gref R, et al. Biodistribution of long-circulating PEG-grafted nanocapsules in mice: effects of PEG chain length and density. Pharm. Res. 2001;18(10):1411–9.

92. Sadzuka Y, Nakade A, Hirama R, Miyagishima A, Nozawa Y, Hirota S, et al. Effects of mixed polyethyleneglycol modification on fixed aqueous layer thickness and antitumor activity of doxorubicin containing liposome. Int. J. Pharm. 2002;238(1–2):171–80.

93. Allen TM. The use of glycolipids and hydrophilic polymers in avoiding rapid uptake of liposomes by the mononuclear phagocyte system. Adv. Drug Deliv. Rev. 1994;13(3):285–309.

94. Moghimi SM, Hedeman H, Christy NM, Illum L, Davis SS. Enhanced hepatic clearance of intravenously administered sterically stabilized microspheres in zymosan-stimulated rats. J. Leukoc. Biol. 1993;54(6):513–7.

95. Tirosh O, Barenholz Y, Katzhendler J, Priev A. Hydration of polyethylene glycol-grafted liposomes. Biophys. J. 1998;74(3):1371–9.

96. Xu H, Deng YH, Chen DW. Recent advances in the study of cleavable PEG-lipid derivatives modifying liposomes [in Chinese]. Yao Xue Xue Bao. 2008;43(1):18–22.

97. Torchilin VP, Papisov MI. Why do polyethylene glycol-coated liposomes circulate so long? Molecular mechanism of liposome steric protection with polyethylene glycol: role of polymer chain flexibility. J. Liposome Res. 1994;4(1):725–39.

98. Baekmark TR, Pedersen S, Jorgensen K, Mouritsen OG. The effects of ethylene oxide containing lipopolymers and tri-block copolymers on lipid bilayers of dipalmitoylphosphatidylcholine. Biophys. J. 1997;73(3):1479–91.

99. Leroux JC, De Jaeghere F, Anner B, Doelker E, Gurny R. An investigation on the role of plasma and serum opsonins on the internalization of biodegradable poly(D,L-lactic acid) nanoparticles by human monocytes. Life Sci. 1995;57(7):695–703.

100. Salmaso S, Caliceti P. Stealth properties to improve therapeutic efficacy of drug nanocarriers. J. Drug Deliv. 2013;2013:19.

101. Li SD, Huang L. Stealth nanoparticles: high density but sheddable PEG is a key for tumor targeting. J. Control. Release. 2010;145(3):178–81.

102. Sheng Y, Yuan Y, Liu C, Tao X, Shan X, Xu F. *In vitro* macrophage uptake and *in vivo* biodistribution of PLA–PEG nanoparticles loaded with hemoglobin as blood substitutes: effect of PEG content. J. Mater. Sci. Mater. Med. 2009;20(9):1881–91.

103. Gref R, Minamitake Y, Peracchia M, Trubetskoy V, Torchilin V, Langer R. Biodegradable long-circulating polymeric nanospheres. Science 1994;263(5153):1600–3.

104. Beletsi A, Panagi Z, Avgoustakis K. Biodistribution properties of nanoparticles based on mixtures of PLGA with PLGA–PEG diblock copolymers. Int. J. Pharm. 2005;298(1):233–41.

105. Vittaz M, Bazile D, Spenlehauer G, Verrecchia T, Veillard M, Puisieux F, et al. Effect of PEO surface density on long-circulating PLA–PEO nanoparticles which are very low complement activators. Biomaterials. 1996;17(16):1575–81.

106. Stolnik S, Illum L, Davis SS. Long circulating microparticulate drug carriers. Adv. Drug Deliv. Rev. 1995;16(2–3):195–214.

107. Woodle MC. Controlling liposome blood clearance by surface-grafted polymers. Adv. Drug Deliv. Rev. 1998;32(1–2):139–52.

108. Klibanov AL, Maruyama K, Torchilin VP, Huang L. Amphipathic polyethyleneglycols effectively prolong the circulation time of liposomes. FEBS Lett. 1990;268(1):235–7.

109. Allen TM, Hansen C, Martin F, Redemann C, Yau-Young A. Liposomes containing synthetic lipid derivatives of poly(ethylene glycol) show prolonged circulation half-lives *in vivo*. Biochim. Biophys. Acta. 1991;1(1):29–36.

110. Romberg B, Hennink W, Storm G. Sheddable coatings for long-circulating nanoparticles. Pharm. Res. 2008;25(1):55–71.

111. Mishra S, Webster P, Davis ME. PEGylation significantly affects cellular uptake and intracellular trafficking of non-viral gene delivery particles. Eur. J. Cell Biol. 2004;83(3):97–111.

112. Ishida T, Wang X, Shimizu T, Nawata K, Kiwada H. PEGylated liposomes elicit an anti-PEG IgM response in a T cell-independent manner. J. Control. Release. 2007;122(3):349–55.

113. Khalil IA, Kogure K, Akita H, Harashima H. Uptake pathways and subsequent intracellular trafficking in non-viral gene delivery. Pharmacol. Rev. 2006;58(1):32–45.

114. Masuda T, Akita H, Niikura K, Nishio T, Ukawa M, Enoto K, et al. Envelope-type lipid nanoparticles incorporating a short PEG-lipid conjugate for improved control of intracellular trafficking and transgene transcription. Biomaterials 2009;30(27):4806–14.

115. Hong RL, Huang CJ, Tseng YL, Pang VF, Chen ST, Liu JJ, et al. Direct comparison of liposomal doxorubicin with or without polyethylene glycol coating in C-26 tumor-bearing mice: is surface coating with polyethylene glycol beneficial? Clin. Cancer Res. 1999;5(11):3645–52.

116. Moghimi SM, Szebeni J. Stealth liposomes and long circulating nanoparticles: critical issues in pharmacokinetics, opsonization and protein-binding properties. Prog. Lipid Res. 2003;42(6):463–78.

117. Laverman P, Boerman OC, Oyen WJG, Corstens FHM, Storm G. *In vivo* applications of PEG liposomes: unexpected observations. Crit. Rev. Ther. Drug Carrier Syst. 2001;18(6):551–66.

118. Laverman P, Brouwers AH, Dams ET, Oyen WJ, Storm G, van Rooijen N, et al. Preclinical and clinical evidence for disappearance of long-circulating characteristics of polyethylene glycol liposomes at low lipid dose. J. Pharmacol. Exp. Ther. 2000;293(3):996–1001.

119. Ishida T, Harada M, Wang XY, Ichihara M, Irimura K, Kiwada H. Accelerated blood clearance of PEGylated liposomes following preceding liposome injection: effects of lipid dose and PEG surface-density and chain length of the first-dose liposomes. J. Control. Release. 2005;105(3):305–17.

120. Ishida T, Kiwada H. Accelerated blood clearance (ABC) phenomenon upon repeated injection of PEGylated liposomes. Int. J. Pharm. 2008;354(1–2):56–62.

121. Zhao Y, Wang C, Wang L, Yang Q, Tang W, She Z, et al. A frustrating problem: accelerated blood clearance of PEGylated solid lipid nanoparticles following subcutaneous injection in rats. Eur. J. Pharm. Biopharm. 2012;81(3):506–13.

122. Armstrong JK, Hempel G, Koling S, Chan LS, Fisher T, Meiselman HJ, et al. Antibody against poly(ethylene glycol) adversely affects PEG-asparaginase therapy in acute lymphoblastic leukemia patients. Cancer 2007;110(1):103–11.

123. Jain D, Athawale R, Bajaj A, Shrikhande S, Goel PN, Gude RP. Studies on stabilization mechanism and stealth effect of poloxamer 188 onto PLGA nanoparticles. Colloids Surf. B Biointerfaces 2013;109:59–67.

124. Norman ME, Williams P, Illum L. Influence of block copolymers on the adsorption of plasma proteins to microspheres. Biomaterials 1993;14(3):193–202.

125. Gulyaev A, Gelperina S, Skidan I, Antropov A, Kivman G, Kreuter J. Significant transport of doxorubicin into the brain with polysorbate 80-coated nanoparticles. Pharm. Res. 1999;16(10):1564–9.

126. Fan L, Li F, Zhang H, Wang Y, Cheng C, Li X, et al. Co-delivery of PDTC and doxorubicin by multifunctional micellar nanoparticles to achieve active targeted drug delivery and overcome multidrug resistance. Biomaterials 2010;31(21):5634–42.

127. Pain D, Das PK, Ghosh P, Bachhawat BK. Increased circulatory half-life of liposomes after conjunction with dextran. J. Biosci. 1984;6(6):811–6.

128. Li YL, Zhu L, Liu Z, Cheng R, Meng F, Cui JH, et al. Reversibly stabilized multifunctional dextran nanoparticles efficiently deliver doxorubicin into the nuclei of cancer cells. Angew. Chem. Int. Ed. Engl. 2009;48(52): 9914–8.

129. Choi KY, Chung H, Min KH, Yoon HY, Kim K, Park JH, et al. Self-assembled hyaluronic acid nanoparticles for active tumor targeting. Biomaterials 2010;31(1):106–14.

130. Wang Y, Xin D, Hu J, Liu K, Pan J, Xiang J. A model ternary heparin conjugate by direct covalent bond strategy applied to drug delivery system. Bioorg. Med. Chem. Lett. 2009;19(1):149–52.

131. Torchilin VP, Levchenko TS, Whiteman KR, Yaroslavov AA, Tsatsakis AM, Rizos AK, et al. Amphiphilic poly-N-vinylpyrrolidones: synthesis, properties and liposome surface modification. Biomaterials 2001;22(22): 3035–44.

132. Torchilin VP, Shtilman MI, Trubetskoy VS, Whiteman K, Milstein AM. Amphiphilic vinyl polymers effectively prolong liposome circulation time in vivo. Biochim. Biophys. Acta. 1994;12(1):181–4.

133. Sartore L, Ranucci E, Ferruti P, Caliceti P, Schiavon O, Veronese FM. Low molecular weight end-functionalized poly(N-vinylpyrrolidinone) for the modification of polypeptide aminogroups. J. Bioact. Comp. Polym. 1994;9(4):411–28.

134. Vermette P, Meagher L. Interactions of phospholipid- and poly(ethylene glycol)-modified surfaces with biological systems: relation to physico-chemical properties and mechanisms. Colloids Surf. B Biointerfaces 2003;28(2–3):153–98.

135. Massenburg D, Lentz BR. Poly(ethylene glycol)-induced fusion and rupture of dipalmitoylphosphatidylcholine large, unilamellar extruded vesicles. Biochemistry 1993;32(35):9172–80.

136. Saez R, Alonso A, Villena A, Goni FM. Detergent-like properties of polyethyleneglycols in relation to model membranes. FEBS Lett. 1982;137(2):323–6.

137. He Y, Hower J, Chen S, Bernards MT, Chang Y, Jiang S. Molecular simulation studies of protein interactions with zwitterionic phosphorylcholine self-assembled monolayers in the presence of water. Langmuir 2008;24(18):10358–64.

138. Cao Z, Zhang L, Jiang S. Superhydrophilic zwitterionic polymers stabilize liposomes. Langmuir 2012;28(31):11625–32.

139. Yang W, Zhang L, Wang S, White AD, Jiang S. Functionalizable and ultra stable nanoparticles coated with zwitterionic poly(carboxybetaine) in undiluted blood serum. Biomaterials 2009;30(29):5617–21.

140. Ladd J, Zhang Z, Chen S, Hower JC, Jiang S. Zwitterionic polymers exhibiting high resistance to nonspecific protein adsorption from human serum and plasma. Biomacromolecules 2008;9(5):1357–61.

141. Cheon Lee S, Kim C, Chan Kwon I, Chung H, Young Jeong S. Polymeric micelles of poly(2–ethyl-2-oxazoline)-block-poly(epsilon-caprolactone) copolymer as a carrier for paclitaxel. J. Control. Release. 2003;89(3):437–46.

IV. NOVEL APPROACHES FOR CANCER THERAPIES

142. Wang CH, Wang WT, Hsiue GH. Development of polyion complex micelles for encapsulating and delivering amphotericin B. Biomaterials 2009;30(19):3352–8.
143. Zalipsky S, Hansen CB, Oaks JM, Allen TM. Evaluation of blood clearance rates and biodistribution of poly(2-oxazoline)-grafted liposomes. J. Pharm. Sci. 1996;85(2):133–7.
144. Romberg B, Metselaar JM, Baranyi L, Snel CJ, Bunger R, Hennink WE, et al. Poly(amino acid)s: promising enzymatically degradable stealth coatings for liposomes. Int. J. Pharm. 2007;331(2):186–9.
145. Romberg B, Oussoren C, Snel CJ, Carstens MG, Hennink WE, Storm G. Pharmacokinetics of poly(hydroxyethyl-l-asparagine)-coated liposomes is superior over that of PEG-coated liposomes at low lipid dose and upon repeated administration. Biochim. Biophys. Acta. 2007;3:737–43.
146. Maruyama K, Okuizumi S, Ishida O, Yamauchi H, Kikuchi H, Iwatsuru M. Phosphatidyl polyglycerols prolong liposome circulation *in vivo*. Int. J. Pharm. 1994;111(1):103–7.
147. Siegers C, Biesalski M, Haag R. Self-assembled monolayers of dendritic polyglycerol derivatives on gold that resist the adsorption of proteins. Chemistry 2004;10(11):2831–8.
148. Banerjee I, Pangule RC, Kane RS. Antifouling coatings: recent developments in the design of surfaces that prevent fouling by proteins, bacteria, and marine organisms. Adv. Mater. 2011;23(6):690–718.
149. Wyszogrodzka M, Haag R. Synthesis and characterization of glycerol dendrons, self-assembled monolayers on gold: a detailed study of their protein resistance. Biomacromolecules 2009;10(5):1043–54.
150. Frey H, Haag R. Dendritic polyglycerol: a new versatile biocompatible-material. J. Biotechnol. 2002;90(3–4): 257–67.
151. Calderon M, Quadir MA, Sharma SK, Haag R. Dendritic polyglycerols for biomedical applications. Adv. Mater. 2010;22(2):190–218.
152. Felder KM, Hoelzle K, Ritzmann M, Kilchling T, Schiele D, Heinritzi K, et al. Hemotrophic mycoplasmas induce programmed cell death in red blood cells. Cell. Physiol. Biochem. 2011;27(5):557–64.
153. Magnani M, Rossi L, Fraternale A, Bianchi M, Antonelli A, Crinelli R, et al. Erythrocyte-mediated delivery of drugs, peptides and modified oligonucleotides. Gene Ther. 2002;9(11):749–51.
154. Magnani M, Pierigè F, Rossi L. Erythrocytes as a novel delivery vehicle for biologics: from enzymes to nucleic acid-based therapeutics. Ther. Deliv. 2012;3(3):405–14.
155. Doshi N, Zahr AS, Bhaskar S, Lahann J, Mitragotri S. Red blood cell-mimicking synthetic biomaterial particles. Proc. Natl. Acad. Sci. U.S.A. 2009;106(51):21495–9.
156. Muzykantov VR, Sakharov DV, Smirnov MD, Samokhin GP, Smirnov VN. Immunotargeting of erythrocyte-bound streptokinase provides local lysis of a fibrin clot. Biochim. Biophys. Acta. 1986;884(2):355–62.
157. Dale GL, Kuhl W, Beutler E. Incorporation of glucocerebrosidase into Gaucher's disease monocytes *in vitro*. Proc. Natl. Acad. Sci. U.S.A. 1979;76(1):473–5.
158. Desilets J, Lejeune A, Mercer J, Gicquaud C. Nanoerythrosomes, a new derivative of erythrocyte ghost. IV. Fate of reinjected nanoerythrosomes. Anticancer Res. 2001;21(3B):1741–7.
159. Merkel TJ, Jones SW, Herlihy KP, Kersey FR, Shields AR, Napier M, et al. Using mechanobiological mimicry of red blood cells to extend circulation times of hydrogel microparticles. Proc. Natl. Acad. Sci. U.S.A. 2011;108(2):586–91.
160. Fan W, Yan W, Xu Z, Ni H. Erythrocytes load of low molecular weight chitosan nanoparticles as a potential vascular drug delivery system. Colloids Surf. B Biointerfaces 2012;95:258–65.
161. Chambers E, Mitragotri S. Long circulating nanoparticles via adhesion on red blood cells: mechanism and extended circulation. Exp. Biol. Med. 2007;232(7):958–66.
162. Bradley AJ, Murad KL, Regan KL, Scott MD. Biophysical consequences of linker chemistry and polymer size on stealth erythrocytes: size does matter. Biochim. Biophys. Acta. 2002;1561(2):147–58.
163. Hu CM, Zhang L, Aryal S, Cheung C, Fang RH. Erythrocyte membrane-camouflaged polymeric nanoparticles as a biomimetic delivery platform. Proc. Natl. Acad. Sci. U.S.A. 2011;108(27):10980–5.
164. Hamidi M, Zarrin A, Foroozesh M, Mohammadi-Samani S. Applications of carrier erythrocytes in delivery of biopharmaceuticals. J. Control. Release 2007;118(2):145–60.
165. Hamidi M, Tajerzadeh H. Carrier erythrocytes: an overview. Drug Deliv. 2003;10(1):9–20.
166. Muzykantov VR. Drug delivery by red blood cells: vascular carriers designed by mother nature. Expert Opin. Drug Deliv. 2010;7(4):403–27.
167. Clark MR, Shohet SB. Red cell senescence. Clin. Haematol. 1985;14(1):223–57.
168. Kazatchkine MD, Fearon DT, Austen KF. Human alternative complement pathway: membrane-associated sialic acid regulates the competition between B and β1H for cell-bound C3b. J. Immunol. 1979;122(1):75–81.

169. C eh B, Winterhalter M, Frederik PM, Vallner JJ, Lasic DD. Stealth® liposomes: from theory to product. Adv. Drug Deliv. Rev. 1997;24(2–3):165–77.
170. Surolia A, Bachhawat BK. Monosialoganglioside liposome-entrapped enzyme uptake by hepatic cells. Biochim. Biophys. Acta. 1977;497(3):760–5.
171. Yamauchi H, Kikuchi H, Yachi K, Sawada M, Tomikawa M, Hirota S. Effects of glycophorin and ganglioside GM3 on the blood circulation and tissue distribution of liposomes in rats. Int. J. Pharm. 1993;90(1):73–9.
172. Allen TM, Hansen C, Rutledge J. Liposomes with prolonged circulation times: factors affecting uptake by reticuloendothelial and other tissues. Biochim. Biophys. Acta. 1989;981(1):27–35.
173. Leonhard V, Alasino RV, Bianco ID, Garro AG, Heredia V, Beltramo DM. Self-assembled micelles of monosialo-gangliosides as nanodelivery vehicles for taxanes. J. Control. Release. 2012;162(3):619–27.
174. Liu D, Mori A, Huang L. Role of liposome size and RES blockade in controlling biodistribution and tumor uptake of GM1–containing liposomes. Biochim. Biophys. Acta. 1992;17(1):95–101.
175. Yamauchi H, Yano T, Kato T, Tanaka I, Nakabayashi S, Higashi K, et al. Effects of sialic acid derivative on long circulation time and tumor concentration of liposomes. Int. J. Pharm. 1995;113(2):141–8.
176. Oldenborg PA. Role of CD47 in erythroid cells and in autoimmunity. Leuk. Lymphoma 2004;45(7):1319–27.
177. Hu C-MJ, Fang RH, Luk BT, Chen KNH, Carpenter C, Gao W, et al. "Marker-of-self" functionalization of nanoscale particles through a top-down cellular membrane coating approach. Nanoscale 2013;5(7):2664–8.
178. Parkinson JE, Sanderson CM, Smith GL. The vaccinia virus A38L gene product is a 33-kDa integral membrane glycoprotein. Virology 1995;214(1):177–88.
179. Fang RH, Hu C-MJ, Chen KNH, Luk BT, Carpenter CW, Gao W, et al. Lipid-insertion enables targeting functionalization of erythrocyte membrane-cloaked nanoparticles. Nanoscale 2013;5(19):8884–8.
180. Hsu Y-C, Acuña M, Tahara S, Peng C-A. Reduced phagocytosis of colloidal carriers using soluble CD47. Pharm. Res. 2003;20(10):1539–42.
181. Zhang Y, Hong H, Cai W. Tumor-targeted drug delivery with aptamers. Curr. Med. Chem. 2011;18(27):4185–94.
182. Yu MK, Park J, Jon S. Targeting strategies for multifunctional nanoparticles in cancer imaging and therapy. Theranostics 2012;2(1):3–44.
183. Zhou L, Liang D, He X, Li J, Tan H, Li J, et al. The degradation and biocompatibility of pH-sensitive biodegrad-able polyurethanes for intracellular multifunctional antitumor drug delivery. Biomaterials 2012;33(9):2734–45.
184. Shen M, Huang Y, Han L, Qin J, Fang X, Wang J, et al. Multifunctional drug delivery system for targeting tumor and its acidic microenvironment. J. Control. Release 2012;161(3):884–92.
185. Torchilin V. Multifunctional and stimuli-sensitive pharmaceutical nanocarriers. Eur. J. Pharm. Biopharm. 2009;71(3):431–44.
186. Wu Q, Du F, Luo Y, Lu W, Huang J, Yu J, et al. Poly(ethylene glycol) shell-sheddable nanomicelle prodrug of camptothecin with enhanced cellular uptake. Colloids Surf. B Biointerfaces 2013;105(0):294–302.
187. van der Meel R, Vehmeijer LJC, Kok RJ, Storm G, van Gaal EVB. Ligand-targeted particulate nanomedicines undergoing clinical evaluation: current status. Adv. Drug Deliv. Rev. 2013;65(10):1284–98.
188. Khaw BA, Klibanov A, O'Donnell SM, Saito T, Nossiff N, Slinkin MA, et al. Gamma imaging with negatively charge-modified monoclonal antibody: modification with synthetic polymers. J. Nucl. Med. 1991;32(9):1742–51.
189. Torchilin VP, Klibanov AL, Huang L, O'Donnell S, Nossiff ND, Khaw BA. Targeted accumulation of polyethyl-ene glycol-coated immunoliposomes in infarcted rabbit myocardium. FASEB J. 1992;6(9):2716–9.
190. Sawant RR, Torchilin VP. Design and synthesis of novel functional lipid-based bioconjugates for drug delivery and other applications. Methods Mol. Biol. 2011;751:357–78.
191. Torchilin VP, Levchenko TS, Lukyanov AN, Khaw BA, Klibanov AL, Rammohan R, et al. p-Nitrophenylcarbonyl-PEG-PE-liposomes: fast and simple attachment of specific ligands, including monoclonal antibodies, to distal ends of PEG chains via p-nitrophenylcarbonyl groups. Biochim. Biophys. Acta. 2001;2(2):397–411.
192. Blume G, Cevc G, Crommelin MD, Bakker-Woudenberg IA, Kluft C, Storm G. Specific targeting with poly(ethylene glycol)-modified liposomes: coupling of homing devices to the ends of the polymeric chains combines effective target binding with long circulation times. Biochim. Biophys. Acta. 1993;18(1):180–4.
193. Harding JA, Engbers CM, Newman MS, Goldstein NI, Zalipsky S. Immunogenicity and pharmacokinetic attributes of poly(ethylene glycol)-grafted immunoliposomes. Biochim. Biophys. Acta. 1997;25(2):181–92.
194. Allen TM, Brandeis E, Hansen CB, Kao GY, Zalipsky S. A new strategy for attachment of antibodies to steri-cally stabilized liposomes resulting in efficient targeting to cancer cells. Biochim. Biophys. Acta. 1995;26(2):99–108.

195. Lukyanov AN, Elbayoumi TA, Chakilam AR, Torchilin VP. Tumor-targeted liposomes: doxorubicin-loaded long-circulating liposomes modified with anti-cancer antibody. J. Control. Release 2004;100(1):135–44.

196. Raffaghello L, Pagnan G, Pastorino F, Cosimo E, Brignole C, Marimpietri D, et al. Immunoliposomal fenretinide: a novel antitumoral drug for human neuroblastoma. Cancer Lett. 2003;197(1–2):151–5.

197. Nakase I, Kobayashi S, Futaki S. Endosome-disruptive peptides for improving cytosolic delivery of bioactive macromolecules. Biopolymers 2010;94(6):763–70.

198. Xie J, Ma C, Lin J, Wang G, Kuang A, Zuo S. An anionic long-circulating liposome that improves radioiodinated antisense oligonucleotide delivery *in vitro* and *in vivo*. Adv. Polymer Technol. 2012;31(1):20–8.

199. Fattal E, Couvreur P, Dubernet C. "Smart" delivery of antisense oligonucleotides by anionic pH-sensitive liposomes. Adv. Drug Deliv. Rev. 2004;56(7):931–46.

200. Holland JW, Hui C, Cullis PR, Madden TD. Poly(ethylene glycol)–lipid conjugates regulate the calcium-induced fusion of liposomes composed of phosphatidylethanolamine and phosphatidylserine. Biochemistry 1996;35(8):2618–24.

201. Dharap SS, Wang Y, Chandna P, Khandare JJ, Qiu B, Gunaseelan S, et al. Tumor-specific targeting of an anticancer drug delivery system by LHRH peptide. Proc. Natl. Acad. Sci. U.S.A. 2005;102(36):12962–7.

202. Nishikawa K, Asai T, Shigematsu H, Shimizu K, Kato H, Asano Y, et al. Development of anti-HB-EGF immunoliposomes for the treatment of breast cancer. J. Control. Release 2012;160(2):274–80.

203. Sapra P, Shor B. Monoclonal antibody-based therapies in cancer: advances and challenges. Pharmacol. Ther. 2013;138(3):452–69.

204. Lu Y, Low PS. Folate-mediated delivery of macromolecular anticancer therapeutic agents. Adv. Drug Deliv. Rev. 2002;54(5):675–93.

205. Pan XQ, Lee RJ. *In vivo* antitumor activity of folate receptor-targeted liposomal daunorubicin in a murine leukemia model. Anticancer Res. 2005;25(1A):343–6.

206. Xiong S, Yu B, Wu J, Li H, Lee RJ. Preparation, therapeutic efficacy and intratumoral localization of targeted daunorubicin liposomes conjugating folate-PEG-CHEMS. Biomed. Pharmacother 2011;65(1):2–8.

207. Riviere K, Huang Z, Jerger K, Macaraeg N, Szoka FC Jr. Antitumor effect of folate-targeted liposomal doxorubicin in KB tumor-bearing mice after intravenous administration. J. Drug Target 2011;19(1):14–24.

208. Koopaei MN, Dinarvand R, Amini M, Rabbani H, Emami S, Ostad SN, et al. Docetaxel immunonanocarriers as targeted delivery systems for HER 2-positive tumor cells: preparation, characterization, and cytotoxicity studies. Int. J. Nanomed. 2011;6:1903–12.

209. He Y, Zhang L, Song C. PEGylated liposomes modified with LHRH analogs for tumor targeting. J. Control. Release 2011;152(Suppl. 1):e29–31.

210. Geisert EE Jr, Del Mar NA, Owens JL, Holmberg EG. Transfecting neurons and glia in the rat using pH-sensitive immunoliposomes. Neurosci. Lett. 1995;184(1):40–3.

211. Bae Y, Nishiyama N, Fukushima S, Koyama H, Yasuhiro M, Kataoka K. Preparation and biological characterization of polymeric micelle drug carriers with intracellular pH-triggered drug release property: tumor permeability, controlled subcellular drug distribution, and enhanced *in vivo* antitumor efficacy. Bioconjug. Chem. 2004;16(1):122–30.

212. Tannock IF, Rotin D. Acid pH in tumors and its potential for therapeutic exploitation. Cancer Res. 1989;49(16):4373–84.

213. Ta T, Porter TM. Thermosensitive liposomes for localized delivery and triggered release of chemotherapy. J. Control. Release. 2013;169(1–2):112–25.

214. Zhu L, Huo Z, Wang L, Tong X, Xiao Y, Ni K. Targeted delivery of methotrexate to skeletal muscular tissue by thermosensitive magnetoliposomes. Int. J. Pharm. 2009;370(1–2):136–43.

215. Evjen TJ, Hagtvet E, Moussatov A, Røgnvaldsson S, Mestas J-L, Fowler RA, et al. *In vivo* monitoring of liposomal release in tumours following ultrasound stimulation. Eur. J. Pharm. Biopharm. 2013;84(3):526–31.

216. Lee ES, Na K, Bae YH. Doxorubicin loaded pH-sensitive polymeric micelles for reversal of resistant MCF-7 tumor. J. Control. Release 2005;103(2):405–18.

217. Toncheva V, Schacht E, Ng SY, Barr J, Heller J. Use of block copolymers of poly(ortho esters) and poly (ethylene glycol) micellar carriers as potential tumour targeting systems. J. Drug Target 2003;11(6):345–53.

218. Kim HK, Van den Bossche J, Hyun SH, Thompson DH. Acid-triggered release via dePEGylation of fusogenic liposomes mediated by heterobifunctional phenyl-substituted vinyl ethers with tunable pH-sensitivity. Bioconjug. Chem. 2012;23(10):2071–7.

219. Liu C, Liu F, Feng L, Li M, Zhang J, Zhang N. The targeted co-delivery of DNA and doxorubicin to tumor cells via multifunctional PEI-PEG based nanoparticles. Biomaterials 2013;34(10):2547–64.

220. Heffernan MJ, Murthy N. Polyketal nanoparticles: a new pH-sensitive biodegradable drug delivery vehicle. Bioconjug. Chem. 2005;16(6):1340–2.

221. Oishi M, Nagasaki Y, Itaka K, Nishiyama N, Kataoka K. Lactosylated poly(ethylene glycol)-siRNA conjugate through acid-labile beta-thiopropionate linkage to construct pH-sensitive polyion complex micelles achieving enhanced gene silencing in hepatoma cells. J. Am. Chem. Soc. 2005;127(6):1624–5.

222. Sethuraman VA, Bae YH. TAT peptide-based micelle system for potential active targeting of anti-cancer agents to acidic solid tumors. J. Control. Release 2007;118(2):216–24.

223. Yuan YY, Mao CQ, Du XJ, Du JZ, Wang F, Wang J. Surface charge switchable nanoparticles based on zwitterionic polymer for enhanced drug delivery to tumor. Adv. Mater. 2012;24(40):5476–80.

224. Biswas S, Dodwadkar NS, Sawant RR, Torchilin VP. Development of the novel PEG-PE-based polymer for the reversible attachment of specific ligands to liposomes: synthesis and *in vitro* characterization. Bioconjug. Chem. 2011;22(10):2005–13.

225. Sawant RM, Hurley JP, Salmaso S, Kale A, Tolcheva E, Levchenko TS, et al. "SMART" drug delivery systems: double-targeted pH-responsive pharmaceutical nanocarriers. Bioconjug. Chem. 2006;17(4):943–9.

226. Chen W, Meng F, Cheng R, Zhong Z. pH-Sensitive degradable polymersomes for triggered release of anticancer drugs: a comparative study with micelles. J. Control. Release 2010;142(1):40–6.

227. Guo X, Szoka FC Jr. Steric stabilization of fusogenic liposomes by a low-pH sensitive PEG–diortho ester–lipid conjugate. Bioconjug. Chem. 2001;12(2):291–300.

228. Li W, Huang Z, MacKay JA, Grube S, Szoka FC Jr. Low-pH-sensitive poly(ethylene glycol) (PEG)-stabilized plasmid nanolipoparticles: effects of PEG chain length, lipid composition and assembly conditions on gene delivery. J. Gene Med. 2005;7(1):67–79.

229. Kim D, Gao ZG, Lee ES, Bae YH. *In vivo* evaluation of doxorubicin-loaded polymeric micelles targeting folate receptors and early endosomal pH in drug-resistant ovarian cancer. Mol. Pharm. 2009;6(5):1353–62.

230. Lee ES, Shin HJ, Na K, Bae YH. Poly(L-histidine)–PEG block copolymer micelles and pH-induced destabilization. J. Control. Release 2003;90(3):363–74.

231. Oishi M, Kataoka K, Nagasaki Y. pH-responsive three-layered PEGylated polyplex micelle based on a lactosylated ABC triblock copolymer as a targetable and endosome-disruptive nonviral gene vector. Bioconjug. Chem. 2006;17(3):677–88.

232. Chan C-L, Majzoub RN, Shirazi RS, Ewert KK, Chen Y-J, Liang KS, et al. Endosomal escape and transfection efficiency of PEGylated cationic liposome–DNA complexes prepared with an acid-labile PEG-lipid. Biomaterials 2012;33(19):4928–35.

233. Gialeli C, Theocharis AD, Karamanos NK. Roles of matrix metalloproteinases in cancer progression and their pharmacological targeting. FEBS J. 2011;278(1):16–27.

234. Zhu L, Kate P, Torchilin VP. Matrix metalloprotease 2-responsive multifunctional liposomal nanocarrier for enhanced tumor targeting. ACS Nano. 2012;6(4):3491–8.

235. Hattori Y, Kawakami S, Yamashita F, Hashida M. Controlled biodistribution of galactosylated liposomes and incorporated probucol in hepatocyte-selective drug targeting. J. Control. Release 2000;69(3):369–77.

236. Terada T, Iwai M, Kawakami S, Yamashita F, Hashida M. Novel PEG-matrix metalloproteinase-2 cleavable peptide-lipid containing galactosylated liposomes for hepatocellular carcinoma-selective targeting. J. Control. Release 2006;111(3):333–42.

237. Managit C, Kawakami S, Nishikawa M, Yamashita F, Hashida M. Targeted and sustained drug delivery using PEGylated galactosylated liposomes. Int. J. Pharm. 2003;266(1–2):77–84.

238. Li J, Ge Z, Liu S. PEG-sheddable polyplex micelles as smart gene carriers based on MMP-cleavable peptide-linked block copolymers. Chem. Commun. 2013;49(62):6974–6.

239. Schafer FQ, Buettner GR. Redox environment of the cell as viewed through the redox state of the glutathione disulfide/glutathione couple. Free Radic. Biol. Med. 2001;30(11):1191–212.

240. Carlisle RC, Etrych T, Briggs SS, Preece JA, Ulbrich K, Seymour LW. Polymer-coated polyethylenimine/DNA complexes designed for triggered activation by intracellular reduction. J. Gene Med. 2004;6(3):337–44.

241. Sun H, Guo B, Cheng R, Meng F, Liu H, Zhong Z. Biodegradable micelles with sheddable poly(ethylene glycol) shells for triggered intracellular release of doxorubicin. Biomaterials 2009;30(31):6358–66.

242. Sun Y, Huang Y, Bian S, Liang J, Fan Y, Zhang X. Reduction-degradable PEG-b–PAA-b–PEG triblock copolymer micelles incorporated with MTX for cancer chemotherapy. Colloids Surf. B Biointerfaces 2013;112(0):197–203.

243. Fleige E, Quadir MA, Haag R. Stimuli-responsive polymeric nanocarriers for the controlled transport of active compounds: concepts and applications. Adv. Drug Deliv. Rev. 2012;64(9):866–84.

244. Ren T-B, Xia W-J, Dong H-Q, Li Y-Y. Sheddable micelles based on disulfide-linked hybrid PEG-polypeptide copolymer for intracellular drug delivery. Polymer 2011;52(16):3580–6.

245. Ren T-B, Feng Y, Zhang Z-H, Li L, Li Y-Y. Shell-sheddable micelles based on star-shaped poly(ε-caprolactone)-SS-poly(ethyl glycol) copolymer for intracellular drug release. Soft Matter 2011;7(6):2329–31.

246. Sun H, Guo B, Li X, Cheng R, Meng F, Liu H, et al. Shell-sheddable micelles based on dextran-SS-poly(ε-caprolactone) diblock copolymer for efficient intracellular release of doxorubicin. Biomacromolecules 2010;11(4):848–54.

247. Meyer DE, Shin BC, Kong GA, Dewhirst MW, Chilkoti A. Drug targeting using thermally responsive polymers and local hyperthermia. J. Control. Release 2001;74(1–3):213–24.

248. Ponce AM, Vujaskovic Z, Yuan F, Needham D, Dewhirst MW. Hyperthermia mediated liposomal drug delivery. Int. J. Hyperthermia 2006;22(3):205–13.

249. Kono K. Thermosensitive polymer-modified liposomes. Adv. Drug Deliv Rev. 2001;53(3):307–19.

250. Kono K, Yoshino K, Takagishi T. Effect of poly(ethylene glycol) grafts on temperature-sensitivity of thermosensitive polymer-modified liposomes. J. Control. Release 2002;80(1–3):321–32.

251. Meyer DE, Shin BC, Kong GA, Dewhirst MW, Chilkoti A. Drug targeting using thermally responsive polymers and local hyperthermia. J. Control. Release 2001;74(1–3):213–24.

252. Zhang JX, Zalipsky S, Mullah N, Pechar M, Allen TM. Pharmaco attributes of dioleoylphosphatidylethanolamine/cholesterylhemisuccinate liposomes containing different types of cleavable lipopolymers. Pharmacol. Res. 2004;49(2):185–98.

253. Meers P. Enzyme-activated targeting of liposomes. Adv. Drug Deliv. Rev. 2001;53(3):265–72.

254. Hatakeyama H, Akita H, Kogure K, Oishi M, Nagasaki Y, Kihira Y, et al. Development of a novel systemic gene delivery system for cancer therapy with a tumor-specific cleavable PEG-lipid. Gene Ther. 2007;14(1):68–77.

255. de Graaf AJ, Azevedo Próspero dos Santos II, Pieters EHE, Rijkers DTS, van Nostrum CF, Vermonden T, et al. A micelle-shedding thermosensitive hydrogel as sustained release formulation. J. Control. Release 2012;162(3):582–90.

256. Li L, ten Hagen TL, Hossann M, Suss R, van Rhoon GC, Eggermont AM, et al. Mild hyperthermia triggered doxorubicin release from optimized stealth thermosensitive liposomes improves intratumoral drug delivery and efficacy. J. Control. Release 2013;168(2):142–50.

257. Kong G, Braun RD, Dewhirst MW. Hyperthermia enables tumor-specific nanoparticle delivery: effect of particle size. Cancer Res. 2000;60(16):4440–5.

258. Koning GA, Eggermont AM, Lindner LH, ten Hagen TL. Hyperthermia and thermosensitive liposomes for improved delivery of chemotherapeutic drugs to solid tumors. Pharm. Res. 2010;27(8):1750–4.

Recent Advances and Trends in the Brain Delivery of Small Molecule Based Cancer Therapies

Werner Gladdines, Corine C. Visser, Marco de Boer, Chantal C.M. Appeldoorn, Arie Reijerkerk, Jaap Rip, Pieter J. Gaillard

to-BBB Technologies B.V., Leiden, The Netherlands

OUTLINE

Novel Approaches and Strategies for Biologics, Vaccines and Cancer Therapies. DOI: 10.1016/B978-0-12-416603-5.00019-5

INTRODUCTION

Effective treatment of brain cancer, either primary or metastases from a peripheral location, is a growing challenge. Malignant glioma is the most common type of primary brain cancer in adults and in children. Despite surgical and medical advancements, the 5-year survival rate in the United States for glioblastoma multiforme, the most aggressive glioma, has remained at a dismal 3.4% for the past three decades.[1] After recurrence, rapid tumor progression results in a median progression-free survival and overall survival of 9 weeks and 25 to 28 weeks, respectively.[1,2] In 2007, the latest year for which updated statistics are available, the U.S. incidence rate of brain and other central nervous system (CNS) cancers among adults was 6.4 new cases per 100,000 persons (www.cancer.gov). The estimated deaths from brain and other CNS cancers in 2013 have been estimated to be 14,080. These numbers are approximately 10-fold higher for brain metastases from peripheral tumors, with highest incidences in patients with lung cancer, melanoma, and breast cancer.[3] Consequently, both for primary as well as for brain metastases from solid tumors, multiple experimental therapies are being evaluated in clinical trials and are reviewed elsewhere.[3–6] In our view, advanced drug delivery systems can have a major positive impact on the overall outcomes of the treatment regimens; therefore, we focus this review on the clinical development of liposomal chemotherapeutics for brain cancer (i.e., primary tumors). After a short introduction on currently approved treatment options for brain cancer, we discuss the benefits of liposomal formulations, initially for systemic tumors as most information is available for these indications. Subsequently, we discuss brain-targeted chemotherapies using these formulations, and finally we highlight the issues that are relevant for the clinical development thereof.

Current Treatment Options for Brain Cancer Being Used in Clinical Practice

In the past decades much progress has been made in finding an effective treatment for brain cancer. Treatment of single (large) tumors usually exists of debulking surgery and/or local (focused) radiotherapy followed by chemotherapy. For multiple smaller tumors, for which surgery is not always possible, whole-brain radiation therapy (WBRT) can increase median survival up to 7 months, but with possible consequences with regard to quality of life, such as a decline in cognition and the risk of late detrimental radiation side-effects.[7]

In addition to surgery, local chemotherapy can be indicated. The carmustine wafer (Gliadel®) is indicated in patients with newly diagnosed high-grade malignant glioma or recurrent glioblastoma multiforme, as an adjunct to surgery.[8,9] The biodegradable wafer is implanted after the tumor, or part of it, is removed. This local therapy, however, is only suitable for a single tumor and not for multiple smaller tumors.

Several systemic chemotherapeutic drugs (e.g., temozolomide, bevacizumab) and biologicals (e.g., lomustine, methotrexate, capecitabine, lapatinib, vinorelbine) have been approved and are in clinical practice for brain cancer. A chemotherapeutic drug in clinical practice is exemplified by the oral drug lomustine (CCNU), which was already approved by the U.S. Food and Drug Administration (FDA) in the 1970s. It is prescribed for brain tumors as second-line treatment after surgery and/or radiotherapy and for Hodgkin's disease as a secondary therapy in combination with other approved therapies. In a recent Phase III trial in patients with recurrent glioblastoma where lomustine was included as control, it was shown that when lomustine was given at the time of first recurrence the progression-free survival (PFS) was 42 to 168 days (median, 82), and the median overall survival (OS) was 9.8 months.[10] This trial demonstrated the efficacy of lomustine monotherapy in patients with recurrent glioblastoma previously treated with temozolomide.[10]

In contrast to the old chemotherapeutic drugs in clinical practice, temozolomide (Temodal®, Temodar®, Temcad®) was established as first-line therapy in 2005 and is considered to be the most important therapy for newly diagnosed glioma. As an adjuvant to radiotherapy, it showed a significant, though modest, increase in median survival (14 versus 12 months; $p < 0.001$), 2-year survival, and progression-free survival when compared to radiotherapy alone.[7] In 2009, bevacizumab (Avastin®) as a single-agent angiogenesis inhibitor received an accelerated approval by the FDA as second-line therapy based on a clinically meaningful and durable tumor response rate.[1,12] It should be noted that, particularly due to the infiltrative nature of brain tumors, antiangiogenesis therapy (e.g., bevacizumab) may shift tumor progression from an expansive to an invasive, angiogenesis-independent phenotype that is not affected by the treatment,[13] as was confirmed in orthotopic glioma xenograft models.[14,15] But still, despite major improvement of treatment results over the last decade, brain cancer remains a highly fatal and devastating disease and a cure is extremely rare. Therefore, the development of novel and innovative therapeutic approaches to enhance the delivery of drugs into the brain may hold significant promise for improving the efficiency of brain cancer treatments.

LIPOSOMES FOR THE DELIVERY OF CHEMOTHERAPEUTICS

In general, the objective when developing liposomal formulations is to improve the efficacy and reduce the side effects of a chemotherapy by improving the drug release, pharmacokinetics, and biodistribution profile. For example, free doxorubicin has an elimination half-life of several minutes and an area under the curve (AUC) of 3.5 mg-hr/L, while the PEGylated (polyethylene glycol, or PEG) liposomal formulation of the same drug has a half-life of more than 50 hours and an AUC of more than 2000 mg-hr/L, respectively.[16] These pharmacokinetic parameters are dependent on several factors such as liposomal characteristics and dose, as well as host-associated factors such as age and gender.[16] The distribution across the body and associated toxicity profile was also changed. Although doxorubicin as a free drug is associated with dose-limiting cardiotoxicity, PEGylated liposomal doxorubicin is essentially free of cardiotoxicity but is associated with palmar-plantar erythrodysethesia (hand-foot syndrome).[17] So, although certain side-effects might be reduced due to liposomal formulations, others might increase. Liposomal composition strongly influences blood circulation time and the release profile of the encapsulated drug. For example, this profile is influenced by the selection of lipids used in the liposomal formulation, which can be charged or neutral and have high or low melting temperatures, as well as by the degree of PEGylation; also, the particle size of the liposomes plays an important role.

When looking into the history of liposomal drugs for intravenous anticancer therapy, the first to receive approval from the FDA was PEGylated liposomal doxorubicin (Doxil®) in 1995. The European Medicines Agency (EMA) approved Caelyx® (as Doxil is called in the European Union) a year later, in 1996. Quite recently, in 2013, the FDA approved the first generic PEGylated liposomal doxorubicin product: Lipodox.[18] Currently, several intravenous liposomal products are approved for several cancer indications, but so far none is approved for a brain cancer indication (Table 19.1). DepoCyt®, a liposomal formulation with cytarabine (approved in 1999 by the FDA) for the treatment of lymphomatous meningitis and in clinical trials for recurrent GBM, is a chemotherapy that is administered intrathecally or intraventricularly as a slow release depot formulation. It is not listed in the table, as this review is focusing on intravenous treatments.

In addition to the approved products and the products that are in Phase III clinical trials, much research is ongoing for liposomal chemotherapeutics.[19–22] For example, several paclitaxel formulations have been developed and tested in clinical research. In China, paclitaxel liposomes (Lipusu®; Luye Pharma) are already marketed.[22,23] Two other paclitaxel formulation, LEP-ETU and EndoTAG®, are in Phase II clinical trials.[22] In addition to Lipoplatin™ (see Table 19.1), several other liposomal cisplatin formulations are being evaluated, including aroplatin and SPI-077.[19] The development of SPI-77 was stopped due to the lack of release of cisplatin from the liposomes.[24,25] In addition, the development of LiPlaCis®, another liposomal cisplatin formulation,

TABLE 19.1 Overview of Intravenous Liposomal Cancer Therapies Approved or in Phase III

Encapsulated Compound	Trade Name	Clinical Status	Indication
Doxorubicin[a,b]	Doxil® Caelyx® Lipodox[c]	1995 (U.S.); 1996 (E.U.); 2013 (U.S.)	Kaposi's sarcoma, ovarian/breast cancer
Doxorubicin[d]	Myocet®	2000 (E.U.); 2001 (Canada); Phase III (U.S.)	metastatic breast cancer (combination therapy with cyclophosphamide) metastatic breast cancer (combination therapy with paclitaxel and trastuzumab)
Doxorubicin (heat-sensitive release)[e]	ThermoDox®	Phase II/III	primary liver cancer recurrent chest wall breast cancer and colorectal liver metastases
Daunorubicin	DaunoXome®	1996 (U.S.); 1996 (E.U.)	blood tumors, Kaposi's sarcoma
Vincristine	Marqibo®	2012 (U.S.)	ALL (Philadelphia chromosome-negative (Ph-) acute lymphoblastic leukemia)
Cisplatin[a,f,g]	Lipoplatin™	Phase III	pancreatic cancer, head and neck cancer, mesothelioma, breast cancer, gastric cancer, NSCLC
Irinotecan[h,i]	PEP02	Phase III	pancreatic cancer, colorectal cancer

[a]Pegylated liposome.
[b]Barenholz, Y. Doxil®—the first FDA-approved nano-drug: lessons learned. J. Control. Release. 2012; 160(2): 117–34.
[c]Generic; FDA announcement, 2013 (http://www.fda.gov/newsevents/newsroom/pressannouncements/ucm337872.htm).
[d]http://www.ema.europa.eu.
[e]Harris, E. Industry update: the latest developments in therapeutic delivery. Ther. Deliv. 2013; 4(10): 1229–34.
[f]http://www.lipoplatin.com.
[g]Stathopoulos, G.P. and Boulikas, T. Lipoplatin formulation review article. J. Drug Deliv. 2012; 2012: 581363.
[h]Anon. Studies of nanoliposomal irinotecan (PEP02, MM-398) in late stage pancreatic cancer and gastric cancer published in British Journal of Cancer and Annals of Oncology. BusinessWire. August 27, 2013 (http://www.businesswire.com/news/home/20130827006518/en/Studies-Nanoliposomal-Irinotecan-PEP02-MM-398-Late-Stage).
[i]NCT01494506 (http://clinicaltrials.gov/show/NCT01494506).
Data from Chang and Yeh,[19] Sen and Mandal,[20] and Slingerland et al.[21]

was stopped after a Phase I study when it was found that LiPlaCis did not prevent the renal toxicity of cisplatin and the incidence of acute infusion reactions was relatively high in this trial.[26] Finally, a liposomal formulation of vinorelbine (NanoVNB®)[27] is in clinical development (Phase I/II trials). As we do not want to replicate the earlier reviews by Chang and Yen,[19] Sen and Mandal,[20] Slingeland et al.,[21] and Koudelka and Turanek,[22] we limit our examples to these few.

Systemic Delivery: Enhanced Permeation and Retention Effect

None of the currently approved liposomal formulations is specifically targeted to a tumor site, whereas the liposomal formulations of existing drugs were mostly developed to improve plasma circulation time and to reduce side-effects associated with chemotherapeutics. In addition, it was found that liposomal encapsulation resulted in passive targeting of chemotherapeutics through the so-called enhanced permeation and retention (EPR) effect. The EPR effect, previously observed for macromolecules and polymeric drugs,[28] was observed in humans in the first clinical trial with Doxil/Caelyx.[17,29] The EPR effect is based on leaky blood vessels in tumors (enhanced permeation) and a poor lymphatic drainage in tumors (prolonged retention); any biocompatible macromolecular compound above 40 kDa, including liposomes or other drug particles (up to a size of approximately 800 nm), can easily extravasate, reaching a 10- to 30-fold increase in drug concentration in the tumor compared to plasma concentration.[28] The prolonged retention especially seems to be an important factor, as small molecules easily diffuse back into plasma.[17,30]

Targeted Delivery to Systemic Tumors

In addition to passive (non-targeted) drug delivery, much effort is also being directed toward targeted drug delivery, aiming to improve the efficacy of chemotherapeutic compounds. Various "general" receptors, such as the transferrin receptor, lactoferrin receptor, lectin receptor, folate receptor, human epidermal growth factor receptor (EGFR), scavenger receptor, nuclear receptor, and integrin receptor, are being used as targets because they are overexpressed on the surface of cancer cells.[31] In addition, specific ligands based on the tumor type (e.g., HER2-targeted liposomes) are being investigated. Recently, the marketed anticancer monoclonal antibody trastuzumab (Herceptin®) was used for targeting. Herceptin conjugated to docetaxel liposomes showed an improved efficacy in HER2-positive breast cancer cells *in vitro*. In addition, anti-HER2 liposomal doxorubicin and anti-EGFR liposomal doxorubicin are in Phase I clinical trials (NCT01304797, NCT01702129).[32]

The selection of a target for cancer cells depends on several factors, such as the selectivity of the target and the ability to internalize the ligand-targeted formulation.[33] If the target is also expressed on non-target cells, nonspecific toxicity can limit the use of this target. On the other hand, if the relative degree of expression of the target is higher on cancer cells compared to non-target cells, the selectivity will be improved.[33] Finding a ligand–target combination that is being internalized by the cancer cells is also important for therapeutic efficacy, as Sapra and Allen[34] have shown. Selecting an internalizing ligand (anti-CD19) to target liposomal doxorubicin to human B-lymphoma (Namalwa) cells resulted in a higher efficacy *in vitro* and *in vivo* compared to a non-internalizing ligand (anti-CD20). The efficacy of liposomal doxorubicin with the non-internalizing ligand was comparable to non-targeted liposomes.

In the past years, several papers have been published in which dual-targeted liposomes are used.[33,35–37] The dual targeting of a targeting ligand to the tumors and a cell-penetrating peptide is often used to promote internalization. However, according to the clinicaltrial.gov database, no dual-targeted liposomes are in clinical research and development.

TARGETED DELIVERY OF LIPOSOMAL CHEMOTHERAPEUTICS TO BRAIN TUMORS

The limited efficacy of liposomal chemotherapeutics against brain cancer (see, for example, the studies with liposomal doxorubicin by Fabel et al.,[38] Hau et al.,[39] and Glas et al.[40]) suggests that the EPR effect may play a minor role in the treatment of tumors located in the brain. In a paper in the *Journal of Translational Medicine*, Sarin[41] convincingly demonstrated that the physiologic upper limit of pore size in the blood–tumor barrier of malignant solid tumor microvasculature is approximately 12 nm, which is large enough for contrast agents but too small for conventional liposomes to extravasate. In line with these results is the work by Kawano et al.,[42] who recently demonstrated that liposomal doxorubicin did not display a larger effect compared to free doxorubicin in a mouse model of adrenal neuroblastoma. Immunohistochemical analysis has shown that the adrenal tumor vasculature had abundant pericyte coverage, resulting in a less leaky structure for liposomes.[42] A similar observation was made by Guo et al.,[43] who showed that glioblastomas or fibrosarcomas that overexpress platelet-derived growth factor B (PDGF-B) exhibited an increased pericyte density around blood vessels. According to Maeda et al.,[28] a lack of smooth-muscle layer and pericytes is one of the hallmarks of an abnormal vascular architecture that leads to the EPR effect (Figure 19.1).

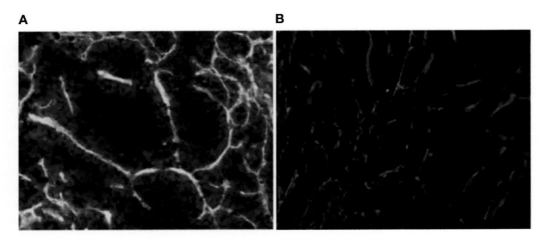

FIGURE 19.1   Coverage of vasculature by pericytes stabilizes vascular structure. The vasculature of the adrenal tumors was found to be relatively stable and non-leaky, thus preventing the enhanced permeation and retention (EPR) effect from taking place in such vascular types. Similar limitations are thought to be of relevance in the brain. Panel A is from transgenic mice and panel B from human patient material. The green signal indicate endothelial cells, and the red signal indicates α-SMA-positive pericytes. *Reproduced from Kawano, K., et al. Combination therapy with gefitinib and doxorubicin inhibits tumor growth in transgenic mice with adrenal neuroblastoma. Cancer Med. 2013; 2(3): 286–95.*

Therefore, the EPR effect is most likely less important or even absent for enhancing the delivery and improving the efficacy of non-targeted liposomal chemotherapeutics in brain cancer.

The Blood–Brain Barrier and Blood–Tumor Barrier Limit Efficacy of Chemotherapeutics

Chemotherapeutic drugs are generally not very effective against brain cancer, partly due to intrinsic resistance but also because of a functional blood–brain barrier (BBB) in the tumor that efficiently restricts the distribution of drugs to tumor cells.[44,45] The BBB, at the interface of blood and brain, maintains homeostasis in the brain by selectively allowing nutrients to enter the brain and, at the same time, keeping harmful substances out. In brain tumors, the BBB can still be intact while parts are interrupted. This is dependent on the tumor type as well as the size of the tumor. High-grade glioblastomas are highly angiogenic tumors; consequently, these tumors harbor new and leaky blood vessels. In fact, this leaky vasculature enables the diagnosis by contrast-enhanced MRI using gadolinium as a contrast agent.[44] However, in the outer rim of the tumor the BBB will still be functional. In contrast to gliomas, brain metastases may form lesions with relatively well-defined boundaries that incorporate leaky blood vessels upon progression due to neovascularization. At the same time, the BBB will still be able to protect smaller metastases from adequate therapy, as these may still reside behind an intact BBB.[44] Palmieri et al.[46] made the same observation; they found that, in mice, in micrometastases smaller than 0.1 mm^2 the blood–tumor barrier was intact, whereas the blood–tumor barrier leaked in larger (>0.4 mm^2) metastases but still excluded therapeutic drugs.[47,48] It is of importance to note that the synergy of combined antiangiogenic therapy and chemotherapeutic agents in other cancers has been partially attributed to normalization of the tumor blood vessels.[49] In the case of brain tumors, however, normalization of the tumor vascular bed through antiangiogenic treatment comes at the expense of restoration of the BBB. In other words, while angiogenesis inhibitors in combination with chemotherapies may be very effective in initial brain tumor reduction, the brain microenvironment will still allow invasion and proliferation of tumor cells behind a functional barrier, even in the presence of chemotherapeutic or other anticancer drugs. This major drawback is supported by published clinical data (for review, see Verhoeff et al.[13]) and confirmed in orthotopic glioma xenograft models of brain cancer as well.[14] As described above, the EPR effect is largely absent in the brain, making conventional drug delivery systems incapable of bringing significant therapeutic benefit. Altogether, it will therefore be extremely important to develop novel and dedicated methods to overcome the BBB and to deliver active drugs into the brain. In particular, such an approach would be beneficial to the efficacy of drugs that display both antiangiogenic and antitumor activities, because otherwise the antitumor effect might get lost.

Safely Enhancing Blood–to–Brain Drug Delivery

To improve the research and clinical development of brain-targeted drugs in general, we have developed ten key criteria for targeted blood–to–brain drug delivery.[50,51] These can be applied to chemotherapeutics for brain cancer as well. The ten key criteria are related to targeting the BBB, drug carriers, and drug development from lab to clinic, and they focus on the safety and efficacy of new treatments for CNS-related disorders. The criteria related to targeting the BBB are focused on the specificity of the ligand (receptor binding), the safety of both the ligand and the receptor, and the applicability of the selected ligand–receptor for both acute and chronic conditions. With regard to drug carriers, the appropriate selection of a drug carrier system is important to improve the drug-like properties and to improve the pharmacokinetic profile of an intravenously administered drug.[50,51] Last, but not least, the criteria related to drug development from lab to clinic address straightforward manufacturing (including low cost), activity in all animals, and strong intellectual property (IP) protection.

Brain-Targeted Chemotherapy Products in Clinical Research

There are currently two brain-targeted chemotherapy products in clinical research: ANG1005, a conjugate with paclitaxel as the active compound, and 2B3-101, a glutathione PEGylated liposomal formulation with doxorubicin as the active compound (Figure 19.2).

The targeting ligand of ANG1005, angiopep-2, has a high affinity for the lipoprotein-related protein 1 (LRP1) receptor at the BBB and is considered a safe targeting ligand due to the fact that the peptide sequence is derived from a protein of human origin.[52] Both the lipoprotein-related protein 1 and 2 receptors are closely related to the low-density lipoprotein (LDL) receptors.[53,54] LRP1 and 2 receptors are also involved in many ligand-specific signaling functions at the BBB and elsewhere in the body, making this an interesting but complex targeting receptor to work with from a safety and drug development perspective.[50]

The Phase II clinical trial with ANG1005 (or GRN1005, as it was also called; NCT01480583) was discontinued after an interim analysis at the end of 2012.[55] The analysis showed that there were no confirmed intracranial responses among the first 30 evaluable patients with brain metastases arising from breast cancer. The Phase II study in patients with brain metastases from non-small-cell lung cancer (NCT01497665) was also stopped because of the inability to successfully enroll the trial. Recently, Angiochem has indicated that it will continue to develop ANG1005 based on additional Phase II data showing that the compound produced responses in breast cancer patients with brain metastases.[56] In 80 HER2-positive and HER2-negative patients in the intent-to-treat (ITT) population of the trial, ANG1005 produced 14 partial responses and 35 cases of stable disease.[57] In addition, ANG1005 will be evaluated in a Phase II trial in patients with recurrent high-grade gliomas (NCT01967810) and in a Phase II trial in HER2-positive breast cancer patients with brain metastases.[56]

Glutathione, the ligand that is used to target 2B3-101 to the brain, has an FDA Generally Recognized as Safe (GRAS) status; it is used as a food supplement and as supportive therapy in cancer and Parkinson's disease (in high intravenous doses). CNS-specific active (sodium-dependent) transport of glutathione across the BBB was first shown by Kannan et al.[58] and was further supported by additional studies.[59,60] The exact mechanism of glutathione-targeted liposomal transport has yet to be elucidated, and it is not known whether the glutathione transporter is an internalizing receptor or a membrane carrier in this configuration.

Results from a Phase I trial with 2B3-101 were recently presented.[61] 2B3-101 is a brain-targeted formulation based on already marketed Doxil/Caelyx. The safety evaluation

A

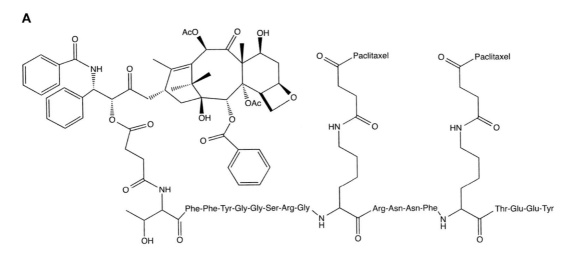

B

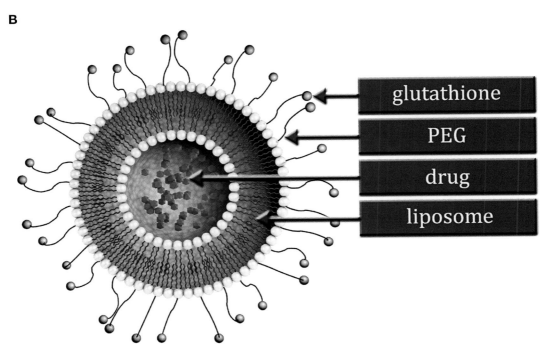

FIGURE 19.2 Brain-targeted chemotherapy products in clinical research. (A) ANG1005, a conjugate with angiopep-2 as targeting ligand and paclitaxel as active compound. (B) 2B3-101, a PEGylated liposomal formulation with glutathione as targeted ligand and doxorubicin as active compound. Please note that these products are not to scale.

of 2B3-101 showed that adverse events were mainly related to transient bone marrow suppression, skin lesions, and mild to moderate infusion reactions. No signs of drug-related neurotoxicity and cardiotoxicity were observed. In addition, at the higher dose levels tested, promising signs of antitumor activity were observed. Therefore, the Phase IIA part of the trial, including patients with recurrent malignant gliomas and patients with brain metastases from breast cancer, small-cell lung cancer, or melanomas, was recently begun.[62]

PRACTICAL ISSUES IN THE DEVELOPMENT OF LIPOSOMAL FORMULATIONS OF CHEMOTHERAPEUTIC DRUGS

Liposomes have matured as a delivery system for therapeutic agents.[63,64] It has taken two decades to develop the liposome carrier concept to a pharmaceutical product level, but such a long incubation time is typical for a front-runner product. There was little understanding of the behavior and therapeutic potential of liposomes *in vivo*, and several pharmaceutical problems had to be solved. The development of commercial liposomal products has never failed for pharmaceutical reasons. Where it has failed, it was for therapeutic or economic reasons.

An important take-home message from the liposome story is the critical importance of multidisciplinary research teams; only through such an approach can liposomes be developed that are both therapeutically beneficial and pharmaceutically acceptable.[64] The ability to be creative and to adapt what we have learned thus far will determine the success of new brain-targeted liposomal products in the future. Some examples of these lessons learned from the past our summarized below.

Liposomal Formulation

Encapsulation

The therapeutic index of many drugs can be significantly enhanced by the use of liposomes. Although many liposomal formulations are FDA approved, most liposomal drug candidates fail in the developmental stage due to poor drug encapsulation efficiency and rapid drug leakage. Over the last decades several approaches have been developed to encapsulate and retain drugs in liposomes. Liposomes can be loaded with drug by either passive or active (or remote) loading. The liposome lipid bilayer is a semipermeable barrier that blocks the diffusion of charged and larger non-charged hydrophilic molecules, while small non-charged substances, which are lipophilic, can penetrate freely. In passive loading, a membrane-impermeable drug is dissolved in the hydration solution during the liposome manufacturing process. Upon addition of the aqueous solution to a lipid mixture, lipid bilayers form and partially encapsulate the drug solution to form liposomes. Most of the drug solution remains in the external solution and must be removed by dialysis or chromatography. Passive encapsulation is limited by the liposomal-trapped volume and drug solubility. Therefore, loading efficiency is low and usually does not exceed 5%.[65]

Alternatively, drugs can be encapsulated by active methods after formation of the liposomes, which can result in loading efficiencies approaching 100%.[66–68] Importantly, not all drugs can be encapsulated in a remote manner, as this requires intrinsic amphiphilic weak acid or basic properties. Efficient encapsulation of such drugs is based on their pH-dependent charge and/or lipophilicity. Thus, a pH gradient is the driving force to translocate and retain the amphiphilic weak bases and acids. Generally, pH gradients are produced by a gradient of the salt of a weak acid (usually acetate)[69] or a weak base (usually ammonium)[70] over the liposome lipid bilayer. Liposomes exhibiting weak acid or base gradients can be employed for loading a second amphipathic weak acid or base, respectively (Figure 19.3), including therapeutically active compounds. In solution, ionized and non-charged forms of weak acids or bases form an equilibrium, which is dependent on the pKa of the drug.

Remote loading protocols take advantage of the fact that non-charged lipophilic molecules can cross a lipid bilayer and enter the internal compartment of liposomes. Upon reaching the internal compartment, the proton gradient induces the ionization of the molecule, shifting the equilibrium toward the impermeable charged species and resulting in the drug being trapped in the liposome.[71] Acetate and ammonium thus act as proton shuttles to maintain the pH gradient and to facilitate additional drug encapsulation. Ideally, the acetate or ammonium counter ion can be selected in such a way it controls the state of precipitation of the ionized drug-counter ion salt. Precipitation of the drug causes a further decrease in the available internal drug pool and thereby a shift in equilibrium, increasing encapsulation efficiency and delaying drug release. In some cases, drug derivatization was applied to enable active encapsulation of hydrophobic drugs, previously not reported to encapsulate, by active or remote loading.

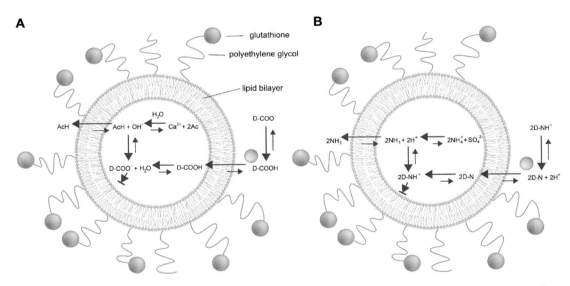

FIGURE 19.3 Remote loading of drug in liposomes with internal aqueous solution containing (A) ammonium sulfate or (B) calcium acetate. High internal, low external ammonium or acetate gradients induce pH gradients that can be employed for the remote loading of weak base or acid drugs respectively. The pH gradient induces the (de) protonation of the drug in the internal compartment forming the charged, impermeable species, thereby inducing a net flux of the drug to the internal compartment. The (de)protonation of the drug in the liposome causes a change in internal pH. This change induces the deionization of acetate or ammonium, which then act as proton shuttles to maintain the pH gradient and the loading potential of the liposome. Moreover, the counter ion of the gradient forming ion can be chosen to precipitate the drug, shifting the equilibrium further toward the charged drug species and increasing the stability of the formulation. *Adapted from Clerc, S. and Barenholz, Y. Loading of amphipathic weak acids into liposomes in response to transmembrane calcium acetate gradients. Biochim. Biophys. Acta. 1995; **1240**(2): 257–65.*

Stability

Phospholipids in the liposomal membrane can slowly become oxidized or hydrolyzed, and this can induce fusion of liposomes, leakage of the encapsulated drug, and/or a change in liposome morphology affecting targeting/efficiency. These oxidation and hydrolysis processes can take place when the liposomes are stored in solution. Removing water by freeze drying (FD) can increase stability by preventing oxidation and hydrolysis. The FD process includes three steps: (1) freezing of the liposome solution, (2) primary drying (sublimation), and (3) secondary drying (desorption). Lyoprotectant agents (LPAs) are required to prevent damage in the FD process. Examples of LPAs used in FD are glycerol, disaccharides (sucrose, lactose, and trehalose), and cyclodextrins.[72] Most authors claim that LPAs should be both inside and outside the bilayer, which means that possible *in vivo* effects of the LPAs used should be carefully monitored. The FD process can induce change in liposome morphology (size and membrane composition) and liposomal efficiency, as well as drug release profiles and pharmacological performance.[73] Chen et al.[74] found that FD induced no change in liposomal size but had an effect on molecular arrangement in the bilayer membrane. This could impair targeting efficiency, so the FD product should be carefully monitored. Other FD consequences can include (1) a negative impact on production costs and an impact on upscaling and production procedures, and (2) a positive impact on storage and logistics. Currently, there are only FD liposomal products on the market involving hydrophobic compounds and where liposomal size/features are less important. A key question remains as to whether or not it will be feasible to make FD targeted liposomes with hydrophilic cargo.

Regulatory Aspects: Pharmaceuticals

Besides the general chemistry, manufacturing, and controls (CMC) documentation supplied by the FDA,[75] the Draft Guidance FDA document on liposome drug products provides the most extensive regulatory information on liposomes.[76] For liposomes, the size, particle size distribution, and charge are often the first characterization steps after preparation. The use of dynamic light scattering (DLS) techniques allows relatively easy measurements of these parameters. In addition, the drug loading efficiency is important to determine for all batches. This requires validated analytical assays of the active substance and its possible metabolites as well as the liposomal components, targeting moiety, and other excipients. In addition, for the definition of the product as well as determination of its stability (shelf-life), it is important that the analytical assay is able to discriminate between encapsulated and the released or non-encapsulated (free) drug substance. The National Characterization Lab has a free service, funded by the U.S. National Cancer Institute, to help the developers of promising nanotech cancer therapies get their products into clinical trials (http://ncl.cancer.gov). Other critical issues to take into account are related to upscaling from animal trial material to clinical trial material, including batch-to-batch consistency. Finally, the regulatory requirements for the validation steps of the use of new excipients and lipids can be quite substantial.

Efficacy and Proof-of-Concept

Translation from Animals to Humans

Proof-of-concept studies in animal tumor models are needed for the development of drug delivery technologies such as the G-Technology®. The translation of results from animal studies to the human situation may be influenced by the drug delivery technology used. Drug development is facilitated if the technology has activity in all animal models,[51] which means that the selected drug delivery ligand should be conserved across all species. It is then possible to select already established models for early proof-of-concept and safety studies, allowing for faster development. When using a monoclonal antibody (mAb) as a ligand for drug delivery, for example, the mAb can have different affinities for the target receptors in different species. This may limit the choice of animal models that can be used. An example is the use of a humanized antibody as brain delivery ligand that needs to be tested separately in rhesus monkeys.[77]

Pharmacokinetics and Biodistribution

Although pharmacokinetic (PK) and biodistribution data may be available for a free drug, this PK biodistribution will change when the drug is administered as a liposomal formulation. The methods used, therefore, require attention.[51,78] Additional questions are related to release of the drug, the possible formation of (toxic) degradation products, and the fate of the liposomes. When the PK and biodistribution are determined *in vivo* in brain tumor models, the tissue and tumor distribution patterns will be different compared to when free drug is compared with drug in a liposomal formulation. When investigating the PK and distribution of liposomes the bioanalytical methods used should preferably be able to discriminate between the free or released drug and the liposome-encapsulated drug.

When investigating liposomes for drug delivery to the brain, brain uptake is of course an important hallmark of biodistribution studies. Most commonly used are measurements of drug in brain homogenates, often after whole body perfusion to remove blood from the brain. Although this method is useful, there will always be some blood contamination in the brain homogenates, which may lead to false-positive results, especially when long circulating liposomes are used. Therefore, other methods have been developed to quantify drug delivery to the brain. Commonly used methods are *in situ* brain perfusion, *in vivo* brain microdialysis, and cerebrospinal fluid (CSF) sampling. The choice of the method to use depends on the particular drug and the liposomes used because all methods have their own limitations, as reviewed elsewhere.[79]

Efficacy Models

Drugs that are already in the clinical phase for peripheral tumors and do not reach the brain in sufficient quantities may be good candidates to be combined with drug delivery technologies. The availability of data from preclinical efficacy studies is of importance. For some drugs, results from proof-of-concept studies in animals models with brain cancer have been published. Sometimes intravenous and intracerebroventricular injections are compared, providing useful information. All of this information may increase the chances of successful therapy improvement through the use of a particular drug delivery approach.

We would like to point out that tumor models should be validated and the appropriate controls (free drug, targeted versus non-targeted liposomes) should be used to compare the efficacy of the investigated liposome-encapsulated drug. Because liposomes influence the PK and biodistribution of a drug, one should take into account that the efficacy parameters might then also change. For example, in efficacy studies the dosing and administration frequency should be adapted based on the results from the PK studies, and the time points at which the efficacy is measured should be adapted based on investigations into the free compound.

Safety Profile

Upon systemic delivery, chemotherapeutic drugs can have serious side-effects because they can also reach off-target tissue. Liposomal encapsulation of these drugs can decrease these safety risks, as it can prevent unwanted non-target tissue distribution. A well-known example is Doxil/Caelyx, where the cardiotoxicity of doxorubicin is reduced due to the liposomal encapsulation, leading to lower concentration in the heart. It is important to realize that differences in distribution to organs (including the CNS) after liposomal encapsulation can possibly also lead to increased toxicity. Available data about the distribution and safety profile of the drug may give insight into possible improvement of the toxicity profile by liposomal encapsulation.

Regulatory Aspects

Based on FDA and EMA recommendations, product quality and product safety are most important to receive approval for clinical research. This is fully in line with the World Medical Association (WMA) *Declaration of Helsinki*, in which it is stated that, "Every medical research study involving human subjects must be preceded by careful assessment of predictable risks and burdens to the individuals and communities involved in the research in comparison with foreseeable benefits to them and to other individuals or communities affected by the condition under investigation."[80] For all human drugs, and especially for neurotherapeutics, it is important to demonstrate the safety of the drug with respect to the central nervous system.[81]

General Safety Testing

To develop a liposomal formulation for clinical use, it is necessary to adhere to FDA and EMA guidelines. The approval of PEGylated liposomal doxorubicin has paved the way but the guidelines are still susceptible to change as research progresses. In the end, the liposomal formulation should be a "definable product" that is made according to a reproducible method with reproducible outcomes related to pharmaceuticals, pharmacology, and safety. We have discussed this extensively in an earlier review.[79]

Because most publicly available information focuses on the content of liposomes (i.e., the active substance), only limited information is available with regard to possible adverse effects of the liposome components themselves. Szebeni and colleagues[82,83] have investigated complement activation by liposomes that could occur after intravenous administration. In most people, the symptoms remain subclinical, even though significant complement activation may occur.[82] The addition of PEG did not decrease complement activation in pigs,[84] although opsonization by proteins and scavenging by the reticuloendothelial system (RES) were decreased.[85] Complement activation-related pseudoallergy (CARPA), an acute hypersensitivity or infusion reaction, occurs not only with liposomal nanocarriers but also with other (polymeric) nanocarriers such as dendrimers, PEGs, and polaxamers; its severity usually declines after repeated administration.[86] Clinically, infusion reactions are often managed by dilution, a longer infusion time, or patient premedication; however, it is still important to predict potential problems and, if possible, to eliminate them.[87]

Other immunological risks include antibody formation against any of the substituents of the liposome, including the targeting ligand and the active drug, and these antibodies can lead to either an accelerated blood clearance (reducing the bioavailability and efficacy) or to a burst-release through complement-mediated lysis of the liposome (resulting in increased blood concentration and possibly toxicity).[86] An immune response in itself does not need to be a problem as long as it is rapidly deactivated; however, a severe pathology can occur when the defense response is anomalous in extent or duration.[88]

CNS-Related Toxicity

For treatments that are being developed for brain diseases it is also important to show that, next to general toxicities, there are no particle or drug-induced CNS-related toxicities, such as behavioral effects. It is important to appreciate that toxicity may lead to a temporary BBB opening that will influence the delivery of drug to the brain and potentially even lead to neurotoxicity.[89] In the preclinical development of 2B3-101, we included electroencephalography (EEG) measurements and a modified Irwin test to demonstrate that there was no change in neurobehavior.[90]

Dosing and Administration Frequency and Therapeutic Window

It is important to realize that liposomal formulations have to be administered intravenously. When combining liposomes with existing drugs this may have consequences for administration and dosage. For example, a drug that is normally given orally will be administered intravenously, which will be less convenient for the patient. Drugs that are given in very high dosages may not match with a delivery strategy using liposomes because the amount of drug that can be encapsulated is limited.

Directly related to the dosing and delivery method is the safety profile of a certain drug. Next to the pharmaceutical parameters, the therapeutic window (or therapeutic index) should be determined by selecting the relevant pharmacology and safety studies. It is important to determine whether the drug delivered to the brain by a liposome can exert an effect at a concentration that is below the maximum tolerated dose. Furthermore, side-effects of the drug under investigation should be acceptable with respect to the severity of the disease. To obtain regulatory approval and continue the development of liposomal treatments for brain tumors, the therapeutic index is therefore a very important decision point.

G-Technology as Example of a Successfully Translated Brain-Targeted Liposomal Platform

2B3-101 is based not only on the already marketed Doxil/Caelyx, but also on our clinical-stage innovative liposomal CNS drug delivery technology called G-Technology. This technology is based on novel use of the antioxidant glutathione, which is actively transported across the BBB to the CNS. Glutathione (GSH) is an endogenous tripeptide with antioxidant activity that is involved in intracellular neutralization of reactive oxygen radicals. Ligation of GSH to the PEG molecules of sterically stabilized liposomes can greatly enhance the delivery of the liposomal contents to the brain, compared to non-targeted PEG liposomes.[91] Thus, GSH–PEG liposomes have been shown to significantly increase efficacy of CNS-disorder treatment compared to conventional delivery systems as was already shown for the anticancer agent doxorubicin[90] and the antiinflammatory methylprednisolone.[92] In short, G-Technology ensures an increased drug half-life, thereby requiring lower total dose levels and dosing frequency, and a reduction in bodily drug exposure. Altogether, fewer side effects and improvement in the therapeutic window of selected compounds result.

CONCLUSIONS AND RECOMMENDATIONS

Much progress has been made toward the clinical development of liposomes since the approval of PEGylated liposomal doxorubicin in 1995. Still, brain-targeted delivery of small-molecule drugs for brain cancer using similar liposomes is lagging behind. This is mainly because of the added challenges associated with delivery across the blood–brain barrier and other inherent difficulties in CNS drug development. By combining safe targeting ligands and receptors with well-known and safe liposome technologies, brain-targeted liposomes may soon become able to enhance drug delivery to the brain and impact clinical treatment. Several examples are underway in clinical trials.

To further strengthen research in clinically applicable liposomes for drug delivery to the brain a continued scientific discussion among researchers from industry and academia is required. These discussions could focus on ensuring the safety of liposomes and targeting ligands to enhance their clinical applicability, while also taking in account the cost and feasibility of the production process.

Momentum is clearly growing for the development of new technologies to enhance the delivery of drugs to the brain within a beneficial therapeutic window. With the ten key development criteria discussed in this paper, we hope to help bridge this gap so that more patients suffering from devastating CNS disorders will be better served in the future.

References

1. Bidros DS, Vogelbaum MA. Novel drug delivery strategies in neuro-oncology. Neurotherapeutics 2009;6(3): 539–46.
2. Nieder C, Grosu AL, Molls M. A comparison of treatment results for recurrent malignant gliomas. Cancer Treat. Rev. 2000;26(6):397–409.
3. Fokas E, Steinbach JP, Rodel C. Biology of brain metastases and novel targeted therapies: time to translate the research. Biochim. Biophys. Acta. 2013;1835(1):61–75.
4. Lu-Emerson C, Eichler AF. Brain metastases. Continuum (Minneap. Minn.) 2012;18(2):295–311.
5. Anton K, Baehring JM, Mayer T. Glioblastoma multiforme: overview of current treatment and future perspectives. Hematol. Oncol. Clin. North Am. 2012;26(4):825–53.
6. Badhiwala J, Decker WK, Berens ME, Bhardwaj RD. Clinical trials in cellular immunotherapy for brain/CNS tumors. Expert Rev Neurother. 2013;13(4):405–24.
7. Stupp R, Mason WP, van den Bent MJ, Weller M, Fisher B, Taphoorn MJ, et al. Radiotherapy plus concomitant and adjuvant temozolomide for glioblastoma. N. Engl. J. Med. 2005;352(10):987–96.
8. La Rocca RV, Rezazadeh A. Carmustine-impregnated wafers and their impact in the management of high-grade glioma. Expert Opin Pharmacother. 2011;12(8):1325–32.
9. Perry J, Chambers A, Spithoff K, Laperriere N. Gliadel wafers in the treatment of malignant glioma: a systematic review. Curr. Oncol. 2007;14(5):189–94.
10. Batchelor TT, Mulholland P, Neyns B, Nabors LB, Campone M, Wick A, et al. Phase III randomized trial comparing the efficacy of cediranib as monotherapy, and in combination with lomustine, versus lomustine alone in patients with recurrent glioblastoma. J. Clin. Oncol. 2013;31(26):3212–8.
11. Reardon DA, Turner S, Peters KB, Desjardins A, Gururangan S, Sampson JH, et al. A review of VEGF/VEGFR-targeted therapeutics for recurrent glioblastoma. J. Natl. Compr. Canc. Netw. 2011;9(4):414–27.

12. U.S. Food and Drug Administration, *FDA Approval for Bevacizumab*, July 1, 2013, http://www.cancer.gov/cancertopics/druginfo/fda-bevacizumab#Anchor-Glioblastoma.
13. Verhoeff JJ, van Tellingen O, Claes A, Stalpers LJ, van Linde ME, Richel DJ, et al. Concerns about anti-angiogenic treatment in patients with glioblastoma multiforme. BMC Cancer 2009;9:444.
14. Claes A, Wesseling P, Jeuken J, Maass C, Heerschap A, Leenders WP. Antiangiogenic compounds interfere with chemotherapy of brain tumors due to vessel normalization. Mol. Cancer Ther. 2008;7(1):71–8.
15. Leenders WP, Kusters B, Verrijp K, Maass C, Wesseling P, Heerschap A, et al. Antiangiogenic therapy of cerebral melanoma metastases results in sustained tumor progression via vessel co-option. Clin. Cancer Res. 2004;10(18, Pt. 1):6222–30.
16. Song G, Wu H, Yoshino K, Zamboni WC. Factors affecting the pharmacokinetics and pharmacodynamics of liposomal drugs. J. Liposome Res. 2012;22(3):177–92.
17. Barenholz Y. Doxil®—the first FDA-approved nano-drug: lessons learned. J. Control. Release 2012;160(2):117–34.
18. U.S. Food and Drug Administration, FDA Approval of Generic Version of Cancer Drug Doxil Is Expected to Help Resolve Shortage [news release], February 4, 2013 (http://www.fda.gov/newsevents/newsroom/pressannouncements/ucm337872.htm).
19. Chang HI, Yeh MK. Clinical development of liposome-based drugs: formulation, characterization, and therapeutic efficacy. Int. J. Nanomed. 2012;7:49–60.
20. Sen K, Mandal M. Second generation liposomal cancer therapeutics: transition from laboratory to clinic. Int. J. Pharm. 2013;448(1):28–43.
21. Slingerland M, Guchelaar HJ, Gelderblom H. Liposomal drug formulations in cancer therapy: 15 years along the road. Drug Discov. Today 2012;17(3-4):160–6.
22. Koudelka S, Turanek J. Liposomal paclitaxel formulations. J. Control. Release 2012;163(3):322–34.
23. Luye Pharma, http://www.luye.cn/en/products/?fid=1013&id=55.
24. Harrington KJ, Lewanski CR, Northcote AD, Whittaker J, Wellbank H, Vile RG, et al. Phase I–II study of pegylated liposomal cisplatin (SPI-077) in patients with inoperable head and neck cancer. Ann. Oncol. 2001;12(4):493–6.
25. Bandak S, Goren D, Horowitz A, Tzemach D, Gabizon A. Pharmacological studies of cisplatin encapsulated in long-circulating liposomes in mouse tumor models. Anticancer Drugs 1999;10(10):911–20.
26. de Jonge MJ, Slingerland M, Loos WJ, Wiemer EA, Burger H, Mathijssen RH, et al. Early cessation of the clinical development of LiPlaCis, a liposomal cisplatin formulation. Eur. J. Cancer 2010;46(16):3016–21.
27. Yang SH, Lin CC, Lin ZZ, Tseng YL, Hong RL. A phase I and pharmacokinetic study of liposomal vinorelbine in patients with advanced solid tumor. Invest. New Drugs 2012;30(1):282–9.
28. Maeda H, Bharate GY, Daruwalla J. Polymeric drugs for efficient tumor-targeted drug delivery based on EPR-effect. Eur. J. Pharm. Biopharm. 2009;71(3):409–19.
29. Gabizon A, Catane R, Uziely B, Kaufman B, Safra T, Cohen R, et al. Prolonged circulation time and enhanced accumulation in malignant exudates of doxorubicin encapsulated in polyethylene-glycol coated liposomes. Cancer Res. 1994;54(4):987–92.
30. Maeda H, Wu J, Sawa T, Matsumura Y, Hori K. Tumor vascular permeability and the EPR effect in macromolecular therapeutics: a review. J. Control. Release 2000;65(1-2):271–84.
31. Mehra NK, Mishra V, Jain NK. Receptor-based targeting of therapeutics. Ther. Deliv. 2013;4(3):369–94.
32. Gray BP, McGuire MJ, Brown KC. A liposomal drug platform overrides peptide ligand targeting to a cancer biomarker, irrespective of ligand affinity or density. PLoS ONE 2013;8(8):e72938.
33. Sawant RR, Torchilin VP. Challenges in development of targeted liposomal therapeutics. AAPS J. 2012;14(2):303–15.
34. Sapra P, Allen TM. Internalizing antibodies are necessary for improved therapeutic efficacy of antibody-targeted liposomal drugs. Cancer Res. 2002;62(24):7190–4.
35. Sugiyama T, Asai T, Nedachi YM, Katanasaka Y, Shimizu K, Maeda N, et al. Enhanced active targeting via cooperative binding of ligands on liposomes to target receptors. PLoS ONE 2013;8(6):e67550.
36. Tang J, Zhang L, Liu Y, Zhang Q, Qin Y, Yin Y, et al. Synergistic targeted delivery of payload into tumor cells by dual-ligand liposomes co-modified with cholesterol anchored transferrin and TAT. Int. J. Pharm. 2013;454(1):31–40.
37. Zhang X, Guo S, Fan R, Yu M, Li F, Zhu C, et al. Dual-functional liposome for tumor targeting and overcoming multidrug resistance in hepatocellular carcinoma cells. Biomaterials 2012;33(29):7103–14.
38. Fabel K, Dietrich J, Hau P, Wismeth C, Winner B, Przywara S, et al. Long-term stabilization in patients with malignant glioma after treatment with liposomal doxorubicin. Cancer 2001;92(7):1936–42.

IV. NOVEL APPROACHES FOR CANCER THERAPIES

39. Hau P, Fabel K, Baumgart U, Rummele P, Grauer O, Bock A, et al. Pegylated liposomal doxorubicin-efficacy in patients with recurrent high-grade glioma. Cancer 2004;100(6):1199–207.
40. Glas M, Koch H, Hirschmann B, Jauch T, Steinbrecher A, Herrlinger U, et al. Pegylated liposomal doxorubicin in recurrent malignant glioma: analysis of a case series. Oncology 2007;72(5-6):302–7.
41. Sarin H. Recent progress towards development of effective systemic chemotherapy for the treatment of malignant brain tumors. J. Transl. Med. 2009;7:77.
42. Kawano K, Hattori Y, Iwakura H, Akamizu T, Maitani Y. Combination therapy with gefitinib and doxorubicin inhibits tumor growth in transgenic mice with adrenal neuroblastoma. Cancer Med. 2013;2(3):286–95.
43. Guo P, Hu B, Gu W, Xu L, Wang D, Huang HJ, et al. Platelet-derived growth factor-B enhances glioma angiogenesis by stimulating vascular endothelial growth factor expression in tumor endothelia and by promoting pericyte recruitment. Am. J. Pathol. 2003;162(4):1083–93.
44. de Vries NA, Beijnen JH, Boogerd W, van Tellingen O. Blood–brain barrier and chemotherapeutic treatment of brain tumors. Expert Rev. Neurother. 2006;6(8):1199–209.
45. Muldoon LL, Soussain C, Jahnke K, Johanson C, Siegal T, Smith QR, et al. Chemotherapy delivery issues in central nervous system malignancy: a reality check. J. Clin. Oncol. 2007;25(16):2295–305.
46. Palmieri D, Chambers AF, Felding-Habermann B, Huang S, Steeg PS. The biology of metastasis to a sanctuary site. Clin. Cancer Res. 2007;13(6):1656–62.
47. Agarwal S, Manchanda P, Vogelbaum MA, Ohlfest JR, Elmquist WF. Function of the blood–brain barrier and restriction of drug delivery to invasive glioma cells: findings in an orthotopic rat xenograft model of glioma. Drug Metab Dispos. 2013;41(1):33–9.
48. Fidler IJ. The role of the organ microenvironment in brain metastasis. Semin. Cancer Biol. 2011;21(2):107–12.
49. Jain RK, di Tomaso E, Duda DG, Loeffler JS, Sorensen AG, Batchelor TT. Angiogenesis in brain tumours. Nat. Rev. Neurosci. 2007;8(8):610–22.
50. Gaillard PJ, Visser CC, Appeldoorn CCM, Rip J. Blood–to-brain drug delivery: 10 key development criteria. Curr. Pharm. Biotechnol. 2012;13:2328–39.
51. Gaillard PJ, Visser CC, Appeldoorn CCM, Rip J. Enhanced brain drug delivery: safely crossing the blood–brain barrier. Drug Discov. Today Technol. 2012;9(2):e155–60.
52. Demeule M, Regina A, Che C, Poirier J, Nguyen T, Gabathuler R, et al. Identification and design of peptides as a new drug delivery system for the brain. J. Pharmacol. Exp. Ther. 2008;324(3):1064–72.
53. Gaillard PJ, Visser CC, de Boer AG. Targeted delivery across the blood–brain barrier. Expert Opin. Drug Deliv. 2005;2(2):299–309.
54. Jones AR, Shusta EV. Blood–brain barrier transport of therapeutics via receptor-mediation. Pharm. Res. 2007;24(9):1759–71.
55. Geron, Geron Discontinues GRN1005 and Restructures to Focus on Imetelstat Development in Hematologic Malignancies and Solid Tumors with Short Telomeres [press release], December 3, 2012 (http://ir.geron.com/phoenix.zhtml?c=67323&p=irol-newsArticle&ID=1763907&highlight=).
56. Anon. Phase 2 clinical data for Angiochem's lead drug candidate, ANG1005, in breast cancer patients with brain metastases, revealed. BusinessWire; October 21, 2013 (http://www.businesswire.com/news/home/20131021005437/en/Phase-2-Clinical-Data-Angiochem's-Lead-Drug).
57. Lin, N.U., Schwartzberg, L., Kesari, S., Elias, A., Anders, C.K., Raizer, J., et al. A Phase II study of ANG1005, a novel, brain-penetrant taxane derivative, in breast cancer patients with brain metastases. In: *Proceedings of the 2013 AACR-NCI-EORTC International Conference on Molecular Targets and Cancer Therapeutics*, Boston, MA, October 19-23, 2013, Abstract no. B76.
58. Kannan R, Kuhlenkamp JF, Jeandidier E, Trinh H, Ookhtens M, Kaplowitz N. Evidence for carrier-mediated transport of glutathione across the blood–brain barrier in the rat. J. Clin. Invest. 1990;85(6):2009–13.
59. Kannan R, Chakrabarti R, Tang D, Kim KJ, Kaplowitz N. GSH transport in human cerebrovascular endothelial cells and human astrocytes: evidence for luminal localization of Na+-dependent GSH transport in HCEC. Brain Res. 2000;852(2):374–82.
60. Zlokovic BV, Mackic JB, McComb JG, Weiss MH, Kaplowitz N, Kannan R. Evidence for transcapillary transport of reduced glutathione in vascular perfused guinea-pig brain. Biochem. Biophys. Res. Commun. 1994;201(1):402–8.
61. Milojkovic-Kerklaan B, Aftimos P, Altintas S, Jager A, Lonnqvist F, Soetekouw P, et al. Phase I dose escalating study of 2B3-101, glutathione PEGylated liposomal doxorubicin, in patients with solid tumors and brain metastases or recurrent malignant glioma. Presented at the European Cancer Congress 2013 Amsterdam, the Netherlands, 27 September–1 October 2013. Eur. J. Cancer 2013;49(Suppl. 2):S789–790.

62. to-BBB press release: 26 September 2013. (http://www.tobbb.com/content/nieuws/2013_09_26_to-bbb_presents_clinical_data_on_lead_product_2b3-101.pdf).
63. Drummond DC, Meyer O, Hong K, Kirpotin DB, Papahadjopoulos D. Optimizing liposomes for delivery of chemotherapeutic agents to solid tumors. Pharmacol. Rev. 1999;51(4):691–743.
64. Storm G, Crommelin DJA. Liposomes: *quo vadis*? Pharm. Sci. Technol. Today 1998;1(1):19–31.
65. Akbarzadeh A, Rezaei-Sadabady R, Davaran S, Joo SW, Zarghami N, Hanifehpour Y, et al. Liposome: classification, preparation, and applications. Nanoscale Res. Lett. 2013;8(1):102.
66. Fritze A, Hens F, Kimpfler A, Schubert R, Peschka-Suss R. Remote loading of doxorubicin into liposomes driven by a transmembrane phosphate gradient. Biochim. Biophys. Acta. 2006;1758(10):1633–40.
67. Lewrick F, Suss R. Remote loading of anthracyclines into liposomes. Methods Mol. Biol. 2010;605:139–45.
68. Gubernator J. Active methods of drug loading into liposomes: recent strategies for stable drug entrapment and increased *in vivo* activity. Expert Opin. Drug Deliv. 2011;8(5):565–80.
69. Clerc S, Barenholz Y. Loading of amphipathic weak acids into liposomes in response to transmembrane calcium acetate gradients. Biochim. Biophys. Acta. 1995;1240(2):257–65.
70. Lasic DD, Frederik PM, Stuart MC, Barenholz Y, McIntosh TJ. Gelation of liposome interior. A novel method for drug encapsulation. FEBS Lett. 1992;312(2-3):255–8.
71. Zucker D, Marcus D, Barenholz Y, Goldblum A. Liposome drugs' loading efficiency: a working model based on loading conditions and drug's physicochemical properties. J. Control. Release 2009;139(1):73–80.
72. van den Hoven JM, Metselaar JM, Storm G, Beijnen JH, Nuijen B. Cyclodextrin as membrane protectant in spray-drying and freeze-drying of PEGylated liposomes. Int. J. Pharm. 2012;438(1-2):209–16.
73. Stark B, Pabst G, Prassl R. Long-term stability of sterically stabilized liposomes by freezing and freeze-drying: effects of cryoprotectants on structure. Eur. J. Pharm. Sci. 2010;41(3-4):546–55.
74. Chen C, Han D, Cai C, Tang X. An overview of liposome lyophilization and its future potential. J. Control. Release 2010;142(3):299–311.
75. U.S. Food and Drug Administration. *Drugs: Chemistry, Manufacturing, and Controls* (CMC), 2014 (http://www.fda.gov/Drugs/GuidanceComplianceRegulatoryInformation/Guidances/ucm064979.htm).
76. U.S. Food and Drug Administration. *Guidance for Industry: Liposome Drug Products: Chemistry, Manufacturing, and Controls; Human Pharmacokinetics and Bioavailability; and Labeling Documentation*, 2002 (http://www.fda.gov/downloads/Drugs/GuidanceComplianceRegulatoryInformation/Guidances/ucm070570.pdf).
77. Boado RJ, Zhang Y, Wang Y, Pardridge WM. GDNF fusion protein for targeted-drug delivery across the human blood–brain barrier. Biotechnol. Bioeng. 2008;100(2):387–96.
78. Nystrom AM, Fadeel B. Safety assessment of nanomaterials: implications for nanomedicine. J. Control. Release 2012;161(2):403–8.
79. Gaillard PJ, Visser CC, de Boer M, Appeldoorn CCM, Rip J. Blood-to-brain drug delivery using nanocarriers. In: Hammarlund-Udenaes M, de Lange E, Thorne R, editors. Drug Delivery to the Brain: Physiological Concepts, Methodologies and Approaches. Arlington, VA: American Association of Pharmaceutical Scientists; 2014. p. 433–54.
80. WMA. *World Medical Association Declaration of Helsinki: Ethical Principles for Medical Research Involving Human Subjects*. Ferney-Voltaire, France: World Medical Association; 2008. (http://www.wma.net/en/30publications/10policies/b3/17c.pdf).
81. U.S. Food and Drug Administration. *Guidance for Industry: S7A Safety Pharmacology Studies for Human Pharmaceutic*als, 2001 (http://www.fda.gov/downloads/Drugs/GuidanceComplianceRegulatoryInformation/Guidances/ucm074959.pdf).
82. Szebeni J, Alving CR, Baranyi L, Bunger R. Interaction of liposomes with complement leading to adverse reactions. In: Gregoriadis G, editor. Liposome Technology. Vol. III. Interactions of Liposomes with the Biological Milieu. 3rd ed. New York: Informa Healthcare; 2007. p. 1–23.
83. Szebeni J, Muggia F, Gabizon A, Barenholz Y. Activation of complement by therapeutic liposomes and other lipid excipient-based therapeutic products: prediction and prevention. Adv. Drug Deliv. Rev. 2011;63(12):1020–30.
84. Szebeni J, Bedocs P, Rozsnyay Z, Weiszhar Z, Urbanics R, Rosivall L, et al. Liposome-induced complement activation and related cardiopulmonary distress in pigs: factors promoting reactogenicity of Doxil and AmBisome. Nanomedicine 2012;8(2):176–84.
85. Gabizon AA. Stealth liposomes and tumor targeting: one step further in the quest for the magic bullet. Clin. Cancer Res. 2001;7(2):223–5.

86. Jiskoot W, van Schie RM, Carstens MG, Schellekens H. Immunological risk of injectable drug delivery systems. Pharm. Res. 2009;26(6):1303–14.

87. Duncan R, Gaspar R. Nanomedicine(s) under the microscope. Mol. Pharm. 2011;8(6):2101–41.

88. Boraschi D, Costantino L, Italiani P. Interaction of nanoparticles with immunocompetent cells: nanosafety considerations. Nanomedicine (Lond.) 2012;7(1):121–31.

89. Rempe R, Cramer S, Huwel S, Galla HJ. Transport of poly(*n*-butylcyano-acrylate) nanoparticles across the blood–brain barrier *in vitro* and their influence on barrier integrity. Biochem. Biophys. Res. Commun. 2011;406(1):64–9.

90. Gaillard, P.J., Gladdines, W., Appeldoorn, C.C.M., Rip, J., Boogerd, W.J., Beijnen, J.H., et al. Development of glutathione pegylated liposomal doxorubicin (2B3-101) for the treatment of brain cancer. In: *Proceedings of the 103rd Annual Meeting of the American Association for Cancer Research*, Chicago, IL, March 31–April 4, 2010, Abstract no. 5687.

91. Rip, J., Appeldoorn, C.C.M., Manca, F.M., Dorland, R., van Kregten, J.M.R., and Gaillard, P.J. Receptor-mediated delivery of drugs across the blood–brain barrier. Paper presented at Pharmacology and Toxicology of the Blood–Brain Barrier: State of the Art, Needs for Future Research and Expected Benefits for the EU, Brussels, Belgium, February 11-12, 2010.

92. Gaillard PJ, Appeldoorn CC, Rip J, Dorland R, van der Pol SM, Kooij G, et al. Enhanced brain delivery of liposomal methylprednisolone improved therapeutic efficacy in a model of neuroinflammation. J. Control. Release 2012;164(3):364–9.

Index